# Understanding Autoimmune Diseases

# Understanding Autoimmune Diseases

Editor: Dallas Lynch

FOSTER
ACADEMICS
www.fosteracademics.com

www.fosteracademics.com

FOSTER ACADEMICS

**Cataloging-in-Publication Data**

Understanding autoimmune diseases / edited by Dallas Lynch.
p. cm.
Includes bibliographical references and index.
ISBN 978-1-63242-847-9
1. Autoimmune diseases. 2. Autoimmunity. 3. Immunologic diseases. I. Lynch, Dallas.
RC600 .U53 2019
616.978--dc23



Foster Academics,
118-35 Queens Blvd., Suite 400,
Forest Hills, NY 11375, USA

ISBN 978-1-63242-847-9 (Hardback)



Printed and bound in China.

# Contents

# Preface

The diseases arising from abnormal immune responses to normal body parts are called autoimmune diseases. Tiredness and fever are two of the most common symptoms of such diseases. Other symptoms include altered organ function, damage to the tissues and altered organ growth. There is no known cause of autoimmune diseases. Graves' disease, multiple sclerosis, celiac disease, rheumatoid arthritis, diabetes mellitus Type 1, systemic lupus erythematosus and psoriasis are some of the common types of autoimmune diseases. Treatment methods include the use of immunosuppressants, nonsteroidal anti-inflammatory drugs (NSAIDs) and intravenous immunoglobulin. The topics included in this book on autoimmune diseases are of utmost significance and bound to provide incredible insights to readers. It includes some of the vital pieces of work being conducted across the world, on various topics related to such diseases. The extensive content of this book provides the readers with a thorough understanding of the subject.

This book has been the outcome of endless efforts put in by authors and researchers on various issues and topics within the field. The book is a comprehensive collection of significant researches that are addressed in a variety of chapters. It will surely enhance the knowledge of the field among readers across the globe.

It gives us an immense pleasure to thank our researchers and authors for their efforts to submit their piece of writing before the deadlines. Finally in the end, I would like to thank my family and colleagues who have been a great source of inspiration and support.

**Editor**

# 1

# Association between Secondary and Primary Sjögren's Syndrome in a Large Collection of Lupus Families

**Rachna Aggarwal,[1,2] Juan-Manuel Anaya,[3] Kristi A. Koelsch,[1,2] Biji T. Kurien,[1,2] and R. Hal Scofield[1,2,4]**

[1] *Department of Medicine, University of Oklahoma Health Sciences Center, Oklahoma City, OK 73104, USA*
[2] *Arthritis & Immunology Program, Oklahoma Medical Research Foundation, Oklahoma City, OK 73104, USA*
[3] *Center for Autoimmune Diseases Research (CREA), Universidad del Rosario, Bogotá, Colombia*
[4] *Medical Service, Department of Veterans Affairs Medical Center, Oklahoma City, OK 73104, USA*

Correspondence should be addressed to R. Hal Scofield; hal-scofield@omrf.ouhsc.edu

Academic Editor: Ricard Cervera

*Objective.* Systemic lupus erythematosus (SLE) and Sjögren's syndrome (SS) share clinical and immunogenetic features and may occur together. We undertook this study to determine the risk of primary SS among SLE-unaffected relatives of SLE patients and whether or not primary and secondary SS tended to occur in the same families. *Methods.* We collected clinical and serological data on 2694 SLE patients, 7390 SLE-unaffected relatives of the SLE patients, and 1470 matched controls. *Results.* Of the 2694 subjects with SLE, 548 had secondary SS, while 71 of their 7390 SLE-unaffected relatives had primary SS. None of the 1470 controls had SS as defined herein ($p = 5 \times 10^{-5}$ compared to SLE-unaffected relatives). Of the 71 SLE-unaffected relatives with primary SS, 18 (25.3%) had an SLE-affected family member with secondary SS, while only 530 of the 7319 (7.2%) SLE-unaffected relatives without SS did so ($p = 1 \times 10^{-8}$). *Conclusion.* Among families identified for the presence of SLE, primary and secondary SS tend to occur within the same families. These results highlight the commonalities between these two forms of SS, which in fact correspond to the same disease.

## 1. Introduction

Sjögren's syndrome (SS) is a chronic autoimmune disease that characteristically affects salivary and lacrimal glands such that patients have severe dry eyes and dry mouth [1]. Pathology in these glands consists of lymphocytic infiltration, commonly with germinal center formation [2]. The disease may also involve numerous other organs, including the lungs, kidneys, joints, skin, peripheral nerves, and brain. Patients with SS are at high risk for mucosal-associated lymphoid tissue (MALT) lymphoma [3]. The diagnosis of SS is based on the combination of symptoms (sicca symptoms) and the presence of the autoimmune characteristics: activation of T cells (confirmed in practice by a positive salivary gland biopsy) or B cells (i.e., presence of autoantibodies). The most common specificities are anti-Ro (or SSA) and anti-La (or SSB) [4]. SS may be the second only to rheumatoid arthritis in terms of prevalence of the inflammatory rheumatic illnesses [5].

In most of the cases, SS occurs without any other inflammatory, autoimmune illness. In this case, the disease is still termed primary. Meanwhile, SS can also occur in association with another autoimmune disease (i.e., polyautoimmunity), the most frequent being autoimmune thyroid disease, rheumatoid arthritis (RA), and systemic lupus erythematosus (SLE) [6]. When this occurs, the disease is designated secondary. The classification criteria for SS are those of the American-European Consensus Group (AECG), which require one of either salivary gland pathology showing foci of lymphocytic infiltration or positive serology in the form of anti-Ro or anti-La [7]. Recently, new criteria have been proposed [8] and compared to the AECG criteria [9].

Among those with SLE, about 20% of patients have secondary SS. SLE and SS can share clinical features such as nondeforming, inflammatory arthritis, photosensitivity, and lymphopenia [10]. In addition, anti-Ro and anti-La are also found in the sera of patients with SLE, although at a lower rate than in SS [7].

Risk of SLE and SS clearly has a genetic component [11]. However, the study of the genetics of SLE is much farther along than that of SS. There are now multiple genome-wide association studies reported for the former with genetic association reported and confirmed for many dozens of genes [12]. On the other hand, two genome-wide association studies have been reported for SS and show some associations in common with SLE while others are unique to SS [13, 14]. Other reported genetic associations for SS are from small cohorts in which candidate genes already known to be associated with SLE were studied [11].

We have collected a large cohort of patients with SLE and have data concerning the presence of sicca symptoms, autoantibodies, and a past diagnosis of SS in both the SLE patients and their SLE-unaffected relatives. Thus, we undertook this study to determine whether there is a familial relationship between putative "primary" and "secondary" SS.

## 2. Methods

*2.1. Lupus Family Registry and Repository.* We collected data and biological samples from families with SLE for over two decades. The methods of this resource have been presented in depth [15]. Briefly, putative SLE patients completed an extensive questionnaire, underwent an interview, and had medical records reviewed to ensure that all patients met the American College of Rheumatology SLE classification criteria [10, 16]. Family members also completed a questionnaire about their health status and were interviewed by trained personnel if there were any answers suggesting a diagnosis of SLE. Unrelated controls were also recruited and by questionnaire and interview were determined not to have SLE, as defined by classification criteria.

*2.2. Serology.* All subjects underwent serological testing for SLE-associated autoantibodies in the Oklahoma Medical Research Foundation Clinical Immunology Laboratory, a CLIA-approved facility. For purposes of the present study, this included determination of anti-Ro60 and anti-La by double immunodiffusion [17, 18].

*2.3. Putative Sjögren's Syndrome.* SS was defined in part by the presence of dry mouth and dry eye symptoms. All subjects, both SLE patients and their SLE-unaffected relatives, were asked the following questions: (1) have you had daily, persistent, troublesome dry eyes for more than three months?; (2) do you have a recurrent sensation of sand or gravel in the eyes?; (3) do you use tear substitutes more than three times a day?; (4) have you had a daily feeling of dry mouth for more than three months?; (5) have you had recurrently or persistently swollen salivary glands as an adult?; (6) do you frequently drink liquids to aid in swallowing dry foods?; and (7) have you ever been told by a doctor that you have Sjögren's syndrome? The first six questions allow classification as to presence or absence of the American-European Consensus Group SS classification criteria for subjective dry eyes and dry mouth [7]. These questions also correspond to those asked in the Connective Disease Screening Questionnaire, a validated tool with high sensitivity and specificity for SS [19]. Thus, SLE patients were classified as "secondary" SS if dry eyes, dry mouth, and anti-Ro were present. SLE-unaffected relatives were classified as "primary" SS if they gave a history of a diagnosis of the disease or if at least one dry eye and at least one dry mouth were answered positively and anti-Ro was present.

*2.4. Statistics.* Categorical data were compared by a chi square analysis. A $p$ value less than 0.05 was considered statistically significant.

## 3. Results

A total of 2694 subjects meeting the ACR SLE classification criteria [10, 16] were considered in the analyses. There were 2400 (89.1%) women and 294 (10.9%) men. Among these, 45.2% self-identified as white Americans, 36.4% as black Americans, 9.3% as Hispanic Americans, 0.4% as Asian Americans, and 6% as Native Americans. There were 7390 relatives of these lupus patients who entered the study, none of whom met these same criteria for the classification of SLE. There were 2459 (33.3%) male relatives and 4931 (66.7%) female relatives. The unrelated controls numbered 1470 and were matched for age, sex, and ethnicity/race to the SLE patients.

Among the 2694 SLE patients, there were 548 (20.3%) who had dry eyes, dry mouth, and anti-Ro, that is, putative "secondary" SS as we have defined it. Of these, 507 (92.5%) were women. A plurality, 228 (41%), was white Americans, with 218 (39.7%) black, 3 (0.5%) Asian, 45 (8.2%) Hispanic, and 35 (6.3%) Native Americans. Among the 7390 SLE-unaffected relatives, there were 71 who met our criteria for putative SS. None of the 1470 unrelated controls met these criteria, which was less common compared to the SLE-unaffected relatives ($\chi^2 = 16.8$, $p = 0.00004$).

We then considered the distribution of "primary" and "secondary" SS among the subjects with SLE as well as their SLE-unaffected relatives. Of the 548 with "secondary" SS, 18 had a relative with "primary" SS. Meanwhile, of those with SLE but no "secondary" SS, only 53 of 2146 had a non-SLE-affected relative with "primary" SS ($\chi^2 = 1.3$, $p$ = NS, odds ratio = 1.4). Thus, SLE patients with "secondary" SS were about ~1.5 times more likely to have a family member with "primary" SS, compared to those SLE-affected subjects without "secondary" SS, but this difference did not reach statistical significance.

Alternatively, we considered the presence of "secondary" SS within the families with "primary" SS. There were 71 "primary" SS patients, of whom 18 (25.3%) had a relative with "secondary" SS, while, among 7319 lupus-unaffected relatives without SS, 530 (7.1%) had a lupus-affected relative with SS ($\chi^2 = 34$, $p < 1\times10^{-8}$, odds ratio = 4.4). Thus, SLE-unaffected relatives with "primary" SS were almost 5 times more likely

TABLE 1: Distribution of secondary Sjögren's syndrome among relatives of those with systemic lupus erythematosus with and without primary Sjögren's syndrome.

| | SLE-unaffected relatives | |
|---|---|---|
| | pSS | No pSS |
| SLE with sSS | 18 | 530 |
| SLE without sSS | 53 | 6789 |

$\chi^2 = 34$; $p < 0.00000001$; odds ratio = 4.4.
sSS: secondary Sjögren's syndrome; SLE: systemic lupus erythematosus.

to have a SLE-affected relative with "secondary" SS than were those relatives without "primary" SS (see Table 1).

## 4. Discussion

SLE and SS are autoimmune diseases that share clinical and serological features. The majority of Sjögren's patients have anti-Ro and about half of these same patients have anti-La antibodies. Both anti-Ro and anti-La also occur in those with SLE with less frequency, but anti-La is associated with lack of renal and central nervous system disease [20]. The diseases share clinical features as described and some patients present with both phenotypes (i.e., polyautoimmunity) [6, 21].

While much less research has been done on SS, thus far at least, the genetics of these two diseases are similar [11]. We found that among families recruited for the presence of SLE about 1% of SLE-unaffected relatives had SS, while none of over 1400 controls had this disease. Although it is well to remember that the controls were matched with the SLE patients, not the SLE-unaffected relatives, our data demonstrate that SLE and SS tend to occur in the same families.

We have defined SS in this study by the presence of dry eyes, dry mouth, and anti-Ro. This definition, of course, does not meet the usual research classification criteria [7] and is thus a potential weakness. On the other hand, we have used this same definition in this cohort previously with success [22]. Furthermore, combinations of clinical symptoms such as dry mouth, dry eyes, and painful mouth predict classification by the research criteria very well [23]. The Connective Disease Screening Questionnaire has a sensitivity of 85% and a specificity of 83% for Sjögren's syndrome [19]. Furthermore, a strategy combining this screening tool with autoantibody testing produced 95% sensitivity and 99% specificity along with 71% positive predictive value and 98% negative predictive value for RA [24]. Thus, these data support those in SS [23] where a screening questionnaire combined with autoantibody testing is useful for case finding. Nonetheless, we have likely misclassified some individuals, but there is no reason to suspect that such misclassification occurred in a way that biased the association result we found between "primary" and "secondary" SS in these families with SLE.

Our data also demonstrate that "secondary" SS among the SLE patients and "primary" SS are found within the same families such that individuals with "primary" SS were 4.4 times more likely to have a lupus-affected relative with "secondary" SS than were those without "primary" SS (Table 1). The data generated by the present work imply that there might be not only common genetic factors leading to these diseases but also common environmental (nongenetic) factors putting persons at risk (i.e., the autoimmune tautology) [25].

## Conflict of Interests

The authors declare that there is no conflict of interests regarding the publication of this paper.

## Acknowledgments

This work was supported in part by NIH Grants AR053483, AI082714, GM104938, and AR060804 and NAIMS funding for the Lupus Family Registry and Repository.

## References

[1] R. I. Fox, "Sjögren's syndrome," *The Lancet*, vol. 366, no. 9482, pp. 321–331, 2005.

[2] M. V. Jonsson, K. Skarstein, R. Jonsson, and J. G. Brun, "Serological implications of germinal center-like structures in primary Sjögren's syndrome," *The Journal of Rheumatology*, vol. 34, no. 10, pp. 2044–2049, 2007.

[3] M. N. Lazarus, D. Robinson, V. Mak, H. Møller, and D. A. Isenberg, "Incidence of cancer in a cohort of patients with primary Sjögren's syndrome," *Rheumatology*, vol. 45, no. 8, pp. 1012–1015, 2006.

[4] H. Nakamura, A. Kawakami, and K. Eguchi, "Mechanisms of autoantibody production and the relationship between autoantibodies and the clinical manifestations in Sjögren's syndrome," *Translational Research*, vol. 148, no. 6, pp. 281–288, 2006.

[5] C. G. Helmick, D. T. Felson, R. C. Lawrence et al., "Estimates of the prevalence of arthritis and other rheumatic conditions in the United States. Part I," *Arthritis & Rheumatism*, vol. 58, no. 1, pp. 15–25, 2008.

[6] M. J. Amador-Patarroyo, J. G. Arbelaez, R. D. Mantilla et al., "Sjögren's syndrome at the crossroad of polyautoimmunity," *Journal of Autoimmunity*, vol. 39, no. 3, pp. 199–205, 2012.

[7] C. Vitali, S. Bombardieri, R. Jonsson et al., "Classification criteria for Sjögren's syndrome: a revised version of the European criteria proposed by the American-European Consensus Group," *Annals of the Rheumatic Diseases*, vol. 61, no. 6, pp. 554–558, 2002.

[8] S. C. Shiboski, C. H. Shiboski, L. A. Criswell et al., "American College of rheumatology classification criteria for Sjögren's syndrome: a data-driven, expert consensus approach in the Sjögren's International Collaborative Clinical Alliance cohort," *Arthritis Care & Research*, vol. 64, no. 4, pp. 475–487, 2012.

[9] A. Rasmussen, J. A. Ice, H. Li et al., "Comparison of the American-European Consensus Group Sjögren's syndrome classification criteria to newly proposed American College of Rheumatology criteria in a large, carefully characterised sicca cohort," *Annals of the Rheumatic Diseases*, vol. 73, no. 1, pp. 31–38, 2014.

[10] E. M. Tan, A. S. Cohen, J. F. Fries et al., "The 1982 revised criteria for the classification of systemic lupus erythrematosus," *Arthritis and Rheumatism*, vol. 25, no. 11, pp. 1271–1277, 1982.

[11] R. H. Scofield, "Genetics of systemic lupus erythematosus and Sjögren's syndrome," *Current Opinion in Rheumatology*, vol. 21, no. 5, pp. 448–453, 2009.

[12] R. R. Graham, G. Hom, W. Ortmann, and T. W. Behrens, "Review of recent genome-wide association scans in lupus," *Journal of Internal Medicine*, vol. 265, no. 6, pp. 680–688, 2009.

[13] C. J. Lessard, I. Adrianto, J. A. Ice et al., "Identification of IRF8, TMEM39A, and IKZF3-ZPBP2 as susceptibility loci for systemic lupus erythematosus in a large-scale multiracial replication study," *American Journal of Human Genetics*, vol. 90, no. 4, pp. 648–660, 2012.

[14] Y. Li, K. Zhang, H. Chen et al., "A genome-wide association study in Han Chinese identifies a susceptibility locus for primary Sjogren's syndrome at 7q11.23," *Nature Genetics*, vol. 45, no. 11, pp. 1361–1365, 2013.

[15] A. Rasmussen, S. Sevier, J. A. Kelly et al., "The lupus family registry and repository," *Rheumatology*, vol. 50, no. 1, pp. 47–59, 2011.

[16] M. C. Hochberg, "Updating the American College of Rheumatology revised criteria for the classification of systemic lupus erythematosus," *Arthritis and Rheumatism*, vol. 40, no. 9, article 1725, 1997.

[17] G. Clark, M. Reichlin, and T. B. Tomasi Jr., "Characterization of a soluble cytoplasmic antigen reactive with sera from patients with systemic lupus erythmatosus," *Journal of Immunology*, vol. 102, no. 1, pp. 117–122, 1969.

[18] R. G. Hamilton, J. B. Harley, W. B. Bias et al., "Two Ro (SS-A) autoantibody responses in systemic lupus erythematosus: correlation of HLA-DR/DQ specificities with quantitative expression of Ro (SS-A) autoantibody," *Arthritis & Rheumatism*, vol. 31, no. 4, pp. 496–505, 1988.

[19] E. W. Karlson, J. Sanchez-Guerrero, E. A. Wright et al., "A connective tissue disease screening questionnaire for population studies," *Annals of Epidemiology*, vol. 5, no. 4, pp. 297–302, 1995.

[20] S. Malik, G. R. Bruner, C. Williams-Weese et al., "Presence of anti-La autoantibody is associated with a lower risk of nephritis and seizures in lupus patients," *Lupus*, vol. 16, no. 11, pp. 863–866, 2007.

[21] T. T. Provost, R. Watson, and E. Simmons-O'Brien, "Anti-Ro(SS-A) antibody positive Sjogren's/lupus erythematosus overlap syndrome," *Lupus*, vol. 6, no. 2, pp. 105–111, 1997.

[22] R. H. Scofield, G. R. Bruner, J. B. Harley, and B. Namjou, "Autoimmune thyroid disease is associated with a diagnosis of secondary Sjögren's syndrome in familial systemic lupus," *Annals of the Rheumatic Diseases*, vol. 66, no. 3, pp. 410–413, 2007.

[23] I. Al-Hashimi, S. Khuder, N. Haghighat, and M. Zipp, "Frequency and predictive value of the clinical manifestations in Sjögren's syndrome," *Journal of Oral Pathology and Medicine*, vol. 30, no. 1, pp. 1–6, 2001.

[24] K. D. Deane, C. C. Striebich, B. L. Goldstein et al., "Identification of undiagnosed inflammatory arthritis in a community health fair screen," *Arthritis Care and Research*, vol. 61, no. 12, pp. 1642–1649, 2009.

[25] J.-M. Anaya, "The autoimmune tautology," *Arthritis Research & Therapy*, vol. 12, no. 6, article 147, 2010.

# 2

# Current Understanding on the Role of Standard and Immunoproteasomes in Inflammatory/Immunological Pathways of Multiple Sclerosis

**Elena Bellavista,[1,2] Aurelia Santoro,[2] Daniela Galimberti,[3] Cristoforo Comi,[4] Fabio Luciani,[5] and Michele Mishto[6,7]**

[1] *Interdepartmental Center for Studies on Biophysics, Bioinformatics and Biocomplexity "L. Galvani" (CIG), University of Bologna, 40126 Bologna, Italy*
[2] *Department of Experimental, Diagnostic and Specialty Medicine (DIMES), University of Bologna, 40126 Bologna, Italy*
[3] *Neurology Unit, Department of Pathophosiology and Transplantation, University of Milan, Centro Dino Ferrari, Fondazione IRCCS Cà Granda, Ospedale Maggiore Policlinico, 20122 Milan, Italy*
[4] *Interdisciplinary Research Center of Autoimmune Diseases (IRCAD), University of Eastern Piedmont, "Amedeo Avogadro," 28100 Novara, Italy*
[5] *Inflammation and Infection Research Centre, School of Medical Sciences, University of New South Wales, Sydney, NSW 2052, Australia*
[6] *Institut für Biochemie, Charité Universitätsmedizin Berlin, 10117 Berlin, Germany*
[7] *Centro Interdipartimentale di Ricerca sul Cancro "Giorgio Prodi," University of Bologna, 40126 Bologna, Italy*

Correspondence should be addressed to Michele Mishto; michele.mishto@charite.de

Academic Editor: Umberto Dianzani

The ubiquitin-proteasome system is the major intracellular molecular machinery for protein degradation and maintenance of protein homeostasis in most human cells. As ubiquitin-proteasome system plays a critical role in the regulation of the immune system, it might also influence the development and progression of multiple sclerosis (MS). Both *ex vivo* analyses and animal models suggest that activity and composition of ubiquitin-proteasome system are altered in MS. Proteasome isoforms endowed of immunosubunits may affect the functionality of different cell types such as $CD8^+$ and $CD4^+$ T cells and B cells as well as neurons during MS development. Furthermore, the study of proteasome-related biomarkers, such as proteasome antibodies and circulating proteasomes, may represent a field of interest in MS. Proteasome inhibitors are already used as treatment for cancer and the recent development of inhibitors selective for immunoproteasome subunits may soon represent novel therapeutic approaches to the different forms of MS. In this review we describe the current knowledge on the potential role of proteasomes in MS and discuss the *pro et contra* of possible therapies for MS targeting proteasome isoforms.

## 1. Multiple Sclerosis and Proteasome Isoforms

Multiple sclerosis (MS) is a chronic disease of the central nervous system (CNS) characterized by the presence of inflammation, myelin damage, and axonal degeneration. There are two main clinical courses of multiple sclerosis: about 90% of MS patients experience the relapsing-remitting MS phase (RRMS), characterized by disability episodes followed by a complete or partial recovery. Multifocal lesions are found by magnetic resonance imaging, typically but not exclusively, in the white matter of the optic nerve, brain stem, cerebellum, and spinal cord. Some lesions are enhanced after intravenous administration of gadolinium, indicating breakdown of the blood-brain barrier (BBB) as a result of active inflammation. The majority of RRMS patients enter into a secondary progressive phase (SPMS), characterized by a variable degree of inflammation and a continuous and progressive neurological decline in disability state (with or without superimposed relapses) [1, 2]. A minor percentage (10%) of MS patients shows a primary progressive form of MS

(PPMS), characterized by progression of neurological disability from onset. Clinically relevant factors differentiating RRMS and PPMS are age at disease onset (a decade later in PPMS) and gender (1 : 1.3 male/female in PPMS versus 1 : 2 in RRMS) [3]. Although the initial course of RRMS and PPMS is very different, both proceed at remarkably similar rates during the progressive phase. However, it is still an ongoing debate whether the RRMS and the progressive forms of MS are the same disease observed at different stages or whether they are pathogenetically different.

One of the factors characterising MS is the autoimmune response against self-antigens and the immune-mediated demyelination which contribute, at least in part, to the neurological manifestations. Based on scientific evidence, it has been proposed that a predisposing genetic background, in combination with environmental factors such as infection, diet, sun exposure, and smoking, drives the immune system to mount an immune response towards a yet unknown myelin antigen, eventually resulting in myelin disruption [4]. Indeed, genetic associations of HLA class II (HLA-DRB1*15) and HLA class I (HLA-A*02, -A*03, and -B*07) with MS, as well as the presence of autoreactive $CD4^+$ and $CD8^+$ T lymphocytes, together with other inflammatory cells and cytokines in active MS lesions, suggest an autoimmune pathogenesis [5, 6]. Several studies support the view that an immune response in MS subjects starts and is maintained in the periphery, and specifically in the lymphatic system, although the most lethal cytotoxic effect occurs in the brain with oligodendrocytes, neuron loss, and plaque formation (outside-in model) [2]. A competing view argues that the initial malfunction occurs within the CNS, similarly to other neurodegenerative diseases, by cytodegeneration, possibly focused on the oligodendrocyte-myelin complex, and a release of highly antigenic constituents that secondarily promote an autoimmune and inflammatory response in predisposed individuals [2, 7].

In the last few years, additional players have emerged in the MS pathogenic cascade, including proteasome and gut microbiota (for the latter see Section 3). The proteasome is the central catalytic unit of the ubiquitin-proteasome system, which plays several crucial functions for cell metabolism (Figure 1). By eliminating obsolete, misfolded, or aberrant proteins, the ubiquitin-proteasome system accomplishes housekeeping functions and maintains cellular homeostasis and the physiological levels of intracellular proteins. It has been demonstrated that proteasome inactivation leads to cellular death by apoptosis or necrosis [8–10]. The central role of ubiquitin-proteasome system in inflammatory responses is supported by evidence of its involvement in the on/off switching of many cellular pathways through the time-specific cleavage of short-life proteins, like transcription factors or molecules regulating the cell cycle [11]. Accordingly, the proteasome is crucial in several inflammatory processes by regulating cytokine signalling, cell proliferation, and clearance of potentially deleterious products of inflammation and is involved in the major histocompatibility complex (MHC) class I-mediated antigen presentation (Figure 1) [12]. Therefore, proteasome modulation can alter at different levels

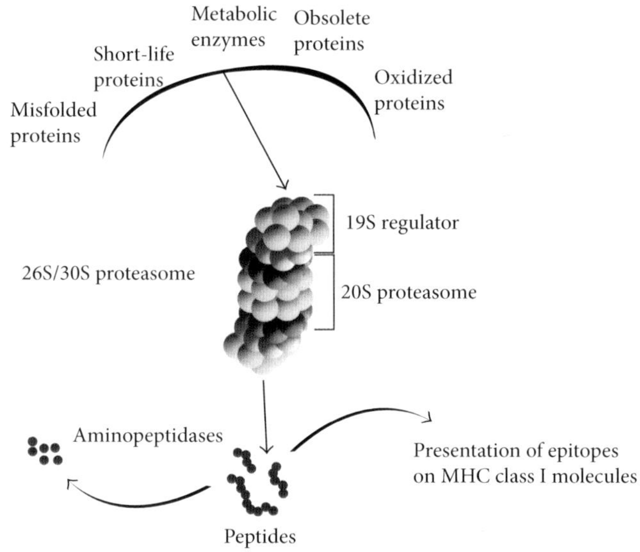


FIGURE 1: Schematic representation of the proteasome degradation pathways.

both the physiological and pathological processes of the immune system.

Different forms of proteasomes are known in eukaryotes. They vary in terms of catalytic subunits and regulatory complexes. The core 20S standard proteasome (s-proteasome) is a cylinder-shaped complex, that is, composed of four stacked rings, each consisting of seven protein subunits. Among them the $\beta 1$, $\beta 2$, and $\beta 5$ subunits harbour the proteolytic active sites. The result of the association of the 20S proteasome core to the PA700 regulators is the 26S/30S proteasomes, which cleave polyubiquitylated proteins in an ATP-dependent manner. 20S proteasome can also bind the PA28 regulator, which alters proteasome catalytic activities [13, 14].

The immunoproteasome (i-proteasome) is an isoform of the 20S proteasome. It carries specific catalytic subunits, that is, $\beta 1i$, $\beta 2i$, and $\beta 5i$ (also known as LMP2, MECL-1, and LMP7, resp.), which confer to the i-proteasome quantitative differences in cleavage preferences and substrate degradation rates compared to the s-proteasome. I-proteasome is generally synthesized upon interferon-$\gamma$ (IFN-$\gamma$) stimuli, but tumor necrosis factor-$\alpha$ (TNF-$\alpha$) or lipopolysaccharide has also been found to be involved in its inducible expression [15, 16]. The vast majority of endogenous peptides that are presented by the MHC class I molecules at the cell surface and recognised by $CD8^+$ T cells are generated by proteasomes. I-proteasome is generally linked to its high efficiency in the generation of the MHC class I-restricted epitopes. In support of this, i-proteasomes are predominantly expressed by professional antigen presenting cells (APCs), such as dendritic cells (DCs) and B cells, or in other cell types during inflammation, thereby indicating the i-proteasome as a major player of the MHC class I antigen presentation (Figure 1) [11, 17].

Preliminary observations on white and grey matter of MS patients suggested that the degradation rates of short fluorogenic peptides by 20S proteasomes are decreased when compared to brain-tissue controls [18]. These results, however, cannot be interpreted as a general decrease of the proteasome-mediated proteolytic activity, as recently shown in [19–21]. Furthermore, an accumulation of i-proteasome and its regulator PA28$\alpha\beta$ has been observed in different cell types affected by MS, such as oligodendrocytes, astrocytes, macrophages/microglia, infiltrating lymphocytes, and weakly neurons [22]. Such disease-related expression of i-proteasome is in agreement with recent observations in the experimental model of MS, that is, the experimental autoimmune encephalomyelitis (EAE). In this model, the cerebral expression of i-proteasome and PA28$\alpha\beta$ was increased as compared with baseline levels during the acute phase of EAE. Of note, i-proteasomes were also detected in neurons, infiltrated T lymphocytes, and microglia in EAE mice [23]. However, in this study by Zheng et al., an equal expression of s- and i-proteasome subunits has been described in control mouse brain, contrasting with other studies on rodents and humans which reported a faint expression of i-proteasome in young/adult brains [21, 24, 25]. Furthermore, Zheng et al. reported no differences in the i-proteasome expression by comparing young and old control mouse brains, which is in contrast to studies on other mammals such as rats [21, 26] and humans [27], but in agreement with a study conducted on nonhuman primates [28].

The expression of i-proteasome in MS lesions or in cells involved in MS mechanisms is important because this isoform has been recently linked to different inflammatory processes. Indeed, i-proteasomes are specifically implicated in cytokine-mediated inflammation, cell growth, and differentiation in mice [11]. I-proteasome depletion alters the T cell antigen receptor (TCR) repertoire formation, the number and differentiation of $CD8^+$ T cells, and the production of proinflammatory cytokines [29]. In addition, i-proteasome depletion during IFN-$\gamma$-mediated oxidative stress is consistent with a deficient clearance of oxidized proteins and aggresomes [30, 31]. These events have been associated with worsening of EAE clinical score in $\beta$5i −/− mice [31], although discordant results have also been reported by others [32].

In the following sections we will discuss these and additional data suggesting an involvement of proteasomes in specific pathways underlying MS.

## 2. I-Proteasome and $CD8^+$ T Cells in MS

$CD4^+$ and $CD8^+$ T lymphocytes reactive against myelin have been found in peripheral blood, cerebrospinal fluid (CSF), and CNS plaques of MS patients, but their role in MS pathogenesis is still a matter of debate. Antimyelin $CD4^+$ T cells in MS have been widely studied because of their role in regulating cell-mediated inflammation, their ability in inducing EAE, and the identification of HLA-DRB1*15 allele as the most significant genetic risk factor associated with MS [33]. EAE can also be triggered by the administration of $CD8^+$ T cells specific against myelin antigens in mice. In MS, $CD8^+$ T cells exceed $CD4^+$ T cells by 3–10-fold in regions of demyelination, and the degree of axonal damage within MS lesions correlates with the number of $CD8^+$ T cells [33]. Furthermore, several studies described an increased prevalence of $CD8^+$ cytotoxic T cells reactive against specific myelin epitopes in peripheral blood of MS patients compared to healthy controls [34–36]. These observations, in addition to the genetic associations of HLA class I alleles with MS risk, suggest an involvement of $CD8^+$ T cells in MS [33].

Because i-proteasome is a major player in the processing of MHC class I-restricted epitopes in professional APCs or in inflamed conditions, it is likely that it is also involved in the presentation of myelin antigens in the MS brain. For instance, i-proteasome expression is induced in oligodendrocytes of MS patients [22]. These cells are the main producers of myelin, and hence likely to be the target of $CD8^+$ T cells in MS. Indeed, $CD8^+$ T cells were observed in close proximity to oligodendrocytes and demyelinated axons in brain tissue, towards which cytolytic granules were polarized [33]. The expression of i-proteasome in oligodendrocytes might therefore alter the presentation onto the MHC class I molecules of myelin antigens and the cytotoxic activity of specific $CD8^+$ T cells towards these cells.

Although the abovementioned scenario lacks experimental validation, there is substantial support for this theory. For instance, our group has previously observed *in vitro* that i-proteasome carrying a polymorphic variant at codon 60 (i.e., HH60) of $\beta$1i subunit produces less amount of the myelin basic protein epitope $MBP_{111-119}$ [22]. This epitope is presented on the HLA-A*02 molecule, although with moderate affinity [22] and memory $CD8^+$ cytotoxic T cells specific for this epitope are more prevalent in the blood of MS patients than controls [35–37]. We also described a lower prevalence of the $\beta$1i HH60 variant among MS females with HLA-A*$02^+$ genotype when compared to a matched control population. These observations led us to hypothesize that the lower risk of developing MS in HLA-A*$02^+$ subjects carrying the $\beta$1i HH60 variant could be—at least in part—due to a lower production of $MBP_{111-119}$ by oligodendrocytes or APCs in these subjects [22].

The key role of i-proteasomes in autoreactive $CD8^+$ T cell response has been recently confirmed by the observation that mice lacking i-proteasome $\beta$5i-$\beta$2i subunits developed a multitissue autoimmune disorder mediated by $CD8^+$ T cells *via* altered MHC class I-restricted self-antigen presentation [38]. The authors of the study speculated that a relatively high percentage of MHC class I molecules present "dangerous" epitopes in presence of inflammation and in the absence of i-proteasome. These self-peptides are low-affinity binders to the MHC class I complexes (as the epitope $MBP_{111-119}$ [22]) and are better produced by s-proteasomes. Hence, in the absence of an appropriate i-proteasome activity these "dangerous" self-epitopes may be generated and targeted by autoreactive $CD8^+$ cytotoxic T cells, thereby triggering an autoimmune response [38]. It is attractive to hypothesize that a similar mechanism is at work in MS and would imply that i-proteasome might hamper MS development by reducing the amount of "dangerous" self-peptides presented by APCs in periphery.

Another matter of debate relies on the mechanisms causing the disruption of the immune system tolerance and the activation of autoreactive CD4+ and CD8+ T lymphocytes towards CNS cells. Different studies suggest that molecular mimicry could be involved in the immune system disruption. This phenomenon describes the reaction of a single T cell clone to epitopes derived from both pathogen and human proteomes. It has been proposed that MS is triggered by a viral infection that, in the presence of (unknown) additional environmental and genetic factors, leads to an uncontrolled activation of autoreactive T cells. Such theory could explain in part the geographic distribution of the risk of developing MS [4] and is supported by several studies showing an increase of EBV-specific cellular immune responses in the blood and in the CSF of subjects with MS [5, 39–42], although the association with other viruses has also been found [4]. Conflicting results however exist about the role of molecular mimicry in driving pathological disorders associated with CD8+ T cells, as a comprehensive analysis on a broad range of CD8+ cytotoxic T cell clones showed a very limited number of cross-reactive T cells recognising both viral and self-epitopes [43].

The mechanisms of molecular mimicry related to CD8+ T cells in autoimmune disorders could be further investigated bearing in mind another proteasome-mediated process, named proteasome-catalyzed peptide splicing (PCPS). PCPS occurs through the binding of separate peptide fragments originating from a single protein, that is, *cis*-PCPS, or from two distinct protein segments, that is, *trans*-PCPS (Figure 2) [44–46]. The role of PCPS in MS has not been investigated yet, although it might be relevant for several reasons. Firstly, PCPS is more prone to generate MHC class I-restricted potential epitopes than the simple proteasomal peptide hydrolysis because of specific biochemical features of PCPS [47]. In addition, PCPS highly increases the diversity of MHC class I-restricted epitopes from self- and viral-antigens as the number of potential peptides presented on MHC molecules is several times higher than the number of peptides encoded in the proteome [48]. Consequently, through the PCPS there could be a significant increase of MHC class I-restricted epitopes with high sequence homology to viral and human proteomes. This phenomenon implies that the activation of CD8+ T cells specific for "spliced" viral epitopes with high or even complete homology with myelin antigens could represent a threat against myelin-producing cells and eventually take part in the development of MS.

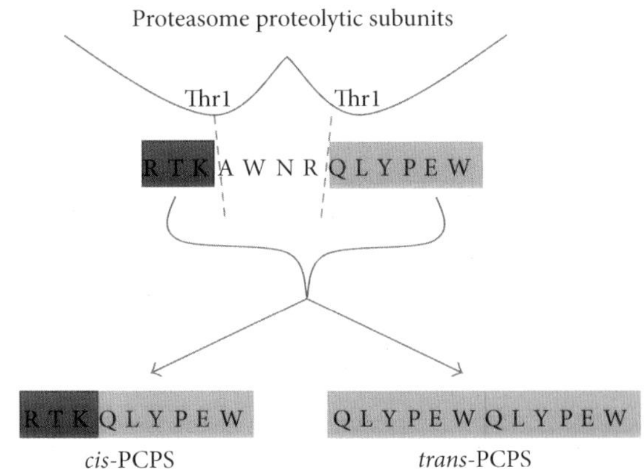


FIGURE 2: Proteasome-catalyzed peptide splicing (PCPS). PCPS can occur by ligation of two fragments of the same substrate molecule (*cis*-PCPS) or derived from two distinct protein molecules (*trans*-PCPS). Shown here are the representative cleavages (depicted by dotted lines) of the peptide $gp100_{40-52}$ (sequence: RTKAWN-RQLYPEW) by two distinct proteasome catalytic subunits, which generate the fragments RTK, AWNR, and QLYPEW. According to the PCPS model [44, 47], the protein is first cleaved by the active site residue Thr1 of the proteasome proteolytic subunits, thereby producing a protein fragment. The latter peptide stays attached to the catalytic centre where, subsequently, it is ligated to a second peptide generating the proteasome-generated spliced peptide.

## 3. Th17 Cells, Gut Microbiota, and Proteasome in MS

CD4+ T cells become activated by recognising antigens presented onto the MHC class II molecules, which are only expressed on professional APCs (such as DCs, macrophages, and B cells). Upon antigen stimulus, CD4+ T lymphocytes differentiate into two main subpopulations, T helper type 1 (Th1) cells and T helper type 2 (Th2) cells. Activated CD4+ T cells can also differentiate into regulatory T (Treg) cells, which are characterised by the expression of the forkhead box P3 (FoxP3) transcription factor [49].

More recently, a new T cell subpopulation, the Th17 cells, which secretes IL-17, IL-21, and IL-22, has been described and associated with the control of extracellular pathogens [50]. Th17 cells and their cytokines are associated with several autoimmune and inflammatory diseases, such as rheumatoid arthritis, systemic lupus erythematosus, MS, psoriasis, inflammatory bowel disease, allergy, and asthma [51]. In MS patients, IL-17 expression is increased in blood mononuclear cells and in CSF as well as at the site of lesions [52]. IL-17 and IL-22 promote blood-brain barrier permeability and CNS inflammation by inducing chemokine production in endothelial cells and by downregulating tight junction proteins. IL-17 also stimulates astrocytes to produce CXC chemokines that can attract neutrophils to the BBB and activate them to release vasoactive substances [53]. It has been shown that myelin-specific Th17 cells directly interact with neuronal cells in demyelinating lesions [54]. Either deficiency or neutralization of IL-17 delay the onset and reduce the severity of EAE [55]. Furthermore, IL-23 expands Th17 cells and is critical for the induction of EAE. In contrast, a recent paper reported that overexpression of IL-2 *in vivo* reverses EAE pathology by decreasing the Th1 and Th17 infiltration. Notably, under inflammatory conditions (such as in EAE), Th17 cells display plasticity because these cells can change phenotype in inflamed tissues and secrete proinflammatory cytokines such as IFN-$\gamma$ instead of IL-17 [56].

A modifier of Th17 cell response in MS may be gut bacteria, which play an important role in shaping intestinal CD4+ T cell responses [57] and in affecting brain inflammation, as suggested by evidence on gut-brain communication [58, 59].

The mammalian gastrointestinal track harbors a highly heterogeneous population of microbial organisms, which vary across geographical areas and are essential for the complete development of the immune system. The gut microbes or "microbiota" also drive a swarm of T cell responses in the gut. For instance, segmented filamentous bacteria trigger intestinal Th17 cell responses; indeed when these bacteria are used to monocolonize germ-free mice they restore Th17 cell responses in the lamina propria of the small intestine [60]. Gut bacteria are also critically involved in the differentiation of some Treg cell subsets [61] as these specific microbial organisms have developed distinct ways to promote effector T cells or Treg cell differentiation in the gut [62]. The Treg/Th17 ratio and also the Treg cell frequency have been negatively correlated with MS severity [63], thereby suggesting that the measure of their balance could be an informative biomarker for evaluating or comparing the effectiveness of MS therapies.

In the context of MS models, it has been reported that the treatment of EAE mice with probiotics reduces neuroinflammation [64] and that different gut microbiota could induce [34, 65] or tackle CNS inflammation [66]. In addition, antibiotic-mediated depletion of the gut microbiota reduces the EAE severity and the levels of proinflammatory cytokines and chemokines, whereas it increases the levels of the anti-inflammatory cytokines IL-10 and IL-13. Moreover, IL-10-producing FoxP3+ Treg cells accumulate in the cervical lymph nodes of antibiotic-treated mice and protect *naïve* recipients against the transfer of EAE [65].

The tight connection between commensal gut microbiota, EAE, and Th17 lymphocytes has been recently investigated in two different models of EAE. Lee and colleagues [67] studied the induction of EAE by immunizing germ-free bacteria, specific-pathogen-free and control mice with $MOG_{35-55}$ peptide + *Mycobacterium tuberculosis*. They observed that germ-free mice are highly resistant to EAE development and have a lower prevalence of Th17 and Th1 cells leading to the conclusion that there is a hampering of the systemic and neuronal proinflammatory Th17 and Th1 response during EAE in absence of commensal microbiota in mice. This phenomenon seems to be reversible because intestinal colonization with segmented filamentous bacteria in germ-free mice promotes EAE development. They concluded that the microbiota dynamically and reversibly impacts the programming of pathogenic immune response during autoimmunity and that microbial colonization may provide proinflammatory signals that affect the reciprocal development of Th and Treg cells both in gut and in CNS [67].

In a second article, Berer and colleagues [68] reported that germ-free mice develop less frequently EAE, a phenomenon accompanied by a reduced number of Th17 cells in the lamina propria and reduced secretion of IL-17 and IFN-$\gamma$ by splenic T cells in response to cognate antigen stimulation. In this latter study, a spontaneous remitting-relapsing EAE mouse model has been used. These mice express, in a large proportion of their $CD4^+$ T cells, a transgenic TCR that recognizes $MOG_{92-106}$ peptide in the context of MHC class II molecules [68]. The fact that two independent studies described, in different models of EAE, an impairment of Th17-mediated induction of EAE in germ-free mice supports the hypothesis that gut microbiota may influence MS *via* Th17 cell activity.

Another modifier of the Th17 cell response in MS may be the i-proteasome. Indeed, it has been shown that the *in vitro* administration of i-proteasome $\beta$5i subunit inhibitor prevents the early activation of $CD4^+$ T cells, their differentiation into Th17 cells, and the secretion of TNF-$\alpha$, IL-23, and IL-6 [69]. *In vivo*, $\beta$5i inhibition or deficiency results in reduced Th1 and Th17 cell expansion and Treg cell development through STAT3/STAT1/SMAD phosphorylation [70]. The treatment with $\beta$5i subunit inhibitor also attenuates the progression of the experimental arthritis in mice [69]. Because this phenomenon acts on the Th17 differentiation pathway and it is not observed by inhibiting s-proteasome activity, we may speculate that a selective block of i-proteasome $\beta$5i subunit in mice might also tackle the development of EAE. Preliminary evidence in dextran sodium sulfate-induced colitis indirectly support such speculation, since this animal model mimics inflammatory bowel diseases, such as Crohn's disease and ulcerative colitis, which are characterized by a marked mucosal infiltration of T cells that secrete Th1 and Th17 cytokines and alterations of faecal and mucosal bacterial communities [71]. Interestingly, in $\beta$5i subunit −/− mice and in wild type mice treated with a proteasome inhibitor, there is a reduction in the secretion of proinflammatory cytokines and chemokines, the infiltration into the colon by neutrophils, and the expansion of Th1 and Th17 cells, thereby preventing excessive tissue damage [72]. These observations are in agreement with the results of Basler et al. [73], which showed a role of $\beta$5i subunit inhibition in reducing the production of proinflammatory cytokines, inflammation, tissue destruction, and consequently pathological symptoms of experimental colitis.

These data suggest that in EAE the activity of Th17 cells could be regulated by gut microbiota and i-proteasomes. Therefore, both of them may be potential targets for the treatment of MS, although there are no studies that investigated the direct interaction between gut microbiota and i-proteasome in EAE.

## 4. Humoral Immunity, Proteasomes, and MS

The understanding of MS pathogenesis has been mostly driven by studies on T cells and their inflammatory cytokines produced in damaged tissues [74]. The interest regarding the antibody-dependent as well as antibody-independent B cell involvement has received a strong boost from the success of clinical trials targeting B cells in MS and other autoimmune diseases [75, 76].

Beyond their ability to produce antibodies, B cells function as APC, thereby contributing to T cells activation in the CNS [77]. They also influence the immune response through the production of effector cytokines, such as those involved in immune regulation (e.g., anti-inflammatory IL-10), polarization (IL-4), and cytokines involved in lymphoid tissue organization (e.g., TNF-$\alpha$ and leukotrienes) [78]. Remarkably, decreased levels of IL-10 and increased concentrations of TNF-$\alpha$ and leukotrienes have been described in patients affected by MS [79], thus contributing to abnormal T-cell activation. This fact provides a conceivable mechanism of action to explain why B cell depletion may be relevant, both in the periphery and in the CNS, in diminishing new MS activity [79]. Indeed, Rituximab, a monoclonal antibody against CD20 molecules, exerts its therapeutic effect through a rapid and profound depletion of peripheral B cell, along with a significant reduction in the volume of T2 lesions and clinical relapse in the RRMS patients, and a reduced disease progression in PPMS [80, 81]. Additionally, in a small cohort of PPMS, it has been shown that Rituximab temporarily suppresses the activation of B cells in CSF [82]. However, the presence of regulatory B cell subsets (B regs), which could either induce or inhibit immune response, accounts for the variable effects that targeting B cells may have *in vivo* [77–80]. At present, new monoclonal antibodies (i.e., Ocrelizumab, Ofatumumab) targeting CD20 or specific surface markers of B cell subset (i.e, Atacicept) are under investigation in phase II/II trials [83, 84].

Although at present there is no data available on proteasome isoforms, B cell regulation, and MS, the recent observation of Hensley et al. [85] is relevant to connect all these three topics. Indeed, the authors reported that i-proteasome $\beta$1i subunit −/− mice have a defect in B cells maturation and Ig isotope switch upon viral infection as well as in $CD4^+$ T cell survival and DC activation. They identified in the NF-$\kappa$B activation one of the pathways affected by the presence of intermediate type proteasomes instead of the i-proteasome, which is normally present in these cells. A role of i-proteasome in modulating NF-$\kappa$B signalling has also been observed by Maldonado and coworkers [86] in retinal pigment epithelial cells of $\beta$1i subunit −/− mice. In knockout mice a higher content and a diminished activation of the NF-$\kappa$B alternative pathway, as well as a delayed termination of the classical pathway, after *in vitro* stimulation by TNF-$\alpha$, has been observed compared to wild type littermates [86].

Concerning the role and significance of antibodies in MS patients, the presence of CSF oligoclonal bands and increased immunoglobulin IgG synthesis is a frequent feature of MS [87] as well as other localized autoimmune diseases of the CNS [88]. These pathogenic autoantibodies (autoAbs) can induce tissue damage and thus be involved in plaque initiation and demyelination by recruiting macrophages and by complement deposition in white matter lesion of MS patients [89]. However, the antigenic targets of these antibodies and their potential use as biomarkers of MS are still a matter of debate. Indeed, autoAbs against antigens not specific for the CNS have also been associated with MS, although it is unclear if they are pathogenic effectors instead of being secondary products of the release of antigens upon CNS tissue damage. Proteasome Abs, for example, are elevated in sera of RR-, PP-, and SP-MS patients compared to other autoimmune diseases or healthy controls [90–92]. It has been shown *in vitro* that autoAbs against 20S proteasome block the proteasome activation by PA28 regulator, thereby suggesting that these autoAbs might have a regulatory function towards extracellular proteasomes such as circulating proteasomes [93]. Notably, although proteasomes are mainly studied as intracellular proteases, extracellular circulating proteasomes are normally present in peripheral blood, and their levels are significantly increased in a variety of pathological conditions, including autoimmune diseases and tumours [94]. In particular, as biomarkers of ongoing pathological mechanisms, circulating proteasomes have demonstrated to have prognostic power as regards therapy outcome and survival in multiple myeloma patients [95]. Although cells originating extracellular proteasomes detected in peripheral blood and in the CSF have not been identified, an active release of circulating proteasomes has been recently proposed [96] as they have been copurified with exosomes [97]. In line with this hypothesis, the immunological activity rather than the cellular damage has been suggested as the causative mechanism for increased circulating proteasome levels in sepsis and sever injury [98]. Recently, a preliminary study carried out on a limited number of patients affected by RRMS has shown that circulating proteasome amount increases in MS and even further in MS patients treated with IFN-$\beta$. The authors have also described a specific proteasome activity pattern in plasma of MS patients although they have not reported appropriate control experiments with proteasome inhibitors [99]. This preliminary observation, however, might be relevant for future studies. Indeed, a fascinating speculation is that circulating proteasomes in peripheral blood are not only simple biomarkers of inflammatory status, but also active proteases that might control cytokine levels, cell-mediated cytotoxicity, and plasma membrane permeability [94] and synergize with other component to ameliorate tissue damage [97].

## 5. Maintenance of Cellular Homeostasis during Inflammation-Mediated Oxidative Stress in MS

The pathological mechanisms of neurodegeneration, although largely unknown, are often mediated by oxidative stress and excitotoxicity (degenerative cascade), two processes that are closely interactive [100, 101]. The increased production of reactive oxygen and nitrogen species induces oxidative damage to different cellular components including lipid, DNA, and proteins [102]. Accordingly, in MS patients, oxidized DNA is present in a small number of reactive astrocytes as well as in oligodendrocyte nuclei, with evidence of apoptosis [103]. Similarly, lipid peroxidation-derived structures (malondialdehyde and oxidized phospholipid epitopes) can be detected in the cytoplasm of oligodendrocytes and some astrocytes as well as in degenerating neurons within grey matter lesions [103]. Oxidized proteins are more prevalent in cerebellar astrocytes as well as in spinal cord neurons of EAE mice [104, 105]. In such scenario, an effective removal of oxidized proteins seems to be a key element to maintain cellular homeostasis during neuroinflammation.

Studies performed on neuronal cell lines have suggested that proteasome plays a central role in mitochondria homeostasis. Proteasome inhibition decreases the activity of complexes I and II and increases the production of reactive oxygen species and the accumulation of lipofuscin, a highly oxidized cross-linked aggregate of oxidized protein and lipid [106, 107]. In addition, proteasome is essential in maintaining cell homeostasis by degrading obsolete, damaged, and oxidized proteins [108–112]. Notably, the 20S proteasomes are more resistant to oxidative stress than 26S proteasomes and seem to be able to degrade oxidized proteins in an ATP-independent manner [113, 114]. Furthermore, i-proteasome expression is induced during oxidative stress in several inflammatory-based diseases in the CNS and in peripheral organs [30, 115, 116] and it provides enhanced cellular resistance to oxidative stress, at least in part by an increased degradation rate of oxidized proteins compared to s-proteasome [117]. Indeed, the blocked expression of $\beta$1i subunit by siRNA significantly reduces the adaptive response to mild oxidative stress in mouse embryonic fibroblasts [116], $\beta$5i-depleted retinal pigment epithelial cell viability is more compromised than wild type cells [30], and $\beta$1i subunit −/− mice exhibit higher levels of protein carbonyls in brain and liver upon aging than those of their wild type littermates [118]. Accordingly, Seifert and coworkers [31] have shown an accumulation of oxidized and polyubiquitylated proteins and aggresome-like induced structures upon INF-$\gamma$ stimuli in the liver and brain of i-proteasome $\beta$5i subunit −/− mice. Moreover, $\beta$5i subunit deficient cells and tissues are not only more sensitive to apoptosis but also have a delayed activation of NF-$\kappa$B after TNF-$\alpha$ stimulation [31]. This dependence of protein oxidation clearance on i-proteasome activity might be pivotal for MS because i-proteasome $\beta$5i subunit −/− mice showed an earlier onset and worse clinical score than wild type mice in an EAE model [31] although this fact, recently, has been disputed by Nathan and colleagues [32].

Overall, these results suggest that i-proteasomes may influence onset and progression of MS by affecting the response of different cell types to the inflammatory aggression in the CNS.

## 6. Is Proteasome Inhibition a Potential Therapy of MS?

The administration of immunomodulatory drugs (glatiramer acetate and IFN-$\beta$) represents the first line therapy for RRMS, but these drugs are seldom useful towards the progressive form of MS [119]. The partial or total inefficacy of the common MS treatments in SPMS and PPMS patients demands the identification of novel therapies. The progressive forms of MS seem to be characterized by peculiar immunological mechanisms that differ from RRMS. In PPMS and SPMS the whole brain is affected and inflammation as well as axonal injury is diffuse, whereas in RRMS inflammation and tissue damage are more focalized in plaques [120]. In the progressive forms of MS, the $CD4^+$ and $CD8^+$ T cells and the B cells seem to be part of the pathological mechanisms, although with characteristics that differ from those observed in RRMS and without a clear correlation between immune cell activation and clinical measures of disease duration and severity, especially in PPMS [121]. Considering the complex pathogenic mechanisms at the basis of MS development, further studies would be needed to better characterize the role of different immune system players, including proteasomes, autoAbs as well as specific Th17 and $CD8^+$ T cells, in the different forms of MS. These studies are likely to support the discovery of new diagnostic and prognostic biomarkers for different MS forms and to generate novel therapeutic drugs such as the specific proteasome inhibitors. Indeed, proteasome inhibitors have been utilised as therapeutic approach towards other diseases, such as multiple myeloma, and selective inhibitors for s- or i-proteasome have been recently developed [122].

Two factors could influence the success of novel therapies based on proteasome inhibitors: their toxicity profiles and their delivery pathways to the CNS and/or the periphery. Regarding the former, the experience of the first proteasome inhibitor, named Bortezomib, approved for clinical treatment of hematologic malignancies, showed that the toxicity could be a limiting factor [122]. However, this disadvantage can be controlled with new inhibitors specific for i-proteasome subunits that can therefore block proteasome activity only in specific cells or pathological conditions [122]. In such contest, the induction of i-proteasome expression in specific cell types upon MS onset—reviewed in Section 1—is a pivotal element ought to be borne in mind.

An additional critical issue is drug delivery. Indeed, the inhibition of i-proteasome is detrimental in tackling the oxidative stress during inflammation, leading to the accumulation of oxidised proteins [11]; this has been linked to the disputed observation that the depletion of $\beta$5i subunit anticipated EAE onset [31, 32] (Table 1). However, further investigations have to be performed since the blockage of i-proteasome activity resulted in a decreased expression of inflammatory biomarkers in *ex vivo* analyses of microglia of a mouse model of Alzheimer's disease [19]. Conversely, an inhibition of i-proteasomes limited to the periphery and towards immune system components such as B and Th17 lymphocytes might be beneficial in treating MS. Noteworthy, the promising results of the clinical trials with the monoclonal antibody Rituximab for the treatment of MS (see Section 4) are consistent with the hypothesis that also a depletion of B cells might ameliorate MS disease. In mice, such depletion could be achieved by a defect in $\beta$1i subunit expression [85] (Table 1).

Furthermore, Th17 cells could be targeted for ameliorating MS course. As i-proteasome inhibition decreases the activation of Th17 cells in mice [69, 70], it can be envisaged that i-proteasome inhibitors could be used to limit Th17 cell activation and EAE progression in mice (Table 1). The first test of this hypothesis could be obtained by treating EAE mice with inhibitors of the i-proteasome $\beta$5i subunit, as it has been already done for other experimental disease models [69, 73]. Notably, a blockage of the i-proteasome activity along the Th17 cell pathway could be coupled to the therapeutic administration of probiotics (live beneficial bacteria) or prebiotics (compounds that stimulate the growth of beneficial bacteria) in EAE mice, given their common action on Th17 lymphocytes [67, 68]. Nonetheless, whether the modulation of gut microbiota could have similar beneficial effects also on MS is largely unknown. In EAE, the depletion or the strong modification of gut microbiota showed beneficial effects on the development of the disease [67, 68]. However, unlike

Table 1: Proteasome isoforms as potential targets of immunological pathways. The table summarizes the major results that may help future studies to understand how the inhibition of distinct proteasome isoforms may affect the development and progression of MS.

| Final targets[a] | Anatomic area | Proteasome subunits inhibited[b] | MS forms | Potential effects[c] | References |
|---|---|---|---|---|---|
| $CD8^+$ T cells | Thymus, lymph nodes, CNS | $\beta$1i, $\beta$2i, $\beta$5i | NA | +/− | [22, 29, 38, 123, 124] |
| $CD4^+$ Th17 cells | Thymus, lymph nodes, CNS, gut | $\beta$1i, $\beta$2i, $\beta$5i | NA | + | [51, 67, 68, 70, 72, 73] |
| B cells | Thymus, lymph nodes, CNS | $\beta$1i | RR, PP, SP | + | [80, 81, 85] |
| Proteasome Abs | Serum | NA | RR, PP, SP | NA | [90] |
| Circulating proteasome | Serum | NA | NA | NA | [94, 99] |
| CNS parenchyma | CNS | $\beta$5i | NA | − | [31] |

[a]Pathways that are directly or indirectly affected by treatment with proteasome inhibitors; [b]evidence from studies where the inhibition/depletion of specific proteasome subunit provided hints about their potential effect on MS; [c]these effects also include speculative arguments on how the proteasome subunit inhibition may affect specific pathways. The detrimental or beneficial effects are marked as "−" or "+," respectively; NA = not available evidence.

mouse models, the human being has a broad variety of diet, environment, genetics, and early microbial exposure features that lead to highly diversified microbiota, which is furthermore extremely adaptable and variable over time [125, 126]. Therefore, the identification of a beneficial or detrimental microbiota towards MS might be strenuous.

While the potential inhibition of i-proteasome activity in B and Th17 cells points towards a beneficial effect against MS, the knowledge of the role of circulating proteasome and of proteasome Abs remains poor. Because of high levels of circulating proteasomes and proteasome Abs in the serum of MS patients [90, 99] a tempting speculation is that the production of proteasome Abs might aim to affect the circulating proteasome activity, although the role of circulating proteasomes in MS and more in general in the peripheral blood is largely unknown (Table 1). Further studies are mandatory to investigate such an issue because a therapy with proteasome inhibitors delivered through peripheral blood would immediately affect circulating proteasomes.

The potential effects of an i-proteasome inhibition within the $CD8^+$ T cell-mediated immune response are still unclear. This inhibition could affect therapy outcome depending on whether the drug is delivered in the periphery only or also in the CNS. Indeed, i-proteasome could influence the presentation of endogenously produced myelin antigens in oligodendrocytes (i.e., in CNS) and in bone marrow-derived APCs (i.e., in periphery) [123, 127], although the outcome of the activation of antimyelin $CD8^+$ T cells is still a matter of debate. For instance, in transgenic mice the induction of EAE by HLA-A*03-restricted myelin epitope was hampered by the overexpression of HLA-A*02 molecules, confirming the opposite (and interacting) action of MHC class I-restricted myelin epitopes on EAE onset [124]. Furthermore, it has been hypothesized that the expression of i-proteasome limits the generation of self-epitopes associated with autoimmune responses [38] and we have proposed that a link exists between a genetic protection toward MS and an i-proteasome polymorphism that impairs the generation of a specific MBP epitope [22]. We therefore conclude that i-proteasomes could play a role in the $CD8^+$ T cell-mediated immune response in MS, and further studies shall better define the role of $CD8^+$ T cells in this pathology and identify which epitopes trigger a deleterious autoimmune $CD8^+$ T cell reaction and how they are generated by different proteasome isoforms.

## Abbreviations

| | |
|---|---|
| APC: | Antigen presenting cells |
| AutoAbs: | Autoantibodies |
| BBB: | Blood-brain barrier |
| CNS: | Central nervous system |
| CSF: | Cerebrospinal fluid |
| DCs: | Dendritic cells |
| EAE: | Experimental autoimmune encephalitis |
| FoxP3: | Forkhead box P3 |
| IFN: | Interferon |
| Ig: | Immunoglobulin |
| IL: | Interleukin |
| I-proteasome: | Immunoproteasome |
| MHC: | Major histocompatibility complex |
| MBP: | Myelin basic protein |
| MOG: | Myelin oligodendrocyte glycoprotein |
| MS: | Multiple sclerosis |
| PPMS: | Primary progressive MS |
| PCPS: | Proteasome-catalyzed peptide splicing |
| RRMS: | Relapsing-remitting MS |
| SPMS: | Secondary progressive phase MS |
| S-proteasome: | Standard proteasome |
| TcR: | T cell antigen receptor |
| Th: | T helper cells |
| TNF-$\alpha$: | Tumor necrosis factor-$\alpha$ |
| Treg: | Regulatory T cells |
| UPS: | Ubiquitin-proteasome system. |

## Conflict of Interests

The authors declare that there is no conflict of interests regarding the publication of this paper.

## Acknowledgments

This work was financed in part by the grant Giovani Ricercatori 2007 from the Italian Ministry of Health, by the grant AICE-FIRE 2012 from AICE FIRE Onlus Emilia Romagna, and by Onyx Pharmaceuticals to MM.

## References

[1] E. M. Frohman, M. K. Racke, and C. S. Raine, "Multiple sclerosis. The plaque and its pathogenesis," *The New England Journal of Medicine*, vol. 354, no. 9, pp. 942–955, 2006.

[2] P. K. Stys, G. W. Zamponi, J. van Minnen, and J. J. Geurts, "Will the real multiple sclerosis please stand up?" *Nature Reviews Neuroscience*, vol. 13, no. 7, pp. 507–514, 2012.

[3] A. Compston and A. Coles, "Multiple sclerosis," *The Lancet*, vol. 372, no. 9648, pp. 1502–1517, 2008.

[4] G. Giovannoni and G. Ebers, "Multiple sclerosis: the environment and causation," *Current Opinion in Neurology*, vol. 20, no. 3, pp. 261–268, 2007.

[5] S. Jilek, M. Schluep, A. Harari et al., "HLA-B7-restricted EBV-specific CD8+ T cells are dysregulated in multiple sclerosis," *Journal of Immunology*, vol. 188, no. 9, pp. 4671–4680, 2012.

[6] L. Fugger, M. A. Friese, and J. I. Bell, "From genes to function: the next challenge to understanding multiple sclerosis," *Nature Reviews Immunology*, vol. 9, no. 6, pp. 408–417, 2009.

[7] B. D. Trapp and K.-A. Nave, "Multiple sclerosis: an immune or neurodegenerative disorder?" *Annual Review of Neuroscience*, vol. 31, pp. 247–269, 2008.

[8] A. L. Goldberg, "Functions of the proteasome: from protein degradation and immune surveillance to cancer therapy," *Biochemical Society Transactions*, vol. 35, no. 1, pp. 12–17, 2007.

[9] B. Dahlmann, "Role of proteasomes in disease," *BMC Biochemistry*, vol. 8, no. 1, article S3, 2007.

[10] F. Schmidt, B. Dahlmann, H. K. Hustoft et al., "Quantitative proteome analysis of the 20S proteasome of apoptotic Jurkat T cells," *Amino Acids*, vol. 41, no. 2, pp. 351–361, 2011.

[11] F. Ebstein, P.-M. Kloetzel, E. Krüger, and U. Seifert, "Emerging roles of immunoproteasomes beyond MHC class I antigen processing," *Cellular and Molecular Life Sciences*, vol. 69, no. 15, pp. 2543–2558, 2012.

[12] A. M. Weissman, N. Shabek, and A. Ciechanover, "The predator becomes the prey: regulating the ubiquitin system by ubiquitylation and degradation," *Nature Reviews Molecular Cell Biology*, vol. 12, no. 9, pp. 605–620, 2011.

[13] M. Bochtler, L. Ditzel, M. Groll, C. Hartmann, and R. Huber, "The proteasome," *Annual Review of Biophysics and Biomolecular Structure*, vol. 28, pp. 295–317, 1999.

[14] D. Voges, P. Zwickl, and W. Baumeister, "The 26S proteasome: a molecular machine designed for controlled proteolysis," *Annual Review of Biochemistry*, vol. 68, pp. 1015–1068, 1999.

[15] C. Pintado, M. P. Gavilán, E. Gavilán et al., "Lipopolysaccharideinduced neuroinflammation leads to the accumulation of ubiquitinated proteins and increases susceptibility to neurodegeneration induced by proteasome inhibition in rat hippocampus," *Journal of Neuroinflammation*, vol. 9, no. 1, article 87, 2012.

[16] D. A. Ferrington and D. S. Gregerson, "Immunoproteasomes: structure, function, and antigen presentation," *Progress in Molecular Biology and Translational Science*, vol. 109, pp. 75–112, 2012.

[17] N. Qureshi, D. C. Morrison, and J. Reis, "Proteasome protease mediated regulation of cytokine induction and inflammation," *Biochimica et Biophysica Acta*, vol. 1823, no. 11, pp. 2087–2093, 2012.

[18] J. Zheng and O. A. Bizzozero, "Decreased activity of the 20S proteasome in the brain white matter and gray matter of patients with multiple schlerosis," *Journal of Neurochemistry*, vol. 117, no. 1, pp. 143–153, 2011.

[19] M. Orre, W. Kamphuis, S. Dooves et al., "Reactive glia show increased immunoproteasome activity in Alzheimer's disease," *Brain*, vol. 136, no. 5, pp. 1415–1431, 2013.

[20] S. Gohlke, M. Mishto, K. Textoris-Taube et al., "Molecular alterations in proteasomes of rat liver during aging result in altered proteolytic activities," *Age*, 2013.

[21] C. Giannini, A. Kloss, S. Gohlke et al., "Poly-ub-substrate-degradative activity of 26S proteasome is not impaired in the aging rat brain," *PLoS ONE*, vol. 8, no. 5, Article ID e64042, 2013.

[22] M. Mishto, E. Bellavista, C. Ligorio et al., "Immunoproteasome LMP2 60HH variant alters MBP epitope generation and reduces the risk to develop multiple sclerosis in Italian female population," *PLoS ONE*, vol. 5, no. 2, Article ID e9287, 2010.

[23] J. Zheng, A. Dasgupta, and O. A. Bizzozero, "Changes in 20S subunit composition are largely responsible for altered proteasomal activities in experimental autoimmune encephalomyelitis," *Journal of Neurochemistry*, vol. 121, no. 3, pp. 486–494, 2012.

[24] M. Mishto, C. Ligorio, E. Bellavista et al., "Immunoproteasome expression is induced in mesial temporal lobe epilepsy," *Biochemical and Biophysical Research Communications*, vol. 408, no. 1, pp. 65–70, 2011.

[25] M. Kremer, A. Henn, C. Kolb et al., "Reduced immunoproteasome formation and accumulation of immunoproteasomal precursors in the brains of lymphocytic choriomeningitis virus-infected mice," *Journal of Immunology*, vol. 185, no. 9, pp. 5549–5560, 2010.

[26] M. P. Gavilán, A. Castaño, M. Torres et al., "Age-related increase in the immunoproteasome content in rat hippocampus: molecular and functional aspects," *Journal of Neurochemistry*, vol. 108, no. 1, pp. 260–272, 2009.

[27] M. Mishto, E. Bellavista, A. Santoro et al., "Immunoproteasome and LMP2 polymorphism in aged and Alzheimer's disease brains," *Neurobiology of Aging*, vol. 27, no. 1, pp. 54–66, 2006.

[28] E. Bellavista, M. Mishto, A. Santoro, C. Bertoni-Freddari, R. B. Sessions, and C. Franceschi, "Immunoproteasome in Macaca fascicularis: no age-dependent modification of abundance and activity in the brain and insight into an in silico structural model," *Rejuvenation Research*, vol. 11, no. 1, pp. 73–82, 2008.

[29] M. Groettrup, C. J. Kirk, and M. Basler, "Proteasomes in immune cells: more than peptide producers?" *Nature Reviews Immunology*, vol. 10, no. 1, pp. 73–78, 2010.

[30] S. A. Hussong, R. J. Kapphahn, S. L. Phillips, M. Maldonado, and D. A. Ferrington, "Immunoproteasome deficiency alters retinal proteasome's response to stress," *Journal of Neurochemistry*, vol. 113, no. 6, pp. 1481–1490, 2010.

[31] U. Seifert, L. P. Bialy, F. Ebstein et al., "Immunoproteasomes preserve protein homeostasis upon interferon-induced oxidative stress," *Cell*, vol. 142, no. 4, pp. 613–624, 2010.

[32] J. A. Nathan, V. Spinnenhirn, G. Schmidtke, M. Basler, M. Groettrup, and A. L. Goldberg, "Immuno- and constitutive proteasomes do not differ in their abilities to degrade ubiquitinated proteins," *Cell*, vol. 152, no. 5, pp. 1184–1194.

[33] M. A. Friese and L. Fugger, "Autoreactive CD8+ T cells in multiple sclerosis: a new target for therapy?" *Brain*, vol. 128, no. 8, pp. 1747–1763, 2005.

[34] H. Yokote, S. Miyake, J. L. Croxford, S. Oki, H. Mizusawa, and T. Yamamura, "NKT cell-dependent amelioration of a mouse model of multiple sclerosis by altering gut flora," *The American Journal of Pathology*, vol. 173, no. 6, pp. 1714–1723, 2008.

[35] T. Tsuchida, K. C. Parker, R. V. Turner, H. F. McFarland, J. E. Coligan, and W. E. Biddison, "Autoreactive CD8+ T-cell responses to human myelin protein-derived peptides," *Proceedings of the National Academy of Sciences of the United States of America*, vol. 91, no. 23, pp. 10859–10863, 1994.

[36] A. Jurewicz, W. E. Biddison, and J. P. Antel, "MHC class I-restricted lysis of human oligodendrocytes by myelin basic protein peptide-specific CD8 T lymphocytes," *Journal of Immunology*, vol. 160, no. 6, pp. 3056–3059, 1998.

[37] Y. C. Q. Zang, S. Li, V. M. Rivera et al., "Increased CD8+ cytotoxic T cell responses to myelin basic protein in multiple sclerosis," *Journal of Immunology*, vol. 172, no. 8, pp. 5120–5127, 2004.

[38] D. M. W. Zaiss, C. P. J. Bekker, A. Gröne, B. A. Lie, and A. J. A. M. Sijts, "Proteasome immunosubunits protect against the development of CD8 T cell-mediated autoimmune diseases," *Journal of Immunology*, vol. 187, no. 5, pp. 2302–2309, 2011.

[39] J. D. Lünemann, N. Edwards, P. A. Muraro et al., "Increased frequency and broadened specificity of latent EBV nuclear antigen-1-specific T cells in multiple sclerosis," *Brain*, vol. 129, no. 6, pp. 1493–1506, 2006.

[40] S. Jilek, M. Schluep, P. Meylan et al., "Strong EBV-specific CD8+ T-cell response in patients with early multiple sclerosis," *Brain*, vol. 131, no. 7, pp. 1712–1721, 2008.

[41] P. Höllsberg, H. J. Hansen, and S. Haahr, "Altered CD8+ T cell responses to selected Epstein-Barr virus immunodominant epitopes in patients with multiple sclerosis," *Clinical and Experimental Immunology*, vol. 132, no. 1, pp. 137–143, 2003.

[42] S. Cepok, D. Zhou, R. Srivastava et al., "Identification of Epstein-Barr virus proteins as putative targets of the immune response in multiple sclerosis," *Journal of Clinical Investigation*, vol. 115, no. 5, pp. 1352–1360, 2005.

[43] J. Ishizuka, K. Grebe, E. Shenderov et al., "Quantitating T cell cross-reactivity for unrelated peptide antigens," *Journal of Immunology*, vol. 183, no. 7, pp. 4337–4345, 2009.

[44] N. Vigneron, V. Stroobant, J. Chapiro et al., "An antigenic peptide produced by peptide splicing in the proteasome," *Science*, vol. 304, no. 5670, pp. 587–590, 2004.

[45] A. Dalet, N. Vigneron, V. Stroobant, K.-I. Hanada, and B. J. Van Den Eynde, "Splicing of distant peptide fragments occurs in the proteasome by transpeptidation and produces the spliced antigenic peptide derived from fibroblast growth factor-5," *Journal of Immunology*, vol. 184, no. 6, pp. 3016–3024, 2010.

[46] J. Liepe, M. Mishto, K. Textoris-Taube et al., "The 20S proteasome splicing activity discovered by SpliceMet," *PLoS Computational Biology*, vol. 6, no. 6, Article ID e1000830, 2010.

[47] M. Mishto, A. Goede, K. T. Taube et al., "Driving forces of proteasome-catalyzed peptide splicing in yeast and humans," *Molecular and Cellular Proteomics*, vol. 11, no. 10, pp. 1008–1023, 2012.

[48] H.-G. Rammensee, "Protein surgery," *Nature*, vol. 427, no. 6971, pp. 203–204, 2004.

[49] K. Mori, M. Itoi, N. Tsukamoto, H. Kubo, and T. Amagai, "The perivascular space as a path of hematopoietic progenitor cells and mature T cells between the blood circulation and the thymic parenchyma," *International Immunology*, vol. 19, no. 6, pp. 745–753, 2007.

[50] E. Bettelli, Y. Carrier, W. Gao et al., "Reciprocal developmental pathways for the generation of pathogenic effector TH17 and regulatory T cells," *Nature*, vol. 441, no. 7090, pp. 235–238, 2006.

[51] M. S. Maddur, P. Miossec, S. V. Kaveri, and J. Bayry, "Th17 cells: biology, pathogenesis of autoimmune and inflammatory diseases, and therapeutic strategies," *The American Journal of Pathology*, vol. 181, no. 1, pp. 8–18, 2012.

[52] J. S. Tzartos, M. A. Friese, M. J. Craner et al., "Interleukin-17 production in central nervous system-infiltrating T cells and glial cells is associated with active disease in multiple sclerosis," *The American Journal of Pathology*, vol. 172, no. 1, pp. 146–155, 2008.

[53] T. Carlson, M. Kroenke, P. Rao, T. E. Lane, and B. Segal, "The Th17-ELR+ CXC chemokine pathway is essential for the development of central nervous system autoimmune disease," *Journal of Experimental Medicine*, vol. 205, no. 4, pp. 811–823, 2008.

[54] V. Siffrin, H. Radbruch, R. Glumm et al., "In Vivo imaging of partially reversible Th17 cell-induced neuronal dysfunction in the course of encephalomyelitis," *Immunity*, vol. 33, no. 3, pp. 424–436, 2010.

[55] Y. Komiyama, S. Nakae, T. Matsuki et al., "IL-17 plays an important role in the development of experimental autoimmune encephalomyelitis," *Journal of Immunology*, vol. 177, no. 1, pp. 566–573, 2006.

[56] L. Cosmi, L. Maggi, V. Santarlasci et al., "Identification of a novel subset of human circulating memory CD4+ T cells that produce both IL-17A and IL-4," *Journal of Allergy and Clinical Immunology*, vol. 125, no. 1–3, pp. 222-30.e1–222-30.e4, 2010.

[57] K. Berer and G. Krishnamoorthy, "Commensal gut flora and brain autoimmunity: a love or hate affair?" *Acta Neuropathologica*, vol. 123, no. 5, pp. 639–651, 2012.

[58] J. Bienenstock and S. Collins, "99th Dahlem Conference on Infection, Inflammation and Chronic Inflammatory Disorders: psycho-neuroimmunology and the intestinal microbiota: clinical observations and basic mechanisms," *Clinical and Experimental Immunology*, vol. 160, no. 1, pp. 85–91, 2010.

[59] S. M. Collins, M. Surette, and P. Bercik, "The interplay between the intestinal microbiota and the brain," *Nature Reviews Microbiology*, vol. 10, no. 11, pp. 735–742, 2012.

[60] I. I. Ivanov, K. Atarashi, N. Manel et al., "Induction of intestinal Th17 cells by segmented filamentous bacteria," *Cell*, vol. 139, no. 3, pp. 485–498, 2009.

[61] C. O'Mahony, P. Scully, D. O'Mahony et al., "Commensal-induced regulatory T cells mediate protection against pathogen-stimulated NF-κB activation," *PLoS Pathogens*, vol. 4, no. 8, Article ID e1000112, 2008.

[62] K. Atarashi, T. Tanoue, T. Shima et al., "Induction of colonic regulatory T cells by indigenous Clostridium species," *Science*, vol. 331, no. 6015, pp. 337–341, 2011.

[63] A. Jamshidian, V. Shaygannejad, A. Pourazar, S. H. Zarkesh-Esfahani, and M. Gharagozloo, "Biased Treg/Th17 balance away from regulatory toward inflammatory phenotype in relapsed multiple sclerosis and its correlation with severity of symptoms," *Journal of Neuroimmunology*, vol. 262, no. 1-2, pp. 106–112, 2013.

[64] S. Lavasani, B. Dzhambazov, M. Nouri et al., "A novel probiotic mixture exerts a therapeutic effect on experimental autoimmune encephalomyelitis mediated by IL-10 producing

regulatory T cells," *PLoS ONE*, vol. 5, no. 2, Article ID e9009, 2010.

[65] J. Ochoa-Repáraz, D. W. Mielcarz, L. E. Ditrio et al., "Role of gut commensal microflora in the development of experimental autoimmune encephalomyelitis," *Journal of Immunology*, vol. 183, no. 10, pp. 6041–6050, 2009.

[66] J. Ochoa-Repáraz, D. W. Mielcarz, Y. Wang et al., "A polysaccharide from the human commensal Bacteroides fragilis protects against CNS demyelinating disease," *Mucosal Immunology*, vol. 3, no. 5, pp. 487–495, 2010.

[67] Y. K. Lee, J. S. Menezes, Y. Umesaki, and S. K. Mazmanian, "Proinflammatory T-cell responses to gut microbiota promote experimental autoimmune encephalomyelitis," *Proceedings of the National Academy of Sciences of the United States of America*, vol. 108, supplement 1, pp. 4615–4622, 2011.

[68] K. Berer, M. Mues, M. Koutrolos et al., "Commensal microbiota and myelin autoantigen cooperate to trigger autoimmune demyelination," *Nature*, vol. 479, no. 7374, pp. 538–541, 2011.

[69] T. Muchamuel, M. Basler, M. A. Aujay et al., "A selective inhibitor of the immunoproteasome subunit LMP7 blocks cytokine production and attenuates progression of experimental arthritis," *Nature Medicine*, vol. 15, no. 7, pp. 781–787, 2009.

[70] K. W. Kalim, M. Basler, C. J. Kirk, and M. Groettrup, "Immunoproteasome subunit LMP7 deficiency and inhibition suppresses Th1 and Th17 but enhances regulatory T cell differentiation," *Journal of Immunology*, vol. 189, no. 8, pp. 4182–4193, 2012.

[71] W. Strober, I. Fuss, and P. Mannon, "The fundamental basis of inflammatory bowel disease," *Journal of Clinical Investigation*, vol. 117, no. 3, pp. 514–521, 2007.

[72] N. Schmidt, E. Gonzalez, A. Visekruna et al., "Targeting the proteasome: partial inhibition of the proteasome by bortezomib or deletion of the immunosubunit LMP7 attenuates experimental colitis," *Gut*, vol. 59, no. 7, pp. 896–906, 2010.

[73] M. Basler, M. Dajee, C. Moll, M. Groettrup, and C. J. Kirk, "Prevention of experimental colitis by a selective inhibitor of the immunoproteasome," *Journal of Immunology*, vol. 185, no. 1, pp. 634–641, 2010.

[74] S. Oh, C. Cudrici, T. Ito, and H. Rus, "B-cells and humoral immunity in multiple sclerosis. Implications for therapy," *Immunologic Research*, vol. 40, no. 3, pp. 224–234, 2008.

[75] P. Engel, J. A. Gómez-Puerta, M. Ramos-Casals, F. Lozano, and X. Bosch, "Therapeutic targeting of B cells for rheumatic autoimmune diseases," *Pharmacological Reviews*, vol. 63, no. 1, pp. 127–156, 2011.

[76] A. C. Chan, "B cell immunotherapy in autoimmunity: 2010 update," *Molecular Immunology*, vol. 48, no. 11, pp. 1344–1347, 2011.

[77] B. Serafini, B. Rosicarelli, R. Magliozzi, E. Stigliano, and F. Aloisi, "Detection of ectopic B-cell follicles with germinal centers in the meninges of patients with secondary progressive multiple sclerosis," *Brain Pathology*, vol. 14, no. 2, pp. 164–174, 2004.

[78] M. Duddy, M. Niino, F. Adatia et al., "Distinct effector cytokine profiles of memory and naive human B cell subsets and implication in multiple sclerosis," *Journal of Immunology*, vol. 178, no. 10, pp. 6092–6099, 2007.

[79] A. Bar-Or, L. Fawaz, B. Fan et al., "Abnormal B-cell cytokine responses a trigger of T-cell-mediated disease in MS?" *Annals of Neurology*, vol. 67, no. 4, pp. 452–461, 2010.

[80] K. Hawker, P. O'Connor, M. S. Freedman et al., "Rituximab in patients with primary progressive multiple sclerosis: results of a randomized double-blind placebo-controlled multicenter trial," *Annals of Neurology*, vol. 66, no. 4, pp. 460–471, 2009.

[81] S. L. Hauser, E. Waubant, D. L. Arnold et al., "B-cell depletion with rituximab in relapsing-remitting multiple sclerosis," *The New England Journal of Medicine*, vol. 358, no. 7, pp. 676–688, 2008.

[82] N. L. Monson, P. D. Cravens, E. M. Frohman, K. Hawker, and M. K. Racke, "Effect of rituximab on the peripheral blood and cerebrospinal fluid B cells in patients with primary progressive multiple sclerosis," *Archives of Neurology*, vol. 62, no. 2, pp. 258–264, 2005.

[83] L. Kappos, D. Li, P. A. Calabresi et al., "Ocrelizumab in relapsing-remitting multiple sclerosis: a phase 2, randomised, placebo-controlled, multicentre trial," *The Lancet*, vol. 378, no. 9805, pp. 1779–1787, 2011.

[84] S. Lulu and E. Waubant, "Humoral-targeted immunotherapies in multiple sclerosis," *Neurotherapeutics*, vol. 10, no. 1, pp. 34–43, 2013.

[85] S. E. Hensley, D. Zanker, B. P. Dolan et al., "Unexpected role for the immunoproteasome subunit LMP2 in antiviral humoral and innate immune responses," *Journal of Immunology*, vol. 184, no. 8, pp. 4115–4122, 2010.

[86] M. Maldonado, R. J. Kapphahn, M. R. Terluk et al., "Immunoproteasome deficiency modifies the alternative pathway of NFkappaB signaling," *PLoS ONE*, vol. 8, no. 2, Article ID e56187, 2013.

[87] M. W. Lin, D. Suan, K. Lenton et al., "Differentiating patterns of oligoclonal banding in the cerebrospinal fluid improves diagnostic utility for multiple sclerosis," *Pathology*, vol. 44, no. 3, pp. 248–250, 2012.

[88] O. Stich, S. Jarius, B. Kleer, C. Rasiah, R. Voltz, and S. Rauer, "Specific antibody index in cerebrospinal fluid from patients with central and peripheral paraneoplastic neurological syndromes," *Journal of Neuroimmunology*, vol. 183, no. 1-2, pp. 220–224, 2007.

[89] M. K. Storch, S. Piddlesden, M. Haltia, M. Iivanainen, P. Morgan, and H. Lassmann, "Multiple sclerosis: in situ evidence for antibody- and complement-mediated demyelination," *Annals of Neurology*, vol. 43, no. 4, pp. 465–471, 1998.

[90] I. Mayo, J. Arribas, P. Villoslada et al., "The proteasome is a major autoantigen in multiple sclerosis," *Brain*, vol. 125, no. 12, pp. 2658–2667, 2002.

[91] H. Thuy-Tien, M. Haugen, J. Aarseth, A. Storstein, and C. A. Vedeler, "Proteasome antibodies in patients with cancer or multiple sclerosis," *Scandinavian Journal of Immunology*, vol. 67, no. 4, pp. 400–403, 2008.

[92] N. H. Beyer, J. Milthers, B. A.-M. Lauridsen, G. Houen, and L. J. Frederiksen, "Autoantibodies to the proteasome in monosymptomatic optic neuritis may predict progression to multiple sclerosis," *Scandinavian Journal of Clinical and Laboratory Investigation*, vol. 67, no. 7, pp. 696–706, 2007.

[93] M. Brychcy, U. Kuckelkorn, G. Hausdorf et al., "Anti-20S proteasome autoantibodies inhibit proteasome stimulation by proteasome activator PA28," *Arthritis and Rheumatism*, vol. 54, no. 7, pp. 2175–2183, 2006.

[94] S. U. Sixt and B. Dahlmann, "Extracellular, circulating proteasomes and ubiquitin: incidence and relevance," *Biochimica et Biophysica Acta*, vol. 1782, no. 12, pp. 817–823, 2008.

[95] C. Jakob, K. Egerer, P. Liebisch et al., "Circulating proteasome levels are an independent prognostic factor for survival in multiple myeloma," *Blood*, vol. 109, no. 5, pp. 2100–2105, 2007.

[96] O. Mueller, T. Anlasik, J. Wiedemann et al., "Circulating extracellular proteasome in the cerebrospinal fluid: a study on concentration and proteolytic activity," *Journal of Molecular Neuroscience*, vol. 46, no. 3, pp. 509–515, 2012.

[97] R. C. Lai, S. S. Tan, B. J. Teh et al., "Proteolytic potential of the MSC exosome proteome: implications for an exosome-mediated delivery of therapeutic proteasome," *International Journal of Proteomics*, vol. 2012, Article ID 971907, 14 pages, 2012.

[98] G. A. Roth, B. Moser, C. Krenn et al., "Heightened levels of circulating 20S proteasome in critically ill patients," *European Journal of Clinical Investigation*, vol. 35, no. 6, pp. 399–403, 2005.

[99] A. Minagar, W. Ma, X. Zhang et al., "Plasma ubiquitin-proteasome system profile in patients with multiple sclerosis: correlation with clinical features, neuroimaging, and treatment with interferon-beta-1b," *Journal of Neurology Research*, vol. 34, no. 6, pp. 611–618, 2012.

[100] C. Stadelmann, C. Wegner, and W. Brück, "Inflammation, demyelination, and degeneration: recent insights from MS pathology," *Biochimica et Biophysica Acta*, vol. 1812, no. 2, pp. 275–282, 2011.

[101] R. E. Gonsette, "Neurodegeneration in multiple sclerosis: the role of oxidative stress and excitotoxicity," *Journal of the Neurological Sciences*, vol. 274, no. 1-2, pp. 48–53, 2008.

[102] H. Lassmann and J. van Horssen, "The molecular basis of neurodegeneration in multiple sclerosis," *FEBS Letters*, vol. 585, no. 23, pp. 3715–3723, 2011.

[103] L. Haider, M. T. Fischer, J. M. Frischer et al., "Oxidative damage in multiple sclerosis lesions," *Brain*, vol. 134, no. 7, pp. 1914–1924, 2011.

[104] S. M. Smerjac and O. A. Bizzozero, "Cytoskeletal protein carbonylation and degradation in experimental autoimmune encephalomyelitis," *Journal of Neurochemistry*, vol. 105, no. 3, pp. 763–772, 2008.

[105] J. Zheng and O. A. Bizzozero, "Accumulation of protein carbonyls within cerebellar astrocytes in murine experimental autoimmune encephalomyelitis," *Journal of Neuroscience Research*, vol. 88, no. 15, pp. 3376–3385, 2010.

[106] L. Papa and P. Rockwell, "Persistent mitochondrial dysfunction and oxidative stress hinder neuronal cell recovery from reversible proteasome inhibition," *Apoptosis*, vol. 13, no. 4, pp. 588–599, 2008.

[107] P. G. Sullivan, N. B. Dragicevic, J.-H. Deng et al., "Proteasome inhibition alters neural mitochondrial homeostasis and mitochondria turnover," *Journal of Biological Chemistry*, vol. 279, no. 20, pp. 20699–20707, 2004.

[108] C. T. Aiken, R. M. Kaake, X. Wang, and L. Huang, "Oxidative stress-mediated regulation of proteasome complexes," *Molecular and Cellular Proteomics*, vol. 10, no. 5, Article ID R110.006924, 2011.

[109] S. Grimm, A. Höhn, and T. Grune, "Oxidative protein damage and the proteasome," *Amino acids*, vol. 42, no. 1, pp. 23–38, 2012.

[110] T. Jung and T. Grune, "The proteasome and its role in the degradation of oxidized proteins," *IUBMB Life*, vol. 60, no. 11, pp. 743–752, 2008.

[111] T. Grune, K. Merker, G. Sandig, and K. J. A. Davies, "Selective degradation of oxidatively modified protein substrates by the proteasome," *Biochemical and Biophysical Research Communications*, vol. 305, no. 3, pp. 709–718, 2003.

[112] L. Farout and B. Friguet, "Proteasome function in aging and oxidative stress: implications in protein maintenance failure," *Antioxidants and Redox Signaling*, vol. 8, no. 1-2, pp. 205–216, 2006.

[113] T. Reinheckel, N. Sitte, O. Ullrich, U. Kuckelkorn, K. J. A. Davies, and T. Grune, "Comparative resistance of the 20 S and 26 S proteasome to oxidative stress," *Biochemical Journal*, vol. 335, no. 3, pp. 637–642, 1998.

[114] M. Kästle and T. Grune, "Proteins bearing oxidation-induced carbonyl groups are not preferentially ubiquitinated," *Biochimie*, vol. 93, no. 6, pp. 1076–1079, 2011.

[115] S. Kotamraju, S. Matalon, T. Matsunaga, T. Shang, J. M. Hickman-Davis, and B. Kalyanaraman, "Upregulation of immunoproteasomes by nitric oxide: potential antioxidative mechanism in endothelial cells," *Free Radical Biology and Medicine*, vol. 40, no. 6, pp. 1034–1044, 2006.

[116] A. M. Pickering, A. L. Koop, C. Y. Teoh, G. Ermak, T. Grune, and K. J. A. Davies, "The immunoproteasome, the 20S proteasome and the PA28$\alpha\beta$ proteasome regulator are oxidative-stress-adaptive proteolytic complexes," *Biochemical Journal*, vol. 432, no. 3, pp. 585–594, 2010.

[117] A. M. Pickering and K. J. Davies, "Differential roles of proteasome and immunoproteasome regulators Pa28alphabeta, Pa28gamma and Pa200 in the degradation of oxidized proteins," *Archives of Biochemistry and Biophysics*, vol. 523, no. 2, pp. 181–190, 2012.

[118] Q. Ding, S. Martin, E. Dimayuga, A. J. Bruce-Keller, and J. N. Keller, "LMP2 knock-out mice have reduced proteasome activities and increased levels of oxidatively damaged proteins," *Antioxidants and Redox Signaling*, vol. 8, no. 1-2, pp. 130–135, 2006.

[119] D. Bates, "Treatment effects of immunomodulatory therapies at different stages of multiple sclerosis in short-term trials," *Neurology*, vol. 76, supplement 1, no. 1, pp. S14–S25, 2011.

[120] C. F. Lucchinetti, J. Parisi, and W. Bruck, "The pathology of multiple sclerosis," *Neurologic Clinics*, vol. 23, no. 1, pp. 77–105, 2005.

[121] G. Frisullo, D. Plantone, A. Marti et al., "Type 1 immune response in progressive multiple sclerosis," *Journal of Neuroimmunology*, vol. 249, no. 1-2, pp. 112–116, 2012.

[122] E. Bellavista, F. Andreoli, M. Parenti et al., "Immunoproteasome in cancer and neuropathologies: a new therapeutic target?" *Current Pharmaceutical Design*, vol. 19, no. 4, pp. 702–718, 2013.

[123] A. Perchellet, I. Stromnes, J. M. Pang, and J. Goverman, "CD8+ T cells maintain tolerance to myelin basis protein by 'epitope theft'," *Nature Immunology*, vol. 5, no. 6, pp. 606–614, 2004.

[124] M. A. Friese, K. B. Jakobsen, L. Friis et al., "Opposing effects of HLA class I molecules in tuning autoreactive CD8 + T cells in multiple sclerosis," *Nature Medicine*, vol. 14, no. 11, pp. 1227–1235, 2008.

[125] Human Microbiome Project Consortium, "Structure, function and diversity of the healthy human microbiome," *Nature*, vol. 486, no. 7402, pp. 207–214, 2012.

[126] M. Candela, E. Biagi, S. Maccaferri, S. Turroni, and P. Brigidi, "Intestinal microbiota is a plastic factor responding to environmental changes," *Trends in Microbiology*, vol. 20, no. 8, pp. 385–391, 2012.

[127] A. Perchellet, T. Brabb, and J. M. Goverman, "Crosspresentation by nonhematopoietic and direct presentation by hematopoietic cells induce central tolerance to myelin basic protein," *Proceedings of the National Academy of Sciences of the United States of America*, vol. 105, no. 37, pp. 14040–14045, 2008.

# 3

# Association of IFN-$\gamma$ : IL-10 Cytokine Ratio with Nonsegmental Vitiligo Pathogenesis


**Yaswanth Ala,[1] Mohammed Khalid Pasha,[1] Raja Narasimha Rao,[2] Prasanna Latha Komaravalli,[1] and Parveen Jahan[1,3]**

[1]*Department of Genetics, Osmania University, Hyderabad, Telangana 500007, India*
[2]*Central Railway Hospital, Lallaguda, Hyderabad, Telangana 500017, India*
[3]*Department of Zoology, School of Sciences, Maulana Azad National Urdu University, Gachibowli, Hyderabad, Telangana 500032, India*

Correspondence should be addressed to Parveen Jahan; dr.pjahan@gmail.com



Academic Editor: Xu-Jie Zhou



*Background and Objectives.* Cytokines regulate immune response and inflammation and play a crucial role in depigmentation process of vitiligo. The present study aimed to estimate the serum levels of pro- and anti-inflammatory cytokines, IFN-$\gamma$ and IL-10, and their ratios in nonsegmental vitiligo patients and healthy individuals from India. *Methods.* Blood samples were collected from 280 subjects and serum IFN-$\gamma$ and IL-10 levels were measured using standard ELISA. *Results.* Nonsegmental vitiligo patients showed increased levels of IFN-$\gamma$ ($12.4 \pm 3.2$ versus $9.9 \pm 4.4$ pg/mL) and decreased levels of IL-10 ($9.3 \pm 1.7$ versus $11.5 \pm 5$ pg/mL) compared to controls. Ratio of IFN-$\gamma$ : IL-10 differed significantly from patients to controls ($p < 0.05$). IFN-$\gamma$ concentrations and IFN-$\gamma$ : IL-10 ratio varied significantly with respect to clinical variants, disease stability, and social habits (smoking and alcohol consumption) and showed a positive correlation with disease duration. Family history of vitiligo was significantly associated with IFN-$\gamma$ : IL-10 ratio but not with their individual levels. *Conclusion.* The ratio of IFN-$\gamma$ : IL-10 serum levels may be considered as one of the promising immunological markers in nonsegmental vitiligo. This is the first study considering multiple aspects in relation to ratio of cytokine levels. Similar studies with large samples are warranted to confirm our observations.


## 1. Introduction

Vitiligo is defined as an acquired cutaneous complex disorder resulting from functional loss of melanocytes in epidermis, characterized by milky white macules of various sizes and shapes that tend to enlarge peripherally in the course of time [1]. It is an inflammatory disorder associated with increased expression of inflammatory cytokines in the skin and blood [2]. The melanocytes are targeted by multiple aggressions leading to marked reduction and destruction of pigment cells in vitiligo patients [3]. The prevalence of the disease is estimated to be <0.1% to >8% of the world population and is found to be 0.5–2.5% in India with a high prevalence of 8.8% in Gujarat and Rajasthan states [4, 5]. The pathogenesis of vitiligo includes both intrinsic defects within melanocytes that activate cellular stress response and the autoimmune mechanisms targeting the melanocytes involving both humoral and cell mediated immunity [5–7]. Infiltration of cytotoxic T cells in perilesional lesions is the characteristic hallmark of vitiligo [8]. There is growing evidence that cytokines are important in the depigmentation process and show a cytokine imbalance in the skin of vitiligo patients suggesting their prominent role in autoimmune pathogenesis [9, 10]. Systemic biological therapies used for treating psoriasis and other autoimmune diseases by targeting cytokines indicate that a similar approach might be effective for vitiligo [6].

Cytokines are protein molecules that include Interferons (IFNs), Interleukins (ILs), various Colony Stimulating Factors (CSFs), and Tumor Necrosis Factors (TNFs) which are key molecules in mediating inflammatory and cytokine reactions. Their response due to imbalance or deficiency in the cytokine network may largely determine autoimmune disease susceptibility and severity. Alteration in the concentration of various proinflammatory and anti-inflammatory cytokines such as IL-6, IL-8, IL-10, IL-2, TNF-$\alpha$, and IFN-$\gamma$ has been associated with various autoimmune disorders [11–13]. IL-10 is a potent regulator of anti-inflammatory immune responses and is hence considered to be a downregulator of cytokine production by Th1 cells and macrophages [14, 15]. On the other hand, elevated concentrations of IFN-$\gamma$ initiate apoptosis and it has been suggested that melanocyte death is mediated by apoptosis in the context of autoimmunity [16]. In view of the above literature, we aimed to assess the balance between the proinflammatory IFN-$\gamma$ and anti-inflammatory IL-10 cytokine serum levels in NSV patients and healthy controls from India.

## 2. Materials and Methodology

The present study enrolled a total of 280 subjects that included 130 patients (mean age 27.6 ± 6.9 years) and 150 healthy controls (mean age 26.9 ± 5.6 years) from Central Railway Hospital, Hyderabad, India, in the period of April 2012 to March 2014. Approval for the study was obtained from the Institutional Ethical Committee, Osmania University, Hyderabad, India. The subjects were enrolled after providing informed consent and detailed information was procured from all the subjects regarding demographic, clinical, and family history of vitiligo. The patients enrolled were either on no drug treatment or in the washout period of three months.

Information was recorded in a pro forma with respect to clinical presentation of the disease, age, gender, age at onset, family history, dietary habits, occupation, socioeconomic background, associated diseases, and clinical parameters. Five millilitres (mL) of blood sample was collected from each of the enrolled patients and controls. An inclusion criterion of patients was presence of nonsegmental vitiligo without any other associated disorder as well as not being under any treatment. Patients with segmental vitiligo, known allergies, other skin diseases, or other autoimmune disorders such as Hashimoto's thyroiditis, Graves' disease, type 1 insulin-dependent diabetes mellitus, Addison's disease, psoriasis, rheumatoid arthritis, and thyroid dysfunction which are known to have altered levels of cytokines were excluded from the study [11, 17].

Based upon the spreading of the lesions or white macules at the time of sample collection, the patients were categorized into active vitiligo (existing lesions are spreading and/or new lesions had appeared within the previous six months) and stable vitiligo (no increase in the size or number of lesions within 6 months or more) [18]. The duration of the disease was considered as the time between initial appearance of the clinical symptoms of the disease and sample collection.

*2.1. Determination of Serum IL-10 and IFN-$\gamma$ Levels.* Analysis was performed on blood serum using sandwich ELISA method (eBioscience Inc., San Diego, CA, USA). In brief, the antibody was coated onto a 96-well plate by adding 100 $\mu$L of capture antibody (1X) to each well and incubated overnight at 4°C. The wells were blocked with 200 $\mu$L/well of 1X assay diluent and incubated for 1 hour at room temperature (RT). After that, 100 $\mu$L/well of serum samples and standards was added to the wells and incubated for 2 hours at RT. After incubation, detection antibody (100 $\mu$L/well) was added and incubated for 1 hour. Then 100 $\mu$L/well of avidin-HRP (Horseradish Peroxidase) was added and incubated at RT for another 30 minutes. The plate was incubated with substrate (100 $\mu$L/well) for 15 minutes at RT followed by (50 $\mu$L/well) stop solution. Each of the above steps was interspersed by 5–7 washes to ensure no carryover and absorbance was measured at 450 nm and 540 nm. The concentrations were calculated using MPM software version 6.1.

*2.2. Statistical Analysis.* Data was analysed using descriptive statistics to calculate the percentages, mean values, and standard deviation. Student's "$t$-" test, one-way ANOVA, and Pearson correlation were carried out to analyse the variation between patients and controls, clinical variants of vitiligo, and association among the variables, respectively. A $p$ value less than 0.05 was considered as statistically significant.

## 3. Results

A total of 130 vitiligo patients with a mean age of 27.6 ± 6.9 years and 150 healthy controls with a mean age of 26.9 ± 5.6 years were enrolled in this study. Approximately, equal numbers of males and females were observed in both of the study groups. The mean age at onset of the disease was 23.3±7.0 years (23.2±7.8 years in females and 23.4±6.5 years in males) and the duration of the disease ranged from 1 to 14 years with a mean of 4.2 ± 3.1 years (4.6 ± 3.5 years in females and 3.8 ± 2.8 years in males). In the present study 63.8% of the patients showed active vitiligo and 36.2% stable vitiligo; family history of NSV was seen in 40% of patients and 32% of male patients had the social habits of smoking and alcohol consumption (Table 1).

*3.1. IFN-$\gamma$ Serum Concentrations.* The proinflammatory cytokine IFN-$\gamma$ levels were noted to be significantly elevated in vitiligo patients compared to healthy controls (12.4 ± 3.2 pg/mL versus 9.9 ± 4.4 pg/mL; $p < 0.05$). Analysis of variance (ANOVA) showed a significant difference with respect to serum IFN-$\gamma$ levels among the clinical variants of vitiligo (nondermatomal, acrofacial, mucosal, and focal) ($p < 0.05$). Increased amounts of IFN-$\gamma$ were observed in active vitiligo patients compared to patients with the stable condition of the disease ($p < 0.05$). With respect to social habits (smoking and alcohol consumption), the cytokine levels were analysed for only male patients and controls as none of our female subjects were with these social habits.

Significantly elevated concentrations of IFN-$\gamma$ were noticed in patients compared to controls ($p = 0.001$) and in patients with social habits compared to patients without social habits ($p = 0.04$). However, the levels were not significant between controls with and without social habits ($p = 0.156$). IFN-$\gamma$ levels were nearly similar in patients with and without family history of vitiligo ($p > 0.05$) (Table 2) (Figure 1). A positive correlation was observed between the

TABLE 1: Demographic and clinical characteristics of subjects included in the study.

| | Patients ($n = 130$) Mean ± SD | Controls ($n = 150$) Mean ± SD | $p$ value |
|---|---|---|---|
| Age in years | 27.6 ± 6.9 years | 26.9 ± 5.6 | **0.34 (NS)** |
| Males | 27.3 ± 6.7 (76) | 27.2 ± 6.0 (85) | **0.92 (NS)** |
| Females | 27.9 ± 7.3 (54) | 26.3 ± 4.7 (65) | **0.15 (NS)** |
| Duration of the disease | 4.2 ± 3.1 years | NA | |
| Males | 3.8 ± 2.8 years | | |
| Females | 4.6 ± 3.5 years | | |
| Age at onset | 23.3 ± 7.0 years | NA | |
| Males | 23.4 ± 6.5 years | | |
| Females | 23.2 ± 7.8 years | | |
| | $n$ (%) | $n$ (%) | |
| Males with social habits | | | |
| Yes | 29 (22.3) | 20 (23.5) | |
| No | 47 (77.7) | 65 (76.5) | |
| Clinical variants of vitiligo | | | |
| Nondermatomal | 58 (44.6) | NA | |
| Acrofacial | 33 (25.4) | — | |
| Mucosal | 22 (17) | — | |
| Focal | 17 (13) | — | |
| Disease status | | | |
| Stable | 47 (36.2) | NA | |
| Active | 83 (63.8) | — | |
| Family history | | | |
| Yes | 52 (40) | | |
| No | 78 (60) | — | |

Note: NS: not significant; $n$ = number of subjects, and SD = standard deviation.

concentration of this proinflammatory cytokine and the duration of the disease (Figure 2).

*3.2. IL-10 Serum Concentrations.* A significant difference was found in the mean serum concentrations of the anti-inflammatory cytokine IL-10 between patients and controls (9.3 ± 1.7 pg/mL versus 11.5 ± 5 pg/mL; $p < 0.05$). However, no difference in the levels of IL-10 with respect to clinical variants, disease stability, social habits, and family history within the patient group was seen ($p > 0.05$) (Table 2, Figure 1). Furthermore, we did not find correlation between the duration of disease and serum levels of IL-10 ($p > 0.05$) (Figure 2).

A positive correlation between the concentrations of the two cytokines IL-10 and IFN-$\gamma$ was seen in patients but not in controls. Similarly, active vitiligo patients exhibited a positive correlation between IL-10 and IFN-$\gamma$ but the stable vitiligo patients did not (Figure 2).

*3.3. Ratio of IFN-$\gamma$ : IL-10 in Serum.* The ratio of IFN-$\gamma$ to IL-10 was detected to be significantly higher in NSV patients compared to controls (1.3 ± 0.3 versus 0.9 ± 0.7; $p < 0.05$). Patients with clinical variants, with active and stable vitiligo, with and without social habits of smoking and alcohol consumption, and with and without family history of nonsegmental vitiligo also exhibited a significantly increased ratio of IFN-$\gamma$ : IL-10 ($p < 0.05$) (Table 2, Figure 1). Further, there was a positive correlation between this ratio and the duration of the disease ($p < 0.05$) (Figure 2).

## 4. Discussion

In the present study, the serum concentration of the proinflammatory cytokine IFN-$\gamma$ was significantly elevated in NSV patients compared to controls. Supporting our observation, Th1 predominance has been reported to be associated with vitiligo from previous studies. Shi and Erf in Smyth line (SL) chicken model for autoimmune vitiligo have shown that IFN-$\gamma$, a proinflammatory cytokine which acts as a signature cytokine of Th1 mediated immunity, has remarkably increased in the Smyth line vitiligo samples proving the central role of this cytokine in the SLV pathomechanism [19]. Rashigi et al. reported that both vitiligo patients and mouse model of vitiligo reflect a uniquely IFN-$\gamma$ specific Th1 cytokine signature in the skin that includes IFN-$\gamma$ dependent chemokines such as CXCL9, CXCL10, and CXCL11 which induces T cell homing into peripheral tissues [6]. Mechanistic studies in mouse model revealed that depigmentation

TABLE 2: Serum concentrations of IFN-$\gamma$, IL-10, and IFN-$\gamma$ : IL-10 ratio in controls and vitiligo patients.

| | IFN-$\gamma$ in pg/mL Mean ± SD | IL-10 in pg/mL Mean ± SD | IFN-$\gamma$ : IL-10 in pg/mL Mean ± SD |
|---|---|---|---|
| Vitiligo patients (130) | 12.4 ± 3.2 | 9.3 ± 1.7 | 1.3 ± 0.3 |
| Controls (150) | 9.9 ± 4.4 | 11.5 ± 5.0 | 0.9 ± 0.7 |
| "$t$-" test $p$ value | **0.0001*** | **0.0001*** | **0.0001*** |
| Clinical variants of vitiligo (%) | | | |
| Nondermatomal (44.6) | 12.5 ± 3.2 | 9.7 ± 1.8 | 1.2 ± 0.2 |
| Acrofacial (25.4) | 14.4 ± 2.7 | 8.9 ± 1.2 | 1.6 ± 0.3 |
| Mucosal (17) | 10.5 ± 3.1 | 9.1 ± 2.1 | 1.1 ± 0.3 |
| Focal (13) | 11.0 ± 2.0 | 8.9 ± 1.7 | 1.2 ± 0.1 |
| One-way ANOVA "$p$" value | **0.000*** | **0.111 (NS)** | **0.000*** |
| Disease status (%) | | | |
| Stable (36.2) | 11.5 ± 2.7 | 9.3 ± 1.8 | 1.2 ± 0.3 |
| Active (63.8) | 13.0 ± 3.3 | 9.3 ± 1.7 | 1.4 ± 0.3 |
| "$t$-" test $p$ value | **0.009*** | **1 (NS)** | **0.0004*** |
| Family history (%) | | | |
| Yes (40) | 12.9 ± 3.4 | 9.1 ± 1.6 | 1.4 ± 0.3 |
| No (60) | 12.1 ± 3.1 | 9.4 ± 1.8 | 1.3 ± 0.3 |
| "$t$-" test $p$ value | **0.1 (NS)** | **0.3 (NS)** | **0.02*** |
| Male patients with SH (%) | | | |
| Yes (42) | 14.2 ± 4.1 | 9.9 ± 2.0 | 1.45 ± 0.3 |
| No (58) | 10.9 ± 2.8 | 9.1 ± 2.0 | 1.2 ± 0.3 |
| "$t$-" test $p$ value | **0.0004*** | **0.09 (NS)** | **0.0008*** |

Note: NS: not significant; $^{*}p < 0.05$, $n$ = number of subjects, SD = standard deviation, and SH = social habits.

requires IFN-$\gamma$, which induces the local accumulation of melanocyte specific $CD8^+$ T cells within the skin supporting the critical role of IFN-$\gamma$ in vitiligo [20]. Further, Nigam et al. also reported an increased number of $CD8^+$ T cells in patients with vitiligo compared to controls [21]. Gregg et al. suggested that vitiligo is entirely dependent on $CD8^+$ T cells, while $CD4^+$ T cells exert a negative regulatory effect and the genetic ablation of IFN-$\gamma$ resulted in scarce $CD8^+$ T cell infiltration into the skin [22]. Skin explant model studies reported that the stronger the $CD8^+$ T cell response the more elaborate the vitiligo [8]. IFN-$\gamma$ indirectly increases the expression of intercellular adhesion molecule-1 (ICAM-1) on melanocytes and enhances T cell-melanocyte attachment in the skin and thus establishes a link between cytokine and T cell mediated destruction of melanocytes in vitiligo [23, 24].

Decreased serum concentrations of the anti-inflammatory cytokine IL-10 were observed in patients compared to controls suggesting low Th2 cytokine profile in the pathogenesis of vitiligo. Shi and Erf suggested that the physiological inducer of T regulatory cells (Tregs) function and proliferation, IL-10 cytokine, was found to be decreased in active vitiligo lesions [19]. Taher et al. and Tembhre et al. had reported increased levels of this immunosuppressive cytokine in vitiligo patients who showed the repigmentation process upon treatment with tacrolimus and narrow band ultraviolet B (NB-UVB), respectively [17, 25]. This indicates that upregulation of IL-10 may be responsible for the drug response which indirectly supports the decreased levels of IL-10 in vitiligo pathogenesis observed in our study.

Contrary to the serum levels observed at systemic level in the present study, Grimes et al. reported increased IL-10 mRNA levels in involved and uninvolved tissue of vitiligo [26]. Estimation of the cytokines in the involved tissue and circulating levels together in the same patients and comparison with normal healthy controls may help in understanding the discrepancy in the results.

The higher IFN-$\gamma$ : IL-10 ratio noted in our patients compared to controls corroborates the cell based studies of Dwivedi et al. and Nigam et al. from India who observed a decrease in the ratio of $CD4^+/CD8^+$ T cells in vitiligo patients compared to controls signifying the role of T cell mediated pathogenesis in vitiligo [18, 21]. The impaired cytokine network might contribute to the reduction and loss of functional Tregs which are involved in immune tolerance [27]. This implies that the balance between pro- and anti-inflammatory cytokines may play an important role in the pathogenesis of NSV.

Another significant observation of the present study was increase in the anti-inflammatory cytokine with an increase in the proinflammatory cytokine exhibiting a positive correlation between IL-10 concentrations and the IFN-$\gamma$ levels in NSV patients indicating that there might be a concomitant

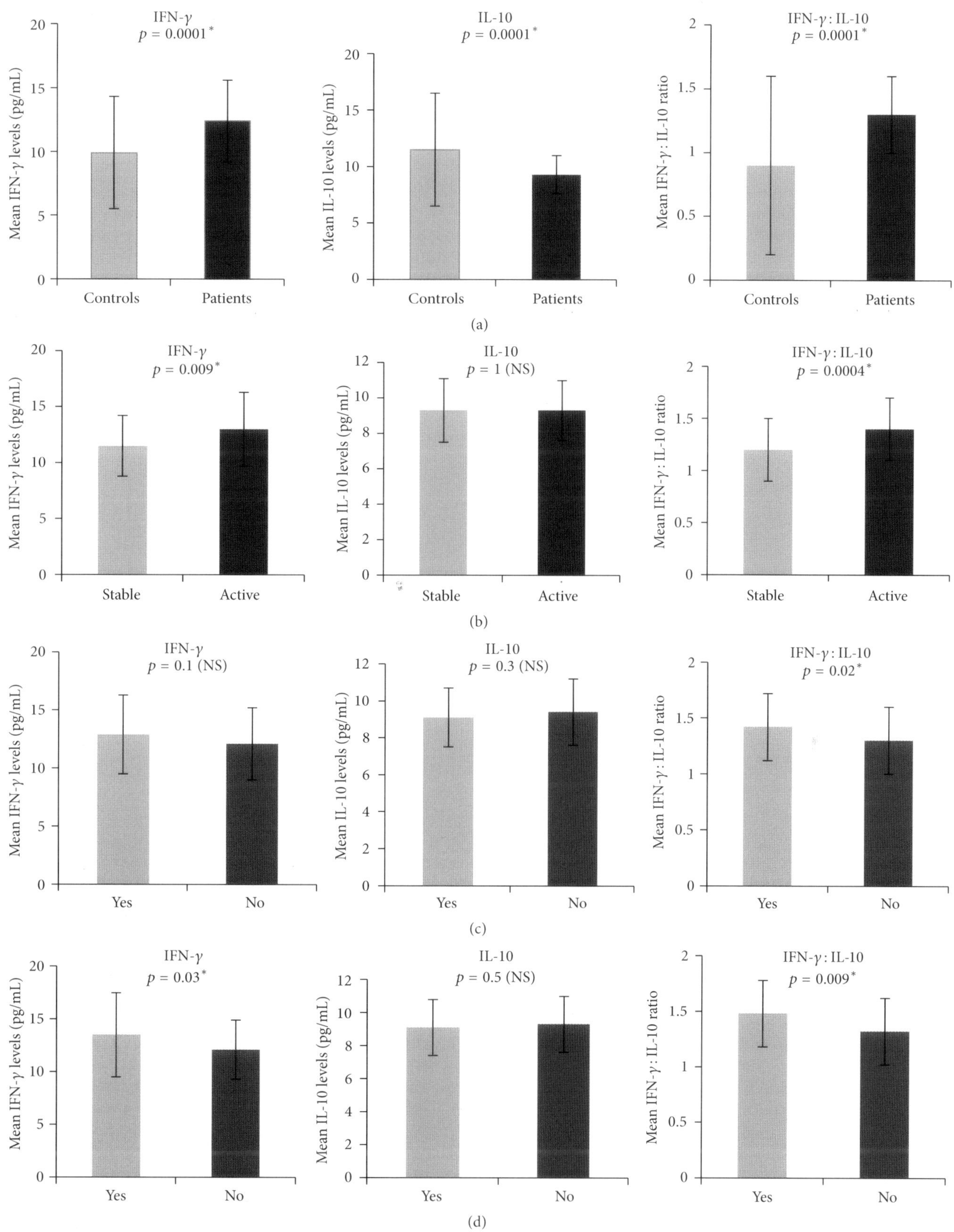


FIGURE 1: Representing mean IFN-γ, IL-10, and IFN-γ : IL-10 ratio in (a) patients and controls, (b) patients with active and stable vitiligo, (c) patients with family history of vitiligo, and (d) patients with a habit of smoking and alcohol consumption.

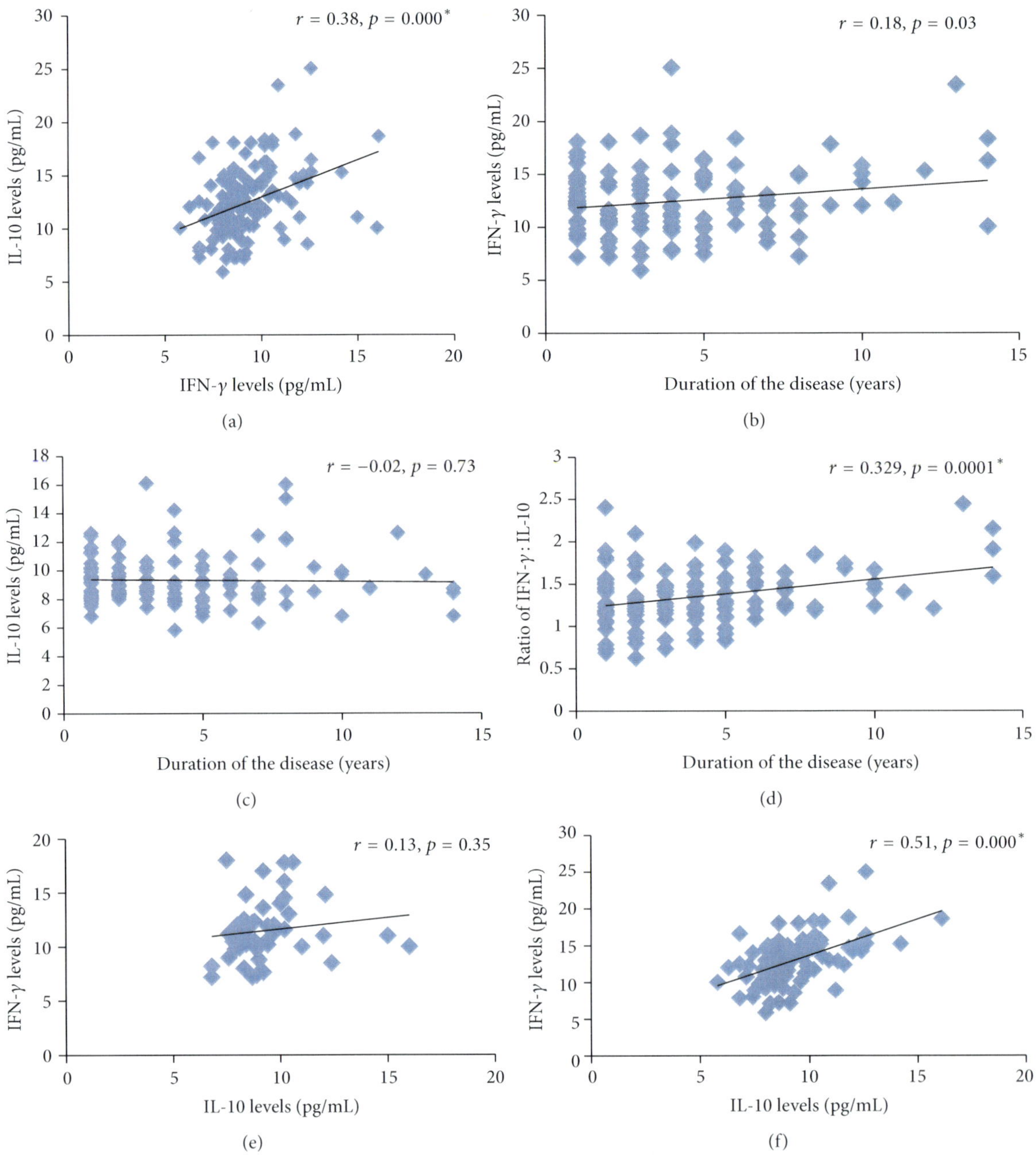


FIGURE 2: Representing correlation of (a) IL-10 and IFN-$\gamma$ levels in patients, (b) duration of the disease with IFN-$\gamma$ levels, (c) duration of the disease with IL-10 levels, (d) duration of the disease with IFN-$\gamma$ : IL-10 ratio, (e) IL-10 with IFN-$\gamma$ levels in stable vitiligo patients, and (f) IL-10 with IFN-$\gamma$ levels in active vitiligo patients.

increase in IL-10 and IFN-$\gamma$ levels at the individual patient level. Shi and Erf showed a strong association of IFN-$\gamma$ with a parallel increase in IL-10 suggesting the Th1 polarization in Smyth line chickens. The amount of the anti-inflammatory cytokine IL-10 might have increased to be a counterpart of the proinflammatory effect which could be insufficient to control the proinflammatory cascade of events that are responsible for melanocyte destruction [19].

The basis behind various clinical presentations of NSV such as nondermatomal, acrofacial, mucosal, and focal variants at the time of diagnosis is not well understood. In the present study, evaluation of serum IFN-$\gamma$ levels and the ratio of IFN-$\gamma$ : IL-10 among clinical variants of NSV exhibited a significant difference. However, no difference was observed in relation to serum concentrations of IL-10 alone. Acrofacial vitiligo showed the highest IFN-$\gamma$ and the least IL-10 concentrations among the variants. These observations may gain support by the findings of Gupta et al. and Shah et al. who stated that acrofacial and nondermatomal vitiligo conditions are very difficult to treat [28, 29], which indirectly indicates the relation between higher proinflammatory environment and clinical presentation. The ratio of IFN-$\gamma$ : IL-10 may reflect the state of inflammation in NSV pathogenesis. However, in order to support our observation, studies with a large sample size in relation to clinical variants should be taken up.

In addition, the data was evaluated by taking the duration of the disease into consideration, which showed a positive correlation with IFN-$\gamma$ and IFN-$\gamma$ : IL-10 ratio but not with IL-10 levels. It gives a hint that systemic proinflammatory environment may increase with increase in the duration of the disease. Due to lack of literature in this aspect, we claim indirect support from another study that showed higher grades of response to UVB treatment in patients with recent vitiligo compared to those with long-standing disease [30].

Appraisal of proinflammatory and anti-inflammatory cytokines in relation to active and stable vitiligo revealed significantly elevated amounts of IFN-$\gamma$ and IFN-$\gamma$ : IL-10 ratio and no variation in the serum concentrations of IL-10. Similar to our observation, another Indian study has also reported higher IFN-$\gamma$ serum concentrations in active vitiligo compared to the stable one [23]. Further, our results are supported by the cell based studies which showed an increased number of $CD8^+$ T cells compared to $CD4^+$ T cells in the blood samples of active vitiligo compared to the stable one. Our observation of elevated IFN-$\gamma$ : IL-10 ratio in the former group compared to the latter also goes hand in hand with the report of Dwivedi et al. showing decreased ratio of $CD4^+/CD8^+$ count [18]. Further, *in vitro* direct analysis of margins of vitiliginous skin showed polarized type 1 T cells ($CD4^+$ and particularly $CD8^+$) that predominantly secrete IFN-$\gamma$ and TNF-$\alpha$ cytokines that are associated with the destruction of melanocytes during active vitiligo [31].

Significantly elevated concentrations of IFN-$\gamma$ and the ratio of IFN-$\gamma$ : IL-10 in male patients with social habits suggest smoking and alcohol may contribute to increased inflammatory response. Smoking and alcohol consumption are known to affect the balance between oxidants and antioxidants [32, 33].

Six to thirty-eight percent of patients with this complex disorder were reported to be associated with family background of vitiligo [34]. The present study was comprised of 40% of the patients with the familial history of NSV. Hence, it was felt that the analysis should be carried out taking this aspect into consideration in relation to cytokines. Interestingly, we found that the patients with familial history of NSV exhibited significantly elevated concentrations of IFN-$\gamma$ : IL-10 ratio compared to those without. Further, there was a lack of variation with respect to individual levels of IFN-$\gamma$ and IL-10 between the two subgroups of patients. There are no reports available in the literature in alliance with cytokine levels in vitiligo patients with familial background of vitiligo. We took an initiation to correlate the link between familial history and cytokine levels and their ratio. Based on our present observations, it can be explored towards the potentiality of the ratio as an immunological marker for identifying the high risk individuals from unaffected sibs of NSV patients. In addition, tracing the cosegregation of genetic variants of IFN-$\gamma$ and IL-10 through family studies may provide the role of these cytokines in NSV pathogenesis.

In conclusion, further studies assessing other pro- and anti-inflammatory cytokines and their ratios at systemic as well as epidermal cytokines (lesional and perilesional) before and after the treatment with a large sample size in various ethnic groups are warranted to confirm our results and to open up the new therapeutic options.

## Conflict of Interests

The authors declare no conflict of interests regarding the publication of this paper.

## Acknowledgment

The authors thank the Department of Science and Technology (DST), New Delhi, for providing the financial support no. SR/SO/HS/0151/2010.

## References

[1] R. V. Koranne, D. Derm, and K. G. Sachdeva, "Vitiligo," *International Journal of Dermatology*, vol. 27, no. 10, pp. 676–681, 1988.

[2] B. Esmaeili, S. A. R. Rezaee, P. Layegh et al., "Expression of IL-17 and COX2 gene in peripheral blood leukocytes of vitiligo patients," *Iranian Journal of Allergy, Asthma and Immunology*, vol. 10, no. 2, pp. 81–89, 2011.

[3] J. J. Nordlund and J. P. Ortonne, "Vitiligo vulgaris," in *The Pigmentary System: Physiology and Pathophysiology*, pp. 513–551, Oxford University Press, New York, NY, USA, 1988.

[4] P. Jahan, R. Cheruvu, S. Tippisetty, P. L. Komaravalli, V. Valluri, and M. Ishaq, "Association of FOXP3 (rs3761548) promoter polymorphism with nondermatomal vitiligo: a study from India," *Journal of the American Academy of Dermatology*, vol. 69, no. 2, pp. 262–266, 2013.

[5] E. M. Shajil, S. Chatterjee, D. Agrawal, T. Bagchi, and R. Begum, "Vitiligo: pathomechanisms and genetic polymorphism of susceptible genes," *Indian Journal of Experimental Biology*, vol. 44, no. 7, pp. 526–539, 2006.

[6] M. Rashigi, P. Agarwal, J. M. Richmond et al., "CXCL10 is critical for the progression and maintenance of depigmentation in a mouse model of vitiligo," *Science Translational Medicine*, vol. 6, no. 223, Article ID 223ra23, 2014.

[7] E. H. Kemp, E. A. Waterman, and A. P. Weetman, "Immunological pathomechanisms in vitiligo," *Expert Reviews in Molecular Medicine*, vol. 3, no. 20, pp. 1–22, 2001.

[8] J. G. van den Boorn, D. Konijnenberg, T. A. M. Dellemijn et al., "Autoimmune destruction of skin melanocytes by perilesional T cells from vitiligo patients," *Journal of Investigative Dermatology*, vol. 129, no. 9, pp. 2220–2232, 2009.

[9] M. Feldmann, F. M. Brennan, and R. Maini, "Cytokines in autoimmune disorders," *International Reviews of Immunology*, vol. 17, no. 1–4, pp. 217–228, 1998.

[10] S. Moretti, A. Spallanzani, L. Amato et al., "New insights into the pathogenesis of vitiligo: imbalance of epidermal cytokines at sites of lesions," *Pigment Cell Research*, vol. 15, no. 2, pp. 87–92, 2002.

[11] S. Singh, U. Singh, and S. S. Pandey, "Serum concentration of IL-6, IL-2, TNF-$\alpha$, and IFN$\gamma$ in vitiligo patients," *Indian Journal of Dermatology*, vol. 57, no. 1, pp. 12–14, 2012.

[12] A. Alkhateeb, P. R. Fain, A. Thody, D. C. Bennett, and R. A. Spritz, "Epidemiology of vitiligo and associated autoimmune diseases in Caucasian probands and their families," *Pigment Cell Research*, vol. 16, no. 3, pp. 208–214, 2003.

[13] F. Paolieri, C. Salmaso, M. Battifora et al., "Possible pathogenetic relevance of interleukin-1$\beta$ in 'destructive' organ-specific autoimmune disease (Hashimoto's thyroiditis)," *Annals of the New York Academy of Sciences*, vol. 876, pp. 221–228, 1999.

[14] K. W. Moore, R. de Waal Malefyt, R. L. Coffman, and A. O'Garra, "Interleukin-10 and the interleukin-10 receptor," *Annual Review of Immunology*, vol. 19, pp. 683–765, 2001.

[15] D. F. Fiorentino, A. Zlotnik, P. Vieira et al., "IL-10 acts on the antigen presenting cell to inhibit cytokine production by Th1 cells," *The Journal of Immunology*, vol. 146, no. 10, pp. 3444–3451, 1991.

[16] C. L. Huang, J. J. Nordlund, and R. Boissy, "Vitiligo: a manifestation of apoptosis?" *American Journal of Clinical Dermatology*, vol. 3, no. 5, pp. 301–308, 2002.

[17] M. K. Tembhre, V. K. Sharma, A. Sharma, P. Chattopadhyay, and S. Gupta, "T helper and regulatory T cell cytokine profile in active, stable and narrow band ultraviolet B treated generalized vitiligo," *Clinica Chimica Acta*, vol. 424, pp. 27–32, 2013.

[18] M. Dwivedi, N. C. Laddha, P. Arora, Y. S. Marfatia, and R. Begum, "Decreased regulatory T cells and $CD4^+/CD8^+$ ratio correlate with disease onset and progression in patients with generalized vitiligo," *Pigment Cell & Melanoma Research*, vol. 26, no. 4, pp. 586–591, 2013.

[19] F. Shi and G. F. Erf, "IFN-$\gamma$, IL-21, and IL-10 co-expression in evolving autoimmune vitiligo lesions of smyth line chickens," *Journal of Investigative Dermatology*, vol. 132, no. 3, pp. 642–649, 2012.

[20] J. E. Harris, T. H. Harris, W. Weninger, E. J. Wherry, C. A. Hunter, and L. A. Turka, "A mouse model of vitiligo with focused epidermal depigmentation requires IFN-$\gamma$ for autoreactive $CD8^+$ T-cell accumulation in the skin," *Journal of Investigative Dermatology*, vol. 132, no. 7, pp. 1869–1876, 2012.

[21] P. K. Nigam, P. K. Patra, P. K. Khodiar, and J. Gual, "A study of blood CD3+, CD4+, and CD8+ T cell levels and CD4+:CD8+ ratio in vitiligo patients," *Indian Journal of Dermatology, Venereology and Leprology*, vol. 77, no. 1, p. 111, 2011.

[22] R. K. Gregg, L. Nichols, Y. Chen, B. Lu, and V. H. Engelhard, "Mechanisms of spatial and temporal development of autoimmune vitiligo in tyrosinase-specific tcr transgenic mice," *The Journal of Immunology*, vol. 184, no. 4, pp. 1909–1917, 2010.

[23] M. Dwivedi, N. C. Laddha, K. Shah, B. J. Shah, and R. Begum, "Involvement of interferon-gamma genetic variants and intercellular adhesion molecule-1 in onset and progression of generalized Vitiligo," *Journal of Interferon and Cytokine Research*, vol. 33, no. 11, pp. 646–659, 2013.

[24] J. J. Yohn, M. M. Critelli, B. Lyons, and D. A. Norris, "Modulation of melanocyte intercellular adhesion molecule-1 by immune cytokines," *Journal of Investigative Dermatology*, vol. 95, no. 2, pp. 233–237, 1990.

[25] Z. A. Taher, G. Lauzon, S. Maguiness, and M. T. Dytoc, "Analysis of interleukin-10 levels in lesions of vitiligo following treatment with topical tacrolimus," *British Journal of Dermatology*, vol. 161, no. 3, pp. 654–659, 2009.

[26] P. E. Grimes, R. Morris, E. Avaniss-Aghajani, T. Soriano, M. Meraz, and A. Metzger, "Topical tacrolimus therapy for vitiligo: therapeutic responses and skin messenger RNA expression of proinflammatory cytokines," *Journal of the American Academy of Dermatology*, vol. 51, no. 1, pp. 52–61, 2004.

[27] R. Colucci, F. Dragoni, and S. Moretti, "Oxidative stress and immune system in vitiligo and thyroid diseases," *Oxidative Medicine and Cellular Longevity*, vol. 2015, Article ID 631927, 7 pages, 2015.

[28] S. Gupta, T. Narang, M. J. Olsson, and J. P. Ortonne, "Surgical management of vitiligo and other leukodermas: evidence-based practice guidelines," in *Surgical Management of Vitiligo*, S. Gupta, M. J. Olsson, A. J. Kanwar, and J.-P. Ortonne, Eds., chapter 9, Blackwell Publishing, Oxford, UK, 2007.

[29] B. H. Shah, S. P. Joshipura, and J. K. Thakkar, "Surgical treatment in acrofacial vitiligo," *Indian Journal of Dermatology, Venereology and Leprology*, vol. 60, no. 1, pp. 26–27, 1994.

[30] Z. Hallaji, M. Ghiasi, A. Eisazadeh, and M. Rayati Damavandi, "Evaluation of the effect of disease duration in generalized vitiligo on its clinical response to narrowband ultraviolet B phototherapy," *Photodermatology Photoimmunology and Photomedicine*, vol. 28, no. 3, pp. 115–119, 2012.

[31] A. Wańkowicz-Kalińska, R. M. J. G. J. van den Wijngaard, B. J. Tigges et al., "Immunopolarization of $CD4^+$ and $CD8^+$ T cells to type-1-like is associated with melanocyte loss in human vitiligo," *Laboratory Investigation*, vol. 83, no. 5, pp. 683–695, 2003.

[32] B. Isik, A. Ceylan, and R. Isik, "Oxidative stress in smokers and non-smokers," *Inhalation Toxicology*, vol. 19, no. 9, pp. 767–769, 2007.

[33] J. W. Shin, K. M. Nam, H. R. Choi et al., "Erythrocyte malondialdehyde and glutathione levels in vitiligo patients," *Annals of Dermatology*, vol. 22, no. 3, pp. 279–283, 2010.

[34] J. P. Ortonne, D. B. Mosher, and T. B. Fitzpatrick, "Vitiligo and other hypomelanoses of hair and skin," in *Topics in Dermatology*, J. P. Ortonne, D. B. Mosher, and T. B. Fitzpatrick, Eds., pp. 257–258, Plenum Medical Book, New York, NY, USA, 1983.

# 4

# Role of Autoimmune Responses in Periodontal Disease

**Soumya Nair,[1] Mohamed Faizuddin,[2] and Jayanthi Dharmapalan[2]**

[1] *Om Dental Clinic, No. 1554, Hebbal 2nd Stage, Mysore 570017, India*
[2] *M.R. Ambedkar Dental College and Hospital, No. 1/37, Cline Road, Cooke Town, Bangalore 560005, India*

Correspondence should be addressed to Soumya Nair; soumyak_nair@yahoo.com

Academic Editor: Corrado Betterle

Periodontal diseases are characterized by localized infections and inflammatory conditions that directly affect teeth supporting structures which are the major cause of tooth loss. Several studies have demonstrated the involvement of autoimmune responses in periodontal disease. Evidences of involvement of immunopathology have been reported in periodontal disease. Bacteria in the dental plaque induce antibody formation. Autoreactive T cells, natural killer cells, ANCA, heat shock proteins, autoantibodies, and genetic factors are reported to have an important role in the autoimmune component of periodontal disease. The present review describes the involvement of autoimmune responses in periodontal diseases and also the mechanisms underlying these responses. This review is an attempt to throw light on the etiopathogenesis of periodontal disease highlighting the autoimmunity aspect of the etiopathogenesis involved in the initiation and progression of the disease. However, further clinical trials are required to strengthen the role of autoimmunity as a cause of periodontal disease.

## 1. Introduction

Periodontal diseases are characterized by localized infections and inflammatory conditions where anaerobic Gram-negative bacteria are mainly involved and directly affect teeth-supporting structure. Periodontal disease affects one or more of the periodontal tissues—alveolar bone, periodontal ligament, cementum, and gingiva. The pathogenesis of this disease involves immunological responses leading to tissue destruction and bone loss [1].

Autoimmunity can be defined as breakdown of mechanism responsible for self-tolerance and induction of an immune response against components of the self. Such an immune response may not always be harmful (e.g., anti-idiotype antibodies). However, in numerous (autoimmune) diseases it is well recognized that products of the immune system cause damage to the self (Jiang and Lechler 2003) [2].

In 1965, Brandtzaeg and Kraus were the first to postulate the autoimmune basis in the pathogenesis of periodontal disease. It has been more than 30 years since the concept of autoimmunity has been considered for periodontal disease. An increasing number of reports in the past decade have lent support to the concept of an autoimmune component of periodontal disease [1]. The review is an attempt to focus on the concepts dealing with autoimmunity in periodontal diseases.

## 2. Autoimmunity in Periodontal Disease

*2.1. Evidence of Autoimmunity in Periodontal Disease: See [3].* There are records of both human as well as animal studies documenting the role of autoimmunity in periodontal disease. The majority of reports deal with the detection of antibodies to host components, in particular, collagen, although antibodies to DNA and aggregated IgG have also been reported (Table 1).

*2.2. Possible Causes of Autoimmunity [3, 4]*

(1) Enhanced presentation of self-antigens through increased expression of the molecule associated with antigen presentation, namely, the IgA antigen;

(2) altered T helper or T suppressor cell function;

(3) polyclonal activation of cells which have the ability, for reasons unclear, to produce autoantibodies;

Table 1

| Humoral | Cellular |
|---|---|
| (1) Antibody to aggregated IgG (rheumatoid factor) detected in gingiva and saliva | (1) Lymphocytotoxicity shown for oral epithelial cells |
| (2) Antibody levels to double stranded DNA were elevated in dog gingival | (2) Histological damage observed in gingival human fibroblasts with associated mononuclear cells |
| (3) Elevated levels of serum antibody to human collagen type I | (3) Lymphocytotoxic killing of autologous fibroblasts with associated mononuclear cells |
| (4) IgM, IgA rheumatoid factor antibody to human collagen types I and III produced by mononuclear cells | (4) Lymphoblastogenesis detected to native and denatured collagen |
| (5) Serum IgG antibodies to native and denatured types I and III bovine collagen detected in juvenile periodontitis | (5) Cellular immunity to proteoglycan detected in periodontal disease patients |

(4) idiosyncrasies of the antigen idiotype network;

(5) bacterial or viral cross reactivity with self-antigens leading to production of cross reactive antibodies;

(6) genetic predisposition factors.

*2.2.1. Increased IgA Expression.* In several autoimmune diseases, increase in autoantibody is associated with an increase in molecules which are involved in antigen presentation, in particular on cells which do not normally express these molecules. When these cells which are normally not involved in antigen presentation become involved, it may lead to self-antigen presentation to the immune system and the resultant production of autoantibodies.

*2.2.2. Altered T-Helper and T Suppressor Cell Function.* In relation to periodontal disease, it has been explained as follows: a reduction in the T cell population of lymphocytes from patients with periodontal disease led to an increase in the B cell component of the spontaneous lymphoblastic proliferation. This would suggest that T suppressor activity would increase in patients with periodontal disease.

*2.2.3. Polyclonal Expansion of B Cell Pool: See [4, 5].* Natural autoantibodies (Nab), to a range of self-components, are found in the absence of disease and are presumed to be a natural phenomenon. Such a pool of Nab may be expanded polyclonally by one of the polyclonal B cell activators found in periodontal plaque (LPS) or selectively antigenically by the release of tissue components which expose these natural antigens to the immune system to a greater extent than usual.

*2.2.4. Autoantigen Presentation and Autoreactive T Cells: See [3].* All nucleated cells of the body possess class I MHC molecules so that gingival epithelial cell and fibroblast killing reported to occur in periodontal disease in vitro could be mediated by this mechanism of presentation of antigen, in association with class I MHC molecules, to cytotoxic T cells. However, in the lymphocytotoxicity seen in periodontal disease, both allogeneic and syngeneic target cells have been used with similar results. Increased expression of class II MHC molecules has been observed in the surface of basal and suprabasal gingival sulcular epithelial cells in inflamed tissues.

*2.2.5. Idiosyncrasies of the Antigen Idiotypic Network [3].* Jerne proposed a network theory of the immune response in which the antigen stimulated the production of antibody exhibiting an idiotype that elicited the formation of an anti-idiotype bearing an "internal image" of that antigen. This latter antibody in turn stimulated the production of anti-anti-idiotype antibody leading to an open ended network.

In periodontal disease there is so far no evidence for existence of anti-idiotype antibodies. The antibodies to immunoglobulin detected in humans and experimental animal periodontal disease are directed to the Fc end of the molecule not the idiotype region.

*2.2.6. Viral and Bacterial Infection and the Immune System: See [3, 6].* Viral and bacterial infections may play a role as an exogenous factor triggering an autoimmune response. Activation and clonal expansion of autoreactive lymphocytes is a critical step in the pathogenesis of autoimmune diseases. In experimental models of autoimmunity, disease can be transferred by activated, but not resting, autoreactive T cells [6], indicating that activation of autoreactive T cells is required for the development of autoimmune diseases.The infectious agents act as a stimulating factor such responses. Thus the existence of such a microorganism in periodontal pocket may not only stimulate the production of antibody to this microbe but also stimulate autoantibody production to serum components or degenerated host periodontal tissues.

*2.2.7. Genetic Predisposing Factors: See [7–10].* Several investigators have reported an association between a high incidence of selected histocompatibility complex antigens and certain autoimmune diseases, for example, rheumatoid arthritis with HLA-DRw4, systemic lupus erythematosus in association with HLA-DR3 and HLA-B8. This could be an underlying predisposing factor for the development of autoimmune disease. The evidence relating HLA phenotype distribution and the prevalence of periodontal disease has been contradictory. Reports relating HLA phenotype and susceptibility to periodontal disease are mainly associated with HLA class I antigen distribution. A possible role of HLA class I antigens in the development of periodontal disease might be either in relation to cell mediated cytotoxicity and the T cell response or in association with the structural features of the antigens themselves.

Patients with periodontitis juveniles and patient with periodontitis were tissue typed. In the juvenile group, frequencies of tissue type specificities HLA-A9, HLA-A28, and HLABJ'V15 were significantly increased as compared to the findings in the general population. In the periodontitis groups, no significant tissue type deviations were found as discussed by Reinholdt et al. Several theories have been advanced to explain the associations between HLA and a variety of diseases [7].

*2.2.8. Role of Antibodies [11].* Perhaps the most pertinent aspect of the antibodies detected in periodontal disease is their role: protective, destructive, or inconsequential. Pathologic changes appear to occur in those circumstances where the otherwise physiologic autoimmune response leads to the initiation of further humoral and or cellular immune activity capable of causing tissue damage or disease. It should be noted that "natural" autoantibody is generally of the IgM class. In adult periodontitis local antibody to collagen type I is predominantly IgG rather than IgM, a reversal of the situation in serum, suggesting that continued antigenic stimulation has led to class switch. In periodontal disease there is alteration in the various subclasses of antibodies, with increasing severity of the disease, such that IgG1 and IgG3 decrease and IgG4 increase. The latter antibody is protective in nature, as it does not form complexes with antigen which activate complement. Studies suggest that the autoantibodies detected in periodontal disease are derived from preexisting natural antibodies and play a physiological role in the elimination of dead cells and damaged tissue constituents that have appeared during the tissue degradation which occurred in periodontal disease. However, the possibility still remains that this system, established to deal with the consequence of tissue damage, may in certain circumstances become excessive and actually contribute to the progress of the disease.

*2.3. Antineutrophil Cytoplasmic Autoantibodies (ANCA) [12, 13].* ANCAs represent a heterogeneous group of antibodies that target antigens that are primarily present in azurophil granules of polymorphonuclear leukocytes (PMNs). Some ANCA associated diseases are known to coexist during periodontitis in humans. Such diseases include the rheumatoid arthritis and to a lesser extent systemic lupus erythematosus (SLE). More studies are required to explore the link between these conditions and a probable common mechanism in these disease processes.

Exposure of the host to the periodontal pathogens, along with a genetic susceptibility, could trigger ANCA by two different mechanisms. The production of TNF-$\alpha$ would sensitize the neutrophils to express its granule contained enzymes, such as MPO and PR-3, which in turn could trigger the production of ANCA. In addition, periodontal pathogens are known to possess a "superantigen" property, where they can directly activate the autoreactive B lymphocytes in a T cell independent and mediated pathway, which can also result in the activation of neutrophils. The activated neutrophils release reactive oxygen radicals, enzymes, and various proinflammatory cytokines, all of which are known to mediate periodontal destruction. ANCA activated neutrophils are also known to delay apoptosis, which can prolong the activity of neutrophils and thereby increase tissue destruction. Delayed apoptosis has been reported in periodontal disease, which can be attributed to ANCA. Furthermore, ANCA is known to have a direct toxic effect on the cells bearing antigens such as endothelial cells, which can result in increased endothelial permeability, a feature common in the inflammatory process.

*2.4. Role of Natural Killer T Cells in Autoimmunity [14–17].* Human CD1d molecules present glycolipid antigens such as galactosylceramide to CD1d-restricted natural killer T cells. The natural killer T cells appear to associate with CD1d cells, and it was suggested that they have a regulatory role to play in periodontal disease. Autoimmunity has been suggested to be a feature of periodontal disease. Cross reactivity of human heat shock protein (HSP) 60 and *P. gingivalis* GroEL, which is the bacterial homologue has been shown in periodontal disease. HSP 60 specific as well as P.g cross reactive T cells have also been demonstrated to accumulate in periodontitis lesions. The study by Yamazaki et al. suggests that an immune response to autoantigens such as collagen type I or HSP60 may be well controlled by natural killer T cells. A relationship between a deficiency in natural killer cell activity and autoimmune diseases has been cited in mice. An impairment of the subtle balance could be involved in the pathogenesis of periodontal disease. The results, however, did show increase of natural killer T cells in periodontitis, suggesting a functional role for these cells, and because of their ability to secrete rapid amounts of cytokines, they may influence the T helper cytokine response. The role of autoimmunity in chronic inflammation is still not clear. It is possible that autoimmunity is a feature of all chronic inflammation. In this context it has been known for many years that gingival fibroblasts are able to phagocytose collagen such as anticollagen; antibodies may facilitate this phagocytosis and hence removal of broken down collagen. At the same time, an anti-HSP response may enhance the removal of dead and dying cells, such that these autoimmune responses may be a natural part of chronic inflammation. Control of these responses would therefore be essential, hence the increase in regulatory natural killer T cells in periodontal tissues. This concept further illustrates that the role of T cells in periodontal disease may be one of immune homeostasis. Further studies are clearly needed to test this hypothesis and to determine the role of regulatory T cells in periodontal inflammation.

*2.5. Oral Microbial Heat Shock Proteins [18–20].* When exposed to a wide range of environmental stressors (temperature, pH, redox potential, etc.), prokaryotic and eukaryotic cells respond by inducing or accelerating the synthesis of specific proteins known as stress proteins, including the heat shock proteins (HSPs) which have a high degree of homology. These HSPs are unregulated under stressful conditions. HSPs act as molecular chaperones in the assembly and folding of proteins, and proteases when damaged or toxic proteins have

to be degraded. HSPs thus protect cells from damaging effects associated with stressful conditions. The GroELs and, to a lesser extent, the DnaKs of several pathogenic bacteria may become major antigens, since they are strongly expressed under stressful conditions. These HSPs are antigenic, and the recognition of specific epitopes on such highly conserved antigens may contribute to protective immunity or may have pathological autoimmune responses. Because of the similarities between microbial and mammalian HSPs, a humoral response against microbial HSPs may be destructive for the host due to antigenic mimicry leading to autoimmune response.

Three models have been proposed to link microbial infections to subsequent autoimmune reactions involving the HSPs. These models are as follows:

(1) molecular mimicry between the microbial HSPs and HSPs or constituent proteins from the host,

(2) inflammation induced exposure of cryptic cell epitopes that could be a target for immune reactions,

(3) antigen presentation in infected sites leading to chronic immunological reactions.

*2.6. Role of Autoreactive B Cells in Autoimmunity of Periodontal Disease [3, 4, 11, 21].* B cells upon activation transform into antibody producing plasma cells. There are reasons to anticipate that immunoglobulins produced by plasma cells directed against subgingival plaque may also be autoantibodies directed to host cells. It was observed that the gingival lesions contained a large number of cells that produce either antibodies directed to type I collagen.

In sites of chronic inflammation, polyclonal B cell activators (PBA) are known to exhibit adjuvant activity when combined with foreign antigens. The adjuvant effect of microbial polyclonal B cell activator may be important in anticollagen antibody production, and thus the localization of PBA in periodontal pockets may explain why anticollagen antibody forming cells are restricted to the chronically inflamed periodontal tissues. Interleukin-10 has been reported to selectively promote the expansion of a B lymphocyte lineage which has the propensity for secreting high levels of autoantibody in type I diabetic individuals.

*2.7. Role of Anti-CCP in Periodontal Disease and RA [22, 23].* Rheumatoid arthritis (RA) is a common, systemic autoimmune disease causing destruction of the joint architecture leading to disability. Etiology of RA remains unknown; accumulating studies have established a strong association between RA and periodontitis (PD). The anti-cyclic citrullinated peptide antibodies (anti-CCP) are produced locally in the inflamed synovium of rheumatoid arthritis (RA) patient. In scientific literature periodontal bacterial DNA in serum and synovial fluid of RA with periodontal disease patients were found. RA and adult periodontitis share common pathogenetic and immunologic mechanisms. One oral pathogen strongly implicated in the pathogenesis of periodontal disease (PD), *Porphyromonas gingivalis*, possesses a unique microbial enzyme, peptidylarginine deiminase (PAD), the human equivalent of which has been identified as a susceptibility factor for RA. *P. gingivalis* is the only oral bacterium that possesses peptidylarginine deiminase activity, which is essential for citrullination of arginine, an RA autoantigen,, leading to the formation of immune complexes involved in inflammation and joint destruction seen in RA. The anti-cyclic citrullinated peptide (anti-CCP) autoantibody and citrullinated peptide have been realized to be involved in the breaking of self-tolerance and development of autoimmune in RA. The citrullinated peptide is generated by posttranslational modification (citrullination) of protein-bound arginine by peptidylarginine deiminase (PAD). *Porphyromonas gingivalis* (*P. gingivalis*), the major aetiological agent of PD and the only bacterium known to express a PAD enzyme, has been reported to be significantly associated with RA. It is also confirmed that bacterial PAD produced by *P. gingivalis* has the capacity of deiminating arginine in fibrin found in the periodontal lesion. What is more, it has been demonstrated that citrullination of HLA binding peptide causes a 100-fold increase in peptide-MHC affinity and leads to the activation of CD4(+) T cells in HLA DRB1 0401 transgenic mice. Therefore, we postulate that *P. gingivalis* may play a crucial role in the pathogenesis of periodontitis-associated RA. *P. gingivalis*, which colonizes in the oral cavity, produces PAD enzyme continuously that leads to the citrullination of RA autoantigen such as fibrin in synovium joint. These PAD engendered antigens, presented in association with major histocompatibility complex (MHC) molecules by antigen-presenting cells (APC), ultimately lead to production of the anti-CCP antibody. The anti-CCP antibodies form immune complexes with citrullinated proteins, which can be bound by inflammatory cells via their Fc receptors. The roles of these immune complexes and inflammatory cells are mediated by a complex cascade involving complement activation. These mechanisms result in a release of mediators of inflammation and joint destruction ultimately leading to the onset of RA. This hypothesis reveals that oral bacterial infection may play a role in peptide citrullination which might be involved in loss of self-tolerance and development of autoimmunity in RA.

## 3. Autoimmunity as a Component in Various Periodontal Diseases

*3.1. Host Immune Response Linked to the High Risk of Periodontal Disease in Diabetics [24–26].* Diabetic patients are at a higher risk of developing periodontitis is a known fact, however the mechanism is not fully understood. An autoimmune component cannot be fully ruled out as per the Mahamed et al. study. This research study shows that the autoimmune environment and CD4+ T cells display an unusual hyperactive response when mounting an antibacterial immunity to oral microbial assaults in the experimental diabetic NOD (non obese diabetic) mice, which is similar to human type 1 diabetes. These findings will lead to a new understanding of the potential causes of the high rates of microbial infections in diabetics and future treatments for both periodontal/dental care and medical risk factor management. This study clearly describes the impact of the autoimmunity environment to

anaerobic infection in an experimental periodontitis model of type1 diabetes. Moreover, these cells in high-risk diabetic patients may open a new door for the therapeutic potential of treating periodontal disease. In another study a cytokine, interleukin (IL)-10, has been reported to selectively promote the expansion of a B lymphocyte lineage (CD5/LY1/B1) which has the propensity for secreting high leves of autoantibody in diabectic patients.

*3.2. Role of Autoimmunity in Aggressive Periodontitis [26].* Aggressive forms of periodontitis have been intensively investigated due to their aggressiveness, quick progression, and occurrence in adolescents and young individuals. Periodontopathogenic bacteria have been implicated in the pathogenic ability of AgP, and there is evidence in literature that bacterial toxins and autoimmune mechanisms are likely involved in the pathogenesis of AgP. In a recent study carried out, the presences of autoantibodies directed against ECM components were found in the sera of patients. However it does not necessarily mean that these autoantibodies primarily participate in the destructive mechanism of periodontal tissue. Their presence could be a coadjuvant factor rather than the cause of these lesions. It was demonstrated that self-antigens may be altered in the course of infection. Furthermore microbial antigens exhibit molecular mimicry with host self-antigens and thus facilitate the production of autoantibodies.

*3.3. Desquamative Gingivitis [1].* It is not a specific disease entity, but a gingival response associated with a variety of conditions. A variety of conditions affect the gingiva, either in part or totally. The gingiva consists of the epithelium, the connective tissue, and the basement membrane separating the two. Consequently, various conditions can involve each component specifically or totally, or, in some cases, can involve specific aspects of each component, such as certain layers of epithelium. In many of these conditions some type of inflammatory process is involved, either acute or chronic. Autoimmune mechanisms appear to be a prominent aspect of etiology in many patients. Thus, similar to periodontal disease, inflammation and the immune response are involved in pathogenesis of the mucocutaneous lesions of the gingiva.

## 4. Discussion

Periodontal disease is characterized by the loss of the normal supporting tissues of the teeth and a humoral and cellular immune response to bacterial antigens of dental plaque which accumulates at the dentogingival junction. However, till date with so much advances made in the field of periodontics, the etiopathogenesis of this infectious disease is still an enigma. It has been more than 30 years since the concept of autoimmune pathogenesis for periodontal disease was considered. An increasing number of reports in the past decades has lent support to the concept of an autoimmune component of periodontal disease. Three aspects of the phenomenon warrant consideration: firstly, the evidence which has accumulated over the past in relation to autoimmunity; secondly, the mechanism by which such autoimmunity may arise; and lastly, the possible role of such an abnormal immune response in the natural history of the disease.

Perhaps the most pertinent aspect of the antibodies detected in periodontal disease is their role: protective role, destructive, or inconsequential part in the pathogenesis of the disease. Just the mere presence of antibodies to self-components does not necessarily lead to disease. Pathologic changes appear to occur in those circumstances where the otherwise physiological autoimmune response leads to initiation of further humoral and/or cellular immune activity capable of causing damage or disease. To some extent the pathologic potential of the autoantibodies can be determined by knowledge of their nature, for example, their class and possibly subclass. It should be noted that natural autoantibodies are generally IgM class. In adult periodontitis there is local antibody to collagen type I, which is predominantly IgG type rather than IgM, a reversal of what is there in serum, suggesting that continued antigenic stimulation could lead to a class switch and further an increase in IgG4 and decrease in IgG1 and IgG3 occurs. IgG4 is protective in nature in that it does not form complexes with antigen to stimulate the complement. These findings suggest that the autoantibodies detected in periodontal disease are derived from preexisting natural antibodies and play a physiological role in elimination of dead cells and tissues that have occurred during tissue degradation. However, the possibility still remains that this system, established to deal with the consequences of tissue damage, may in certain circumstances become aggressive to actually contribute to the disease process [1, 3, 11].

Considering the role of antinuclear cytoplasmic antibodies (ANCA) in periodontal disease, it is seen that exposure of the host to the periodontal pathogens, along with a genetic susceptibility, could trigger ANCA. The production of TNF-a would sensitize or prime the neutrophils which in turn could trigger the production of ANCA. In addition, periodontal pathogens are known to possess a "super-antigen" property, which can also result in the activation of neutrophils. The activated neutrophils release reactive oxygen radicals, enzymes, and various proinflammatory cytokines, all of which are known to mediate periodontal destruction. ANCA activated neutrophils are also known to delay apoptosis, which can prolong the activity of neutrophils and thereby increase tissue destruction. Delayed apoptosis has been reported in periodontal disease. Furthermore, ANCA is known to have a direct toxic effect on the cells bearing antigens such as endothelial cells, which can result in increased endothelial permeability, a feature common in the inflammatory process. All said and done, to evaluate the exact role of ANCA in periodontal disease pathogenesis, further human clinical trials are required [12, 13].

The HSPs are antigenic, and the recognition of specific epitopes on such highly conserved antigens may contribute to protective immunity or may have pathological autoimmune responses. Because of the similarities between microbial and mammalian HSPs, a humoral response against microbial HSPs may be destructive for the host due to antigenic mimicry leading to autoimmune response.

Studies show that an immune response to autoantigens such as collagen type I or HSP60 may be well controlled by natural killer T cells. However downregulation of CD1d in murine T cells by P.g has been demonstrated implying that even though there may be higher numbers of natural killer T cells in periodontitis, they may not be functional. Furthermore the exact role of these natural killer cells in autoimmunity is still not clear [15].

Finally we come to the genetic predisposition towards autoimmunity in terms of HLA [24, 26].

The HLA system probably contains so-called immune response (Ir) genes which control the specific responsiveness toward a variety of antigens. These genes are most likely in linkage disequilibrium with the HLAA and B genes, and, in one instance, it is possible that an Ir gene controlling autoimmunity could explain the findings; in the other instance, absence of a specific Ir gene could lead to chronic infection. Some microbial antigens may resemble some HLA antigens which would make individuals carrying these antigens less capable of reacting immunologically against the microorganisms in question. Finally, it seems as if HLA antigens serve a biological function as receptors for foreign antigens which they present in an adequate way for immunocompetent cells. This mechanism could lead both to autoimmunity and, if the relevant HLA antigen was absent, susceptibility to infection. It is impossible to decide which mechanism operates in the possible association between HLA and juvenile periodontitis.

Just as so many aspects of the etiopathogenesis of periodontal disease remain unsolved, this particular aspect of role of autoimmunity in periodontics is still quite intriguing. Lots of pieces of this jigsaw puzzle still do not fit in accurately. However, our attempt to understand the natural history of this disease process still has a long way to go. Probably once this is properly understood, the etiopathogenesis may become more coherent and help us enhance our cognizance of this chronic inflammatory condition. Understanding the exact role of autoimmunity can have serious therapeutic implications in the treatment of periodontitis either in the form of development of a vaccine or some miracle drug [27–30].

## 5. Conclusion

Periodontal disease being a chronic inflammatory disease has a complex etiopathogenesis which still remains not completely understood. The present review has thrown light on the autoimmune component of the disease, which may be somewhere underplayed or ignored in its role in the etiopathogenesis of this disease. The objective of the review is to highlight this particular aspect of the disease so that further research can be conducted to get a more clear picture of the autoimmune component of this disease and how we can apply it in therapeutics. There is more than enough evidence to quote an autoimmunity aspect to periodontal disease, which could be the main reason why the initiation and progression of this disease is still unclear.

## Conflict of Interests

There is no conflict of interests whatsoever for this work.

## References

[1] M. G. Newman, H. Takei, P. R. Klokkevold, and F. A. Carranza, *Caranza,s Clinical Periodontology*, Elsevier, 10th edition, 2006.

[2] S. Jiang and R. I. Lechler, "Regulatory T cells in the control of transplantation tolerance and autoimmunity," *American Journal of Transplantation*, vol. 3, no. 5, pp. 516–524, 2003.

[3] O. Anusaksathien and A. E. Dolby, "Autoimmunity in periodontal disease," *Journal of Oral Pathology and Medicine*, vol. 20, no. 3, pp. 101–107, 1991.

[4] O. Anusaksathien, G. Singh, N. Matthews, and A. E. Dolby, "Autoimmunity to collagen in adult periodontal disease: immunoglobulin classes in sera and tissue," *Journal of Periodontal Research*, vol. 27, no. 1, pp. 55–61, 1992.

[5] C.L. Hahn, H. A. Schenkein, and J. G. Tew, "Polyclonal B cell acivators and in vitro induction of auto antibody reactive with collagen," *Journal of Periodontal Research*, vol. 32, pp. 608–613, 1997.

[6] K. W. Wucherpfennig, "Mechanisms for the induction of autoimmunity by infectious agents," *Journal of Clinical Investigation*, vol. 108, no. 8, pp. 1097–1104, 2001.

[7] J. Reinholdt, I. Bay, and A. Svejgaard, "Role of HLA antigen in periodontal diseased," *Journal of Dental Research*, vol. 56, no. 10, pp. 1261–1263, 1977.

[8] J. A. Encinas and V. K. Kuchroo, "Mapping and identification of autoimmunity genes," *Current Opinion in Immunology*, vol. 12, no. 6, pp. 691–697, 2000.

[9] J. Klien and A. Sato, "The HLA system," *New England Journal of Medicine*, vol. 43, pp. 782–786, 2000.

[10] H. Wigzell, "Positive autoimmunity," in *Autoimmunity, Genetic, Immunologic, Virologic and Clinical Aspects*, pp. 693–707, Academic Press, New York, NY, USA, 1977.

[11] M. Sugawara, K. Yamashita, H. Yoshie, and K. Hara, "Detection of, and anti-collagen antibody produced by, CD5-positive B cells in inflamed gingival tissues," *Journal of Periodontal Research*, vol. 27, no. 5, pp. 489–498, 1992.

[12] N. V. Rohini, A. R. Pradeep, and M. Faizuddin, "Antineutrophil cytoplasmic antibodies and adult periodontitis," *Journal of Periodontal Research*, vol. 35, no. 6, pp. 374–376, 2000.

[13] C. G. Dileep Sharma and A. R. Pradeep, "Anti nuclear cytoplasmic autoantibodies: a renewed paradigm in periodontal disease pathogenesis?" *Journal of Periodontology*, vol. 77, pp. 1304–1313, 2006.

[14] A. M. Marmount, "Defining Criteria for autoimmune disease," *Immunology Today*, vol. 15, article 338, 1994.

[15] K. Yamazaki, H. Yoshie, and G. J. Seymour, "T cell regulation of the immune response to infection in periodontal diseases: a review," *Histology and Histopathology*, vol. 18, pp. 889–896, 2003.

[16] B. T. Kurien, S. Asfa, C. Li, Y. Dorri, R. Jonsson, and R. H. Scofield, "Induction of oral tolerance in experimental Sjögren's syndrome autoimmunity," *Scandinavian Journal of Immunology*, vol. 61, no. 5, pp. 418–425, 2005.

[17] M. A. lynch, V. J. Brightman, and M. S. Greenberg, *Burkett's Oral Medicine Diagnosis and Treatment*, Lipponcott-Raven, 9th edition, 1997.

[18] T. Ando, T. Kato, K. Ishihara, H. Ogiuchi, and K. Okuda, "Heat shock proteins in the human periodontal disease process," *Microbiology and Immunology*, vol. 39, no. 5, pp. 321–327, 1995.

[19] F. Goulhen, D. Grenier, and D. Mayrand, "Oral microbial heat-shock proteins and their potential contributions to infections," *Critical Reviews in Oral Biology and Medicine*, vol. 14, no. 6, pp. 399–412, 2003.

[20] J.-Y. Lee, N.-N. Yi, U.-S. Kim, J.-S. Choi, S.-J. Kim, and J.-I. Choi, "Porphyromonas gingivalis heat shock protein vaccine reduces the alveolar bone loss induced by multiple periodontopathogenic bacteria," *Journal of Periodontal Research*, vol. 41, no. 1, pp. 10–14, 2006.

[21] T. Berglundh, B. Liljenberg, A. Tarkowski, and J. Lindhe, "The presence of local and circulating autoreactive B cells in patients with advanced periodontitis," *Journal of Clinical Periodontology*, vol. 29, no. 4, pp. 281–286, 2002.

[22] I. Hollan, P. L. Meroni, J. M. Ahearn et al., "Cardiovascular disease in autoimmune rheumatic diseases," *Autoimmunity Reviews*, vol. 12, pp. 1004–1015, 2013.

[23] F. Liao, Z. Li, Y. Wang, B. Shi, Z. Gong, and X. Cheng, "Porphyromonas gingivalis may play an important role in the pathogenesis of periodontitis-associated rheumatoid arthritis," *Medical Hypotheses*, vol. 72, no. 6, pp. 732–735, 2009.

[24] D.A. Mahamed, A. Marleau, M. Alnaeeli et al., "G(-) anaerobes-reactive CD4+ T cells trigger RANKL-mediated enhanced alveolar bone loss in diabetic NOD mice," *Diabetes*, vol. 54, pp. 1477–1486, 2005.

[25] S. H. Stein, T. E. Hart, and W. H. Hoffman, "Interleukin 10 promotes anticollagen antibody production in type I diabetic peripheral B lymphocytes," *Journal of Periodontal Research*, vol. 32, pp. 189–195, 1997.

[26] Y. Takeuchi, H. Yoshie, and K. Hara, "Expression of interleukin-2 receptor and HLA-DR on lymphocyte subsets of gingival crevicular fluid in patients with periodontitis," *Journal of Periodontal Research*, vol. 26, no. 6, pp. 502–510, 1991.

[27] R. Jonsson, J. Mountz, and W. Koopman, "Elucidating the pathogenesis of autoimmune disease: recent advances at the molecular level and relevance to oral mucosal disease," *Journal of Oral Pathology and Medicine*, vol. 19, no. 8, pp. 341–350, 1990.

[28] L. A. de-Gennaro, J. D. Lopes, and M. Mariano, "Autoantibodies directed to extracellular matrix components in patients with different clinical forms of periodontitis," *Journal of Periodontology*, vol. 77, no. 12, pp. 2025–2030, 2006.

[29] D. W. Talmage, "Immunological specificity," *Science*, vol. 129, no. 3364, pp. 1643–1648, 1959.

[30] W. H. Robinson, L. Steinman, and P. J. Utz, "Proteomics technologies for the study of autoimmune disease," *Arthritis and Rheumatism*, vol. 46, no. 4, pp. 885–893, 2002.

# 5

# Slipping through the Cracks: Linking Low Immune Function and Intestinal Bacterial Imbalance to the Etiology of Rheumatoid Arthritis

**Kuniaki Terato,[1] Christopher T. Do,[1] and Hiroshi Shionoya[2]**

[1]*Chondrex, Inc., 2607 151st Place NE, Redmond, WA 98052, USA*
[2]*Asama Chemicals Co., Ltd., 20-3 Nihonbashi Kodenmacho, Chuo-ku, Tokyo 103, Japan*

Correspondence should be addressed to Kuniaki Terato; terato@chondrex.com

Academic Editor: Gabriel J. Tobón

Autoimmune diseases (ADs) are considered to be caused by the host immune system which attacks and destroys its own tissue by mistake. A widely accepted hypothesis to explain the pathogenic mechanism of ADs is "molecular mimicry," which states that antibodies against an infectious agent cross-react with a self-antigen sharing an identical or similar antigenic epitope. However, this hypothesis was most likely established based on misleading antibody assay data largely influenced by intense false positive reactions involved in immunoassay systems. Thus reinvestigation of this hypothesis using an appropriate blocking agent capable of eliminating all types of nonspecific reactions and proper assay design is strongly encouraged. In this review, we discuss the possibility that low immune function may be the fundamental, common defect in ADs, which increases the susceptibility to potential disease causative pathogens located in the gastrointestinal tract (GI), such as bacteria and their components or dietary components. In addition to these exogenous agents, aberrations in the host's physical condition may disrupt the host defense system, which is tightly orchestrated by "immune function," "mucosal barrier function," and "intestinal bacterial balance." These disturbances may initiate a downward spiral, which can lead to chronic health problems that will evolve to an autoimmune disorder.

## 1. Introduction

The pathogenesis and disease causative antigen(s) of autoimmune diseases (ADs) such as rheumatoid arthritis (RA) remain elusive regardless of extensive studies on potential disease causative agents such as the herpes virus gp110 protein [1], heat shock proteins [2], bacterial superantigens [3], and dietary proteins [4, 5]. The search for a disease causative antigen has mainly been based on the longstanding molecular mimicry hypothesis, which states that an exogenous substance produced or possessed by an infectious agent may share sequence or structural similarities with a self-antigen [6, 7]. Based on this hypothesis, numerous studies on antibody responses to autologous components and exogenous pathogenic agents were conducted using immunoassay systems such as ELISA and RIA. Unfortunately, these assay systems were used without recognizing a number of vexing phenomena such as intense false positive reactions caused by hydrophobic binding of immunoglobulin in sample specimens to plastic surfaces as previously reported [8–10]. Thus, we propose here a systematic reinvestigation of this theory using an appropriate assay system, which utilizes a proper blocking agent capable of eliminating all types of nonspecific reactions, as well as proper experimental design that includes antigen noncoated wells to determine the remarkably high nonspecific background noise reactions unique to individual samples [8, 10].

One candidate group of disease causative pathogens is pathogenic intestinal bacteria, which carry pathogen associated molecular patterns (PAMPs) on their surfaces, which are recognized by pattern recognition receptors (PRRs) such as Toll-like receptors (TLRs), and may activate host innate and adaptive immune responses, thus potentially triggering an uncontrollable inflammatory reaction leading to the development of ADs [11–14].

In addition to pathogenic intestinal bacteria, nonpathogenic commensal bacteria and their cellular components may also be involved in the pathogenesis of ADs. Normally, these intestinal bacteria do not affect the host's health but may overcome the host's defenses and exert pathogenic effects under conditions such as immunosenescence, GI disorders, or other events such as physical and psychological stress [15–22] as we will discuss later. Although none of these hypotheses have been confirmed, advanced technologies such as genomic analysis of bacteria [23, 24] and gnotobiological methods [25] are facilitating studies on the potential linkage or association of intestinal bacteria with ADs [13, 14, 26, 27].

Based on our previous studies [5, 10, 28–32] and others [33, 34], we propose here that the imbalance of intestinal bacteria and a consequent increase in toxin levels in the GI tract may directly contribute to the development of ADs in conjunction with low immune function at the gut associated lymphoid tissue (GALT) and an increased mucosal permeability. As a consequence, chronic translocation of excess amounts of disease causative pathogen(s), especially bacterial toxins, into the body through the mucosal barrier system might contribute to the development of inflammatory diseases, which are characterized as progressive and persistent.

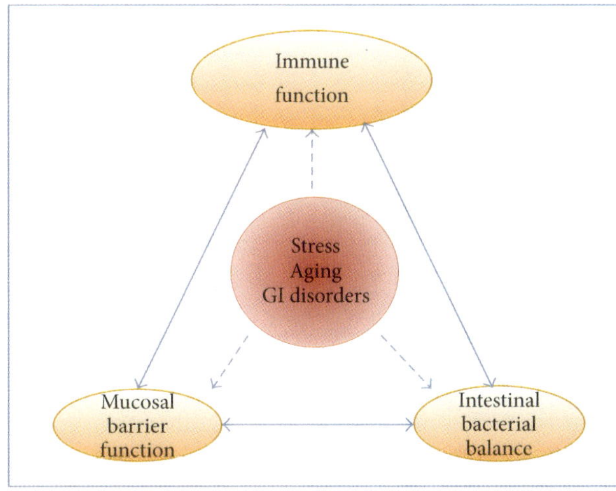


Figure 1: Triangle of three key elements closely linked to maintain host health: immune function is critical to maintaining the balance of these three elements. Once the host's immune function is deteriorated by stress, aging, and other events such as GI disorders, the mucosal barrier system will be deteriorated along with an imbalance of intestinal bacteria, which eventually overcome the GI immune system. As a consequence, hosts with low immune function become more susceptible to these intestinal pathogens and fall into a downward spiral of chronic health problems.

*1.1. Core Contributing Factors to Autoimmune Diseases.* To understand the pathogenesis of ADs, it is important to consider that there is a gender bias in RA and type I diabetics. In fact, recent studies in mouse models suggest that higher susceptibility to arthritis [35] and type I diabetes [36] in female mice could be directly attributed to commensal bacteria. Importantly, intestinal bacteria are influenced by MHC haplotypes, and the guts of arthritis susceptible HLA-DRB1*0401 transgenic mice are dominated by a *Clostridium*-like bacterium, whereas the guts of arthritis resistant DRB1*0402 mice are enriched for members of the Porphyromonadaceae family and *Bifidobacterium* [35]. Moreover, older female *0401 mice exhibit increased intestinal mucosal permeability compared to young *0401 females or old *0402 females. Accordingly, cytokine transcripts in jejuna showed differential TH17 regulatory network gene transcripts in *0401 and *0402 mice. Similarly, Markle et al. [36] show that the commensal microbiota could reinforce the gender bias in the sensitivity of female mice versus resistance of male mice to type 1 diabetes mellitus and alter serum testosterone levels. These observations indicate that intestinal flora linked to gender, age, and genetic background may modulate the gut immune system and enhance proinflammatory conditions in susceptible individuals.

Indeed, RA mainly develops in women older than 40 and men older than 60 years old as reviewed elsewhere [37] and develops long after the emergence of preclinical symptoms such as fatigue, malaise, and diffuse musculoskeletal pain [38]. In fact, we have observed that the majority of RA patients (14/18: 78%) suffer from GI disorders such as constipation (66%) or diarrhea (11%) [32]. These observations indicate that physical and psychological health problems are present in these patients before the onset of clinical RA and highlight the importance of healthy gut function, more specifically the GI immune system.

The GI immune system is exposed to large amounts of countless pathogenic and nonpathogenic foreign substances including dietary proteins and intestinal bacteria. Therefore, in the GI tract, three independent elements, "immune function," "mucosal barrier function," and "intestinal bacterial balance," are tightly orchestrated to protect the host from hazardous pathogenic substances [14, 34, 39] as illustrated in Figure 1. This tight regulation is exemplified by the fact that the GI mucosa is consistently interacting with intestinal bacteria and their components, which stimulate the immune system and induce a state of "controlled physiological inflammation" [40] under healthy conditions. However, it is likely that mucosal barrier function is susceptible to a variety of events such as stress [41–43], GI disorders [44], and immunosenescence associated with aging [45–47], which deteriorate the host immune function and disrupt intestinal bacterial balance. As a consequence, excess amounts of exogenous substances, which may overwhelm the mucosal barrier, penetrate into the mucosa and cause a shift from a controlled inflammation to a pathological inflammation. This phenomenon is similar to the age-related proinflammatory state as characterized by higher levels of interleukin- (IL-) 6, IL-1 receptor antagonist, IL-18, and C-reactive proteins in the elderly with low immune function due to the immunosenescence [48].

In this review, we discuss a possible etiology of RA based on the hypothesis that high intestinal mucosal permeability and imbalance of intestinal bacteria associated with low immune function [10, 49] may be critical disorders in ADs such as RA. We also comment on the legitimacy of molecular mimicry as a mechanism for autoimmunity.

*1.2. Molecular Mimicry in the Search for a Disease Causative Antigen.* Rheumatic fever is considered as a sequela of group A *Streptococcus* infection, as antibodies against this bacterium are believed to cross-react to self-components such as cardiac myosin, resulting in heart valve deterioration [50]. This concept of cross-reactivity between self- and non-self-components became the basis for the hypothesis known as molecular mimicry or the cross-reactivity hypothesis as reviewed elsewhere [6, 50] and has been expanded to explain the pathogenesis of other diseases, such as RA and ankylosing spondylitis (AS). For example, the antibody epitope on the human HLA DR molecule (EQRRAA) is shared with the bacterium *Proteus mirabilis* in RA [51–54], whereas the antibody epitope on the human HLA-B27 molecule (QTDRED or DRDE) is shared with *Klebsiella*, *Shigella*, *Yersinia*, and *Salmonella* in AS [55–58]. Accordingly, numerous studies were conducted based on this hypothesis and concluded that antibodies against a variety of potential pathogenic bacteria, such as *E. coli*, *Klebsiella pneumoniae*, *Proteus mirabilis*, *Serratia marcescens* [7, 17, 59, 60], LPS [61, 62], and *P. gingivalis* [63], were higher in ADs groups than in normal controls. For example, Tani et al. [64] reported that Japanese patients with RA have high IgG antibody titers against *Proteus mirabilis* and *Klebsiella pneumonia*, while Japanese patients with AS have high IgA antibody titers against *Klebsiella pneumonia* but not *Proteus mirabilis*, indicating that a particular strain of bacteria may be involved in different diseases. Although this proposal is very attractive for examining the possible involvement of a variety of bacteria in ADs, a reinvestigation using more appropriate assay protocols and buffer systems with careful consideration on the significant differences in the interactions between individual subclasses and isotypes of serum immunoglobulins from patients with different diseases and individual strains of bacteria is needed, as we briefly discuss below.

These kinds of data and consequently molecular mimicry as a proposed mechanism for ADs have persisted for two reasons. The first is the lack of recognition of intense false positive reactions caused by the sample itself in immunoassays, which are higher in autoimmune patients than in normal controls. In fact, this was clearly addressed by de Vries et al. [9], who ran ELISAs using two additional control wells: blank wells coated only with buffer and wells coated with an irrelevant antigen, in addition to wells coated with a synthetic HLA-B27 peptide to assay serum antibodies in patients with AS and Reiter's syndrome. Indeed, almost identical OD values were observed in all three wells due to the hydrophobic binding of immunoglobulin in sample sera to plastic surfaces of the ELISA plates. Secondly, it is not fully appreciated that human sera, regardless of normal or diseased, contain high levels of IgG and IgA antibodies against virtually all environmental agents, such as dietary proteins, bacteria, and their cellular components, all of which humans are continuously exposed to during their lifetime [10]. Most importantly, it is virtually impossible to differentiate disease groups from healthy controls by the immunoassay systems used in the past and present. This is especially true for low serum dilutions (1:20–1:200), due to the intense false reactions involved in current immunoassay systems. Further discussion on eliminating false positive reactions in immunoassay systems is beyond the scope of this review but has recently been examined [10].

Regardless of these points of criticism, molecular mimicry persists as the main hypothesis for rationalizing the possible association of pathogenic microbes with the development of ADs [7]. Therefore, we believe that it is our obligation to raise questions about the accuracy and reliability of immunoassay systems such as RIA, ELISA, immunoblotting, and immunostaining and ask whether antibodies against these pathogens really cross-react to autologous components.

Nonetheless, the high cross-reactivity of anti-foreign substance antibodies with autologous components should not be disregarded. One example is the strong cross-reactivity of antibodies against heterologous type II collagen, such as chick and bovine, with autologous mouse type II collagen in mice [65, 66] and human type II collagen in RA [5, 29], which share high amino acid sequence homology of more than 85% [67]. Therefore, individual species of type II collagen share multiple common epitopes, while only one epitope is shared by bacteria and the HLA molecule as mentioned above. In fact, antibodies against dietary chick and bovine type II collagen that are cross-reactive with autologous human type II collagen likely play a pathological role in patients with RA [31]. These observations were confirmed by feeding chick type II collagen in an "oral collagen-induced arthritis model" [30]. These data suggest that more detailed studies are required to search for possible pathogenic mimic antigens, which elicit antibodies that are cross-reactive with autologous components by employing an appropriate assay system.

*1.3. Low Immune Function in Patients with Autoimmune Diseases.* The immune system in patients with ADs was considered to be upregulated or overstimulated by autologous components or disease causative pathogens based on antibody assay data influenced by nonspecific reactions as described above. Therefore, the question of whether the host immune system is stimulated by these pathogens or otherwise lowered by the host's conditions such as immunosenescence was addressed by assaying the antibody responses to environmental agents in patients with ADs using ELISA employing a newly developed blocking agent (ChonBlock). In this study, we found that IgG antibody responses to potential pathogenic agents, such as *Escherichia coli* (*E. coli*), *E. coli*-lipopolysaccharide (LPS), and peptidoglycan polysaccharide (PG-PS) from group A *Streptococcus pyogenes*, which is arthritogenic in experimental animals [68–70], as well as nonpathogenic dietary proteins, were significantly lower or tended to be lower in patients with RA and SLE compared to normal controls (Figure 2). On the other hand, IgA antibody responses tended to be higher, and as a consequence, the IgA/IgG antibody ratios were significantly higher in these patients. In contrast, patients with Crohn's disease displayed higher IgG antibody responses to all the antigens tested

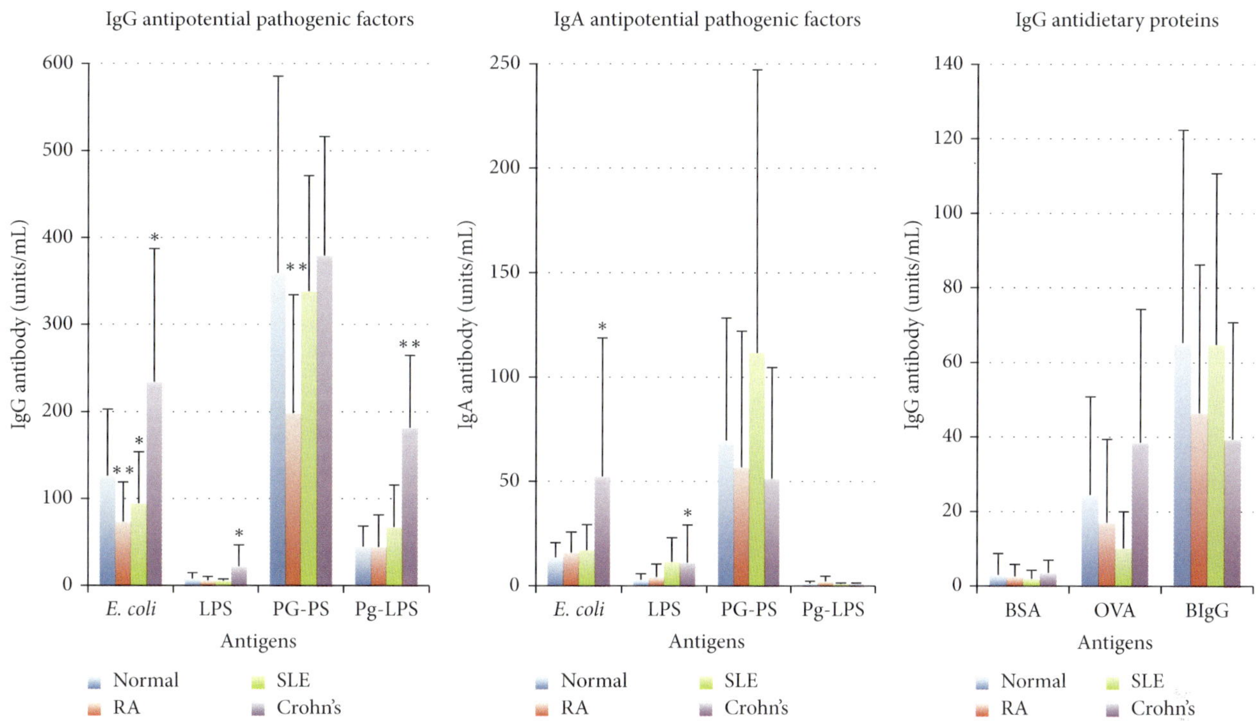


FIGURE 2: Comparison of IgG and IgA antibody responses to potential pathogenic and nonpathogenic environmental agents between normal controls and patients with RA, SLE, and Crohn's disease.

including *Porphyromonas gingivalis* (*P. gingivalis*) LPS (Pg-LPS), indicating that their immune systems are excessively stimulated by these antigens, which have penetrated into the body due to the leakage of the mucosal barrier. These observations indicate that the pathogenic mechanisms and pathogens involved in RA and Crohn's disease are apparently different as discussed later in Section 1.4.

*1.4. Imbalance of Intestinal Bacteria Associated with Low Immune Function.* Intestinal bacterial balance is maintained under the influence of host immune function [71, 72] from childhood through adulthood but starts to change at around 50–60 years of age [73, 74] as illustrated in Figure 3. For example, the relative population of beneficial bacteria such as *Bifidobacterium* declines gradually with aging, whereas the relative population of hazardous bacteria such as *Clostridium perfringens* (*C. perfringens*) and *E. coli* increases. This shift may be attributed to immunosenescence and may increase disease risk in the elderly [45, 73]. Similarly, the imbalance of intestinal bacteria may be due to low immune function associated with stress [41–43] and GI disorders [44]. Consequently, increases in the bacterial toxin levels in the GI tract may not only trigger and exacerbate inflammatory reactions, but also further deteriorate the host's immune system.

In fact, much evidence suggests that changes in the intestinal flora may be a possible etiopathogenic or aggravating factor in RA, and even commensal bacteria may be capable of inducing ADs. Indeed, it was reported that a vegetarian diet modulated the intestinal flora, which was associated with clinical improvement in patients with RA [16, 18, 75].

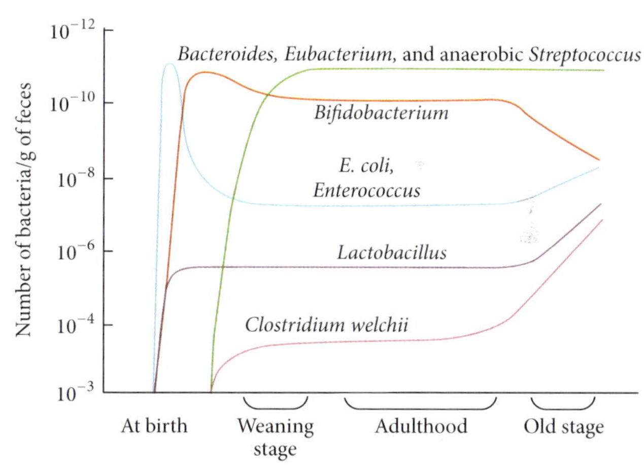


(Provided by Dr. Mitsuoka)

FIGURE 3: Age associated changes of intestinal flora composition.

Furthermore, it was reported that certain strains of bacteria such as *Bifidobacterium*, *Bacteroides-Porphyromonas-Prevotella* group, *Bacteroides fragilis* (*B. fragilis*) subgroup, and *Eubacterium rectale-C. coccoides* group were significantly less numerous in early RA than in controls [21], indicating that these strains may be important in maintaining a barrier for the intestinal wall.

Moreover, the imbalance of intestinal bacteria in inflammatory bowel disease (IBD) has been extensively studied in humans possessing a genetic predisposition for IBD [25, 76]. Indeed, recent phylogenetic comparisons of intestinal bacteria in IBD and non-IBD controls indicated a compositional shift in the bacteria of IBD patients. More specifically, a depletion of commensals such as *Lachnospiraceae* and *Bacteroides* and an enrichment of *Proteobacteria* [77] were observed, whereas other studies indicated a high prevalence of *Bacteroides* and *Prevotella* spp. in ulcerative colitis, a type of IBD [78]. These data demonstrate the importance of intestinal bacterial composition in IBD.

Although compositional changes in intestinal bacteria are observed in patients with RA and IBD, the pathogenic mechanisms involved in RA and IBD apparently differ, as significant differences in antibody responses to environmental pathogens were observed as described in Section 1.3. The differences between RA and IBD may be explained by possible defects in innate immune function, mucosal barrier function, or T-lymphocyte regulatory function in IBD [79]. To distinguish the different types of ADs, detailed studies on possible defects in the host defense system, as well as mucosal barrier function, are required.

*1.5. Pathogenic Role of Intestinal Bacteria in Autoimmunity.* The possible involvement of pathogenic bacteria in ADs has been a prevalent focal point linking bacteria to the etiology of ADs [13, 14]. However, it has been suggested that even nonpathogenic commensal bacteria may be involved in the pathogenesis of ADs. Indeed, it is highly likely that unregulated growth of nonpathogenic commensal bacteria triggers overactivation of innate and adaptive immune responses without precise control by the host immune system [15, 17–22, 25].

For example, the glucose 6-phosphate isomerase (GPI) specific T-cell transgenic K/BxN mouse develops attenuated arthritis in germ-free conditions but develops more severe arthritis when inoculated with commensal bacteria [80]. Moreover, human B-27 transgenic rats [81] and mice [82], developed for studying the contribution of genetic background to developing ankylosing spondylitis (AS), do not develop inflammatory intestinal or peripheral joint disease in germ-free conditions. However, B-27 transgenic rats developed diarrhea and inflammatory changes in the colon after being transferred to a conventional room for 23 days. Similarly, B-27 transgenic mice showed a high incidence of paralysis and mortality following infection with *Yersinia enterocolitica*. Furthermore, the prevalence of the naturally occurring joint disease, ankylosing entheropathy, is higher in conventionally housed mice than their specific pathogen-free (SPF) counterparts [83]. This increased susceptibility to pathogenic and nonpathogenic bacteria in germ-free or SPF housed mice is attributed to an immature immune system. Thus, inoculated intestinal bacteria are capable of invading into the intestinal mucosa and can induce inflammatory reactions at the GI mucosa, as well as other tissues. These observations indicate the importance of the mucosal immune system, which is exposed to a large number of intestinal bacteria and other exogenous substances.

*1.6. Mucosal Permeability Associated with Low Immune Function.* In addition to immune function and intestinal bacterial balance, the third element that is critical to maintaining host health is the mucosal barrier function. Importantly, the mucosal barrier is not completely impermeable, as undigested dietary proteins are absorbed even in healthy normal adults [84]. Moreover, the GI mucosa is susceptible to psychological [41–43] and physical stress [85], nonsteroidal anti-inflammatory drugs [86], and GI disorders [44]. All of these events may increase the mucosal permeability to large molecules such as undigested proteins, bacteria, and bacterial cell components including toxins such as LPS. Indeed, rats under stress exhibit increased translocation of horseradish peroxidase (HRP) and *E. coli* by 4 and 30 times compared to control rats [42]. Similarly, viable gut commensal bacteria were detected in the lymph nodes, spleen, liver, and kidneys of immunodeficient mice [87, 88], suggesting the importance of immune protection against the translocation of macromolecules at the GI mucosa. Finally, degradation products of bacterial cell walls and nucleic acids have been found in joints of RA patients [19], indicating high permeability of the intestinal mucosa in these patients. In fact, some of these bacterial cell components such as a streptococcal proteoglycan polysaccharide (PG-PS) are known to be arthritogenic and capable of inducing arthritis in rodents [68–70], suggesting that bacteria and their components may play a pathological role in humans.

Furthermore, high mucosal permeability along with significant changes in the colonic flora is associated with constipation. Although constipation is not considered as a serious GI disorder, it is still considered as a risk factor for increased susceptibility to pathogenic bacteria and immune disorders [44]. In these patients, (1) serum ovalbumin (OVA) levels are 28 times, (2) anti-*E. coli* antibody levels are 9 times, (3) spontaneous lymphocyte proliferation is 1.5–2.0 times, and (4) serum IgG levels are 1.3 times higher than normal controls, whereas T-cell responses to PHA, a T-cell mitogen, are less than 1/2 of normal controls. These data indicate that increased mucosal permeability, which may be associated with low immune function, is a critical disorder linked to chronic health problems.

*1.7. Pathological Roles of Bacterial Toxins.* LPS is a major component of the outer membrane of gram-negative bacteria representing one of the conserved microbial structures. Interestingly, LPS serves unique functions for the host; one is to stimulate and mature the host immune system, while the other is to trigger and enhance inflammatory reactions. For example, the pathological role of LPS has been demonstrated, as elevated serum LPS levels were observed in patients with type I diabetes [89] and chronic fatigue syndrome [61] and even in healthy men [90, 91]. Moreover, intestinal absorption of LPS is significantly increased by fats such as triolein (olive oil) [92]. In fact, high-fat content meals induce low-grade endotoxemia in an obesity and insulin resistant mouse [93].

Most importantly, LPS absorbed from the intestine is capable of triggering inflammatory reactions. For example, oral administration of LPS (1 mg) into DBA/1 mice older than 1 year old, which previously received a subarthritogenic dose (1 mg) of monoclonal antibody cocktail [66], increased the serum IL-6 levels (Figure 4(a)) and induced severe

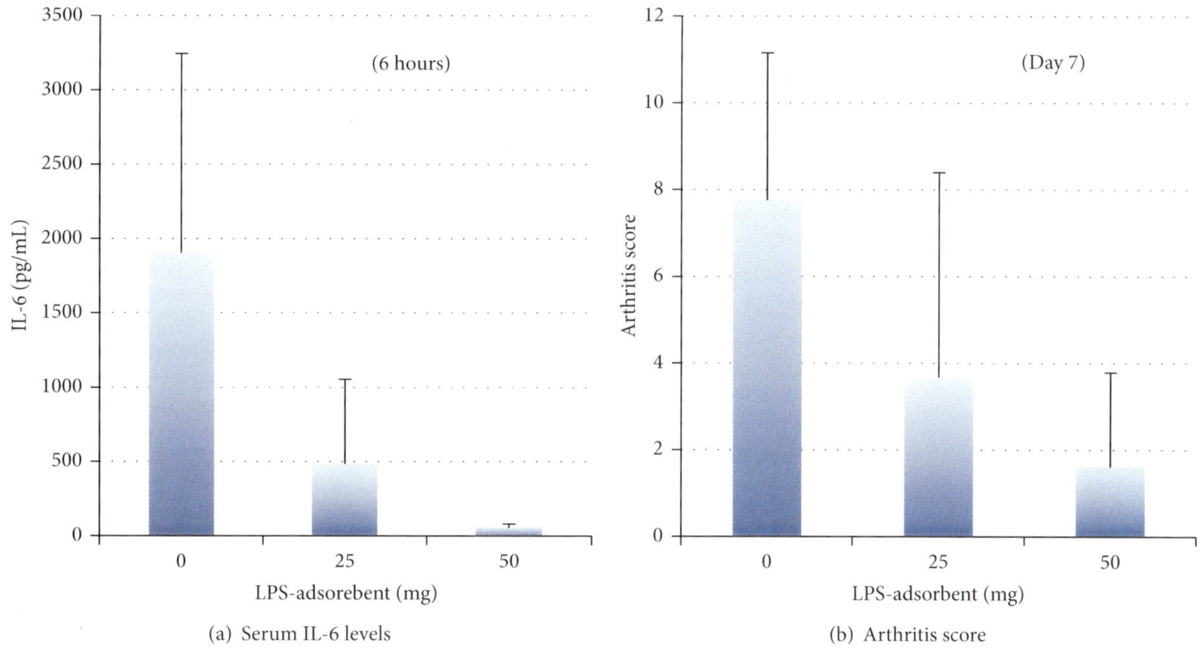


FIGURE 4: Synergistic effect of bacterial toxins and autoantibodies to type II collagen in induction of arthritis in mice. Oral administration of LPS in mice receiving a subarthritogenic dose of monoclonal antibody cocktail displayed an immediate increase in serum IL-6 levels and induced arthritis within 24–48 hours, reaching a maximum score on days 7-8. Co-oral administration of LPS-adsorbent prevents the increase of serum IL-6 and development of arthritis in a dose-dependent manner. *Note*. Serum IL-6 level was increased only in old mice more than 8 months but was not observed in young mice.

arthritis (Figure 4(b)), whereas oral administration of an LPS-adsorbent prevented the increase in serum IL-6 and development of arthritis in a dose-dependent manner. Importantly, young DBA/1 mice (8–14 weeks old) did not respond to oral LPS administration, as serum IL-6 levels were not raised in these animals, indicating that aged mice are more susceptible to bacterial toxins present in the GI tract. This observation supports a possible link between immunosenescence and an age-related proinflammatory state [48], as well as the increased incidence of RA in the elderly [37].

Furthermore, oral coadministration of a low dose of LPS (10 $\mu$g/mouse/day) with chick type II collagen (CII) in DBA/1 mice enhanced not only antibody production, but also CII-specific T-cell responses [30]. Moreover, mice receiving a long-term oral administration of LPS alone developed non-antibody-mediated arthritis, which was characterized by significant deformity of digit and loss of nail, indicating that LPS alone is capable of inducing chronic arthritis without autoantibodies to type II collagen. This evidence supports the observation that chronic stimulation of B cells by mitogenic LPS increased IgG secreting splenocytes, hypergammaglobulinemia, and antibody production, as well as accelerating the development of SLE in MRI/n, BXSB, and NZW female mice [101].

In addition, the proinflammatory effects of LPS and other bacterial toxins have been extensively studied in various types of animal models such as collagen-induced arthritis (CIA) [102], collagen antibody-induced arthritis (CAIA) [28], experimental autoimmune encephalomyelitis (EAE) [97], SLE-nephritis [101, 103], autoimmune thyroiditis [104], autoimmune hemolytic anemia [105, 106], and obesity [93]. Importantly, bacterial toxins, regardless of their B- or T-cell specificities, are not only lethally toxic, but capable of triggering and exacerbating inflammatory reactions. For example, T-cell mitogens, SEB [99, 107], and MAM [98] also trigger and exacerbate severe inflammatory arthritis in CIA and CAIA models, as well as LPS, a B-cell mitogen.

However, bacterial toxins not only are stimulatory, but may even diminish the host immune system [108, 109]. Indeed, T-cell responses to plant mitogens such as PHA, pokeweed, and concanavalin A (ConA) were diminished in patients with RA and constipation [110–112]. These data indicate that B and T cells polyclonally activated by mitogenic bacterial toxins absorbed from the GI tract are no longer responsive to pathogens. Taken together, chronic disturbances of the immune system by intestinal bacterial toxins appear to be an important etiology linked to low immune function and contribute to the development of ADs such as RA.

*1.8. New Approach for Modulating Intestinal Flora and Disease Activities.* Low immune function, compromised mucosal barrier integrity and intestinal bacterial balance may be critical factors in the etiology of RA and other ADs. Thus, one therapeutic approach is to restore the intestinal bacterial balance using antibiotics; however, this approach is not effective for the treatment of infectious diarrhea [95]. On the other hand, *C. difficile*-associated diarrhea, an emerging complication associated with the use of systemic antimicrobials, has been successfully treated using donor stool to normalize the microbiota [113]. Alternatively, passive antibody therapy

Table 1: Internal and exogenous factors possibly involved in the pathogenesis of RA and other ADs: two unrelated types of risk factors apparently contribute to the development of ADs: the first is environmental exogenous factors, and the second is the host's physical condition. In addition, ADs such as RA might be classified into two types, autoantibody-mediated and non-antibody-mediated. Regardless of whether the disease is mediated by autoantibodies or not, bacterial toxins absorbed from the intestine directly trigger and exacerbate an inflammatory reaction.

| Types of risk factors | Antibody-mediated arthritis | Non-antibody-mediated arthritis |
|---|---|---|
| Exogenous factors | Possible risk agents | |
| Mimic antigens | Dietary collagen [29, 30],<br>Cartilage PG [94] | / |
| Pathogenic and nonpathogenic bacteria | PAMPs [13, 14, 95] | PAMPs [13, 14, 95]<br>Arthritogenic PG-PS [96] |
| Bacterial toxins | LPS [28, 97],<br>MAM [28, 98], and SEB [99] | LPS [30], SEB [3] |
| Foods and drugs | High fat diet [90],<br>Proteinase inhibitor, and NSAID [30] | High fat diet [90],<br>Proteinase inhibitor, and NSAID [30] |
| Host's physical condition | Possible risk events | |
| Immune function | Immunosenescence [47, 49]<br>GI disorders [44] | Immunosenescence [47, 49]<br>GI disorders [44] |
| Mucosal barrier function | Stress [41, 42, 100]<br>GI disorders [44] | Stress [41, 42, 100]<br>GI disorders [44] |
| Intestinal bacterial balance | Bacterial imbalance [16, 18, 75]<br>High toxin level in GI tract | Bacterial imbalance [16, 18, 75]<br>High toxin level in GI tract |

using bovine colostrum obtained from cows immunized with specific pathogens was used to treat diarrhea in patients infected with immunodeficiency virus [114, 115] and other infectious agents such as oral candidiasis, *Helicobacter pylori*, rotavirus, *Campylobacter jejuni*, and *C. difficile* [116–118]. To confirm the beneficial effects of milk antibodies, Iwatsuki et al. [119] recently analyzed intestinal bacterial flora in elderly volunteers treated with oral administration of a natural milk antibody product, which contains active antibodies against a wide range of pathogenic bacteria and their toxins [120]. After 8 weeks of treatment, the population of *E. coli*, *C. difficile*, and *C. perfringens* (formerly known as *C. welchii*) decreased significantly, whereas *Lactobacilli, Bacteroides* spp., *Prevotella* spp.,and *B. fragilis* populations increased.

This approach was further applied for the treatment of patients with RA, whose disease activity was uncontrolled by authentic medications [32], resulting in significant reduction of arthritis symptoms and improvement of intestinal disorders in 50% of 18 patients, whereas none of the 20 untreated patients showed improvement in either arthritis or GI symptoms, such as constipation and diarrhea. To confirm the efficacy of this milk antibody product, a multicentered double blind clinical study is currently being conducted. Although not yet mainstream, these alternative medical approaches for the treatment of infectious diseases are gaining traction, as more complications associated with antibiotic resistant bacteria are emerging. Moreover, we are optimistic about these approaches for the successful treatment of ADs.

## 2. Discussion

ADs such as RA may begin with marked systemic symptoms, including fatigue, fever, and weight loss, and slowly progress to classic symptoms such as joint pain and swelling. This progression suggests that a long-term exposure to disease causative pathogens might be the fundamental etiology of RA. In this aspect, we believe that various types of exogenous and internal factors listed in Table 1 are involved in developing health problems, which evolve to progressive, chronic diseases. With regard to mimic antigens, antibodies to heterologous type II collagen apparently contribute to the pathogenesis in the majority of patients with RA and relapsing polychondritis (RP) [5], whereas patients with HLA-DR haplotypes of 0401/0405, 0404, and 0408 are unlikely mediated by autoantibodies [31], but instead mediated by environmental agent(s) such as bacteria and their components, which are chronically absorbed from the GI tract over long periods.

Based on these observations, it is reasonable to consider that host factors such as immunosenescence, stress, and GI disorders, which lower the host's immune function, may play an initial role in disrupting the triangle relationship between the three key elements: "immune function," "mucosal barrier function," and "intestinal bacterial balance." Accordingly, low immune function, which lowers the mucosal defense function in the GI tract, may be the primary and common defects that increase the mucosal permeability and trigger an imbalance in intestinal bacteria, which might increase the toxin levels in the GI tract.

Under these circumstances, nonpathogenic and pathogenic commensal bacteria and their toxins such as LPS may equally contribute to the pathogenesis of ADs. Currently, advanced technologies are available to analyze the complex intestinal bacterial world, and it seems that the time is ripe to study the contribution of intestinal bacteria and

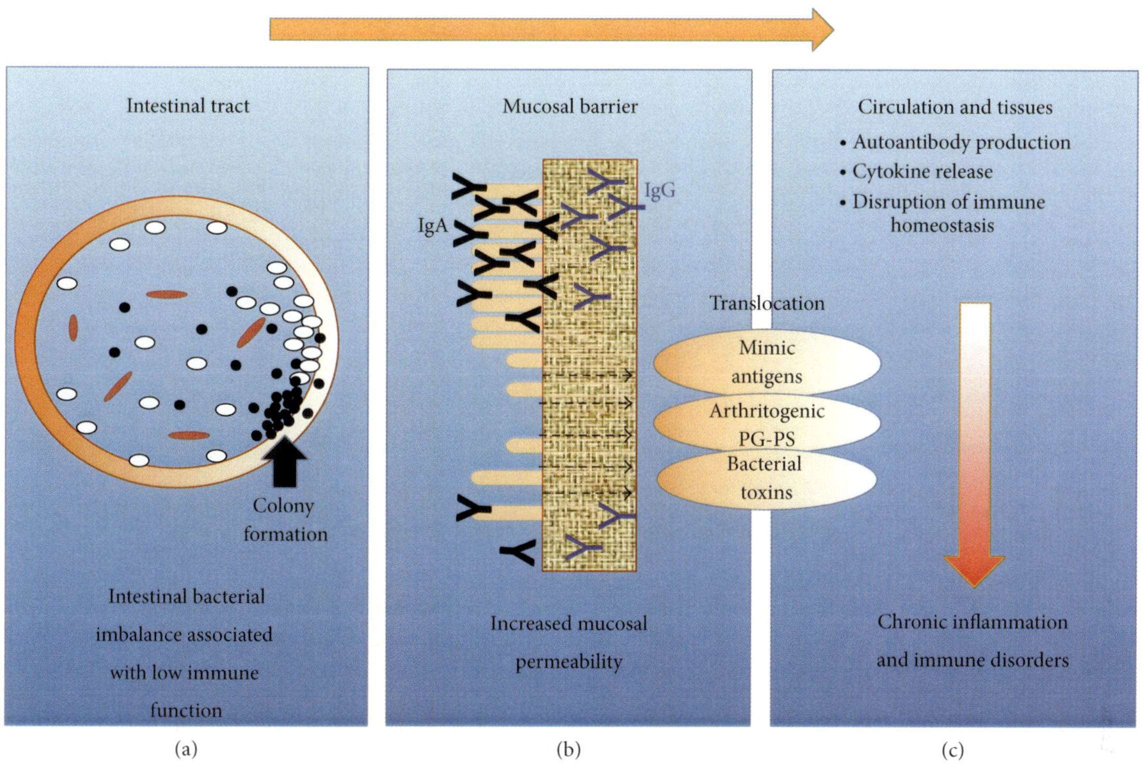


Figure 5: Possible contribution of pathogenic and nonpathogenic environmental factors to autoimmune diseases: low immune function may lead to intestinal bacterial imbalance by failing to prevent the colony formation of pathogenic bacteria (a). In addition decreases in the mucosal barrier function result in increased intestinal mucosal permeability (b). As a result, excess amounts of bacterial components and their toxins and even large molecular, undigested dietary proteins, which share similar amino acid sequences with autologous components such as collagen, cross the mucosal barrier into circulation (c). Some of these exogenous substances can disturb immune homeostasis and result in the development of chronic diseases.

their cellular components in order to reveal the etiologies of RA and other chronic diseases.

## 3. Conclusion

Based on observations in the past and present, we believe that it is important to investigate a possible involvement of intestinal bacteria and their toxins in the development of ADs in conjunction with the host's low immune function as summarized in Figure 5. Patients with low immune function are more susceptible not only to pathogenic intestinal bacteria but also to nonpathogenic commensal bacteria and their toxins, as well as dietary components such as mimic antigens and fats. Importantly, these environmental factors do not affect the host under normal conditions but may affect the global host health and further deteriorate the immune system under conditions such as immunosenescence, GI disorders, or stress. Therefore, to fully appreciate the etiology of ADs, it is important to acknowledge possible low immune function and relating minor disorders or defects, which are observed before the onset of ADs, such as RA.

## Conflict of Interests

Kuniaki Terato and Christopher T. Do declare that they have received financial support by Chondrex, Inc. Hiroshi Shionoya declares that he has no competing interests.

## References

[1] J. Roudier, G. Rhodes, J. Petersen, J. H. Vaughan, and D. A. Carson, "The Epstein-Barr virus glycoprotein gp110, a molecular link between HLA DR4, HLA DR1, and rheumatoid arthritis," *Scandinavian Journal of Immunology*, vol. 27, no. 4, pp. 367–371, 1988.

[2] S. H. E. Kaufmann, "Heat-shock proteins: a link between rheumatoid arthritis and infection?" *Current Opinion in Rheumatology*, vol. 2, no. 3, pp. 430–435, 1990.

[3] C. G. Drake and B. L. Kotzin, "Superantigens: biology, immunology, and potential role in disease," *Journal of Clinical Immunology*, vol. 12, no. 3, pp. 149–162, 1992.

[4] B. Perez-Maceda, J. P. Lopez-Bote, C. Langa, and C. Bernabeu, "Antibodies to dietary antigens in rheumatoid arthritis—possible molecular mimicry mechanism," *Clinica Chimica Acta*, vol. 203, no. 2-3, pp. 153–165, 1991.

[5] K. Terato, Y. Shimozuru, K. Katayama et al., "Specificity of antibodies to type II collagen in rheumatoid arthritis," *Arthritis & Rheumatism*, vol. 33, no. 10, pp. 1493–1500, 1990.

[6] L. Guilherme, J. Kalil, and M. Cunningham, "Molecular mimicry in the autoimmune pathogenesis of rheumatic heart disease," *Autoimmunity*, vol. 39, no. 1, pp. 31–39, 2006.

[7] T. Rashid and A. Ebringer, "Autoimmunity in rheumatic diseases is induced by microbial infections via crossreactivity or molecular mimicry," *Autoimmune Diseases*, vol. 2012, Article ID 539282, 9 pages, 2012.

[8] K. Fujii, M. Tsuji, K. Murota, K. Terato, Y. Shimozuru, and Y. Nagai, "An improved enzyme-linked immunosorbent assay of anti-collagen antibodies in human serum," *Journal of Immunological Methods*, vol. 124, no. 1, pp. 63–70, 1989.

[9] D. D. de Vries, A. J. Dekker-Saeys, E. Gyodi, U. Bohm, and P. Ivanyi, "Absence of autoantibodies to peptides shared by HLA-B27.5 and *Klebsiella pneumoniae* nitrogenase in serum samples from HLA-B27 positive patients with ankylosing spondylitis and Reiter's syndrome," *Annals of the Rheumatic Diseases*, vol. 51, no. 6, pp. 783–789, 1992.

[10] K. Terato, C. T. Do, D. Cutler, T. Waritani, and H. Shionoya, "Preventing intense false positive and negative reactions attributed to the principle of ELISA to re-investigate antibody studies in autoimmune diseases," *Journal of Immunological Methods*, vol. 407, pp. 15–25, 2014.

[11] K. S. Midwood, A. M. Piccinini, and S. Sacre, "Targeting toll-like receptors in autoimmunity," *Current Drug Targets*, vol. 10, no. 11, pp. 1139 1155, 2009.

[12] M. Li, Y. Zhou, G. Feng, and S. B. Su, "The critical role of toll-like receptor signaling pathways in the induction and progression of autoimmune disease," *Current Molecular Medicine*, vol. 9, no. 3, pp. 365–374, 2009.

[13] P. J. Sansonetti, "To be or not to be a pathogen: that is the mucosally relevant question," *Mucosal Immunology*, vol. 4, no. 1, pp. 8–14, 2011.

[14] J. C. Clemente, L. K. Ursell, L. W. Parfrey, and R. Knight, "The impact of the gut microbiota on human health: an integrative view," *Cell*, vol. 148, no. 6, pp. 1258–1270, 2012.

[15] R. B. Sartor, "Importance of intestinal mucosal immunity and luminal bacterial cell wall polymers in the aetiology of inflammatory joint diseases," *Bailliere's Clinical Rheumatology*, vol. 3, no. 2, pp. 223–245, 1989.

[16] R. Peltonen, J. Kjeldsen-Kragh, M. Haugen et al., "Changes of faecal flora in rheumatoid arthritis during fasting and one-year vegetarian diet," *British Journal of Rheumatology*, vol. 33, no. 7, pp. 638–643, 1994.

[17] S. Aoki, K. Yoshikawa, T. Yokoyama et al., "Role of enteric bacteria in the pathogenesis of rheumatoid arthritis: evidence for antibodies to enterobacterial common antigens in rheumatoid sera and synovial fluids," *Annals of the Rheumatic Diseases*, vol. 55, no. 6, pp. 363–369, 1996.

[18] R. Peltonen, M. Nenonen, T. Helve, O. Hänninen, P. Toivanen, and E. Eerola, "Faecal microbial flora and disease activity in rheumatoid arthritis during a vegan diet," *British Journal of Rheumatology*, vol. 36, no. 1, pp. 64–68, 1997.

[19] I. M. van der Heijden, B. Wilbrink, I. Tchetverikov et al., "Presence of bacterial DNA and bacterial peptidoglycans in joints of patients with rheumatoid arthritis and other arthritides," *Arthritis & Rheumatism*, vol. 43, no. 3, pp. 593–598, 2000.

[20] P. Toivanen, "Normal intestinal microbiota in the aetiopathogenesis of rheumatoid arthritis," *Annals of the Rheumatic Diseases*, vol. 62, no. 9, pp. 807–811, 2003.

[21] J. Vaahtovuo, E. Munukka, M. Korkeamäki, R. Luukkainen, and P. Toivanen, "Fecal microbiota in early rheumatoid arthritis," *The Journal of Rheumatology*, vol. 35, no. 8, pp. 1500–1505, 2008.

[22] C. J. Edwards, "Commensal gut bacteria and the etiopathogenesis of rheumatoid arthritis," *The Journal of Rheumatology*, vol. 35, no. 8, pp. 1477–1478, 2008.

[23] E. F. DeLong, G. S. Wickham, and N. R. Pace, "Phylogenetic stains: ribosomal RNA-based probes for the identification of single cells," *Science*, vol. 243, no. 4896, pp. 1360–1363, 1989.

[24] R. I. Amann, L. Krumholz, and D. A. Stahl, "Fluorescent-oligonucleotide probing of whole cells for determinative, phylogenetic, and environmental studies in microbiology," *Journal of Bacteriology*, vol. 172, no. 2, pp. 762–770, 1990.

[25] H. Tlaskalová-Hogenová, R. Tpánková, H. Kozáková et al., "The role of gut microbiota (commensal bacteria) and the mucosal barrier in the pathogenesis of inflammatory and autoimmune diseases and cancer: contribution of germ-free and gnotobiotic animal models of human diseases," *Cellular and Molecular Immunology*, vol. 8, no. 2, pp. 110–120, 2011.

[26] N. Cerf-Bensussan and V. Gaboriau-Routhiau, "The immune system and the gut microbiota: friends or foes?" *Nature Reviews Immunology*, vol. 10, no. 10, pp. 735–744, 2010.

[27] D. Mathis and C. Benoist, "Microbiota and autoimmune disease: the hosted self," *Cell Host & Microbe*, vol. 10, no. 4, pp. 297–301, 2011.

[28] K. Terato, D. S. Harper, M. M. Griffiths et al., "Collagen-induced arthritis in mice: synergistic effect of *E. coli* lipopolysaccharide bypasses epitope specificity in the induction of arthritis with monoclonal antibodies to type II collagen," *Autoimmunity*, vol. 22, no. 3, pp. 137–147, 1995.

[29] K. Terato, D. A. Dearmey, X. J. Ye, M. M. Griffiths, and M. A. Cremer, "The mechanism of autoantibody formation to cartilage in rheumatoid arthritis: possible cross-reaction of antibodies to dietary collagens with autologous type II collagen," *Clinical Immunology and Immunopathology*, vol. 79, no. 2, pp. 142–154, 1996.

[30] K. Terato, X. J. Ye, H. Miyahara, M. A. Cremer, and M. M. Griffiths, "Induction of chronic autoimmune arthritis in DBA/1 mice by oral administration of type II collagen and *Escherichia coli* lipopolysaccharide," *British Journal of Rheumatology*, vol. 35, no. 9, pp. 828–838, 1996.

[31] K. Terato, C. Do, B. Comstock, and J. Zabrecky, "A hypothesis: two distinct factors, autoantibody to type II collagen elicited by mimic antigens and intestinal bacterial toxins, are involved independently and synergistically in the development of autoimmune arthritis," in *Proceedings of the 11th Asia Pacific League of Associations for Rheumatology Congress*, MediMedia Korea, Jeju, Republic of Korea, 2004.

[32] K. Katayama, T. Matsuno, T. Waritani, K. Terato, and H. Shionoya, "Supplemental treatment of rheumatoid arthritis with natural milk antibodies against enteromicrobes and their toxins: results of an open-labelled pilot study," *Nutrition Journal*, vol. 10, article 2, 2011.

[33] S. O'Mahony and A. Ferguson, "Small intestinal mucosal protection mechanisms and their importance in rheumatology," *Annals of the Rheumatic Diseases*, vol. 50, no. 3, pp. 331–336, 1991.

[34] A. Fasano, "Leaky gut and autoimmune diseases," *Clinical Reviews in Allergy and Immunology*, vol. 42, no. 1, pp. 71–78, 2012.

[35] A. Gomez, D. Luckey, C. J. Yeoman et al., "Loss of sex and age driven differences in the gut microbiome characterize arthritis-susceptible *0401 mice but not arthritis-resistant *0402 mice," *PLoS ONE*, vol. 7, no. 4, Article ID e36095, 2012.

[36] J. G. M. Markle, D. N. Frank, S. Mortin-Toth et al., "Sex differences in the gut microbiome drive hormone-dependent regulation of autoimmunity," *Science*, vol. 339, no. 6123, pp. 1084–1088, 2013.

[37] G. Nesher and T. L. Moore, "Rheumatoid arthritis in the aged," *Drugs & Aging*, vol. 3, no. 6, pp. 487–501, 1993.

[38] H. Harris Jr., "Clinical features of rheumatoid arthritis," in *Text Book of Rheumatology*, W. N. Kelley, E. D. Harris, S. Ruddy, and C. B. Sledge, Eds., pp. 898–932, W.B. Sauders, Philadelphia, Pa, USA, 5th edition, 1997.

[39] J. Ermann and C. G. Fathman, "Autoimmune diseases: genes, bugs and failed regulation," *Nature Immunology*, vol. 2, no. 9, pp. 759–761, 2001.

[40] C. Fiocchi, "What is "physiological" intestinal inflammation and how does it differ from "pathological" inflammation?" *Inflammatory Bowel Diseases*, vol. 14, supplement 2, pp. S77–S78, 2008.

[41] P. Anderlik, I. Szeri, Z. Bános, and Z. Barna, "Bacterial translocation after cold stress in young and old mice," *Acta Microbiologica Hungarica*, vol. 37, no. 3, pp. 289–294, 1990.

[42] Å. K. Velin, A.-C. Ericson, Y. Braaf, C. Wallon, and J. D. Söderholm, "Increased antigen and bacterial uptake in follicle associated epithelium induced by chronic psychological stress in rats," *Gut*, vol. 53, no. 4, pp. 494–500, 2004.

[43] G. A. Selkirk, T. M. McLellan, H. E. Wright, and S. G. Rhind, "Mild endotoxemia, NF-$\kappa$B translocation, and cytokine increase during exertional heat stress in trained and untrained individuals," *American Journal of Physiology—Regulatory Integrative and Comparative Physiology*, vol. 295, no. 2, pp. R611–R623, 2008.

[44] I. L. Khalif, E. M. M. Quigley, E. A. Konovitch, and I. D. Maximova, "Alterations in the colonic flora and intestinal permeability and evidence of immune activation in chronic constipation," *Digestive and Liver Disease*, vol. 37, no. 11, pp. 838–849, 2005.

[45] D. L. Schmucker, K. Thoreux, and R. L. Owen, "Aging impairs intestinal immunity," *Mechanisms of Ageing and Development*, vol. 122, no. 13, pp. 1397–1411, 2001.

[46] K. Tiihonen, A. C. Ouwehand, and N. Rautonen, "Human intestinal microbiota and healthy ageing," *Ageing Research Reviews*, vol. 9, no. 2, pp. 107–116, 2010.

[47] A. Larbi, P. Rymkiewicz, A. Vasudev et al., "The immune system in the elderly: a fair fight against diseases?" *Aging Health*, vol. 9, no. 1, pp. 35–47, 2013.

[48] L. Ferrucci, A. Corsi, F. Lauretani et al., "The origins of age-related proinflammatory state," *Blood*, vol. 105, no. 6, pp. 2294–2299, 2005.

[49] T. Pritz, B. Weinberger, and B. Grubeck-Loebenstein, "The aging bone marrow and its impact on immune responses in old age," *Immunology Letters*, vol. 162, no. 1, pp. 310–315, 2014.

[50] M. Cunningham, "Streptococcus and rheumatic fever," *Current Opinion in Rheumatology*, vol. 24, no. 4, pp. 408–416, 2012.

[51] F. Takeuchi, E. Kosuge, K. Matsuta et al., "Antibody to a specific HLA-DR$\beta$1 sequence in Japanese patients with rheumatoid arthritis," *Arthritis & Rheumatism*, vol. 33, no. 12, pp. 1867–1868, 1990.

[52] C. Wilson, A. Ebringer, K. Ahmadi et al., "Shared amino acid sequences between major histocompatibility complex class II glycoproteins, type XI collagen and *Proteus mirabilis* in rheumatoid arthritis," *Annals of the Rheumatic Diseases*, vol. 54, no. 3, pp. 216–220, 1995.

[53] H. Tiwana, C. Wilson, A. Alvarez, R. Abuknesha, S. Bansal, and A. Ebringer, "Cross-reactivity between the rheumatoid arthritis-associated motif EQKRAA and structurally related sequences found in *Proteus mirabilis*," *Infection and Immunity*, vol. 67, no. 6, pp. 2769–2775, 1999.

[54] M. M. Newkirk, R. Goldbach-Mansky, B. W. Senior, J. Klippel, H. R. Schumacher Jr., and H. S. El-Gabalawy, "Elevated levels of IgM and IgA antibodies to *Proteus mirabilis* and IgM antibodies to *Escherichia coli* are associated with early rheumatoid factor (RF)-positive rheumatoid arthritis," *Rheumatology*, vol. 44, no. 11, pp. 1433–1441, 2005.

[55] P. L. Schwimmbeck, D. T. Y. Yu, and M. B. A. Oldstone, "Autoantibodies to HLA B27 in the sera of HLA B27 patients with ankylosing spondylitis and Reiter's syndrome. Molecular mimicry with *Klebsiella pneumoniae* as potential mechanism of autoimmune disease," *The Journal of Experimental Medicine*, vol. 166, no. 1, pp. 173–181, 1987.

[56] N. Tsuchiya, G. Husby, R. C. Williams Jr., H. Stieglitz, P. E. Lipsky, and R. D. Inman, "Autoantibodies to the HLA-B27 sequence cross-react with the hypothetical peptide from the arthritis-associated Shigella plasmid," *The Journal of Clinical Investigation*, vol. 86, no. 4, pp. 1193–1203, 1990.

[57] R. Lahesmaa, M. Skurnik, M. Vaara et al., "Molecular mimickry between HLA B27 and *Yersinia, Salmonella, Shigella* and *Klebsiella* within the same region of HLA $\alpha_1$-helix," *Clinical and Experimental Immunology*, vol. 86, no. 3, pp. 399–404, 1991.

[58] T. Rashid, M. Leirisalo-Repo, Y. Tani et al., "Antibacterial and antipeptide antibodies in Japanese and Finnish patients with rheumatoid arthritis," *Clinical Rheumatology*, vol. 23, no. 2, pp. 134–141, 2004.

[59] L. B. Zapata-Quintanilla, P. Palmeira, M. Tino-De-Franco, J. A. Amaral, C. B. Carbonare, and S. B. Carbonare, "Systemic antibody response to diarrheagenic *Escherichia coli* and LPS O111, O157 and O55 in healthy Brazilian adults," *Scandinavian Journal of Immunology*, vol. 64, no. 6, pp. 661–667, 2006.

[60] C. A. Hitchon, F. Chandad, E. D. Ferucci et al., "Antibodies to *Porphyromonas gingivalis* are associated with anticitrullinated protein antibodies in patients with rheumatoid arthritis and their relatives," *The Journal of Rheumatology*, vol. 37, no. 6, pp. 1105–1112, 2010.

[61] M. Maes, F. N. M. Twisk, M. Kubera, K. Ringel, J.-C. Leunis, and M. Geffard, "Increased IgA responses to the LPS of commensal bacteria is associated with inflammation and activation of cell-mediated immunity in chronic fatigue syndrome," *Journal of Affective Disorders*, vol. 136, no. 3, pp. 909–917, 2012.

[62] M. Arabski, R. Fudala, A. Koza et al., "The presence of anti-LPS antibodies and human serum activity against *Proteus mirabilis* S/R forms in correlation with *TLR4* (Thr399Ile) gene polymorphism in rheumatoid arthritis," *Clinical Biochemistry*, vol. 45, no. 16-17, pp. 1374–1382, 2012.

[63] T. R. Mikuls, J. B. Payne, R. A. Reinhardt et al., "Antibody responses to *Porphyromonas gingivalis* (*P. gingivalis*) in subjects with rheumatoid arthritis and periodontitis," *International Immunopharmacology*, vol. 9, no. 1, pp. 38–42, 2009.

[64] Y. Tani, H. Tiwana, S. Hukuda et al., "Antibodies to *Klebsiella, Proteus*, and HLA-B27 peptides in Japanese patients with ankylosing spondylitis and rheumatoid arthritis," *The Journal of Rheumatology*, vol. 24, no. 1, pp. 109–114, 1997.

[65] K. Terato, K. A. Hasty, M. A. Cremer, J. M. Stuart, A. S. Townes, and A. H. Kang, "Collagen-induced arthritis in mice. Localization of an arthritogenic determinant to a fragment of the type II collagen molecule," *The Journal of Experimental Medicine*, vol. 162, no. 2, pp. 637–646, 1985.

[66] K. Terato, K. A. Hasty, R. A. Reife, M. A. Cremer, A. H. Kang, and J. M. Stuart, "Induction of arthritis with monoclonal antibodies to collagen," *The Journal of Immunology*, vol. 148, no. 7, pp. 2103–2108, 1992.

[67] J. M. Seyer, K. A. Hasty, and A. H. Kang, "Covalent structure of collagen. Amino acid sequence of an arthritogenic cyanogen bromide peptide from type II collagen of bovine cartilage," *European Journal of Biochemistry*, vol. 181, no. 1, pp. 159–173, 1989.

[68] C. Chetty, R. R. Brown, and J. H. Schwab, "Edema-producing activity of group A streptococcal polysaccharide and its possible role in the pathogenesis of cell wall-induced polyarthritis," *The Journal of Experimental Medicine*, vol. 157, no. 4, pp. 1089–1100, 1983.

[69] T. Koga, K. Kakimoto, T. Hirofuji et al., "Acute joint inflammation in mice after systemic injection of the cell wall, its peptidoglycan, and chemically defined peptidoglycan subunits from various bacteria," *Infection and Immunity*, vol. 50, no. 1, pp. 27–34, 1985.

[70] A. F. Wells, J. A. Hightower, C. Parks, E. Kufoy, and A. Fox, "Systemic injection of group A streptococcal peptidoglycan-polysaccharide complexes elicits persistent neutrophilia and monocytosis associated with polyarthritis in rats," *Infection and Immunity*, vol. 57, no. 2, pp. 351–358, 1989.

[71] P. Toivanen, J. Vaahtovuo, and E. Eerola, "Influence of major histocompatibility complex on bacterial composition of fecal flora," *Infection and Immunity*, vol. 69, no. 4, pp. 2372–2377, 2001.

[72] J. A. Stewart, V. S. Chadwick, and A. Murray, "Investigations into the influence of host genetics on the predominant eubacteria in the faecal microflora of children," *Journal of Medical Microbiology*, vol. 54, no. 12, pp. 1239–1242, 2005.

[73] T. Mitsuoka, "Intestinal flora and human health," *Asia Pacific Journal of Clinical Nutrition*, vol. 5, no. 1, pp. 2–9, 1996.

[74] M. J. Hopkins, R. Sharp, and G. T. Macfarlane, "Age and disease related changes in intestinal bacterial populations assessed by cell culture, 16S rRNA abundance, and community cellular fatty acid profiles," *Gut*, vol. 48, no. 2, pp. 198–205, 2001.

[75] J. Kjeldsen-Kragh, "Rheumatoid arthritis treated with vegetarian diets," *The American Journal of Clinical Nutrition*, vol. 70, no. 3, supplement, pp. 594S–600S, 1999.

[76] R. Sartor and S. Mazmanian, "Intestinal microbes in inflammatory bowel diseases," *The American Journal of Gastroenterology*, vol. 1, supplement 1, pp. 15–21, 2012.

[77] D. N. Frank, A. L. St. Amand, R. A. Feldman, E. C. Boedeker, N. Harpaz, and N. R. Pace, "Molecular-phylogenetic characterization of microbial community imbalances in human inflammatory bowel diseases," *Proceedings of the National Academy of Sciences of the United States of America*, vol. 104, no. 34, pp. 13780–13785, 2007.

[78] K. Lucke, S. Miehlke, E. Jacobs, and M. Schuppler, "Prevalence of *Bacteroides* and *Prevotella* spp. in ulcerative colitis," *Journal of Medical Microbiology*, vol. 55, no. 5, pp. 617–624, 2006.

[79] S. Nell, S. Suerbaum, and C. Josenhans, "The impact of the microbiota on the pathogenesis of IBD: lessons from mouse infection models," *Nature Reviews Microbiology*, vol. 8, no. 8, pp. 564–577, 2010.

[80] I. I. Ivanov, K. Atarashi, N. Manel et al., "Induction of intestinal Th17 cells by segmented filamentous bacteria," *Cell*, vol. 139, no. 3, pp. 485–498, 2009.

[81] J. D. Taurog, J. A. Richardson, J. T. Croft et al., "The germfree state prevents development of gut and joint inflammatory disease in HLA-B27 transgenic rats," *The Journal of Experimental Medicine*, vol. 180, no. 6, pp. 2359–2364, 1994.

[82] C. L. Nickerson, H. S. Luthra, S. Savarirayan, and C. S. David, "Susceptibility of HLA-B27 transgenic mice to *Yersinia enterocolitica* infection," *Human Immunology*, vol. 28, no. 4, pp. 382–396, 1990.

[83] Z. Řeháková, J. Čapková, R. Štěpánková et al., "Germ-free mice do not develop ankylosing enthesopathy, a spontaneous joint disease," *Human Immunology*, vol. 61, no. 6, pp. 555–558, 2000.

[84] S. Husby, J. C. Jensenius, and S. E. Svehag, "Passage of undegraded dietary antigen into the blood of healthy adults. Further characterization of the kinetics of uptake and the size distribution of the antigen," *Scandinavian Journal of Immunology*, vol. 24, no. 4, pp. 447–455, 1986.

[85] C. J. O'Boyle, J. MacFie, C. J. Mitchell, D. Johnstone, P. M. Sagar, and P. C. Sedman, "Microbiology of bacterial translocation in humans," *Gut*, vol. 42, no. 1, pp. 29–35, 1998.

[86] G. Sigthorsson, J. Tibble, J. Hayllar et al., "Intestinal permeability and inflammation in patients on NSAIDs," *Gut*, vol. 43, no. 4, pp. 506–511, 1998.

[87] W. E. Owens and R. D. Berg, "Bacterial translocation from the gastrointestinal tract of athymic (nu/nu) mice," *Infection and Immunity*, vol. 27, no. 2, pp. 461–467, 1980.

[88] M. D. Gautreaux, F. B. Gelder, E. A. Deitch, and R. D. Berg, "Adoptive transfer of T lymphocytes to T-cell-depleted mice inhibits *Escherichia coli* translocation from the gastrointestinal tract," *Infection and Immunity*, vol. 63, no. 10, pp. 3827–3834, 1995.

[89] M. Nymark, P. J. Pussinen, A. M. Tuomainen, C. Forsblom, P.-H. Groop, and M. Lehto, "Serum lipopolysaccharide activity is associated with the progression of kidney disease in finnish patients with type 1 diabetes," *Diabetes Care*, vol. 32, no. 9, pp. 1689–1693, 2009.

[90] C. Erridge, T. Attina, C. M. Spickett, and D. J. Webb, "A high-fat meal induces low-grade endotoxemia: evidence of a novel mechanism of postprandial inflammation," *The American Journal of Clinical Nutrition*, vol. 86, no. 5, pp. 1286–1292, 2007.

[91] J. Amar, R. Burcelin, J. B. Ruidavets et al., "Energy intake is associated with endotoxemia in apparently healthy men," *The American Journal of Clinical Nutrition*, vol. 87, no. 5, pp. 1219–1223, 2008.

[92] S. Ghoshal, J. Witta, J. Zhong, W. de Villiers, and E. Eckhardt, "Chylomicrons promote intestinal absorption of lipopolysaccharides," *The Journal of Lipid Research*, vol. 50, no. 1, pp. 90–97, 2009.

[93] P. D. Cani, J. Amar, M. A. Iglesias et al., "Metabolic endotoxemia initiates obesity and insulin resistance," *Diabetes*, vol. 56, no. 7, pp. 1761–1772, 2007.

[94] T. T. Glant, K. Mikecz, A. Arzoumanian, and A. R. Poole, "Proteoglycan-induced arthritis in BALB/c mice. Clinical features and histopathology," *Arthritis & Rheumatism*, vol. 30, no. 2, pp. 201–212, 1987.

[95] C. Ubeda and E. G. Pamer, "Antibiotics, microbiota, and immune defense," *Trends in Immunology*, vol. 33, no. 9, pp. 459–466, 2012.

[96] A. Fox, R. R. Brown, and S. K. Anderle, "Arthropathic properties related to the molecular weight of peptidoglycan-polysaccharide polymers of streptococcal cell walls," *Infection and Immunity*, vol. 35, no. 3, pp. 1003–1010, 1982.

[97] A. Nogai, V. Siffrin, K. Bonhagen et al., "Lipopolysaccharide injection induces relapses of experimental autoimmune encephalomyelitis in nontransgenic mice via bystander activation of autoreactive $CD4^+$ cells," *The Journal of Immunology*, vol. 175, no. 2, pp. 959–966, 2005.

[98] B. C. Cole and M. M. Griffiths, "Triggering and exacerbation of autoimmune arthritis by the *Mycoplasma arthritidis* superantigen MAM," *Arthritis & Rheumatism*, vol. 36, no. 7, pp. 994–1002, 1993.

[99] H. Nagai, Y. Takaoka, H. Kamada, and H. Mori, "The model of arthritis induced by superantigen in mice," *Life Sciences*, vol. 55, no. 12, pp. PL233–PL237, 1994.

[100] H. H. Balch and O. H. Ganley, "Observations on the pathogenesis of *Clostridium welchii* myonecrosis," *Annals of Surgery*, vol. 146, no. 1, pp. 86–97, 1957.

[101] L. Hang, J. H. Slack, C. Amundson, S. Izui, A. N. Theofilopoulos, and F. J. Dixon, "Induction of murine autoimmune disease by chronic polyclonal B cell activation," *The Journal of Experimental Medicine*, vol. 157, no. 3, pp. 874–883, 1983.

[102] S. Yoshino, E. Sasatomi, Y. Mori, and M. Sagai, "Oral administration of lipopolysaccharide exacerbates collagen-induced arthritis in mice," *The Journal of Immunology*, vol. 163, no. 6, pp. 3417–3422, 1999.

[103] T. Cavallo and N. A. Granholm, "Bacterial lipopolysaccharide induces long-lasting IgA deficiency concurrently with features of polyclonal B cell activation in normal and in lupus-proned mice," *Clinical and Experimental Immunology*, vol. 84, no. 1, pp. 134–138, 1991.

[104] W. J. Penhale and P. R. Young, "The influence of the normal microbial flora on the susceptibility of rats to experimental autoimmune thyroiditis," *Clinical and Experimental Immunology*, vol. 72, no. 2, pp. 288–292, 1988.

[105] M. Murakami, T. Tsubata, R. Shinkura et al., "Oral administration of lipopolysaccharides activates B-1 cells in the peritoneal cavity and lamina propria of the gut and induces autoimmune symptoms in an autoantibody transgenic mouse," *The Journal of Experimental Medicine*, vol. 180, no. 1, pp. 111–121, 1994.

[106] M. Murakami, K. Nakajima, K.-I. Yamazaki, T. Muraguchi, T. Serikawa, and T. Honjo, "Effects of breeding environments on generation and activation of autoreactive B-1 cells in anti-red blood cell autoantibody transgenic mice," *The Journal of Experimental Medicine*, vol. 185, no. 4, pp. 791–794, 1997.

[107] P. H. Wooley and B. Cingel, "Staphylococcal enterotoxin B increases the severity of type II collagen induced arthritis in mice," *Annals of the Rheumatic Diseases*, vol. 54, no. 4, pp. 298–304, 1995.

[108] A. Facchinetti, M. Panozzo, P. Pertile, L. Tessarollo, and G. Biasi, "*In vivo* and *in vitro* death of mature T cells induced by separate signals to CD4 and $\alpha\beta$TCR," *Immunobiology*, vol. 185, no. 2–4, pp. 380–389, 1992.

[109] S. Webb and N. Gascoigne, "T-cell activation by superantigens," *Current Opinion in Immunology*, vol. 6, no. 3, pp. 467–475, 1994.

[110] R. S. Panush, "Nonspecific suppressor function in rheumatoid arthritis," *Journal of Clinical and Laboratory Immunology*, vol. 9, no. 1, pp. 59–64, 1982.

[111] M. D. Lockshin, A. C. Eisenhauer, R. Kohn, M. Weksler, S. Block, and S. B. Mushlin, "Cell mediated immunity in rheumatic diseases. II. Mitogen responses in RA, SLE, and other illnesses: correlation with T and B lymphocyte populations," *Arthritis & Rheumatism*, vol. 18, no. 3, pp. 245–250, 1975.

[112] A. J. Rawson and T. C. Huang, "Lymphocyte populations in rheumatoid arthritis," *Arthritis & Rheumatism*, vol. 19, no. 4, pp. 720–724, 1976.

[113] E. van Nood, A. Vrieze, M. Nieuwdorp et al., "Duodenal infusion of donor feces for recurrent clostridium difficile," *The New England Journal of Medicine*, vol. 368, no. 5, pp. 407–415, 2013.

[114] J. A. Rump, R. Arndt, A. Arnold et al., "Treatment of diarrhoea in human immunodeficiency virus-infected patients with immunoglobulins from bovine colostrum," *Clinical Investigator*, vol. 70, no. 7, pp. 588–594, 1992.

[115] J. T. van Dissel, M. de Groot, C. M. H. Hensgens et al., "Bovine antibody-enriched whey to aid in the prevention of a relapse of *Clostridium difficile*-associated diarrhoea: preclinical and preliminary clinical data," *Journal of Medical Microbiology*, vol. 54, no. 2, pp. 197–205, 2005.

[116] C. Weiner, Q. Pan, M. Hurtig, T. Borén, E. Bostwick, and L. Hammarström, "Passive immunity against human pathogens using bovine antibodies," *Clinical and Experimental Immunology*, vol. 116, no. 2, pp. 193–205, 1999.

[117] M. Warny, A. Fatimi, E. F. Bostwick et al., "Bovine immunoglobulin concentrate-*Clostridium difficile* retains *C difficile* toxin neutralising activity after passage through the human stomach and small intestine," *Gut*, vol. 44, no. 2, pp. 212–217, 1999.

[118] H. Korhonen, P. Marnila, and H. S. Gill, "Bovine milk antibodies for health," *British Journal of Nutrition*, vol. 84, supplement 1, pp. S135–S146, 2000.

[119] S. Iwatsuki, Y. Kijima, and H. Shionoya, "Effect of natural milk antibodies on intestinal flora," *Nippon Shokuhin Kagaku Kogaku Kaishi*, vol. 58, no. 6, pp. 236–244, 2011.

[120] Y. Kijima, S. Iwatsuki, H. Akamatsu et al., "Natural antibodies to pathogenic bacteria and their toxins in whey protein concentrate," *Food Science & Technology Research*, vol. 56, no. 9, pp. 475–482, 2009.

# 6

# Composite Indices Using 3 or 4 Components of the Core Data Set Have Similar Predictive Ability to Measure Disease Activity in RA: Evidence from the DANCER and REFLEX Studies

**Martin J. Bergman,[1] William Reiss,[2] Carol Chung,[2] Pamela Wong,[2] and Adam Turpcu[2]**

[1] *Rheumatology Department, Drexel University College of Medicine and Taylor Hospital, 8 Morton Avenue, Suite 304, Ridley Park, Philadelphia, PA 19078-2216, USA*
[2] *Genentech, Inc., 1 DNA Way, South San Francisco, CA 94080, USA*

Correspondence should be addressed to Martin J. Bergman; mjbergman@prodigy.net

Academic Editor: Kamal D. Moudgil

*Background.* Understanding how disease-assessment indices perform in rheumatoid arthritis (RA) clinical trials can inform their use in routine practice. The study objective was to assess the capacity of combinations of RA Core Data Set measures to distinguish rituximab from control treatment. *Methods.* Post hoc analysis of two randomised clinical trials was used. Composite Efficacy Indices were derived by combining three or four RA Core Data Set measures from three possible sources: physician, patient, and laboratory. *Results.* All 105 Composite Efficacy Indices evaluated significantly distinguished rituximab from control treatment ($P < 10^{-7}$). Generally, indices containing measures from three different sources had a greater capacity to distinguish rituximab from control treatment than indices containing three measures from one source. Composite Efficacy Indices performed as well as validated indices such as DAS28, RAPID3, and CDAI. *Conclusions.* All indices composed of three or four RA Core Data Set measures have a similar capacity to detect treatment differences. These results suggest that the precise measurement used is less important than whether any measurement is performed, although selection should be consistent for each patient. Therefore, the choice of assessment tool should not be limited to a prescribed list and should instead be left to the clinician's discretion.

## 1. Introduction

In an effort to improve patient outcomes, recent consensus guidelines have recommended treating patients with rheumatoid arthritis (RA) to a target of clinical remission [1]. To accomplish this aim, different measurement tools of disease activity have been developed. Recently, the American College of Rheumatology (ACR) has published guidelines listing "preferred" indices to be used in clinical practice, including Disease Activity Score in 28 joints (DAS28), Simplified Disease Activity Index (SDAI), Clinical Disease Activity Index (CDAI), and Routine Assessment of Patient Index Data 3 (RAPID3) [2].

These recommended indices are derived from the ACR RA Core Data Set measures [3] and include data from three sources: (1) health professional: assessor global (DOCGL), tender joint count (TJC), and swollen joint count (SJC); (2) patient questionnaires: patient global estimate (PATGL), pain, and physical function (FN); and (3) laboratory tests: C-reactive protein (CRP) level or erythrocyte sedimentation rate (ESR). Each of the recommended indices has variable complexities, which may serve as a barrier to use in clinical practice. Despite these differences, moderate-to-strong levels of agreement have been observed between the indices [4, 5]. Given this agreement, it is speculated that other indices composed of different combinations of RA Core Data Set measures could also be of use in assessing disease activity.

The objective of this study was to determine whether composite indices of any three or four RA Core Data Set measures, not just the "recommended" indices, have a similar capacity to distinguish rituximab from control treatment.

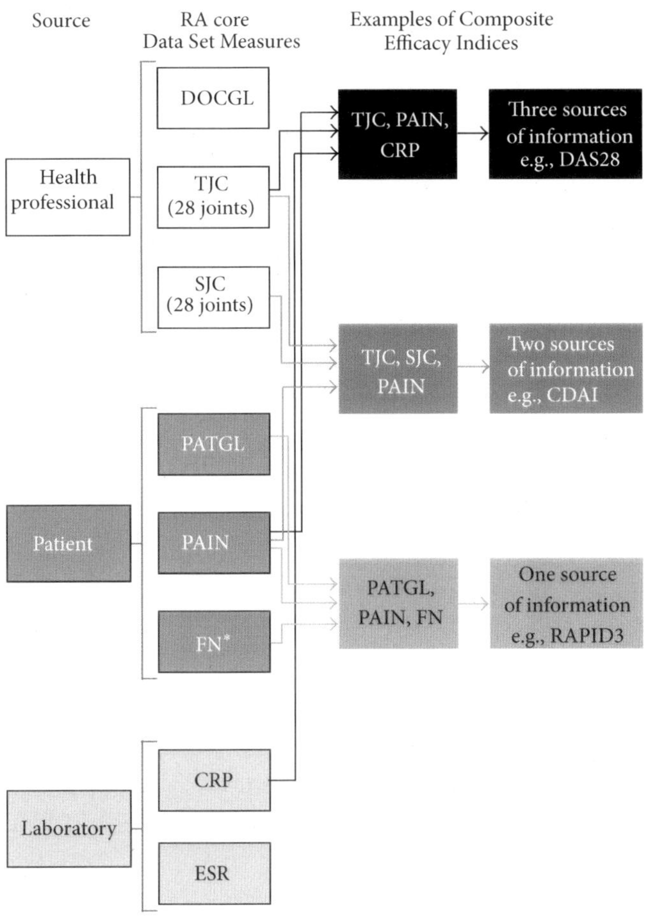


FIGURE 1: Combinations of RA Core Data Set measures used to derive Composite Efficacy Indices. *Measured using the Health Assessment Questionnaire. For comparison, DAS28, CDAI, and RAPID3 are derived using different formulae. DAS28 includes 4 RA Core Data Set measures (TJC, SJC, CRP (or ESR), and PATGL) from three sources. CDAI includes four RA Core Data Set measures (TJC, SJC, DOCGL, and PATGL) from two sources. RAPID3 includes three RA Core Data Set measures (PATGL, PAIN, and FN) from one source. CDAI: Clinical Disease Activity Index; CRP: C-reactive protein; DAS28: Disease Activity Score in 28 joints; DOCGL: assessor global; ESR: erythrocyte sedimentation rate; FN: physical function; PAIN: pain; PATGL: patient global estimate; RAPID3: Routine Assessment of Patient Index Data 3; SJC: swollen joint count; TJC: tender joint count.

## 2. Methods

Patient data from DANCER, a phase IIb study comparing placebo and two doses of rituximab in RA patients who had an inadequate response to methotrexate (MTX) and 1–5 other disease-modifying antirheumatic drugs or biologicals, and REFLEX, a phase III study comparing placebo and rituximab in RA patients with an inadequate response to one or more tumor necrosis factor inhibitors, were used to develop different composite indices [6, 7]. Composite Efficacy Indices were derived by combining 3 or 4 RA Core Data Set measures from 3 possible sources, health professional evaluation, patient questionnaires, and laboratory tests (Figure 1), and no more than one laboratory test (either CRP or ESR). Laboratory test values were log transformed prior to rescaling. Analyses were limited to the approved rituximab dose (2 × 1000 mg) group and placebo group intent-to-treat populations. All RA Core Data Set measures were rescaled from 0–10 and were equally weighted in each possible combination. For each combination, changes from baseline to the last observation on or before week 24 were compared between rituximab and placebo treatment using Kruskal-Wallis tests. Standardized response means (SRMs) were used to estimate a Composite Efficacy Index's ability to distinguish between responsiveness to rituximab and responsiveness to placebo and were calculated [8] using the following formula:

$$\mathrm{SRM} = \left(m_{\mathrm{RTX}} - m_{\mathrm{Placebo}}\right) \times \left(\sqrt{\frac{\left(\left(n_{\mathrm{RTX}} - 1\right) s_{\mathrm{RTX}}^{2} + \left(n_{\mathrm{Placebo}} - 1\right) s_{\mathrm{Placebo}}^{2}\right)}{\left(n_{\mathrm{RTX}} + n_{\mathrm{Placebo}} - 2\right)}}\right)^{-1}, \quad (1)$$

where $m$ is mean; $n$ is number of patients; RTX is rituximab; $s$ is standard deviation of change scores from baseline.

## 3. Results

In general, demographics and clinical characteristics were balanced across both treatment groups and trials and have been described elsewhere [6, 7]. Baseline characteristics of key efficacy indices and RA Core Data Set measures are given in Table 1.

A total of 105 Composite Efficacy Indices, or the maximum number of possible combinations with 3 or 4 Core Data Set measures, were evaluated (Table 2). All indices were found to significantly distinguish rituximab from control treatment. In DANCER, $P$ values ranged from $7 \times 10^{-7}$ to $5 \times 10^{-13}$ for three-measure indices and from $2 \times 10^{-7}$ to $2 \times 10^{-12}$ for four-measure indices. In REFLEX, $P$ values for three- and four-measure indices ranged from $1 \times 10^{-17}$ to $2 \times 10^{-28}$ and $9 \times 10^{-20}$ to $3 \times 10^{-28}$, respectively. Generally, indices containing measures from three different sources had a greater capacity to distinguish rituximab from control treatment than indices containing three measures from one source. Indices showing the greatest SRMs are shown in Figure 2. The best performing index in DANCER (SRM 0.87 (95% CI, 0.65, 1.09)) comprised three measures: SJC, DOCGL, and CRP. In REFLEX, two indices of four measures each performed equally well (SRM 1.13 (95% CI, 0.95, 1.31)): SJC, DOCGL, FN, and CRP and SJC, PATGL, DOCGL, and CRP.

## 4. Discussion

A number of validated and nonvalidated indices are available to assess RA disease status. Identifying those indices that can accurately measure disease activity while requiring less time and resources would be desirable from both physician and patient perspectives. The results of our analysis indicate that any index comprising any three or four RA Core Data

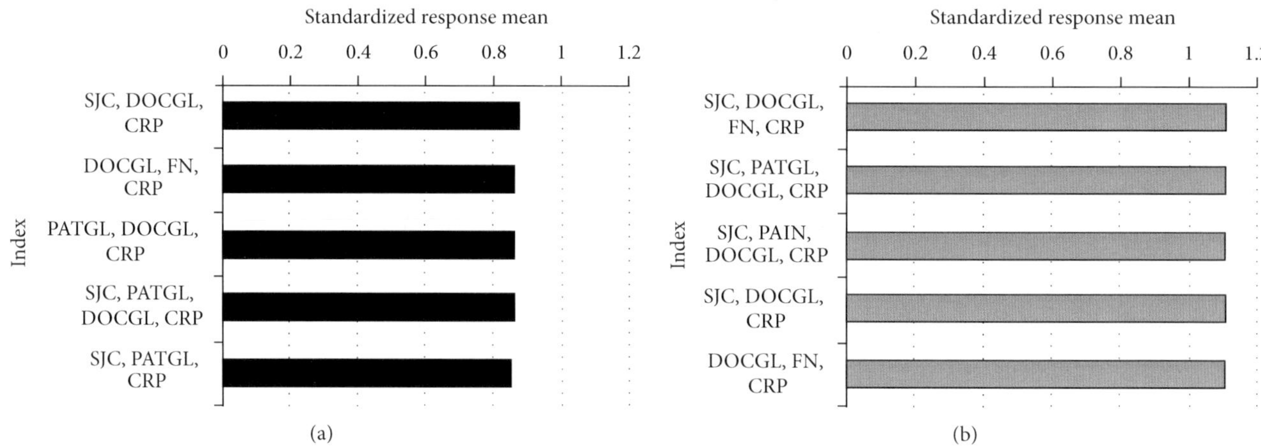


Figure 2: Indices with the greatest standardized response means in (a) DANCER (95% confidence interval for each index was ±0.22. SRMs: DAS28 = 0.77, CDAI = 0.66, and RAPID3 = 0.60) and (b) REFLEX (95% confidence interval for each index was ±0.18. SRMs: DAS28 = 1.04, CDAI = 0.92, and RAPID3 = 0.83). CRP: C-reactive protein; DOCGL: assessor global; FN: physical function; PATGL: patient global estimate; SJC: swollen joint count.

Table 1: Patients' baseline characteristics for key efficacy measurements and rheumatoid arthritis Core Data Set measures in the DANCER [6] and REFLEX [7] clinical trials.

| Mean (SD) | REFLEX | | DANCER | |
|---|---|---|---|---|
| | Placebo ($n = 201$) | RTX ($n = 298$) | Placebo ($n = 143$) | RTX ($n = 185$) |
| DAS28-ESR (0–10) | 6.8 (0.9) | 6.9 (1.0) | 6.8 (0.8) | 6.7 (0.9) |
| DAS28 (3)-ESR (0–10) | 6.5 (0.9) | 6.5 (0.9) | 6.5 (0.7) | 6.4 (0.8) |
| CDAI (0–76) | 44.6 (13.2) | 45.9 (13.7) | 45.9 (11.6) | 43.8 (12.7) |
| RAPID3 (0–10) | 5.8 (1.7) | 5.7 (1.8) | 5.4 (1.6) | 5.3 (1.7) |
| DOCGL (0–10) | 6.7 (1.6) | 6.9 (1.6) | 6.6 (1.5) | 6.6 (1.6) |
| TJC (0–28) | 16.5 (7.0) | 17.2 (7.1) | 18.5 (5.9) | 17.4 (6.5) |
| SJC (0–28) | 14.4 (5.9) | 14.9 (5.9) | 14.2 (5.3) | 13.2 (5.7) |
| PATGL (0–10) | 7.0 (2.0) | 6.9 (2.1) | 6.6 (1.9) | 6.6 (2.0) |
| PAIN (0–10) | 6.4 (2.1) | 6.4 (2.2) | 6.0 (1.9) | 5.9 (2.0) |
| FN (HAQ) (0–3) | 1.9 (0.5)* | 1.9 (0.6) | 1.7 (0.6) | 1.7 (0.6) |
| CRP (mg/dL) | 3.8 (4.1) | 3.7 (3.8) | 3.1 (3.0) | 3.0 (3.5) |
| ESR (mm/h) | 48.4 (27.7) | 47.9 (25.6) | 39.7 (20.8) | 42.0 (23.3) |

*$n = 200$. CDAI: Clinical Disease Activity Index; CRP: C-reactive protein; DAS28: Disease Activity Score in 28 joints; DAS28 (3): Disease Activity Score in 28 joints excluding patient global health component; DOCGL: assessor global; ESR: erythrocyte sedimentation rate; FN: physical function; HAQ: Health Assessment Questionnaire; PAIN: pain; PATGL: patient global estimate; RAPID3: Routine Assessment of Patient Index Data 3; RTX: rituximab; SD: standard deviation; SJC: swollen joint count; TJC: tender joint count.

Set measures was capable of distinguishing rituximab from control treatment at highly statistically significant levels. Furthermore, the Composite Efficacy Indices performed well in comparison to validated indices when assessed by SRM.

The best performing indices were those that included both physician- and laboratory-derived measures suggesting that there may be additional value in including data from multiple domains. However, laboratory results are often unavailable at the time of patient assessment. When using indices that include laboratory tests in a practice setting, immediate calculation of disease activity scores is not always possible. A further consideration is physician resources, particularly the assessment of joint counts, which can be time consuming for the physician [9]. Based on the results of this study, insistence on the inclusion of specific measures, such as TJC or SJC, does not appear to be supported. In fact, a number of 3-component measures without a formal tender or swollen count (e.g., PATGL, DOCGL, and CRP) had better discriminatory value in differentiating rituximab from control treatment ($P = 2 \times 10^{-27}$ and $2 \times 10^{-12}$ in REFLEX and DANCER, resp.) than that of a current "gold standard," CDAI ($P = 8 \times 10^{-23}$ and $4 \times 10^{-9}$ in REFLEX and DANCER, resp.). The clinical importance of such small differences is questionable as even the "worst" measure, RAPID3 (PAIN, PATGL, and FN), had $P$ values significantly below the thresholds that are commonly reported in the medical literature

TABLE 2: Continued.

| Components | Number of components | REFLEX | | DANCER | |
|---|---|---|---|---|---|
| | | SRM | $P$ value | SRM | $P$ value |
| PAIN, PATGL, DOCGL | 3 | 0.92 | $2 \times 10^{-20}$ | 0.68 | $3 \times 10^{-8}$ |
| TJC, PATGL, FN | 3 | 0.89 | $3 \times 10^{-20}$ | 0.64 | $1 \times 10^{-7}$ |
| TJC, PAIN, PATGL | 3 | 0.88 | $1 \times 10^{-19}$ | 0.62 | $6 \times 10^{-7}$ |
| PAIN, PATGL, ESR | 3 | 0.89 | $1 \times 10^{-19}$ | 0.68 | $6 \times 10^{-8}$ |
| PAIN, PATGL, FN | 3 | 0.83 | $1 \times 10^{-17}$ | 0.60 | $7 \times 10^{-7}$ |

SRMs: REFLEX: DAS28 = 1.04, CDAI = 0.92, and RAPID3 = 0.83; DANCER: DAS28 = 0.77, CDAI = 0.66, and RAPID3 = 0.6. Kruskal-Wallis $P$ values compare the changes from baseline to the last observation on or before week 24 between rituximab and placebo treatment. These $P$-values were not adjusted for multiplicity. CRP: C-reactive protein; DOCGL: assessor global; ESR: erythrocyte sedimentation rate; FN: physical function; PAIN: pain; PATGL: patient global estimate; SJC: swollen joint count; TJC: tender joint count.

($P = 1 \times 10^{-17}$ and $7 \times 10^{-7}$ in REFLEX and DANCER, resp.). The effectiveness of patient-derived indices may therefore be worthy of consideration.

## 5. Conclusions

In conclusion, these results suggest that any index using three or four measures from the RA Core Data Set is capable of distinguishing active from control treatment. While certain measurements have been proposed to be preferred, they are not superior to other measures currently in development or in use. Based on our data, it would appear that the precise measurement used may be less important than whether any measurement is performed. While more studies are needed to validate these findings, our results suggest that the choice of measurement tool should not be limited to a prescribed list of "better" or "approved" tools and may instead be left to the discretion of the clinician, allowing for the flexibility to tailor disease activity assessments according to point-of-care time and resource limitations.

Taken together, the results of this study suggest that Composite Efficacy Indices comprised of any combination of three or four measures from the RA Core Data Set perform well in discriminating between treatment responses to rituximab and placebo.

## Conflict of Interests

Martin J. Bergman has received consultancies, speaking fees, and honoraria from Pfizer, UCB, Roche, Abbott, and Bristol-Myers Squibb. William Reiss, Carol Chung, and Adam Turpcu are employees of Genentech, Inc. William Reiss and Adam Turpcu have stock/stock options in F. Hoffmann-La Roche, Ltd. Pamela Wong was an employee of Genentech, Inc., at the time of paper preparation and is currently an employee of Gilead Sciences, Inc.

## Authors' Contribution

All authors designed the study, analysed and interpreted the data, contributed to the development of the paper, and read and approved the final version.

## Acknowledgments

The study was supported by Genentech, Inc. Support for third-party writing assistance for this paper was provided by F. Hoffmann-La Roche Ltd.

## References

[1] J. S. Smolen, D. Aletaha, J. W. J. Bijlsma et al., "Treating rheumatoid arthritis to target: recommendations of an international task force," *Annals of the Rheumatic Diseases*, vol. 69, no. 4, pp. 631–637, 2010.

[2] J. Anderson, L. Caplan, J. Yazdany et al., "Rheumatoid arthritis disease activity measures: American college of rheumatology recommendations for use in clinical practice," *Arthritis Care and Research*, vol. 64, no. 5, pp. 640–647, 2012.

[3] D. T. Felson, J. J. Anderson, M. Boers et al., "The American college of rheumatology preliminary core set of disease activity measures for rheumatoid arthritis clinical trials," *Arthritis and Rheumatism*, vol. 36, no. 6, pp. 729–740, 1993.

[4] T. Pincus, M. J. Bergman, Y. Yazici, P. Hines, K. Raghupathi, and R. Maclean, "An index of only patient-reported outcome measures, routine assessment of patient index data 3 (RAPID3), in two abatacept clinical trials: similar results to disease activity score (DAS28) and other RAPID indices that include physician-reported measures," *Rheumatology*, vol. 47, no. 3, pp. 345–349, 2008.

[5] T. Pincus, C. J. Swearingen, M. Bergman, and Y. Yazici, "RAPID3 (routine assessment of patient index data 3), a rheumatoid arthritis index without formal joint counts for routine care: proposed severity categories compared to disease activity score and clinical disease activity index categories," *Journal of Rheumatology*, vol. 35, no. 11, pp. 2136–2147, 2008.

[6] P. Emery, R. Fleischmann, A. Filipowicz-Sosnowska et al., "The efficacy and safety of rituximab in patients with active rheumatoid arthritis despite methotrexate treatment: results of a phase IIb randomized, double-blind, placebo-controlled, dose-ranging trial," *Arthritis and Rheumatism*, vol. 54, no. 5, pp. 1390–1400, 2006.

[7] S. B. Cohen, P. Emery, M. W. Greenwald et al., "Rituximab for rheumatoid arthritis refractory to anti-tumor necrosis factor therapy: results of a multicenter, randomized, double-blind, placebo-controlled, phase III trial evaluating primary efficacy and safety at twenty-four weeks," *Arthritis and Rheumatism*, vol. 54, no. 9, pp. 2793–2806, 2006.

[8] M. H. Liang, A. H. Fossel, and M. G. Larson, "Comparisons of five health status instruments for orthopedic evaluation," *Medical Care*, vol. 28, no. 7, pp. 632–642, 1990.

[9] Y. Yazici, M. Bergman, and T. Pincus, "Time to score quantitative rheumatoid arthritis measures: 28-joint count, disease activity score, health assessment questionnaire (HAQ), multidimensional HAQ (MDHAQ), and routine assessment of patient index data (RAPID) scores," *Journal of Rheumatology*, vol. 35, no. 4, pp. 603–609, 2008.

7

# The Potential Roles of Bisphenol A (BPA) Pathogenesis in Autoimmunity

**Datis Kharrazian**[1,2]

[1] *1001 Canvasback Court, Carlsbad, CA 92011, USA*
[2] *Division of Sciences, Bastyr University California, 4106 Sorrento Valley Boulevard, San Diego, CA 92121, USA*

Correspondence should be addressed to Datis Kharrazian; datis56@gmail.com

Academic Editor: Aristo Vojdani

Bisphenol A (BPA) is a monomer found in commonly used consumer plastic goods. Although much attention in recent years has been placed on BPA's impact as an endocrine disruptor, it also appears to activate many immune pathways involved in both autoimmune disease development and autoimmune reactivity provocation. The current scientific literature is void of research papers linking BPA directly to human or animal onset of autoimmunity. This paper explores the impact of BPA on immune reactivity and the potential roles these mechanisms may have on the development or provocation of autoimmune diseases. Potential mechanisms by which BPA may be a contributing risk factor to autoimmune disease development and progression include its impact on hyperprolactinemia, estrogenic immune signaling, cytochrome P450 enzyme disruption, immune signal transduction pathway alteration, cytokine polarization, aryl hydrocarbon activation of Th-17 receptors, molecular mimicry, macrophage activation, lipopolysaccharide activation, and immunoglobulin pathophysiology. In this paper a review of these known autoimmune triggering mechanisms will be correlated with BPA exposure, thereby suggesting that BPA has a role in the pathogenesis of autoimmunity.

## 1. Introduction

Bisphenol A [2, 2 bis(4-hydroxyphenyl) propane; BPA] is a monomer used in the manufacture of polycarbonate plastics. BPA is used in diverse forms of plastic products in the food and electronic industries and in various types of commonly used consumer goods, such as plastic containers, utensils, toys, water bottles, and fax paper. BPA has been shown to leach out of products, and high levels of the monomer have been identified in human and animal samples [1]. The extensive use of BPA-containing products has resulted in high human exposure worldwide [2], with studies reporting that more than 90 percent of the US population has detectable levels in urine samples [3]. It appears that increased temperature leaches BPA into food and water products as does acidic pH of liquids [4]. Additionally, dermal contact with sales receipts and printer paper containing BPA compounds can lead to BPA exposure [5].

BPA has been studied extensively as an endocrine disruptor, and numerous papers have shown how BPA may impact perinatal, childhood, and adult health [6]. BPA has the ability to bind to estrogen receptors and promote both agonist and antagonist activity [7]. It also has the ability to bind to aryl hydrocarbon receptors and exert diverse adverse endocrine effects on human physiology [8]. Its impact on hormone signaling and endocrine dysfunction continues to be an area of research.

BPA also has been shown to have potential adverse neurological effects, especially with respect to fetal brain development and promotion of neurodegenerative diseases [9]. Mice models showing perinatal exposure to BPA inhibits synaptogenesis and affects synaptic structural modification after birth [10]. The impact of BPA on brain health and neurodevelopment also continues to be an area of research.

This paper explores the worldwide exposure to BPA and its potential role in the growing epidemic of autoimmune disease. Although no human or animal studies have been published linking BPA to the onset of autoimmune disease, the potential seems very high due to the physiological influences of BPA and current immunological models regarding loss of self-tolerance and autoimmunity. In addition to known immune mechanisms promoted by BPA that overlap with

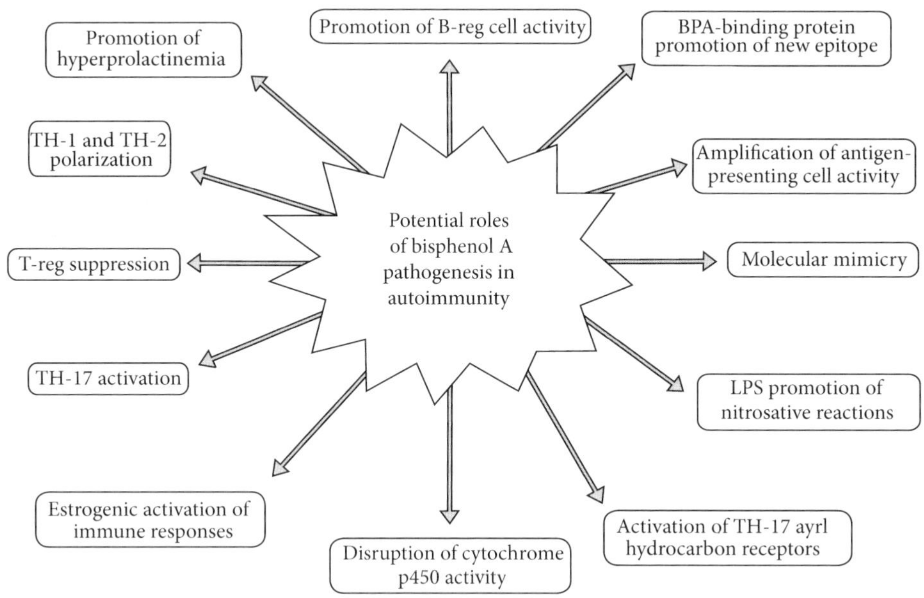


Figure 1: This diagram illustrates the potential mechanisms of bisphenol A's promotion of autoimmunity. BPA: bisphenol A; B-reg cell: regulatory B cell; LPS: lipopolysaccharide; TH: T-helper; T-reg: regulatory T cell.

autoimmune generation, some early evidence also indicates that BPA may contribute to mechanisms that promote autoimmune expression and progression (Figure 1).

## 2. BPA, Hepatic Biotransformation, and Autoimmunity

The hepatic biotransformation of BPA depends on phase I oxidation/reduction involving glutathione and phase II glucuronidation, glutathione, and sulfate conjugation [11]. Healthy humans exposed to BPA appear to have an accumulated body burden of BPA and monitoring studies that measure urinary BPA showed it stored in lipid reservoirs [12]. Despite proper hepatic biotransformation of BPA, the accumulation of BPA in body reservoirs may set the stage for immune reactivity and the onset of autoimmunity. Also, impaired hepatic clearance of circulating immune complexes in response to environmental compounds may induce autoimmunity. In a study of mice exposed to inorganic mercury, those mice that demonstrated reduced hepatic clearance of immune complexes also showed increased levels and altered quality of circulating immune complexes in mercury-induced autoimmunity [13]. Patients with abnormal hepatic biochemistries also have been shown to have a higher frequency of autoimmune disease [14].

A growing body of evidence shows increased toxic loads deplete hepatic tolerance, which leads to over activation of the innate and adaptive immune response and the development of autoimmune disease [15]. Higher BPA concentrations were associated with increased abnormal liver function tests [16]. Animal studies demonstrate that BPA has the ability to generate reactive oxygen species (ROS) and reduce antioxidant reserves and enzymes that are critical for hepatic phase I and II biotransformation, including glutathione, superoxide dismutase, glutathione peroxidase, glutathione S-transferase, glutathione reductase, and catalase activity [17].

BPA disruption of cytochrome P450 enzymes may be a potential mechanism for autoimmune pathophysiology. The cytochrome P450 (CYP) monooxygenases play a crucial role in the liver and various other tissues and are involved with oxidation of organic substances and the bioactivation of drugs and xenoestrogens [18]. CYP activity is necessary for the conversion of xenoestrogens into inactive metabolites that are both noninflammatory and biologically inactive. However, environmental xenoestrogens also have the potential to be metabolized into more reactive and inflammatory metabolites, thereby inducing increased ROS [19]. ROS are involved in apoptosis, activation of antigen presentation cells, and the initiation or amplification of diverse immunologic reactions that may be involved with the pathogenesis of autoimmune disease (Figure 2) [19].

Impairment of hepatic biotransformation of CYP expression may lead to ROS pathophysiology of autoimmunity. ROS have the ability to induce autoreactive molecules that may be involved with both the onset and the exacerbation of autoimmunity [20]. CYP enzymes are involved with metabolizing xenobiotics and producing ROS that may play a role in the pathophysiology of autoimmune disease.

In a study of mice offspring, BPA exposure to 15 and 300 mg/L of drinking water induced cytochrome CYP17 downregulation leading to potential proteomic alterations in immune function [21]. These mechanisms demonstrate the potential for BPA to disrupt proper CYP activity and potentially induce hepatotoxicity by promoting oxidative stress [17]. Increased production of ROS has demonstrated the ability to promote autoimmunity [22]. BPA activity has complex immune-activating reactions throughout the body. The impact of BPA on CYP enzyme expression may be a

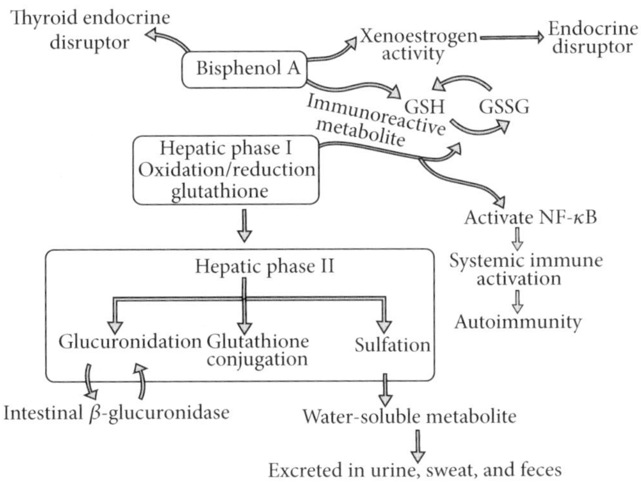


FIGURE 2: This diagram illustrates the hepatic biotransformation of bisphenol A. GSH: reduced glutathione; GSSG: oxidized glutathione.

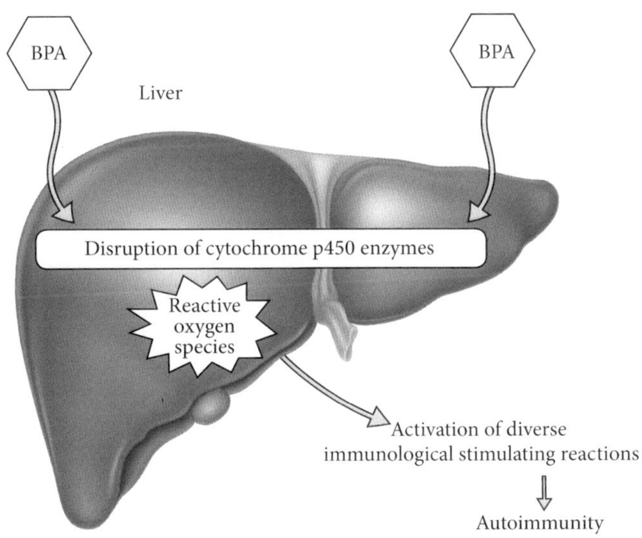


FIGURE 3: This diagram illustrates how bisphenol A can activate autoimmunity by disrupting cytochrome P450 enzymes. BPA: bisphenol A.

contributing mechanism to BPA autoimmune pathophysiology (Figure 3).

## 3. BPA Impact on Prolactin Synthesis and Autoimmunity

Although the peptide hormone prolactin is known primarily for its role in lactation, it also plays a critical role in modulating immune and inflammatory responses through various immune signaling pathways [23]. Prolactin has been shown to play significant roles in antigen presenting functions and in the initiation of the response against major histocompatibility complex (MHC) presenting self-antigens as found in autoimmunity [24].

A review of hyperprolactinemia and autoimmunity has found increased prolactin levels associated with production of anti-DNA antibodies, islet cell antibodies, thyroglobulin antibodies, thyroid peroxidase antibodies, adrenocortical antibodies, and transglutaminase antibodies with individuals suffering from systemic lupus erythematosus (SLE), diabetes mellitus type 1, Hashimoto's disease, Addison's disease, and celiac disease [25]. Prolactin has profound immunological stimulating, enhancing, and proliferative responses to antigens and mitogens by promoting increased cytokine activity and immunoglobin production. It also interferes with B cell tolerance and has autoimmune promoting effects [26].

BPA is an endocrine disruptor with powerful effects on the pituitary lactotroph cells, which are estrogen responsive and promote prolactin release. *In vitro* and *in vivo* studies have found that BPA mimics estradiol and induces hyperprolactinemia [27]. Therefore, BPA has potential impacts on autoimmune disease activation via its impact on increasing the immunostimulatory response of prolactin (Figure 4).

A link between BPA exposure and increased prolactin levels was found in women workers in occupational settings within one year. They demonstrated marked prolactin level increases and a multivariate analysis found BPA exposure was an independent risk factor for increased serum prolactin levels [28].

The correlation between hyperprolactinemia and autoimmune disease promotion has been reported in the literature in multiple papers during the past 20 years [29]. Additionally, recent evidence has found that BPA has major stimulatory impacts on prolactin release. These correlations strongly suggest that BPA may promote autoimmune pathophysiology by increasing prolactin release that then promotes immune-stimulating activity.

## 4. BPA and Estrogenic Activation of Immune Responses

In addition to the impact of BPA on prolactin release through its estrogenic influence on pituitary cells, BPA also appears to directly affect immune cell signaling pathways and thus immune responses [30]. BPA is classified as an endocrine disruptor in the form of a xenoestrogen and has the potential to mimic estrogen activity throughout the body [31]. This is important because increased circulating estrogens have demonstrated relationships with greater autoimmune activity [32]. Furthermore, epidemiological evidence suggests that the significant increase in the prevalence of autoimmune disease may in part be attributed to environmental estrogens (xenoestrogens). A review of the role of estrogens provides reasonable evidence of an association between xenoestrogen exposure and autoimmune disorders [33].

Various estrogen-promoted mechanisms have been found to trigger autoimmune reactivity. The reticulum transmembrane protein UNC93B1, which is essential for trafficking toll-like receptors (TLRs) from endoplasmic reticulum and is found to play a role in autoimmunity, has been shown to be upregulated by estrogenic signaling [34]. Estrogen activity has also been shown to directly and indirectly stimulate

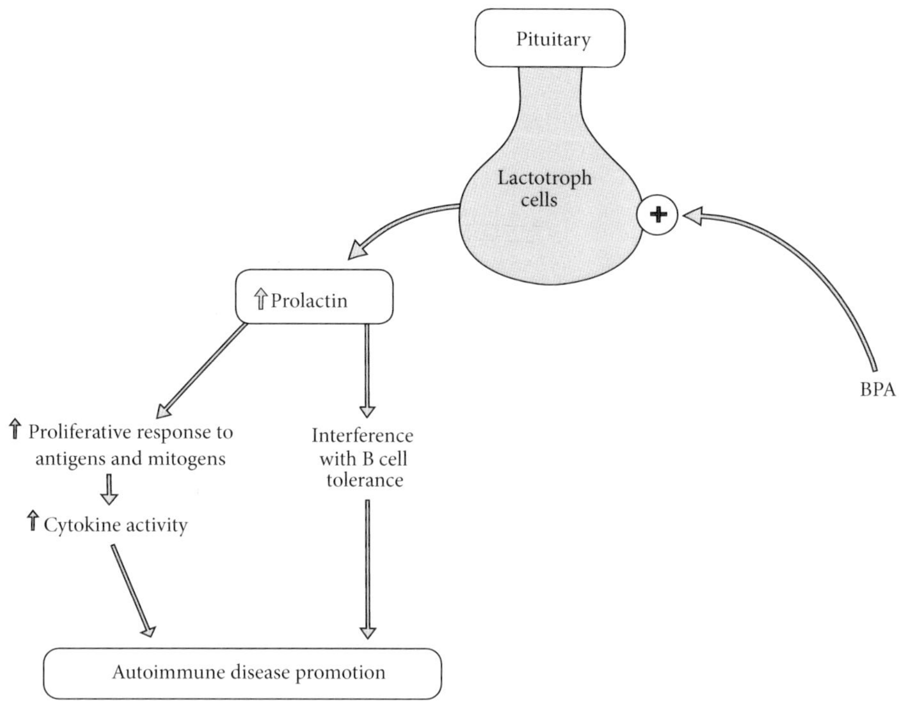


FIGURE 4: This diagram illustrates how bisphenol A can activate hyperprolactinemia and increase immunostimulatory responses, promoting autoimmunity. BPA: bisphenol A.

activation-induced deaminase (AID), leading to immune hyperstimulation. AID plays an important role in immune tolerance and the actual elimination of autoantibodies that may impact autoimmune reactivity [35]. Estrogen activity appears to promote signaling of T cell activation in autoimmunity [36]. Estradiol impacts macrophage production of tumor necrosis factor alpha [37]. Treatment of immune cells with estradiol has been shown to increase levels of B cell activating factor (BAFF) mRNA and protein that are associated with increasing severity of autoimmune disease expression [38]. Estrogen activity appears to impact dendritic cell differentiation and interferon production [39]. In summary, estrogen activity appears to have diverse and complex modulatory and stimulating roles in the immune system [40].

Many of these immune-stimulating responses that perpetuate chronic inflammation and autoimmunity may also be potentiated by the estrogenic activity of BPA [41]. BPA stimulates cell proliferation and induced expression of estrogen responsiveness. It also stimulates uterine, vaginal, and mammary growth and differentiation *in vivo* [42]. BPA treatment in mice induced splenocyte proliferation, a shift of cytokine profiles from Th-2 to Th-1 activity, and hyperstimulation of cellular immunity similar to patterns associated with Th-1 dominant autoimmune disease [43]. Overall, BPA has multiple estrogenic mechanisms in promoting abnormal immune responses that include altering T cell subsets, B cell functions, and dendritic cell activity and inducing abnormal immune signaling via its disruptive impact on estrogen receptor signaling, aryl hydrocarbon receptor signaling, and abnormal signaling of peroxisome proliferator-activated nuclear receptors [44]. These BPA estrogenic impacts on virtually all the major cells of the immune system and critical signaling pathways may be one way in which BPA promotes pathogenesis of autoimmunity (Figure 5).

## 5. BPA Impact on Immune Signaling Pathways

BPA has hapten and estrogenic activity, both of which play roles in activating hyperactive immune responses that may occur in autoimmune pathophysiology.

BPA exposure leads to aquatic animal hemocyte immune dysfunction, potentially increasing its role in induced autoimmunity through immune dysregulation. BPA injected into mussels leads to significant lysosomal membrane destabilization and a dramatic decrease in phosphorylation of the stress-activated p38 mitogen-activated protein kinases (MAPKs) and CREB-like transcription factor (cAMP-responsive element-binding protein) in mussels [45]. These results indicate BPA-induced alteration of hemocyte signal transducers and activator of transcription (STAT). These MAPK and STAT pathways are crucial in normal signaling to prevent upregulation of autoreactive T cells found to induce autoimmune inflammatory reactivity [46].

In addition to turning on gene expression of autoreactive T cells, alterations in these MAPK and STAT signaling pathways lead to chronic activation of antigen-presenting cells (APCs), loss of regulatory T cells (CD4+CD25+), apoptosis of APCs, and inhibition of innate and adaptive immunity wind-up found in the pathogenesis of autoimmunity [47]. The signaling pathways that are activated by BPA exposure have been shown to be the exact signaling pathways of molecular processes in autoimmune disease pathophysiology [48].

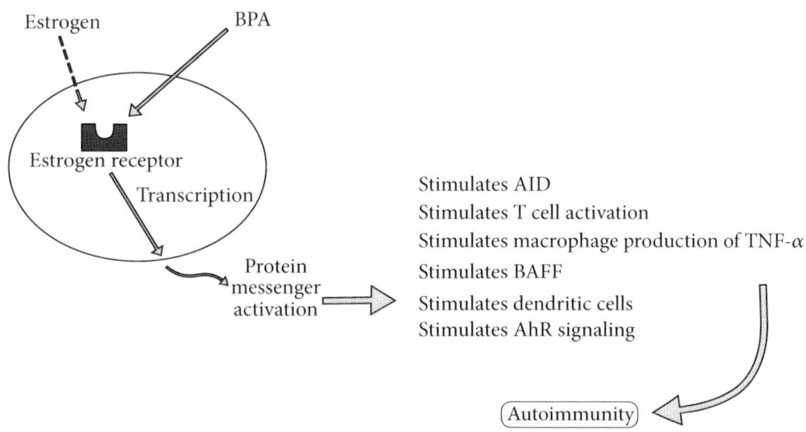


FIGURE 5: This diagram illustrates how bisphenol A can bind to estrogen receptors and promote estrogenic-mediated autoimmunity. AID: activation-induced deaminase; BAFF: B cell activating factor; BPA: bisphenol A; TNF-alpha: tumor necrosis factor alpha; AhR: aryl hydrocarbon.

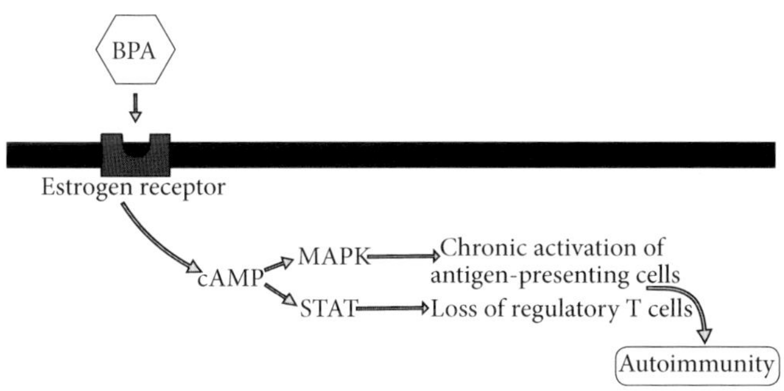


FIGURE 6: This diagram illustrates how bisphenol A can promote autoimmunity by cellular transcription activation. BPA: bisphenol A; cAMP: adenosine $3'5'$-cyclic monophosphate; MARK: mitogen-activated protein kinase; STAT: signal transducer and activator of transcription.

Therefore, BPA activity as either an estrogenic endocrine disruptor or hapten-activating structure seems to specifically disrupt immune signaling pathways found in autoimmune disease (Figure 6).

## 6. BPA and Cytokine Expression

Cytokines have been shown to play a key role in the pathogenesis of autoimmune disease. The shift of cytokines into Th-1/Th-2 dominance and the IL-17/IL-23 (Th-17) axis has been shown to play pivotal roles in the model of autoimmunity and the breakdown of self-tolerance [49]. BPA has been shown to impact the differentiation processes of the dendritic cells that may cause unintended activation of the immune system in the absence of pathological conditions, thus promoting inappropriate polarization of T cells and cytokine profiles and shifting the immune system into an overzealous immunological state [50]. Additionally, BPA exposure prenatally to mice with oral feeding induced upregulation of Th-1 responses in adulthood [51].

The impact of BPA on naïve immune systems using T cell receptor transgenic mice followed by measurement of cytokine responses to antigens suggest that BPA can augment Th-1 reactions when administered orally in low doses (1.5 mg to 1.8 mg/kg weight) in water. Specifically BPA increased antigen-specific interferon gamma production leading to exaggerated T cell activation and polar Th-1 and Th-2 shifts [52]. These mechanisms associated with interferon have been shown to play powerful effector roles in the pathogenesis of autoimmunity, especially system autoimmunity such as systemic lupus erythematosus [53].

Animal studies have also shown that BPA exposure promotes cytokine inflammatory shifts associated with potential autoimmune development. BPA administered to mice in drinking water produced significant shifts of lymphocytes subpopulations. The production of inflammatory Th-1 type cytokines (IFN-gamma) was induced while Th-2 cytokine (IL-4) was suppressed with BPA treatment, promoting the transcription of IRF-1. The mRNA expression of GATA-3 was inhibited in BPA-treated groups in dosages of 0.015, 1.5, and 30 mg/mL for 4 weeks [54]. These responses indicated that BPA has the potential to induce Th-1 polar shifts of transcription factor that lead to exaggerated cellular immune responses leading to an exaggerated Th-1 immune response. The suppression of GATA-3 transcription factors and T cell polarization favoring a Th-1 bias has been shown to be an immune mechanism of multiple sclerosis autoimmunity in animals [55].

A study comparing the effect of BPA exposure on cytokine activity in adulthood and prenatally demonstrated that in adulthood exposure to BPA significantly promoted antigen-stimulated production of IL-4, IL-10, and IL-13, but not IFN-gamma. However, mice exposed prenatally to BPA showed increased production of not only IL-4 but also IFN-gamma. The percentages of T regulatory function (CD4+CD25+) were decreased in both groups exposed to BPA [56]. Loss of regulatory T cell function promotes abnormal cytokine shifts that occur in autoimmune diseases [57]. Suppression of regulatory T cell function leading to impaired

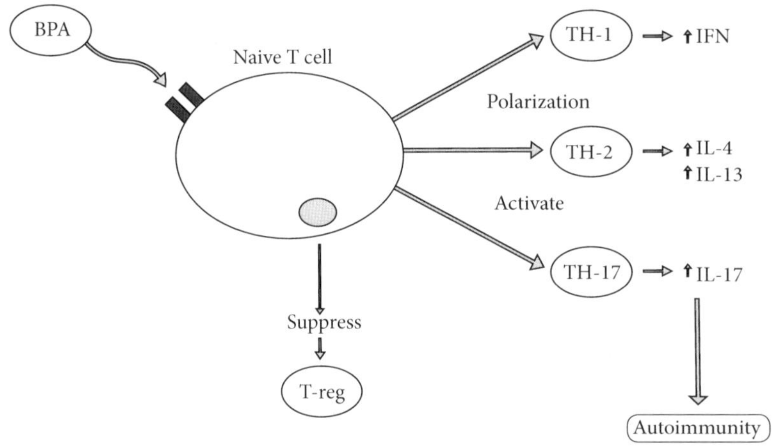


Figure 7: This diagram illustrates how bisphenol A can induce T cell shifts, promoting autoimmunity. BPA: bisphenol A; IFN: interferon; IL: interleukin; TH: T-helper; T-reg: regulatory T cell.

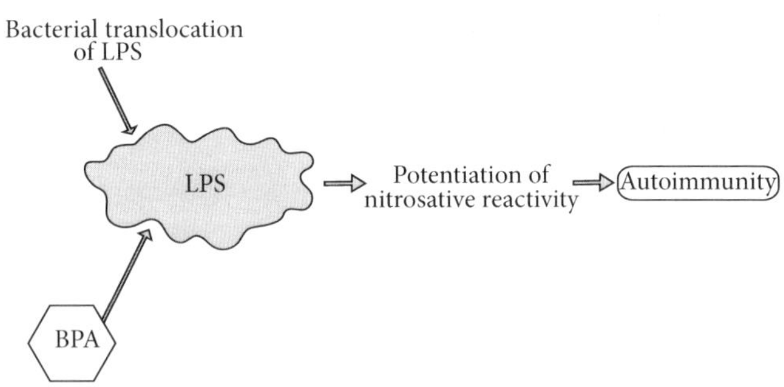


Figure 8: This diagram illustrates how bisphenol A can promote lipopolysaccharide inflammatory sequelae. BPA: bisphenol A; LPS: lipopolysaccharide.

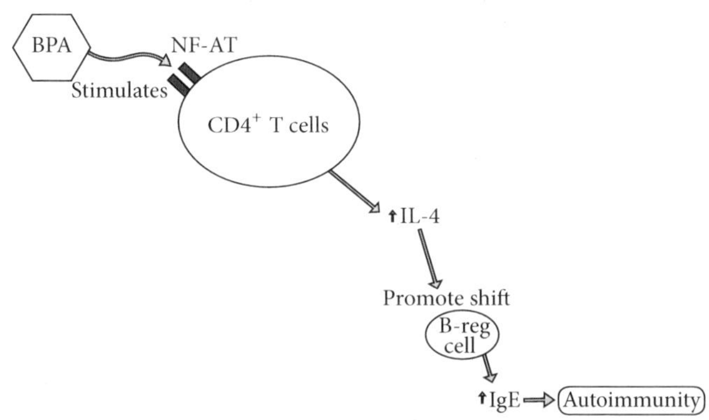


Figure 9: This diagram illustrates how bisphenol A can impact immunoglobulin-promoted autoimmunity. BPA: bisphenol A; B-reg cell: regulatory B cell; IL: interleukin; IgE: immunoglobulin E; NF-AT: $Ca2^+$/calcineurin-dependent nuclear factor binding sites.

cytokine modulation may be part of the immunopathology of BPA autoimmune development.

The delicate interplay between Th-1, Th-2, and Th-17 expression appear to be a key factor in autoimmune pathophysiology. Evidence indicates that BPA may induce polarity in this delicate balance and trigger inflammatory reactions, potentially leading to loss of self-tolerance as noted in subsequent paragraphs. The impact of BPA on the pathogenesis of abnormal cytokine shifts most likely occurs from complex web-like reactions. BPA's role as both a hapten and estrogenic endocrine disruptor appears to promote multiple interwoven pathways involved in adverse cytokine shifts that may play a role in autoimmune pathogenesis (Figure 7).

## 7. BPA and Lipopolysaccharide-Induced Nitric Oxide Production

Bacterial translocation of lipopolysaccharides (LPS) has the ability to activate oxidative and nitrosamine stress pathways associated with the inflammatory responses and pathophysiology of autoimmune responses [58]. BPA directly impacts LPS activation of these pathways, and the role of BPA on LPS activation could likewise play a role in abnormal immune reactivity [59].

Additionally, decreased activation of LPS-induced inflammatory reactions has also demonstrated a reduction in inflammatory sequelae of autoimmune cytokine and chemokine expression. Specifically, mice injected with BPA exhibited increased endotoxin-induced macrophage activation, suggesting that BPA may potentiate infectious autoimmune inflammatory reactions via enhanced tumor necrosis factor and nitric oxide reactivity [60]. Therefore, LPS-induced expression of nitrosative stress reactivity may be a key factor in BPA-promoted models of autoimmunity associated with infectious autoimmune reactions (Figure 8).

## 8. BPA Impacts on Antigen-Presenting Cell Reactivity

Antigen-presenting cells such as dendritic cells and macrophages appear to play a potential role with BPA and autoimmune reactivity. Dendritic cells (DCs) are important antigen-presenting cells that play a critical role in adaptive immunity due to their ability to activate naïve T cells, which, when

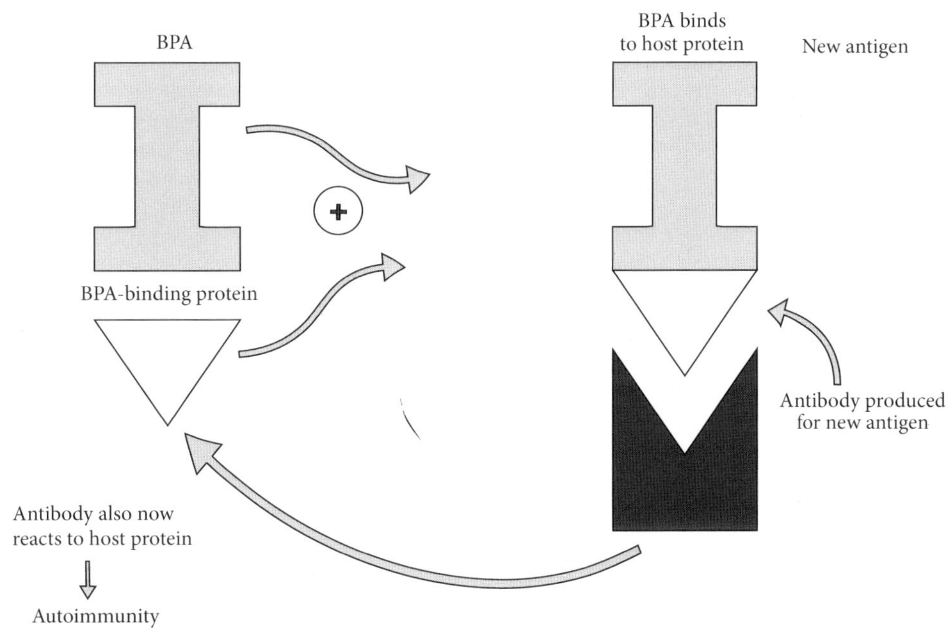


FIGURE 10: This diagram illustrates how bisphenol A can bind to the host protein, leading to a new epitope reaction against the host protein, resulting in autoimmunity. BPA: bisphenol A.

overzealous, could promote autoimmune activity [61]. DCs promote the expressions of Th-1, Th-2, or Th-17 cells that can be switched to express autoimmune inflammatory cascades [62]. DCs exposed to BPA in combination with tumor necrosis factor alpha promote CC chemokine ligand 1 (CCL1) signaling, a chemokine that is known to trigger chemotaxis of CCr8 expressing Th-2 and a subset of T regulatory cells, thereby promoting higher levels of IL-10 relative to those of IL-12p70 on CD40 ligation and preferentially inducing Th-2 deviation [63]. These variant responses from DCs exposed to BPA may play a role in autoimmunity.

Macrophage modulation of nitric oxide release is also critical for the regulation of apoptosis and differentiation of T cells that may lead to progression of autoimmune disease [64]. Additionally, BPA exposure has the ability to exert disruptive effects on macrophages by binding to estrogen receptors and leading to alteration of nitric oxide production and TNF-alpha synthesis in the homeostasis of TH-1 and TH-2 activity [65]. These macrophage expressions from BPA may promote immunological shifts that occur with autoimmunity, linking BPA's potential role to abnormal antigen-presenting cell responses.

## 9. BPA Effects on Immunoglobulin Activity

Increased immunoglobulin reactivity from endocrine disruptors such as BPA may raise concerns about immune hyperactivity associated with autoimmune immunopathology. The activation of immunoglobulins has a potential to promote inflammatory or anti-inflammatory activities through the activation of regulatory B (Breg) cells. Recent research in mice has shown that when B cell expression shifts into IL-10 production, there are suppressive effects on inflammatory responses. However, promotion of IgE-producing B cells plays a direct role in promoting inflammatory responses and the development of immune upregulation associated with most underlying inflammatory conditions, such as allergies and autoimmunity [66].

Recent research has shown that BPA has a direct impact on increasing immunoglobulin expression into the inflammatory IgE response, thereby potentially promoting an inflammatory cascade in autoimmunity. Specifically, exposure to BPA was shown to increase IL-4 production in $CD4^+$ T cells and antigen-specific IgE levels in sera via the stimulation of $Ca^{2+}$/calcineurin-dependent nuclear factor of activated T cells binding sites (NF-AT) [67]. These immune responses have the ability to potentiate allergies and autoimmune reactions in those with autoimmunity. Increased levels of IgE may play a direct role in promoting the inflammatory responses found in autoimmunity [68]. The potential for BPA to increase IL-4 and promote a shift of Breg cells into IgE production may be a mechanism for BPA autoimmune promotion (Figure 9).

In a murine model for SLE, animals implanted with BPA specifically demonstrated B cell activation and promotion of autoimmune disease such as lupus nephritis. BPA implantation enhanced autoantibody production by B1 cells both *in vitro* and *in vivo* in murine models of SLE. The study researchers suggested that BPA exacerbates preexisting autoimmune diseases such as SLE and that continued exposure to endocrine disruptors may potentiate the incidence and severity of autoimmune diseases [69].

Evidence of BPA on expressing B cell activity towards inflammatory expression and autoimmune development may partly explain the complex immune web reactions of this endocrine disruptor. Although inflammatory immunoglobulin reactivity may have a role to play in autoimmune expression, it is most likely part of a larger complex immune

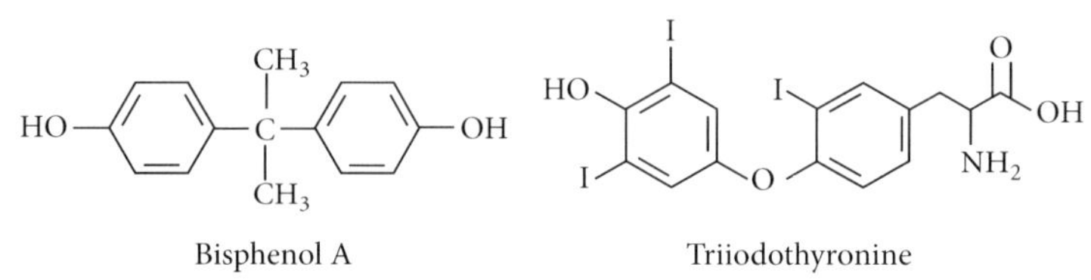


Figure 11: This diagram illustrates the structural similarity between bisphenol A and triiodothyronine, leading to potential cross-reactivity.

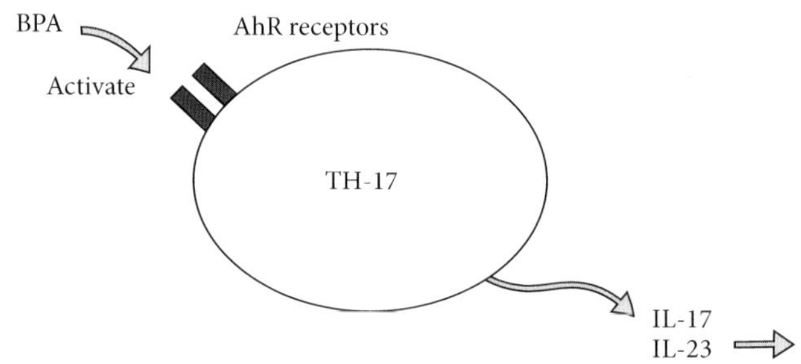


Figure 12: This diagram illustrates how bisphenol A can activate autoimmunity by inducing mRNA expression on aryl hydrocarbon receptors on TH-17 cells. AhR: aryl hydrocarbon; BPA: bisphenol A; IL: interleukin; TH: T-helper.

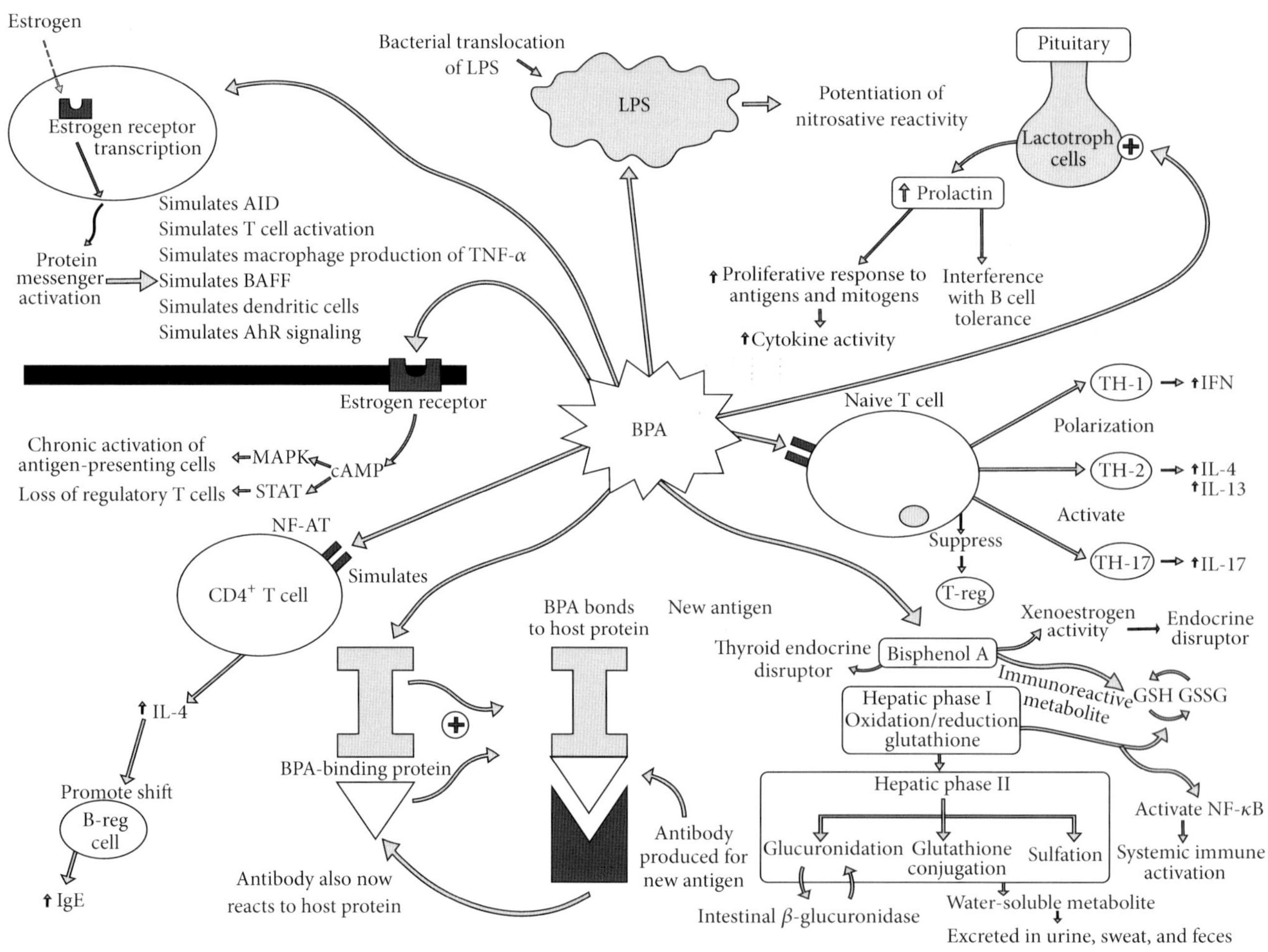


Figure 13: Potential of various autoimmune mechanisms from bisphenol A.

reaction that is linked to this very reactive endocrine disruptor.

## 10. BPA-Binding Protein: A Potential New Epitope

BPA binds to host protein, potentially creating a new epitope for immune reactivity. BPA binds to protein disulfide isomerase (PDI), also known as BPA-binding protein [70], a multifunctional protein involved in diverse cellular functions. This binding protein has been associated with endocrine disruptor mechanisms involving BPA [71]. The binding of environmental BPA to host protein may lead to self-tissue, antigen-antibody interactions associated with environmentally induced molecular mimicry. Autoimmune molecular mimicry requires the similarities of surface topologies leading to antigenic combining sites [72]. The binding of BPA to PDI in host has the potential to lead to new protein epitope activation of autoimmunity (Figure 10).

## 11. BPA and Autoimmune Molecular Mimicry

BPA and triiodothyronine (T3) possess such a degree of molecular structure similarity that BPA may act as an antagonist compound on T3 receptor sites [73]. When compounds have structural similarity, it may potentially lead to autoimmune cross-reactivity with antigen-antibody complexes [74]. In particular, environmental compounds such as hydrocarbon rings found both on BPA and T3 with anchor ring like similarities may induce mimicry [75]. A potential mechanism for the role of BPA in autoimmunity may be structural molecular mimicry, in particular with thyroid hormones (Figure 11).

## 12. BPA and TH-17 Aryl Hydrocarbon Receptors

Aryl hydrocarbon receptors (AhR) are involved with regulating immune responses and the development of TH-17 cells, which are key effector T cells in a variety of human autoimmune diseases. [76] Exposure to low dose BPA has been shown to upregulate mRNA expressions of AhR. AhR activation of TH-17 by BPA may potentiate autoimmunity. The role of chemical contamination and its ability to prompt AhR receptor activation of TH-17 have already been investigated in allergic and autoimmune diseases [77]. Although direct evidence has not been investigated for the role of BPA on AhR activation of TH-17 autoimmune reactivity, the potential mechanism may exist (Figure 12).

## 13. Conclusion

With the growing epidemic of autoimmune disease worldwide and the extensive use of consumer goods containing BPA, we must examine the risk of BPA as a potential triggering compound in autoimmune disease. Although no specific evidence has linked human or animal autoimmune disease development to BPA exposure, many of the mechanisms known to exist in autoimmune pathophysiology also appear to exist with immune reactivity from BPA exposure (Figure 13). Further investigation needs to be conducted correlating autoimmune disease development to BPA exposure. Additionally, the impact of BPA exposure on those already suffering from autoimmunity needs to be investigated further based on potential overlapping pathophysiology.

## Conflict of Interests

The author declares that there is no conflict of interests regarding the publication of this paper.

## References

[1] J. A. McLachlan, "Environmental signaling: what embryos and evolution teach us about endocrine disrupting chemicals," *Endocrine Reviews*, vol. 22, no. 3, pp. 319–341, 2001.

[2] L. N. Vandenberg, I. Chahoud, J. J. Heindel, V. Padmanabhan, F. J. R. Paumgartten, and G. Schoenfelder, "Urinary, circulating, and tissue biomonitoring studies indicate widespread exposure to Bisphenol A," *Ciencia e Saude Coletiva*, vol. 17, no. 2, pp. 407–434, 2012.

[3] A. M. Calafat, X. Ye, L.-Y. Wong, J. A. Reidy, and L. L. Needham, "Exposure of the U.S. population to Bisphenol A and 4-tertiary-octylphenol: 2003-2004," *Environmental Health Perspectives*, vol. 116, no. 1, pp. 39–44, 2008.

[4] W. V. Welshons, S. C. Nagel, and F. S. vom Saal, "Large effects from small exposures. III. Endocrine mechanisms mediating effects of Bisphenol A at levels of human exposure," *Endocrinology*, vol. 147, no. 6, supplement, pp. S56–S69, 2006.

[5] S. Biedermann, P. Tschudin, and K. Grob, "Transfer of Bisphenol A from thermal printer paper to the skin," *Analytical and Bioanalytical Chemistry*, vol. 398, no. 1, pp. 571–576, 2010.

[6] J. R. Rochester, "Bisphenol A and human health: a review of the literature," *Reproductive Toxicology*, vol. 42, pp. 132–155, 2013.

[7] H. Hiroi, O. Tsutsumi, M. Momoeda, Y. Takai, Y. Osuga, and Y. Taketani, "Differential interactions of Bisphenol A and 17$\beta$-estradiol with estrogen receptor $\alpha$ (ER$\alpha$) and ER$\beta$," *Endocrine Journal*, vol. 46, no. 6, pp. 773–778, 1999.

[8] E. C. Bonefeld-Jørgensen, M. Long, M. V. Hofmeister, and A. M. Vinggaard, "Endocrine-disrupting potential of Bisphenol A, Bisphenol A dimethacrylate, 4-*n*-nonylphenol, and 4-*n*-octylphenol *in vitro*: new data and a brief review," *Environmental Health Perspectives*, vol. 115, supplement 1, pp. 69–76, 2007.

[9] K. A. Szychowski and A. K. Wójtowicz, "Components of plastic disrupt the function of the nervous system," *Postępy Higieny i Medycyny Doświadczalnej*, vol. 67, pp. 499–506, 2013.

[10] X. Xu, L. Xie, X. Hong et al., "Perinatal exposure to Bisphenol-A inhibits synaptogenesis and affects the synaptic morphological development in offspring male mice," *Chemosphere*, vol. 91, no. 8, pp. 1073–1081, 2013.

[11] H. Kurebayashi, H. Betsui, and Y. Ohno, "Disposition of a low dose of 14C-Bisphenol A in male rats and its main biliary excreation as BPA glucuronide," *Toxicological Sciences*, vol. 73, no. 1, pp. 17–25, 2003.

[12] K. L. Christensen, M. Lorber, S. Koslitz, T. Brüning, and H. M. Koch, "The contribution of diet to total Bisphenol A body burden in humans: results of a 48 hour fasting study," *Environment International*, vol. 50, pp. 7–14, 2012.

[13] K. Martinsson, T. Skogh, S. Mousavi, T. Berg, J.-I. Jönsson, and P. Hultman, "Deficiency of activating Fc$\gamma$-receptors reduces hepatic clearance and deposition of IC and increases CIC levels in mercury-induced autoimmunity," *PLoS ONE*, vol. 5, no. 10, Article ID e13413, 2010.

[14] A. J. Montaño-Loza, J. C. Crispín-Acuña, J. M. Remes-Troche, and M. Uribe, "Abnormal hepatic biochemistries and clinical liver disease in patients with primary Sjögren's syndrome," *Annals of Hepatology*, vol. 6, no. 3, pp. 150–155, 2007.

[15] P. Invernizzi, "Liver auto-immunology: the paradox of autoimmunity in a tolerogenic organ," *Journal of Autoimmunity*, vol. 46, pp. 1–6, 2013.

[16] M.-R. Lee, H. Park, S. Bae et al., "Urinary Bisphenol A concentrations are associated with abnormal liver function in the elderly: a repeated panel study," *Journal of Epidemiology & Community Health*, 2013.

[17] Z. K. Hassan, M. A. Elobeid, P. Virk et al., "Bisphenol A induces hepatotoxicity through oxidative stress in rat model," *Oxidative Medicine and Cellular Longevity*, vol. 2012, Article ID 194829, 6 pages, 2012.

[18] J. Wang, X. Shi, Y. Du, and B. Zhou, "Effects of xenoestrogens on the expression of vitellogenin (*vtg*) and cytochrome P450 aromatase (*cyp19a* and *b*) genes in zebrafish (*Danio rerio*) larvae," *Journal of Environmental Science and Health A: Toxic/Hazardous Substances and Environmental Engineering*, vol. 46, no. 9, pp. 960–967, 2011.

[19] M. R. Namazi, "Cytochrome-P450 enzymes and autoimmunity: expansion of the relationship and introduction of free radicals as the link," *Journal of Autoimmune Diseases*, vol. 6, article 4, 2009.

[20] L. E. Padgett, K. A. Broniowska, P. A. Hansen, J. A. Corbett, and H. M. Tse, "The role of reactive oxygen species and proinflammatory cytokines in type 1 diabetes pathogenesis," *Annals of the New York Academy of Sciences*, vol. 1281, pp. 16–35, 2013.

[21] H. S. Lee, M. Y. Pyo, and M. Yang, "Set, a putative oncogene, as a biomarker for prenatal exposure to Bisphenol A," *Asian Pacific Journal of Cancer Prevention*, vol. 13, no. 6, pp. 2711–2715, 2012.

[22] L. E. Padgett, K. A. Broniowska, P. A. Hansen, J. A. Corbett, and H. M. Tse, "The role of reactive oxygen species and proinflammatory cytokines in type 1 diabetes pathogenesis," *Annals of the New York Academy of Sciences*, vol. 1281, pp. 16–35, 2013.

[23] L.-Y. Yu-Lee, "Prolactin modulation of immune and inflammatory responses," *Recent Progress in Hormone Research*, vol. 57, pp. 435–455, 2002.

[24] L. Matera, M. Mori, and A. Galetto, "Effect of prolactin on the antigen presenting function of monocyte-derived dendritic cells," *Lupus*, vol. 10, no. 10, pp. 728–734, 2001.

[25] A. de Bellis, A. Bizzarro, R. Pivonello, G. Lombardi, and A. Bellastella, "Prolactin and autoimmunity," *Pituitary*, vol. 8, no. 1, pp. 25–30, 2005.

[26] S. Shelly, M. Boaz, and H. Orbach, "Prolactin and autoimmunity," *Autoimmunity Reviews*, vol. 11, no. 6-7, pp. A465–A470, 2012.

[27] R. Steinmetz, N. G. Brown, D. L. Allen, R. M. Bigsby, and N. Ben-Jonathan, "The environmental estrogen Bisphenol A stimulates prolactin release *in vitro* and *in vivo*," *Endocrinology*, vol. 138, no. 5, pp. 1780–1786, 1997.

[28] J. Hao, J. Wang, W. Zhao, L. Ding, E. Gao, and W. Yuan, "Effect of Bisphenol A exposure on sex hormone level in occupational women," *Wei Sheng Yan Jiu*, vol. 40, no. 3, pp. 312–314, 2011.

[29] S. Shelly, M. Boaz, and H. Orbach, "Prolactin and autoimmunity," *Autoimmunity Reviews*, vol. 11, no. 6-7, pp. A465–A470, 2012.

[30] M. Alizadeh, F. Ota, K. Hosoi, M. Kato, T. Sakai, and M. A. Satter, "Altered allergic cytokine and antibody response in mice treated with Bisphenol A," *The Journal of Medical Investigation*, vol. 53, no. 1-2, pp. 70–80, 2006.

[31] A. Elango, B. Shepherd, and T. T. Chen, "Effects of endocrine disrupters on the expression of growth hormone and prolactin mRNA in the rainbow trout pituitary," *General and Comparative Endocrinology*, vol. 145, no. 2, pp. 116–127, 2006.

[32] L. O. Chailurkit, W. Aekplakorn, and B. Ongphiphadhanakul, "The relationship between circulating estradiol and thyroid autoimmunity in males," *European Journal of Endocrinology*, vol. 170, no. 1, pp. 63–67, 2013.

[33] C. Chighizola and P. L. Meroni, "The role of environmental estrogens and autoimmunity," *Autoimmunity Reviews*, vol. 11, no. 6-7, pp. A493–A501, 2012.

[34] R. Panchanathan, H. Liu, and D. Choubey, "Expression of murine Unc93b1 is up-regulated by interferon and estrogen signaling: implications for sex bias in the development of autoimmunity," *International Immunology*, vol. 25, no. 9, pp. 521–529, 2013.

[35] E. Incorvaia, L. Sicouri, S. K. Petersen-Mahrt, and K. M. Schmitz, "Hormones and AID: balancing immunity and autoimmunity," *Autoimmunity*, vol. 46, no. 2, pp. 128–137, 2013.

[36] M. Cunningham and G. Gilkeson, "Estrogen receptors in immunity and autoimmunity," *Clinical Reviews in Allergy and Immunology*, vol. 40, no. 1, pp. 66–73, 2011.

[37] T.-C. Chao, P. J. van Alten, J. A. Greager, and R. J. Walter, "Steroid sex hormones regulate the release of tumor necrosis factor by macrophages," *Cellular Immunology*, vol. 160, no. 1, pp. 43–49, 1995.

[38] R. Panchanathan and D. Choubey, "Murine BAFF expression is up-regulated by estrogen and interferons: implications for sex bias in the development of autoimmunity," *Molecular Immunology*, vol. 53, no. 1-2, pp. 15–23, 2013.

[39] M. C. Siracusa, M. G. Overstreet, F. Housseau, A. L. Scott, and S. L. Klein, "17$\beta$-estradiol alters the activity of conventional and IFN-producing killer dendritic cells," *The Journal of Immunology*, vol. 180, no. 3, pp. 1423–1431, 2008.

[40] R. S. Bonds and T. Midoro-Horiuti, "Estrogen effects in allergy and asthma," *Current Opinion in Allergy & Clinical Immunology*, vol. 13, no. 1, pp. 92–99, 2013.

[41] J. A. Rogers, L. Metz, and V. W. Yong, "Review: endocrine disrupting chemicals and immune responses: a focus on Bisphenol-A and its potential mechanisms," *Molecular Immunology*, vol. 53, no. 4, pp. 421–430, 2013.

[42] N. Ben-Jonathan and R. Steinmetz, "Xenoestrogens: the emerging story of Bisphenol A," *Trends in Endocrinology and Metabolism*, vol. 9, no. 3, pp. 124–128, 1998.

[43] J.-Y. Youn, H.-Y. Park, J.-W. Lee et al., "Evaluation of the immune response following exposure of mice to Bisphenol A: induction of Th1 cytokine and prolactin by BPA exposure in the mouse spleen cells," *Archives of Pharmacal Research*, vol. 25, no. 6, pp. 946–953, 2002.

[44] J. A. Rogers, L. Metz, and V. W. Yong, "Review: endocrine disrupting chemicals and immune responses: a focus on Bisphenol-A and its potential mechanisms," *Molecular Immunology*, vol. 53, no. 4, pp. 421–430, 2013.

[45] L. Canesi, M. Betti, L. C. Lorusso, C. Ciacci, and G. Gallo, "'In vivo' effects of Bisphenol A in *Mytilus* hemocytes: modulation of kinase-mediated signalling pathways," *Aquatic Toxicology*, vol. 71, no. 1, pp. 73–84, 2005.

[46] G. Wildner and U. Kaufmann, "What causes relapses of autoimmune diseases? The etiological role of autoreactive T cells," *Autoimmunity Reviews*, vol. 12, no. 11, pp. 1070–1075, 2013.

[47] S. André, D. F. Tough, S. Lacroix-Desmazes, S. V. Kaveri, and J. Bayry, "Surveillance of antigen-presenting cells by $CD4^+CD25^+$ regulatory T cells in autoimmunity: immunopathogenesis and therapeutic implications," *The American Journal of Pathology*, vol. 174, no. 5, pp. 1575–1587, 2009.

[48] T. Wu and C. Mohan, "The AKT axis as a therapeutic target in autoimmune diseases," *Endocrine, Metabolic & Immune Disorders—Drug Targets*, vol. 9, no. 2, pp. 145–150, 2009.

[49] K. D. Moudgil and D. Choubey, "Cytokines in autoimmunity: role in induction, regulation, and treatment," *Journal of Interferon & Cytokine Research*, vol. 31, no. 10, pp. 695–703, 2011.

[50] L. Pisapia, G. del Pozzo, P. Barba et al., "Effects of some endocrine disruptors on cell cycle progression and murine dendritic cell differentiation," *General and Comparative Endocrinology*, vol. 178, no. 1, pp. 54–63, 2012.

[51] S. Yoshino, K. Yamaki, X. Li et al., "Prenatal exposure to Bisphenol A up-regulates immune responses, including T helper 1 and T helper 2 responses, in mice," *Immunology*, vol. 112, no. 3, pp. 489–495, 2004.

[52] M. Goto, Y. Takano-Ishikawa, H. Ono, M. Yoshida, K. Yamaki, and H. Shinmoto, "Orally administered Bisphenol A disturbed antigen specific immunoresponses in the naïve condition," *Bioscience, Biotechnology and Biochemistry*, vol. 71, no. 9, pp. 2136–2143, 2007.

[53] K. M. Pollard, D. M. Cauvi, C. B. Toomey, K. V. Morris, and D. H. Kono, "Interferon-$\gamma$ and systemic autoimmunity," *Discovery Medicine*, vol. 16, no. 87, pp. 123–131, 2013.

[54] J.-Y. Youn, H.-Y. Park, J.-W. Lee et al., "Evaluation of the immune response following exposure of mice to Bisphenol A: induction of Th1 cytokine and prolactin by BPA exposure in the mouse spleen cells," *Archives of Pharmacal Research*, vol. 25, no. 6, pp. 946–953, 2002.

[55] A. Weaver, A. Goncalves da Silva, R. K. Nuttall et al., "An elevated matrix metalloproteinase (MMP) in an animal model of multiple sclerosis is protective by affecting Th1/Th2 polarization," *The FASEB Journal*, vol. 19, no. 12, pp. 1668–1670, 2005.

[56] H. Yan, M. Takamoto, and K. Sugane, "Exposure to Bisphenol A prenatally or in adulthood promotes TH2 cytokine production associated with reduction of $CD4^+CD25^+$ regulatory T cells," *Environmental Health Perspectives*, vol. 116, no. 4, pp. 514–519, 2008.

[57] J. S. Ellis, S. H. Hong, H. Zaghouani, and H. Braley-Mullen, "Reduced effectiveness of $CD4^+Foxp3^+$ regulatory T cells in CD28-deficient NOD.H-2h4 mice leads to increased severity of spontaneous autoimmune thyroiditis," *The Journal of Immunology*, vol. 191, no. 10, pp. 4940–4949, 2013.

[58] M. Maes, M. Kubera, J. C. Leunis, M. Berk, M. Geffard, and E. Bosmans, "In depression, bacterial translocation may drive inflammatory responses, oxidative and nitrosative stress (O&NS), and autoimmune responses directed against O&NS-damaged neoepitopes," *Acta Psychiatrica Scandinavica*, vol. 127, no. 5, pp. 344–354, 2013.

[59] A. Igarashi, S. Ohtsu, M. Muroi, and K.-I. Tanamoto, "Effects of possible endocrine disrupting chemicals on bacterial component-induced activation of NF-$\kappa$B," *Biological and Pharmaceutical Bulletin*, vol. 29, no. 10, pp. 2120–2122, 2006.

[60] K. Stechova, R. Pomahacova, J. Hrabak et al., "Reactivity to helicobacter pylori antigens in patients suffering from thyroid gland autoimmunity," *Experimental and Clinical Endocrinology and Diabetes*, vol. 117, no. 8, pp. 423–431, 2009.

[61] J. Banchereau and R. M. Steinman, "Dendritic cells and the control of immunity," *Nature*, vol. 392, no. 6673, pp. 245–252, 1998.

[62] P. Kaliński, C. M. U. Hilkens, E. A. Wierenga, and M. L. Kapsenberg, "T-cell priming by type-1 and type-2 polarized dendritic cells: the concept of a third signal," *Immunology Today*, vol. 20, no. 12, pp. 561–567, 1999.

[63] H. Guo, T. Liu, Y. Uemura et al., "Bisphenol A in combination with TNF-$\alpha$ selectively induces Th2 cell-promoting dendritic cells *in vitro* with an estrogen-like activity," *Cellular and Molecular Immunology*, vol. 7, no. 3, pp. 227–234, 2010.

[64] H. Kolb and V. Kolb-Bachofen, "Nitric oxide in autoimmune disease: cytotoxic or regulatory mediator?" *Immunology Today*, vol. 19, no. 12, pp. 556–561, 1998.

[65] J.-A. Byun, Y. Heo, Y.-O. Kim, and M.-Y. Pyo, "Bisphenol A-induced downregulation of murine macrophage activities in vitro and ex vivo," *Environmental Toxicology and Pharmacology*, vol. 19, no. 1, pp. 19–24, 2005.

[66] H. H. Smits, "B cells in allergic diseases: bad or better?" *Autoimmunity*, vol. 45, no. 5, pp. 415–426, 2012.

[67] M. H. Lee, S. W. Chung, B. Y. Kang et al., "Enhanced interleukin-4 production in $CD4^+$ T cells and elevated immunoglobulin E levels in antigen-primed mice by Bisphenol A and nonylphenol, endocrine disruptors: involvement of nuclear factor-AT and $CA^{2+}$," *Immunology*, vol. 109, no. 1, pp. 76–86, 2003.

[68] S. Altrichter, H.-J. Peter, D. Pisarevskaja, M. Metz, P. Martus, and M. Maurer, "Ige mediated autoallergy against thyroid peroxidase—a novel pathomechanism of chronic spontaneous urticaria?" *PLoS ONE*, vol. 6, no. 4, Article ID e14794, 2011.

[69] H. Yurino, S. Ishikawa, T. Sato et al., "Endocrine disruptors (environmental estrogens) enhance autoantibody production by B1 cells," *Toxicological Sciences*, vol. 81, no. 1, pp. 139–147, 2004.

[70] T. Hiroi, K. Okada, S. Imaoka, M. Osada, and Y. Funae, "Bisphenol A binds to protein disulfide isomerase and inhibits its enzymatic and hormone-binding activities," *Endocrinology*, vol. 147, no. 6, pp. 2773–2780, 2006.

[71] K. Okada, S. Imaoka, S. Hashimoto, T. Hiroi, and Y. Funae, "Over-expression of protein disulfide isomerase reduces the release of growth hormone induced by Bisphenol A and/or T3," *Molecular and Cellular Endocrinology*, vol. 278, no. 1-2, pp. 44–51, 2007.

[72] S. Tapryal, V. Gaur, K. J. Kaur, and D. M. Salunke, "Structural evaluation of a mimicry-recognizing paratope: plasticity in antigen-antibody interactions manifests in molecular mimicry," *The Journal of Immunology*, vol. 191, no. 1, pp. 456–463, 2013.

[73] K. Moriyama, T. Tagami, T. Akamizu et al., "Thyroid hormone action is disrupted by Bisphenol A as an antagonist," *Journal of Clinical Endocrinology and Metabolism*, vol. 87, no. 11, pp. 5185–5190, 2002.

[74] J. M. Davies, "Molecular mimicry: can epitope mimicry induce autoimmune disease?" *Immunology and Cell Biology*, vol. 75, no. 2, pp. 113–126, 1997.

[75] J. D. McKinney and C. L. Waller, "Molecular determinants of hormone mimicry: halogenated aromatic hydrocarbon environmental agents," *Journal of Toxicology and Environmental Health B: Critical Reviews*, vol. 1, no. 1, pp. 27–58, 1998.

[76] N. T. Nguyen, T. Nakahama, and T. Kishimoto, "Aryl hydrocarbon receptor and experimental autoimmune arthritis," *Seminars in Immunopathology*, vol. 35, no. 6, pp. 637–644, 2013.

[77] K. Takahashi, "Chemical contamination of the environment and development of allergic and autoimmune diseases," *Nippon Rinsho*, vol. 68, no. 3, pp. 551–562, 2010.

8

# Chronic Exposure to Oral Pathogens and Autoimmune Reactivity in Acute Coronary Atherothrombosis

**Ivana Burazor[1] and Aristo Vojdani[2]**

[1] *Cardiology Department, Institute for Rehabilitation, Sokobanjska 17, 11000 Belgrade, Serbia*
[2] *Immunosciences Lab Inc, Los Angeles, CA 90035, USA*

Correspondence should be addressed to Ivana Burazor; ivana.burazor@gmail.com

Academic Editor: K. Michael Pollard

*Background.* It has been hypothesized that various infective agents may activate immune reactions as part of the atherosclerotic process. We aimed to investigate the interrelationship between chronic exposure to oral pathogens and immune-inflammatory response in patients with acute coronary atherothrombosis. *Patients and Methods.* The study included 200 participants from Serbia: 100 patients with acute myocardial infarction (MI), and 100 age- and sex-matched controls. Antibodies to oral anaerobes and aerobes were determined as well as autoantibodies to endothelial cells, beta-2 glycoprotein I, platelet glycoprotein IIb/IIIa and anticardiolipin. Interleukin-6 (IL-6) and C-reactive protein (CRP) were measured. *Results.* The mean serum antibodies to oral anaerobes tended to be higher among subjects with MI ($0.876 \pm 0.303$ versus $0.685 \pm 0.172$ OD, $P < 0.001$). Similarly, antibody levels against oral aerobes in patients were significantly different from controls. Antibodies against endothelial cell, beta-2 glycoprotein I, platelet glycoprotein IIb/IIIa, anticardiolipin along with CRP and IL-6 were highly elevated in patients. The levels of antibodies to oral bacteria showed linear correlation with tissue antibodies, CRP and IL-6. *Conclusion.* Antibody response to chronic oral bacterial infections and host immune response against them may be responsible for the elevation of tissue antibodies and biomarkers of inflammation which are involved in acute coronary thrombosis development.

## 1. Introduction

It has been recently hypothesized that various infectious diseases, both bacterial and viral, may activate vessel-associated leucocytes or immune reactions in the atherosclerotic process. Studies have also shown a strong association between poor dental health and cardiovascular diseases [1–3]. There are circumstances in which the presence or absence of teeth and the bacteria that reside on them could be the risk factors for the triggering of cerebrovascular and cardiovascular disorders, such as myocardial infarction. Several hypotheses can explain this scenario, among which asymptomatic bacteremia might play a role. Our body surface is colonized by over $10^{12}$ bacteria. A minuscule proportion of these bacteria gain access to our underlying tissue and are quickly dispatched by the body's immune response [4–7]. The bacteria, typically *Streptococcus sanguis, Streptococcus oralis,* and *Peptostreptococcus anaerobius,* arise in the oral cavity and are believed to enter the bloodstream as a result of trauma as bland as the manipulations of oral hygiene [8]. These bacteremias may infect sites of underlying pathologic changes of heart valves [9, 10]. On the damaged heart valves, adherent bacteria soon become embedded and protected in newly formed thrombi or platelet vegetation. Consequently, streptococci capable of initial adhesion and rapid induction of thrombosis are likely to be more virulent in clinical disease. As many as half of all cases of bacterial endocarditis have been attributed to viridans streptococci, with *S. sanguis* identified as the vector three to four times more frequently than *S. oralis* [11, 12]. This association may reflect the large proportion of these microorganisms in the oral flora and the frequency of these bacteremias in comparison with those that arise from other organs and tissues. The specificity of infection may also reflect special virulence traits of these bacteria. *Porphyromonas gingivalis, Prevotella intermedia,* and *Bacteroides forsythus* are Gram-negative small basil quality obligate anaerobic bacteria and are held directly responsible for the formation of periodontitis. These bacteria usually secrete brown-black pigments and form colonies when they reproduce in blood agar plates used for their cultivation. These bacteria were classified in the *Bacteroides* genus until 1988 and 1990, when they were reclassified to the *Porphyromonas* and *Prevotella* genera, respectively, in accordance with new classification strategies made by Shah and Collins [13, 14].

These anaerobic bacteria, in conjunction with the facultative anaerobic bacteria such as *Streptococcus* mentioned above, can lead to mixed types of infections affecting various tissues, including the joints and the heart [15–20]. An extensive number of virulence factors include fimbriae, degradative enzymes, exopolysaccharide capsules, and atypical lipopolysaccharides; these factors, through various mechanisms of action, including mimicry or citrullination of self-peptide, can inducc inflammation and autoimmunity against various tissue antigens [21–23].

For example, immunological mapping using a library of cyclic citrullinated $\alpha$-enolase peptides led to the identification of a B-cell-dominant epitope comprising amino acids 5-21 of $\alpha$-enolase (KIHAREIFDSRGNPTVE) where arginine-9 and arginine-15 are citrullinated, with an 82% sequence similarity with that of *P. gingivalis* [24]. Immunization with citrullinated human and *P. gingivalis* $\alpha$-enolase and citrullinated fibrinogen causes similar pathology in humanized DR4 transgenic mice. This mechanism may be triggered by the release of different cytokines and prostanoids, such as interleukin-1 (IL-1), IL-6, IL-8, tumor necrosis factor-alpha (TNF-$\alpha$), prostaglandin E2, and different matrix metalloproteinases (MMP). These bacteria and released metabolites beyond this potential local pathogenicity may disseminate systemically and influence directly or indirectly the atheroma pathophysiology. Aside from increasing cytokine production, Gram-negative bacteria may also stimulate hypercoagulability, monocyte activation, and liver activation by releasing acute phase proteins, such as high-sensitivity C-reactive protein (hs-CRP) [4]. This repeated systemic exposure to orally derived bacteria, bacterial endotoxins, and systemic inflammation would eventually directly and/or indirectly affect the vascular walls, inducing a state of endothelial dysfunction.

The purpose of this study, then, is to investigate the potential interrelationship between chronic exposure to oral pathogens, the antibodies produced against them, and elevations in the levels of markers of immune-inflammatory response in patients with acute myocardial atherothrombosis.

## 2. Materials and Methods

*2.1. Study Population.* The study comprised 200 participants from Serbia, of whom 100 were patients admitted due to acute myocardial infarction. 100 were age- and sex-matched controls. In the patients group, the diagnosis of acute myocardial infarction was based on evidence of myocardial necrosis in a clinical setting consistent with acute myocardial ischemia [25]. The inclusion criteria for control groups were absence of known coronary artery diseases (previous stable or unstable angina as well as previous myocardial infarction) or carotid disease; initial electrocardiography (ECG) was recorded to confirm the absence of coronary artery disease. The exclusion criteria for the group of patients and also for controls were concomitant dilated cardiomyopathy, valvular heart disease, atrial fibrillation, major surgery, or trauma within previous months. All patients and controls with known or suspected thrombotic disorders, systemic illness, autoimmune diseases, sepsis, alcohol liver diseases, chronic obstructive pulmonary diseases, acute respiratory infections, current infections of any etiology or infections within previous 3 weeks, and malignancy and inflammatory diseases were also excluded. Study participants were asked about the risk factors for coronary artery disease (CAD), that is, smoking status, family history of CAD, hypertension, dyslipidemia, and diabetes.

The majority of the study participants were males (60% of patients and 58% of controls, $P$ = n.s). The mean age of patients was 59.42 years and 59.03 years in controls ($P$ = n.s).

The investigation conformed to the principles outlined in the Declaration of Helsinki. Signed informed consent or witnessed oral informed consent was obtained from all patients and healthy controls in accordance with the guidelines of the Ethical Review Committee of the Medical Faculty University of Nis, who approved the study protocol.

*2.2. Preparation of Bacterial Antigens.* Oral aerobes or facultative anaerobes (*Streptococcus sanguis*, *Streptococcus oralis*, and *Peptostreptococcus anaerobius*) and oral obligate anaerobes (*Porphyromonas gingivalis*, *Prevotella intermedia*, and *Bacteroides forsythus*) were purchased from American Type Culture Collection (Rockville, Maryland, USA) and cultivated according to the methods described earlier [8, 9]. In brief, bacteria were grown in different media and the cultures were incubated for 48–72 h at 35–37°C. Purity was assessed by colony morphology and gram stain. Bacteria were harvested at the late log phase by centrifugation at 10,000 g for 15 min and then washed twice with 0.15 M sodium chloride. The bacteria were lysed using a sonicator, and after separation of the lysate, the protein concentration was measured and used for coating ELISA plates and antibody measurement.

*2.3. Serum Antibody Assay by Enzyme-Linked Immunosorbent Assay (ELISA).* Pathogen-specific antibody was quantitated by enzyme-linked immunoassay. Wells of microtiter plates were coated with 100 $\mu$L of bacterial antigens (concentration of 10 $\mu$g/mL in 0.1 M of carbonate buffer, pH 9.6). Plates were incubated overnight at 4°C and then washed three times with 200 $\mu$L Tris-buffered saline (TBS) containing 0.05% Tween 20, pH 7.4. The nonspecific binding of immunoglobulins was prevented by adding 2% bovine serum albumin (BSA) to phosphate-buffered saline (PBS) and incubated overnight at 4°C.

Plates were washed as described above, and then serum samples diluted 1 : 200 in 0.1 M PBS Tween containing 2% BSA were added to duplicate wells and incubated for 1 h at room temperature. Plates were washed, and then alkaline phosphatase goat anti-human IgG F(ab′)2 fragments (KPI, Gaithersburg, MD) with optimal dilution of 1 : 400 in serum

diluent were added to each well; plates were incubated for an additional 1 h at room temperature. After washing five times with TBS-Tween buffer, the enzyme reaction was started by adding 100 $\mu$L of paranitrophenylphosphate in 0.1 mL diethanolamine buffer 1 mg/mL containing 1 mM $MgCl_2$ and sodium azide pH 9.8. The reaction was stopped 45 min later with 50 $\mu$L of 1 N NaOH. The optical density (OD) was read at 405 nm by means of a microtiter reader. To detect nonspecific binding, several control wells contained all reagents except human serum, or wells were coated with HSA followed by the addition of human serum and all other reagents to be used for specificity of the antigen-antibody reaction.

*2.4. Autoimmunity and Immunity Markers.* Antibodies against beta-2 glycoprotein I (IgG) were determined by using ELISA method (Calbiochem, La Jolla, CA, USA, Cat# B59407). Anticardiolipin antibodies were determined by using a test kit from Sigma, Cat# P1867. Antiendothelial cell, beta-2 glycoprotein I, and antiplatelet glycoprotein IIb/IIIa (IgG) antibodies were measured by coating each ELISA well plate with one $\mu$g of pure antigen followed by the addition of serum. All additional steps are described in the ELISA section.

*2.5. Markers of Inflammation.* Levels of IL-6 and hs-CRP were measured using kits manufactured by Diagnostic Products Corporation, Los Angeles, CA, on an IMMULITE Automated Immunoassay Analyzer. The IMMULITE system utilizes assay-specific, antibody- or antigen-coated plastic beads as the solid phase, alkaline phosphatase labeled reagent, and a chemiluminescent substrate. The IMMULITE system automates the entire assay process. Light emission was measured by a photomultiplier tube, and the results were calculated for each sample using different calibrators and controls.

The established reference ranges of the lab performing the tests were from 0.7 to 4.6 pg/mL for IL-6 and from 0 to 1 mg/dL for hs-CRP. Values above the established reference ranges were marked as positive.

*2.6. Statistical Analysis.* Results of normally distributed continuous variables are expressed as the mean value ± standard deviation. Analysis of normality of the continuous variables was performed with the Kolmogorov-Smirnov test. Differences between examined groups were assessed by unpaired $t$-test and Mann-Whitney $U$ test and $\chi^2$ testing was used for discrete variables. Relative Risk (RR), odds ratio (OR), and 95% Confidence Interval (CI) for the RR and OR were calculated.

Correlations between continuous variables were analyzed with the two-way Pearson correlation tests. Hs-CRP levels were not of linear nature. Therefore, in order to fulfill the statistical requirement, hs-CRP was logarithmically transformed before entering the analysis. Differences were considered to be significantly important if the null hypothesis could be rejected with > 95% confidence. All $P$ values were two-tailed. The PASW 18.0 statistical software package was used for all calculations.

TABLE 1: Characteristics of patients with acute myocardial infarction.

| Characteristics | (%) |
|---|---|
| ECG abnormalities at entry | |
| ST segment elevation | 45 |
| Without ST segment elevation | 55 |
| Systolic BP, mmHg | |
| <120 | 32.4 |
| 120–139 | 21.6 |
| 140–159 | 15.4 |
| >160 | 30.6 |
| Mean (SD) | 132 ± 35.98 |
| Diastolic BP, mean (SD), mmHg | 79 ± 23.33 |
| Heart rate, heartbeats/min | |
| <70 | 16.3 |
| 70–89 | 38.7 |
| 90–109 | 36.9 |
| >110 | 8.1 |
| Mean (SD), mmHg | 22.73 |
| Previous disease | |
| Previous MI | 29.7 |
| Previous CABG | 17.1 |
| Aspirin before admission | 34.2 |
| Duration of staying in hospital, mean (SD) | 10.8 (5.4) |
| LVEF, mean (SD) | 54.4 (13.30) |
| LVEF < 40 | 16 (16.2) |
| New event | 19.6 |

ECG: electrocardiogram; BP: blood pressure; MI: myocardial infarction; CABG: coronary artery bypass grafting; LVEF: left ventricle ejection fraction. Values are % unless otherwise indicated.

## 3. Results

*3.1. Clinical Characteristics of Patients with Acute Myocardial Infarction.* In this study, we measured the levels of antibodies against oral pathogens as well as antibodies against endothelial cells, beta-2 glycoprotein I, platelet glycoprotein IIb/IIIa, anticardiolipin antibodies, and inflammatory markers such as hs-CRP and interleukin 6, in blood samples of patients with myocardial infarction and compared them to the levels of the same antibodies and markers in samples from control subjects.

Table 1 outlines clinical characteristics of patients with acute myocardial infarction. Mean value of systolic blood pressure was 132 ± 35.98 mm Hg. Patients spent in hospital a period of 10.8 ± 5.4 days to fulfill medical treatment.

*3.2. Antibodies against Oral Pathogens.* IgG antibodies to oral anaerobes were highly present in patients with acute coronary atherothrombosis. A total of 88% of patients with cardiovascular disease had elevated antibodies above the mean of controls, as shown in Figure 1; RR was 1.33 (1.13 to 1.56) 95% CI.

Overall, the mean OD of serum IgG antibodies to oral anaerobes tends to be higher among subjects with coronary

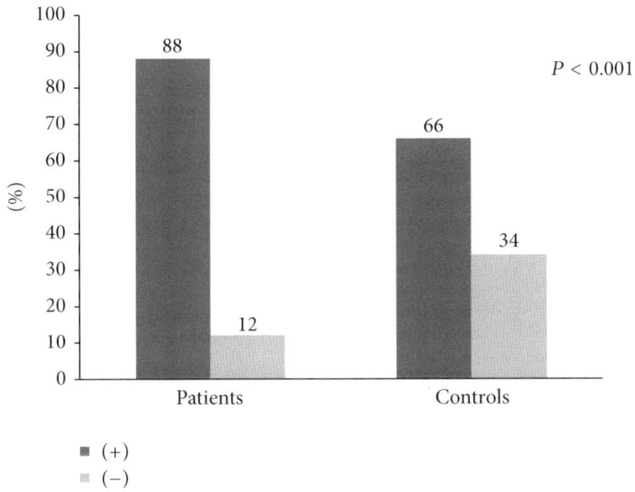


FIGURE 1: Comparison of the levels of IgG antibodies against oral anaerobes within the study participants.

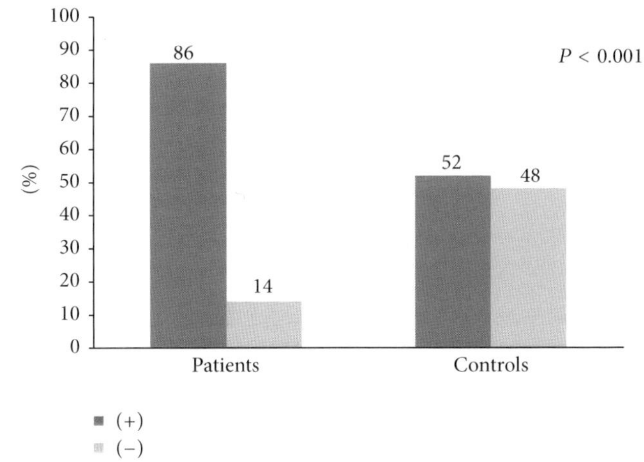


FIGURE 2: Comparison of the levels of IgG antibodies against oral aerobes within the study participants.

artery disease than those without (0.876 ± 0.303 OD versus 0.685 ± 0.172, $P < 0.001$) (Table 2).

IgG antibodies to oral aerobes were highly present in patients with acute coronary atherothrombosis. A total of 86% of patients had antibodies detectable compared to 52% of controls, RR 1.65 (1.34 to 2.02; 95% CI) (Figure 2).

The mean OD of serum IgG antibodies to oral aerobes tends to be higher among subjects with coronary artery disease than those without (0.996 ± 0.323 OD versus 0.769 ± 0.239 OD and $P < 0.001$) (Table 2).

*3.3. Autoimmunity and Inflammation.* Subjects with acute coronary artery atherothrombosis showed very strong autoimmune response with elevation in antiendothelial cell IgG antibodies in the group (45% versus 23%, O.R. 2.73, 95% CI for OR 1.48–5.04, RR 1.95, 95% CI for RR 1.28–2.97, $\chi^2 = 3.14$, $P = 0.001$, Figure 3.

The mean serum antiendothelial cells IgG antibodies were 0.684 ± 0.211 OD in patients versus 0.598 ± 0.193 OD in controls, $P = 0.004$ (Table 3).

Also, anti-beta-2 glycoprotein I antibodies IgG were detected in 25% of patients with acute coronary atherothrombosis compared to 8% of controls (OR 3.91, 95% CI 1.67–9.18, RR 3.12, 95% CI for RR 1.48–6.59, $\chi^2 = 2.992$, $P < 0.001$); see Figure 3. The mean serum titers are shown in Table 3.

Antibodies to platelet glycoprotein IIb/IIIa were detected in 53% of patients and 12% of controls (OR 8.26, 95% CI 4.02–16.98, RR 4.41, 95% CI for RR 2.51–7.74, $\chi^2 = 5.18$, $P < 0.001$), Figure 3.

Anticardiolipin antibodies were detected in 45% of patients and 28% of controls (OR 2.10, 95% CI for OR 1.16–3.78; RR 1.6, 95% CI for RR 1.09–2.35, $\chi^2 = 2.43$, $P < 0.001$). The titers were significantly different between groups, as shown in Table 3.

Our study showed that 46% of patients had elevated levels of circulating IL-6. Statistically, this proportion is significantly higher compared to controls (only 4%), ($\chi^2 =$

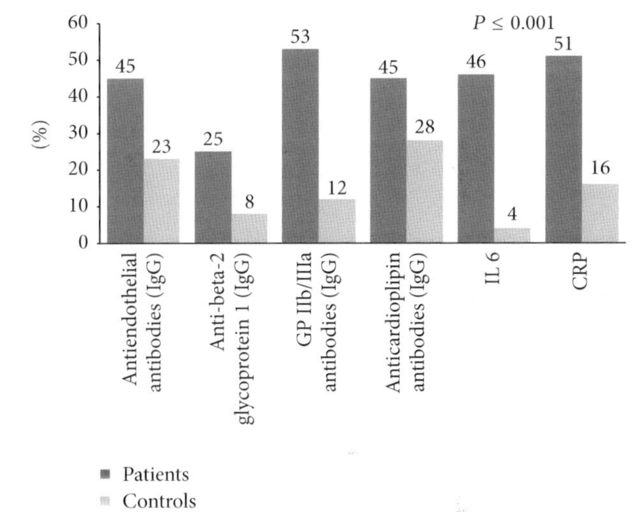


FIGURE 3: Comparison of the levels of IgG antibodies against antigens associated with autoimmunity activation and markers of inflammation in the study participants.

5.53, $P < 0.001$; odds ratio (OR), 20.44; (95% CI, 6.57–59.88); RR 11.5 (4.3 to 30.7). Concentrations of IL-6 were significantly higher in patients compared to controls (9.38 pg/mL (2.00–18.85) versus 1.5 pg/mL (1.2–1.8), $P < 0.001$).

There was a significant difference between patients and controls in regard to CRP; 51% of patients had CRP above reference range compared to 16% of controls, $\chi^2 = 4.65$, $P < 0.001$, RR 3.18 (1.95–5.49): OR 5.46 (2.81–10.63) (Figure 3). The median of this marker of inflammation was 2.67 mg/dL (0.384–20.895) in patients and 0.225 mg/dL (0.075–0.623) in controls, $P < 0.001$.

Antibodies to both oral anaerobes and aerobes showed strong and significant correlation with different parameters of autoimmunity, immunity, and inflammation. Pearson's linear correlation, coefficient of correlation ($r$), and $P$ values are shown in Tables 4 and 5.

TABLE 2: Antibodies against oral pathogens in the study participants.

| ORAL pathogen (Bacterial agent) | Study participants | Mean | SD | 95% CI | | $P$ |
|---|---|---|---|---|---|---|
| | | | | Lower bound | Upper bound | |
| Oral anaerobes (OD) | Patients | 0.876 | 0.303 | 0.662 | 1.035 | <0.001 |
| | Controls | 0.685 | 0.172 | 0.569 | 0.715 | |
| Oral aerobes (OD) | Patients | 0.996 | 0.323 | 0.768 | 1.226 | <0.001 |
| | Controls | 0.769 | 0.239 | 0.622 | 0.873 | |

TABLE 3: Autoantibodies in the study participants.

| Autoantibodies | Group | Mean | S.d. | 95% CI | | Minimum | Maximum | $P$ |
|---|---|---|---|---|---|---|---|---|
| | | | | Lower bound | Upper bound | | | |
| Antiendothelial cells (OD) | Patients | 0.684 | 0.211 | 0.509 | 0.579 | 0.229 | 0.955 | 0.004 |
| | Controls | 0.598 | 0.193 | 0.444 | 0.494 | 0.215 | 0.775 | |
| Beta 2- glycoprotein I (OD) | Patients | 0.665 | 0.344 | 0.595 | 0.1735 | 0.242 | 2.266 | 0.003 |
| | Controls | 0.540 | 0.205 | 0.499 | 0.582 | 0.280 | 1.437 | |
| Platelet glycoprotein IIb/IIIa (OD) | Patients | 0.351 | 0.100 | 0.331 | 0.372 | 0.225 | 0.718 | 0.001 |
| | Controls | 0.306 | 0.074 | 0.290 | 0.321 | 0.176 | 0.499 | |
| Anticardiolipin (OD) | Patients | 0.552 | 0.180 | 0.515 | 0.589 | 0.228 | 1.161 | 0.001 |
| | Controls | 0.415 | 0.097 | 0.396 | 0.435 | 0.237 | 0.704 | |

TABLE 4: Correlations of oral anaerobes IgG with different parameters of autoimmunity and inflammation.

| Autoantibodies and inflammation | Antibodies to oral anaerobes (IgG) | |
|---|---|---|
| | $r$ | $P$ |
| Antiendothelial cells | 0.541 | 0.01 |
| Anti-beta 2 glycoprotein I | 0.459 | 0.01 |
| Antiplatelets glycoprotein IIb/IIIa | 0.499 | 0.01 |
| Anticardiolipin | 0.647 | 0.01 |
| Interleukin 6 | 0.199 | 0.01 |
| hs C-reactive protein | 0.229 | 0.01 |

$r$—coefficient of correlation.

TABLE 5: Correlations of oral aerobes IgG with different parameters of autoimmunity and inflammation.

| Autoantibodies and inflammation | Antibodies to oral aerobes (IgG) | |
|---|---|---|
| | $r$ | $P$ |
| Antiendothelial cells | 0.547 | 0.01 |
| Anti-beta-2 glycoprotein I | 0.443 | 0.01 |
| Antiplatelets glycoprotein IIb/IIIa | 0.546 | 0.01 |
| Anticardiolipin | 0.686 | 0.01 |
| Interleukin 6 | 0.180 | 0.01 |
| hs C-reactive protein | 0.149 | 0.01 |

$r$—coefficient of correlation.

## 4. Discussion

Our understanding of the pathogenesis of the acute thrombotic complications of the atherosclerosis has burgeoned in recent years. We now understand that many acute thrombotic coronary occlusions do not necessarily result from critically stenosed sites in the arteries. This distinction between lesions versus lumen diameter challenges our traditional reliance upon coronary anatomy [26–29]. Atherothrombosis is the major determinant of acute ischemic cardiovascular events, such as myocardial infarction and stroke. Thus, its understanding is essential to enable the development of targeted and more effective therapies. Although related in part to alterations in lipid metabolism, atherosclerosis is now considered a primarily immune-mediated disease [30].

The role of the immune system and autoimmune reactions in atherosclerosis appears to be a double edged-sword, with some of them being proatherogenic, while others can be antiatherogenic depending on what stage in the long-lasting process of atherosclerosis.

The purpose of our study, then, was to investigate the potential interrelationship between chronic exposure to oral pathogens, the antibodies produced against them, and elevations in the levels of markers of immune-inflammatory response in acute, urgent, and lifesaving clinical settings in patients with acute myocardial atherothrombosis.

Our results indicated that IgG antibodies against oral pathogens (oral aerobes/facultative anaerobes) and oral obligate anaerobes were highly present in the patients with acute myocardial infarction, suggesting high exposure to chronic infection. Upon searching the literature, we found that it is has been recently proposed that chronic infections (bacterial *Helicobacter pylori*, *Chlamydia pneumonia,* and periodontitis among many others) can contribute to the development of atheromas either directly (endothelial injury, invasion of endothelial cells, and platelet aggregation) or indirectly (production of antibodies to lipopolysaccharide, cytokines and dysfunction of the immune system) [31].

In response to infection (e.g., oral bacteria among others), the immune system jumps into action, deploying cells as well as antibodies in order to recognize and destroy the invaders. Antibodies are molecules produced by plasma cells and B cells against the "enemy"—the infectious agent. However, owing to molecular mimicry or antigenic similarity between these infectious agents and human tissue structure, in a genetically susceptible individual, components of the body's immune system target one or more types of the person's own tissue, which may result in autoimmunity [18, 32, 33].

Taking these together, evidence indicates that infectious agents play a pivotal role in the induction of autoimmunities. The question of how infectious agents contribute to autoimmunity has continued to be of interest to clinical and basic researchers and immunologists in general [18].

In many cases, it is not a single infection but rather the "burden of infections" from childhood that is responsible for the induction of autoimmunity [18]. Thus, oral pathogens can also give their contribution towards autoimmunity.

An example of this is the case of anti-phospholipid (aPL) syndrome, in which anticardiolipin and anti-beta-2 glycoprotein I pathogenic antibodies are detected. In patients with systemic lupus erythematosus (SLE) or antiphospholipid syndrome, serum complexes and anti-beta-2 glycoprotein-I-oxidized-LDL complex autoantibodies are elevated [34, 35]. Similarly, such complexes and antibodies found in the bloodstream of patients with vascular complications, such as myocardial infarction and unstable angina, strongly associate with arterial thrombosis.

Our results indicated that anti-beta-2 glycoprotein antibodies and anticardiolipin antibodies (aCLs) can be detected in patients with myocardial infarction.

The data is similar from case-control studies that demonstrate the association of aCLs with stroke and acute myocardial infarction [32, 36]. Also, the authors found that IgG/IgM/IgA aCL and IgA for anti-beta-2 glycoprotein I associated with increased risk of ischemic stroke, arterial thrombosis, atherosclerotic immune process, acute myocardial infarction, and peripheral vascular diseases [36]. Although the exact mechanisms remain unknown, anti-beta-2 glycoprotein I was thought to interact with beta 2-glycoprotein I on the endothelial membrane and induce inflammatory reactions [37].

Artenjak et al. [38] reported on the correlation between aPL and cardiovascular risk in nonautoimmune settings. Taken together, these results did not demonstrate a clear association between aPL and acute cardiovascular events.

Beta-2-glycoprotein I is present at high concentrations in the blood stream and is expressed by many cell populations, including endothelial cells, lymphocytes, and monocytes. It binds negatively not only charged molecules, including phospholipids, heparin, and oxLDL, but also the surface of activated platelets and the membrane of apoptotic cells [39–43]. In our study population, those autoantibodies were highly present in patients with acute myocardial infarction. One should have in mind that antiendothelial cell antibodies may cause vasculitis as part of an autoimmune response. This is a heterogeneous family of antibodies. The IgG antibodies are highly present also in the blood sera of SLE patients and may mediate immunologic injury to blood vessel walls.

Finally, significant elevation in the levels of IL-6, CRP and endothelial cell antibody indicates that inflammation driven by oral pathogens plays a significant role in the development of atherothrombosis [44–48].

## 5. Conclusion

Taking together the above presented data, it appears that oral pathogens, through the release of toxins, seem to be capable of inducing changes in the host proteins. These can be recognized by the immune system, triggering an inflammatory process associated with the clinical manifestation of atherosclerosis—acute myocardial infarction. This and other immunopathogenic mechanisms need to be further elucidated.

## Conflict of Interests

The authors declare that there is no conflict of interests regarding the publication of this paper.

## Acknowledgments

The presented results are part of the study protocol designed for a Ph.D. thesis with the title "The role of infectious agents in acute coronary syndromes" which was presented at the Medical Faculty University of Nis and Clinical Center of Nis, Serbia, which were Dr. Burazor's employers at the time. The Ph.D. thesis was successfully defended. Dr. Burazor wants to thank Professor Aristo Vojdani and his employees for all their help and support.

## References

[1] P. Bouchard, P. Boutouyrie, F. D'aiuto et al., "European workshop in periodontal health and cardiovascular disease consensus document," *European Heart Journal, Supplement B*, vol. 12, pp. B13–B22, 2010.

[2] M. Sanz, F. D'aiuto, J. Deanfield, and F. Fernandez-Avilés, "European workshop in periodontal health and cardiovascular disease—scientific evidence on the association between periodontal and cardiovascular diseases: a review of the literature," *European Heart Journal, Supplement B*, vol. 12, pp. B3–B12, 2010.

[3] P. B. Lockhart, A. F. Bolger, P. N. Papapanou et al., "Periodontal disease and atherosclerotic vascular disease: does the evidence support an independent association?: a scientific statement from the american heart association," *Circulation*, vol. 125, pp. 2520–2544, 2012.

[4] W. J. Loesche, "Association of the oral flora with important medical diseases," *Current Opinion in Periodontology*, vol. 4, pp. 21–28, 1997.

[5] L. M. Buja and J. T. Willerson, "Role of inflammation in coronary plaque disruption," *Circulation*, vol. 89, no. 1, pp. 503–505, 1994.

[6] M. Davis, "The birth, growth and consequences of the atherosclerotic plaque," *Dialogues in Cardiovascular Medicine*, vol. 4, pp. 115–178, 1999.

[7] G. K. Hansson, "Immune mechanisms in atherosclerosis," *Arteriosclerosis, Thrombosis, and Vascular Biology*, vol. 21, no. 12, pp. 1876–1890, 2001.

[8] L. T. Lineberger and T. J. DeMarco, "Evaluation of transient bacteremia following routine periodontal procedures," *Journal of Periodontology*, vol. 44, pp. 747–760, 1973.

[9] L. R. Freedman and J. Valone Jr., "Experimental infective endocarditis," *Progress in Cardiovascular Diseases*, vol. 22, no. 3, pp. 169–180, 1979.

[10] R. B. Roberts, A. G. Krieger, N. L. Schiller, and K. C. Gross, "Viridans streptococcal endocarditis: the role of various species, including pyridoxal-dependent streptococci," *Reviews of Infectious Diseases*, vol. 1, no. 6, pp. 955–965, 1979.

[11] C. F. van Reyn, B. S. Levy, and R. D. Arbeit, "Infective endocarditis: an analysis based on strict case definitions," *Annals of Internal Medicine*, vol. 94, no. 4, part 1, pp. 505–518, 1981.

[12] S. E. J. Young, "Aetiology and epidemiology of infective endocarditis in England and Wales," *Journal of Antimicrobial Chemotherapy A*, vol. 20, pp. 7–15, 1987.

[13] H. N. Shah and M. D. Collins, "Proposal for reclassification of *Bacteroides asaccharolyticus, Bacteroides gingivalis*, and *Bacteroides endodontalis* in a new genus, Porphyromonas," *International Journal of Systematic Bacteriology*, vol. 38, no. 1, pp. 128–131, 1988.

[14] H. N. Shah and D. M. Collins, "Prevotella, a new genus to include *Bacteroides melaninogenicus* and related species formerly classified in the genus *Bacteroides*," *International Journal of Systematic Bacteriology*, vol. 40, no. 2, pp. 205–208, 1990.

[15] M. C. Herzberg, K. Gong, G. D. MacFarlane et al., "Phenotypic characterization of *Streptococcus sanguis* virulence factors associated with bacterial endocarditis," *Infection and Immunity*, vol. 58, no. 2, pp. 515–522, 1990.

[16] M. Ogrendik, S. Kokino, F. Ozdemir, P. S. Bird, and S. Hamlet, "Serum antibodies to oral anaerobic bacteria in patients with rheumatoid arthritis," *Medscape General Medicine*, vol. 7, no. 2, article 2, 2005.

[17] C. Cugini, V. Klepac-Ceraj, E. Rackaityte et al., "*Porphyromonas gingivalis*: keeping the pathos out of the biont," *Journal of Oral Microbiology*, 2013.

[18] J. G. Routsias, J. D. Goules, A. Goules, G. Charalampakis, and D. Pikazis, "Autopathogenic correlation of periodontitis and rheumatoid arthritis," *Rheumatology*, vol. 50, no. 7, pp. 1189–1193, 2011.

[19] D. Farquharson, J. P. Butcher, and S. Culshaw, "Periodontitis, *Porphyromonas*, and the pathogenesis of rheumatoid arthritis," *Mucosal Immunology*, vol. 5, no. 2, pp. 112–120, 2012.

[20] M. S. Tonetti, F. D'Aiuto, L. Nibali et al., "Treatment of periodontitis and endothelial function," *The New England Journal of Medicine*, vol. 356, no. 9, pp. 911–920, 2007.

[21] S. C. Holt, L. Kesavalu, S. Walker, and C. A. Genco, "Virulence factors of *Porphyromonas gingivalis*," *Periodontology 2000*, vol. 20, no. 1, pp. 168–238, 1999.

[22] A. J. Kinloch, S. Alzabin, W. Brintnell et al., "Immunization with *Porphyromonas gingivalis* enolase induces autoimmunity to mammalian $\alpha$-enolase and arthritis in DR4-IE-transgenic mice," *Arthritis and Rheumatism*, vol. 63, no. 12, pp. 3818–3823, 2011.

[23] J. A. Hill, D. A. Bell, W. Brintnell et al., "Arthritis induced by posttranslationally modified (citrullinated) fibrinogen in DR4-IE transgenic mice," *Journal of Experimental Medicine*, vol. 205, no. 4, pp. 967–979, 2008.

[24] K. Lundberg, N. Wegner, T. Yucel-Lindberg, and P. J. Venables, "Periodontitis in RA—the citrullinated enolase connection," *Nature Reviews Rheumatology*, vol. 6, no. 12, pp. 727–730, 2010.

[25] K. Thygesen, J. Alpert, M. Simoons et al., "Third universal definition of myocardial infarction," *Circulation*, vol. 126, pp. 2020–2035, 2012.

[26] A. Woods, D. J. Brull, S. E. Humphries, and H. E. Montgomery, "Genetics of inflammation and risk of coronary artery disease: the central role of interleukin-6," *European Heart Journal*, vol. 21, no. 19, pp. 1574–1583, 2000.

[27] D. A. Vorchheimer and V. Fuster, "Inflammatory markers in coronary artery disease: let prevention douse the flames," *Journal of the American Medical Association*, vol. 286, no. 17, pp. 2154–2156, 2001.

[28] G. Hansson, "Inflammation, atherosclerosis and coronary artery disease," *The New England Journal of Medicine*, vol. 352, pp. 1685–1695, 2005.

[29] P. M. Ridker, N. Rifai, M. J. Stampfer, and C. H. Hennekens, "Plasma concentration of interleukin-6 and the risk of future myocardial infarction among apparently healthy men," *Circulation*, vol. 101, no. 15, pp. 1767–1772, 2000.

[30] F. Carbone, A. Neoncini, F. Mach et al., "Evidence on the pathogenic role of autoantibodies in acute cardiovascular disease," *Journal of Thrombosis and Haemostasis*, vol. 109, pp. 854–868, 2013.

[31] A. Pucar, J. Milasin, V. Lekovic et al., "Correlation between atherosclerosis and periodontal putative pathogenic bacterial infections in coronary and internal mammary arteries," *Journal of Periodontology*, vol. 78, no. 4, pp. 677–682, 2007.

[32] S. Kivity, N. Agmon-Levin, M. Blank, and Y. Shoenfeld, "Infections and autoimmunity—friends or foes?" *Trends in Immunology*, vol. 30, no. 8, pp. 409–414, 2009.

[33] M. B. A. Oldstone, M. Nerenberg, P. Southern, J. Price, and H. Lewicki, "Virus infection triggers insulin-dependent diabetes mellitus in a transgenic model: role of anti-self (virus) immune response," *Cell*, vol. 65, no. 2, pp. 319–331, 1999.

[34] G.-P. Shi, "Immunomodulation of vascular diseases: atherosclerosis and autoimmunity," *European Journal of Vascular and Endovascular Surgery*, vol. 39, no. 4, pp. 485–494, 2010.

[35] H. P. McNeil, R. J. Simpson, C. N. Chesterman, and S. A. Krilis, "Anti-phospholipid antibodies are directed against a complex antigen that includes a lipid-binding inhibitor of coagulation: $\beta$2-glycoprotein I (apolipoprotein H)," *Proceedings of the National Academy of Sciences of the United States of America*, vol. 87, no. 11, pp. 4120–4124, 1990.

[36] R. L. Brey, R. D. Abbott, J. D. Curb et al., "$\beta$2-glycoprotein 1-dependent anticardiolipin antibodies and risk of ischemic stroke and myocardial infarction: the Honolulu Heart Program," *Stroke*, vol. 32, no. 8, pp. 1701–1706, 2001.

[37] K. Kobayashi, M. Kishi, T. Atsumi et al., "Circulating oxidized LDL forms complexes with $\beta$2-glycoprotein I: implication as an atherogenic autoantigen," *Journal of Lipid Research*, vol. 44, no. 4, pp. 716–726, 2003.

[38] A. Artenjak, K. Lakota, M. Frank et al., "Antiphospholipid antibodies as non-traditional risk factors in atherosclerosis based cardiovascular diseases without overt autoimmunity. A critical updated review," *Autoimmunity Reviews*, vol. 11, pp. 873–882, 2012.

[39] P. G. de Groot and J. C. M. Meijers, "$\beta$2-glycoprotein I: evolution, structure and function," *Journal of Thrombosis and Haemostasis*, vol. 9, no. 7, pp. 1275–1284, 2011.

[40] J. Fan and T. Watanabe, "Inflammatory reactions in the pathogenesis of atherosclerosis," *Journal of Atherosclerosis and Thrombosis*, vol. 10, no. 2, pp. 63–71, 2003.

[41] R. P. Tracy, R. N. Lemaitre, B. M. Psaty et al., "Relationship of C-reactive protein to risk of cardiovascular disease in the elderly: results from the Cardiovascular Health Study and the Rural Health Promotion Project," *Arteriosclerosis, Thrombosis, and Vascular Biology*, vol. 17, no. 6, pp. 1121–1127, 1997.

[42] W. Koenig, M. Sund, M. Fröhlich et al., "C-reactive protein, a sensitive marker of inflammation, predicts future risk of coronary heart disease in initially healthy middle-aged men: results from the MONICA (monitoring trends and determinants in cardiovascular disease) Augsburg cohort study, 1984 to 1992," *Circulation*, vol. 99, no. 2, pp. 237–242, 1999.

[43] A. D. Pradhan, J. E. Manson, J. E. Rossouw et al., "Inflammatory biomarkers, hormone replacement therapy, and incident coronary heart disease: prospective analysis from the women's health initiative observational study," *Journal of the American Medical Association*, vol. 288, no. 8, pp. 980–987, 2002.

[44] S. E. Epstein, Y. F. Zhou, and J. Zhu, "Infection and atherosclerosis: emerging mechanistic paradigms," *Circulation*, vol. 100, no. 4, pp. e20–e28, 1999.

[45] A. Vojdani, "Antibodies as predictors of autoimmune diseases and cancer," *Expert Opinion on Medical Diagnostics*, vol. 2, no. 6, pp. 593–605, 2008.

[46] J. A. Vita and J. Loscalzo, "Shouldering the risk factor burden: infection, atherosclerosis, and the vascular endothelium," *Circulation*, vol. 106, no. 2, pp. 164–166, 2002.

[47] K. Lundberg, N. Wegner, T. Yucel-Lindberg, and P. J. Venables, "Periodontitis in RA-the citrullinated enolase connection," *Nature Reviews Rheumatology*, vol. 6, no. 12, pp. 727–730, 2010.

[48] T. Dörner and A. Hansen, "Autoantibodies in normals—the value of predicting rheumatoid arthritis," *Arthritis Research and Therapy*, vol. 6, no. 6, pp. 282–284, 2004.

# 9

# Predisposition to Cervical Atypia in Systemic Lupus Erythematosus: A Clinical and Cytopathological Study

**Hend Hilal Al-Sherbeni,[1] Ahmed Mohamed Fahmy,[2] and Nadine Sherif[3]**

[1]*Rheumatology and Rehabilitation Department, Faculty of Medicine, Cairo University, Cairo, Egypt*
[2]*Pathology Department, National Cancer Institute (NCI), Cairo University, Cairo, Egypt*
[3]*Gynecology and Obstetrics Department, Faculty of Medicine, Cairo University, Cairo, Egypt*

Correspondence should be addressed to Ahmed Mohamed Fahmy; ama_fahmy@hotmail.com

Academic Editor: Yehuda Shoenfeld

*Introduction.* Systemic lupus erythematosus (SLE) is a complex disease with variable presentations, course, and prognosis. The female genital tract may be a potential target organ in SLE since cervical inflammation may be associated with disease activity. An increase in cervical dysplasia, a precursor of cervical cancer, has been reported in females with SLE. *Aim of the Work.* This work aimed to study the prevalence of abnormal cervicovaginal smears in patients with systemic lupus erythematosus (SLE) and to correlate abnormal smear findings with exposure to infection with human papilloma virus (HPV) in SLE patients. *Patients and Methods.* Thirty-two patients with SLE, fulfilling the 1997 revised criteria for the classification of SLE, were included in this study. They were subjected to full history taking, clinical examination, laboratory investigations, and cervicovaginal smearing. Twenty healthy subjects not known to suffer from any rheumatological disease were used as controls, and they were subjected to cervicovaginal smearing. *Results.* Four out of 32 SLE patients showed abnormal Pap smears (12.5%) compared to none showing any cervical changes in the control group (0%). Among these 4 patients, 3 were having ASCU and one was having LSIL (HPV). *Conclusion.* Cervicovaginal smearing is an easy, economic, safe, repeatable, and noninvasive technique for screening and early detection of cervical neoplastic lesions in SLE.

## 1. Introduction

Systemic lupus erythematosus (SLE) is an autoimmune disease which is characterized by immune system disturbance. Physicians have been forced to deal with long term complications of SLE disease itself or complications due to its treatment in spite of improved survival rates [1].

Cervical cancer is the second most common cause of death worldwide (after breast cancer) [2]. Cervical cancer constitutes also 25% of female cancers in developing countries and is considered the most common cancer [3]. The association between human papilloma virus (HPV) and cervical squamous cell cancer is higher than the association between smoking and lung cancer [4]. HPV has been implicated for 99.7% of cervical squamous cell cancer worldwide [5].

As HPV cannot be cultured in the laboratory from clinical specimens, the primary diagnostic tools have been cytology and histology in the form of Pap smear [6].

The cervicovaginal smear or Papanicolaou-stained (Pap) smear is named after the pathologist George Papanicolaou, who introduced the method in 1949 before the cause of cervical cancer is known [7]. Since its introduction, the Pap smear has helped in reducing the cervical cancer incidence and mortality rates by half to two-thirds [8]. Pap smear is a screening tool that detects the changes in cells of the transformation zone of the cervix. Mostly, these changes are caused by HPV.

An important complication of SLE is increased incidence of malignancy including cervical cancers [9]. Autoimmune system dysfunction, disease activity, recurrent infections, and immunosuppressive medication exposure may constitute explanations which suggest increased incidence of malignancy in SLE [10].

Women having SLE have a higher rate of infection with HPV than others. And so lupus patients have a higher incidence of abnormal Pap smears than others not having lupus. This rate is significantly higher among women in the first five years following their diagnosis than for those who had lupus for more than 10 years [11].

## 2. Patients and Methods

Thirty-three cases, proven to be SLE patients, fulfilling the ACR criteria for classification of SLE [12], and attending the Inpatient Unit of Rheumatology and Rehabilitation Department, Faculty of Medicine, Cairo University hospitals, in the period between January 2011 and September 2011, were included in this study.

Inclusion criteria included the following:

(i) SLE female patients,

(ii) females in the childbearing period,

(iii) females not pregnant at the time of the Pap smear intake,

(iv) females consenting to be included in the study.

Exclusion criteria included the following:

(i) patients with bleeding,

(ii) pregnant ladies,

(iii) patients refusing examination or participation in the study,

(iv) virgin or menopausal ladies.

Patients included in the study were subjected to full history taking, general examination, local and bimanual examination, speculum examination with Pap smear intake (see Section 2.1), and full laboratory workup. Informed consent was obtained from all patients after full explanation of the aim and procedures of the study; data were collected after informing the patients about the purpose of the study; the patients had the right to withdraw from the study without giving any reasons. Privacy and confidentiality of the obtained data was insured for all participants. The ethical committee of Kasr Al Ainy hospitals approved this study before starting.

*2.1. Technique.* Patients were examined in the examination room, in the lithotomy position, using bimanual examination to determine the size of the uterus, its direction, and any feeling of abnormalities in the uterus or cervix; then exposure of the cervix by Cusco's speculum was done, followed by cleaning with isotonic saline solution and the intake of the Pap smear.

Pap smear test is based on cytological examination of cells shed from the ectocervix. In this study, it was performed using a cytobrush to wipe cells from the ectocervical canal and an Ayre spatula to wipe cells from the surface of the ectocervix. Cells obtained were spread on 4 slides (2 normal slides and another 2 positively charged slides). These cells were then fixed by ethyl alcohol and stained with special stains.

Pap smear is an office procedure, with an accuracy rate > 80%; however, it carries a small percentage of both false positive and false negative results (15–25%) [13, 14]. Smears were stained by hematoxylin and eosin (H&E) stain.

*2.2. Immunostaining.* Smears were immunostained using labeled streptavidin biotin (LSAB Kit, Dako) according to the provided manufacturers' manual. The smear slides were fixed overnight in absolute alcohol. After blocking endogenous peroxidase, human papilloma virus (HBV) ab-3 monoclonal antibody, ready to use (Thermo scientific, USA), was applied and incubated for 30 minutes, followed by secondary biotinylated antibody for 30 minutes. 3,3′-Diaminobenzidine tetrahydrochloride (DAB) solution was used as the final chromogen.

*2.3. Immunostaining Analysis.* Immunostaining results were considered positive nuclear (+) or negative nuclear (−) staining with a positive control used with each run provided by the manufacturer. Negative controls for nonspecific binding, incubated with secondary antibodies only, were processed and revealed no signals.

## 3. Results

This study included 32 patients with SLE; all were females. Their ages ranged from 21 to 50 years with a mean of $31.06 \pm 7.170$ years. Disease duration ranged from 1 year to 16 years with a mean of $6.13 \pm 4.139$ years. A group of 20 age matched females served as control. Their ages ranged from 20 to 45 years with a mean of $30.2 \pm 7.5$ years.

The clinical and laboratory features of SLE patients reported in this study were obtained at time of Pap smears (Tables 1, 2, and 3).

15/32 (46.9%) patients showed positive changes in renal biopsy and they were as follows: one patient showed grade I renal affection, two patients showed grade II, one patient showed grade I-II, one patient showed grade II–V, six patients showed grade III, and one patient showed grade III-IV, while three patients had grade IV renal affection.

21/32 (65.6%) patients were receiving azathioprine (Imuran) with a dose ranging from 50 to 150 mg with a mean of $100 \pm 15.811$. 29/32 (90.6%) patients were receiving hydroxychloroquine (Hydroquine) with a dose ranging from 200 to 400 mg with a mean of $379.31 \pm 61.987$. 17/32 (53.1%) received pulse cyclophosphamide therapy. All patients (100%) were receiving steroids with a dose ranging from 10 to 60 mg with a mean of $25.23 \pm 10.632$.

SLEDAI activity score was performed to SLE patients at study time and was as follows:

(i) 20 out of 32 patients (62.5%) had mild disease activity,

(ii) 10 out of 32 patients (31.25%) had moderate disease activity,

(iii) 2 out of 32 patients (6.25%) had severe activity of SLE.

*3.1. Results of Cervicovaginal Smear Examination.* All cases showed adequate cellular smears with a mixture of superficial, intermediate, and parabasal epithelial cells (Figure 1). Adequacy of smears was determined by the presence of groups

TABLE 1: Showing percentage of each clinical manifestations of SLE patients.

| Clinical feature | Number of patients | % |
|---|---|---|
| Constitutional manifestations | | |
| (Fever and fatigue) | 32 | 100% |
| Mucocutaneous manifestations | | |
| Malar rash | 30 | 93.8% |
| Oral ulcers | 22 | 68.8% |
| Alopecia | 6 | 18.75% |
| Musculoskeletal manifestations | | |
| Arthritis | 31 | 96.9% |
| Vascular manifestations | | |
| Raynaud's phenomenon | 5 | 15.625% |
| Systemic hypertension | 5 | 15.625% |
| Pulmonary manifestations | | |
| Pleurisy | 20 | 62.5% |
| Pleural effusion | 1 | 3.125% |
| Cardiac manifestations | | |
| Pericarditis | 1 | 3.125% |
| Pericardial effusion | 0 | 0% |
| Renal involvement | | |
| Proteinuria | 20 | 62.5% |
| Urinary casts | 8 | 25% |
| Neurological manifestations | | |
| Headache | 12 | 37.5% |
| Seizure | 1 | 3.125% |
| Stroke | 1 | 3.125% |
| Psychosis | 1 | 3.125% |
| Hematological manifestations | | |
| Anemia | 9 | 28.1% |

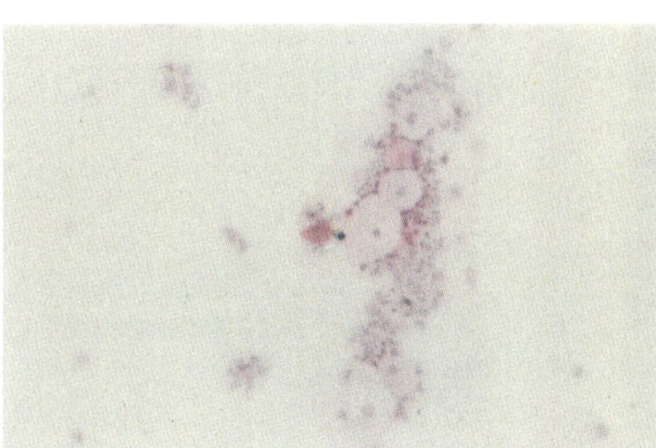

FIGURE 1: Superficial, intermediate, and parabasal epithelial cells (H&E, ×400).

of endocervical cells (Figure 2). Neutrophilic infiltration ranged from mild to marked infiltration with no evidence of specific genital infection in any of the cases. Three cases showed ASCUS cells (Figure 3). One case showed low grade squamous intraepithelial lesion (low grade dysplasia, low grade CIN) with koilocytic changes. This was confirmed by positive nuclear immunostaining for HPV type 16 (Figure 4).

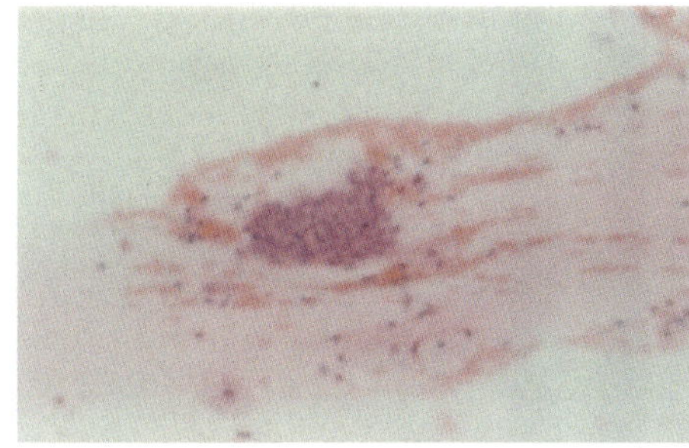

FIGURE 2: Groups of endocervical cells in cervicovaginal smear (HX, ×100).

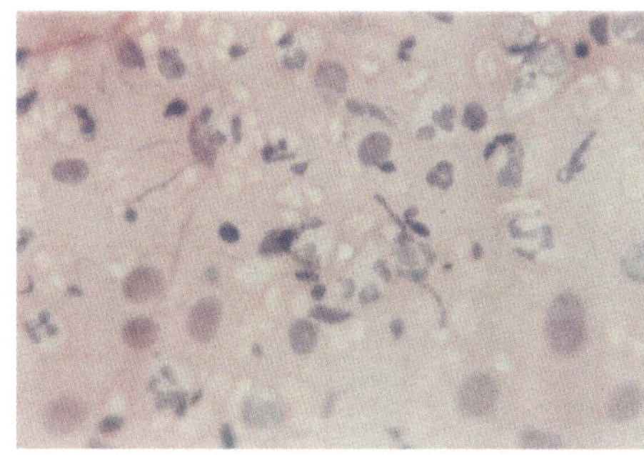

FIGURE 3: Atypical squamous cells of undetermined origin (ASCUS) (H&E, ×400).

*3.2. Cyclophosphamide Exposure.* Despite obvious tendency of SLE patients to develop abnormal cervicovaginal smears, especially after CYC exposure, no statistical significant correlation was found between systemic lupus erythematosus and abnormal cervicovaginal smears nor between CYC and abnormal cervicovaginal smears which could be explained by small number of patients in our study.

## 4. Discussion

In this study, we want to find out whether lupus patients are at increased risk of abnormal Pap smears and whether they are also at increased risk of HPV infections specially the oncogenic subtypes (16, 18). Also we want to highlight the effect of different medications (cyclophosphamide, hydroxychloroquine, and steroids) on Pap smear and cervical changes.

Our study showed that there are 4 out of 32 SLE patients, having abnormal Pap smear (12.5%); this result is comparable with Esmaeili and Ghahremanzadeh who found that the frequency of abnormal Pap smear testing was higher in patients with SLE (8.1%) compared to control group [15].

The present study showed only one case of HPV type 16, having abnormal Pap smear in the form of LSIL (low grade intraepithelial lesion) among the whole 32 cases studied. This cannot be depending on regarding confirming the increased incidence of HPV infection, specially the oncogenic type with SLE disease; however, the study done by Nath et al. in 2007 showed that UK women with a recent SLE diagnosis had disturbingly elevated levels of HPV infections (particularly

TABLE 2: Showing laboratory data of SLE patients.

| Lab | Minimum | Maximum | Mean | ±SD |
|---|---|---|---|---|
| HB | 6 gm/dL | 14.2 | 10.309 | 1.9734 |
| TLC | $1.9 \times 10^3/mm^3$ | $21.3 \times 10^3$ | $7.497 \times 10^3$ | $4.4902 \times 10^3$ |
| PLT | $55 \times 10^3/mm^3$ | $442 \times 10^3$ | $260.59 \times 10^3$ | $93.832 \times 10^3$ |
| ALT | 7 IU/mL | 83 IU/mL | 21.47 IU/mL | 15.110 IU/mL |
| Creatinine | 0.4 | 2.98 | 0.9356 | 0.61415 |

TABLE 3: Showing autoimmune profile and complement.

| | Number of patients | Percentage |
|---|---|---|
| Positive ANA | 27 | 84.4% |
| Positive anti-DNA | 14 | 43.8% |
| Consumed C3 | 5 | 15.6% |

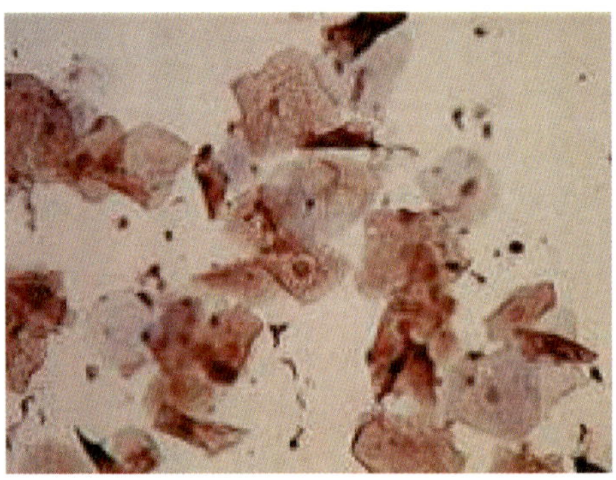

FIGURE 4: A case with HPV type 16 infected cells showing koilocytic changes (CIN I) (×400).

with HPV 16), abnormal cervical cytology, and SIL. Larger sample size in our population may have confirmed the results of Nath study [16]. The same study showed also the higher incidence of abnormal Pap smear in women with SLE, especially in the first 5 years of diagnosis of SLE; in our results, we had 4 patients with abnormal Pap smear in the form of ASCUS and LSIL.

Previous studies showed the effect of different medications used to treat SLE patients on the cervical changes and hence the Pap smear results. Bateman et al. [17] showed that there was a significant decrease in time to dysplasia in patients given IV-C (intravenous cyclophosphamide), with previous dysplasia compared to those without. These preliminary data suggest that IV-C causes an increased number of abnormal Pap smear in SLE patients, particularly those with previous dysplasia. In our study, 17 out of 32 patients were receiving IV-C, and we have 4 patients with cervical dysplasia; one of them was receiving IV-C. So due to these small numbers, we could not state a statistical correlation between IV-C and cervical changes.

Other studies, as Nath et al. [16], stated, similar to us, that it was not possible for them to interpret whether their patients treated with hydroxychloroquine and having cervical changes are having these changes due to the medications used or due to the SLE disease itself, specially that usually the patient is receiving a combination of more than one drug.

Regarding the limitations in our study, the main issue is the small number of the studied population; also they were all receiving medications (21 were receiving azathioprine, 29 were receiving hydroxychloroquine, 17 were receiving cyclophosphamide, and 32 were receiving steroids), so we can never confirm whether the cervical changes were due to the disease SLE itself or due to the medications taken.

Despite its limitation and its small sample size, this study provides further evidence that women having SLE are at increased risk of developing cervical changes which may be HPV of oncogenic subtype compared to their equivalent (4 out of 32 patients with SLE developed cervical changes, compared to none out of 20 control). And as Pap smear is a simple, safe, repeatable procedure, it is recommended regularly to all SLE patients, especially in the first 5 years of diagnosis.

## Conflict of Interests

The authors declare that there is no conflict of interests regarding the publication of this paper.

## References

[1] J. Cibere, J. Sibley, and M. Haga, "Systemic lupus Erythematosus," *Rheumatology*, vol. 48, no. 10, pp. 1222–1226, 2009.

[2] X. W. Jin, J. Cash, and A. W. Kennedy, "Human papillomavirus typing and the reduction of cervical cancer risk," *Cleveland Clinic Journal of Medicine*, vol. 66, no. 9, pp. 533–539, 1999.

[3] C. D. Harro, Y.-Y. S. Pang, R. B. S. Roden et al., "Safety and immunogenicity trial in adult volunteers of a human papillomavirus 16 L1 virus-like particle vaccine," *Journal of the National Cancer Institute*, vol. 93, no. 4, pp. 284–292, 2001.

[4] E. L. Franco, "Cancer causes revisited: human papillomavirus and cervical neoplasia," *Journal of the National Cancer Institute*, vol. 87, no. 11, pp. 779–780, 1995.

[5] J. M. M. Walboomers, M. V. Jacobs, M. M. Manos et al., "Human papillomavirus is a necessary cause of invasive cervical cancer worldwide," *The Journal of Pathology*, vol. 189, no. 1, pp. 12–19, 1999.

[6] P. Holowaty, A. B. Miller, T. Rohan, and T. To, "Natural history of dysplasia of the uterine cervix," *Journal of the National Cancer Institute*, vol. 91, no. 3, pp. 252–258, 1999.

[7] G. N. Papanicolaou, "A survey of the actualities and potentialities of exfoliative cytology in cancer diagnosis," *Annals of internal medicine*, vol. 31, no. 4, pp. 661–674, 1949.

[8] R. J. Kurman, D. E. Henson, A. L. Herbst, K. L. Noller, and M. H. Schiffman, "Interim guidelines for management of abnormal

cervical cytology. The 1992 National Cancer Workshop," *The Journal of the American Medical Association*, vol. 271, no. 23, pp. 1866–1869, 1994.

[9] E. Kriss, L. Kovasc, and P. Szodoray, "Malignancies in systemic lupus erythematosus," *Autoimmunity Reviews*, vol. 9, no. 4, pp. 195–199, 2010.

[10] M. Ciołkiewicz, I. Domysławska, A. Ciołkiewicz, P. A. Klimiuk, and A. Kuryliszyn-Moskal, "Coexistence of systemic sclerosis, scleroderma-like syndromes and neoplastic diseases," *Polskie Archiwum Medycyny Wewnetrznej*, vol. 118, no. 3, pp. 119–126, 2008.

[11] R. Nath, C. Mant, J. Luxton et al., "High risk of human papillomavirus type 16 infections and of development of squamous intraepithelial lesions in systemic lupus erythematosus patients," *Arthritis & Rheumatism*, vol. 57, no. 4, pp. 619–625, 2007.

[12] M. C. Hochberg, "Updating the American College of Rheumatology revised criteria for the classification of systemic lupus erythematosus," *Arthritis and rheumatism*, vol. 40, no. 9, p. 1725, 1997.

[13] A. Vince and S. Z. Lepej, "Diagnostic methods and techniques in cervical cancer prevention part II: molecular diagnostics of HPV infection," *Medicinski Glasnik*, vol. 7, no. 1, pp. 18–25, 2010.

[14] N. Behtash and N. Mehrdad, "Cervical cancer: screening and prevention," *Asian Pacific Journal of Cancer Prevention*, vol. 7, no. 4, pp. 683–686, 2006.

[15] H. Esmaeili and K. Ghahremanzadeh, "Association of pap smear abnormalities with autoimmune disorders," *Pakistan Journal of Biological Sciences*, vol. 14, no. 10, pp. 600–604, 2011.

[16] R. Nath, C. Mant, J. Luxton et al., "High risk of human papillomavirus type 16 infections and of development of cervical squamous intraepithelial lesions in systemic lupus erythematosus patients," *Arthritis Care and Research*, vol. 57, no. 4, pp. 619–625, 2007.

[17] H. Bateman, Y. Yazici, L. Leff, M. Peterson, and S. A. Paget, "Increased cervical dysplasia in intravenous cyclophosphamide-treated patients with SLE: a preliminary study," *Lupus*, vol. 9, no. 7, pp. 542–544, 2000.

# 10

# Serum Leptin Levels in Treatment-Naive Patients with Clinically Isolated Syndrome or Relapsing-Remitting Multiple Sclerosis

**Maria Eleftheria Evangelopoulos, Georgios Koutsis, and Manolis Markianos**

*Department of Neurology, Eginition Hospital, Athens University Medical School, 74 Vassilisis Sophias Avenue, 11528 Athens, Greece*

Correspondence should be addressed to Maria Eleftheria Evangelopoulos; evangelopoulos@yahoo.com

Academic Editor: Dennis Bourdette

Several studies have investigated leptin levels in patients with multiple sclerosis (MS) with somewhat conflicting results. They have all focused on patients with established relapsing-remitting (RR) MS but have not specifically looked at patients with clinically isolated syndrome (CIS) suggestive of MS, in the early stages of disease. In this study, serum leptin levels were measured in 89 treatment-naïve patients with CIS (53 patients) or RRMS (36 patients) and 73 controls searching for differences between the groups and for associations with several disease parameters. The expected significant sexual dimorphism in leptin levels (higher levels in females) was observed in both MS patients and controls. Increased leptin levels were found in female patients with RRMS compared to female controls ($P = .003$) and female CIS patients ($P = .001$). Female CIS patients had comparable levels to controls. Leptin levels correlated positively to disease duration, but not to EDSS, in female patients with RRMS. The results of the present study do not indicate involvement of leptin in the early stages of MS. Normal leptin levels in patients with CIS suggest that leptin does not have a pathogenic role. The ratio leptin/BMI increases during disease course in female MS patients in a time-dependent and disability-independent manner.

## 1. Introduction

Leptin, a cytokine-like hormone released primarily from adipocytes, exhibits neuroendocrine properties influencing energy balance. Serum leptin levels regulate body weight by inhibiting food intake and stimulating energy expenditure and are higher in subjects with a high BMI and body fat [1, 2]. Additionally, leptin has immunomodulatory properties affecting neutrophil chemotaxis and macrophage proinflammatory cytokine expression. It also acts as a proinflammatory cytokine inducing a Th-1 immune response, thus playing a significant role in the pathogenesis of Th-1 mediated autoimmunity such as experimental autoimmune encephalomyelitis (EAE), an experimental model for multiple sclerosis (MS) [3]. In fact, leptin-deficient mice are resistant to the induction of EAE. On the other hand, activated T lymphocytes secrete leptin in active EAE brain lesions [4] indicating a role of leptin in the induction of EAE.

The role of leptin in MS pathogenesis has not yet been fully elucidated and reports have presented to some extent conflicting results. Early studies reported comparable serum leptin levels between relapsing-remitting (RR) MS patients and healthy subjects [5, 6]. Subsequently, Matarese et al. [7] found increased serum leptin in treatment-naïve RRMS patients. Higher serum leptin levels in treatment-naïve RRMS patients were also reported by Frisullo et al. [8]. Recently, two further studies have reported contradictory results. Emamgholipour et al. [9] found increased leptin levels in MS patients, whereas Rotondi et al. [10] found comparable levels with controls. Conflicting results between studies may be partly due to different sample sizes and different inclusion and exclusion criteria. Despite their differences, all studies to date have examined leptin levels in patients with established disease. These have been almost exclusively patients with clinically definite RRMS, with the exception of one study that also included patients with primary or secondary progressive MS [9]. None of these studies evaluated leptin levels at an early stage of the disease, in patients with clinically isolated syndrome (CIS) suggestive of MS, before the establishment of clinically definite MS.

The aim of the present study was to measure serum leptin levels in treatment-naive patients with CIS or RRMS and to evaluate their potential association with several disease parameters.

## 2. Subjects and Methods

Eighty-nine treatment-naïve patients (35 males, 54 females; age range from 20 to 45 years) recruited from year 2005 evenly throughout the years, as part of a larger study of CSF and serum neuroendocrine variables in MS and fulfilling the 2005 McDonald criteria for MS or possible MS were included in the study [11]. Fifty-three patients (21 males, 32 females) had CIS suggestive of MS while 36 (14 males, 22 females) had RRMS. Since there are no reports on serum leptin levels in early MS, patients at first episode (CIS) were separately evaluated in male and female subgroups. All patients had a good clinical status with low EDSS (range 0.0 to 4.0) and were drug-free at assessment, having never received any immunomodulatory therapy or corticosteroid treatment during previous relapse, as either the relapse was mild or underestimated by the patients. None of the patients had an endocrine or metabolic disease. At assessment, 54 patients (22 males) were in relapse [12] and 35 patients (13 males) in remission. Duration of illness ranged from 0.1 to 72 months for patients with CIS and from 2 to 192 months for RRMS patients. All patients were submitted to brain MRI and CSF analysis. Disability was assessed with the Expanded Disability Status Scale [13] (EDSS). Smoking history and numbers of cigarettes per day were registered.

A control group was built from 73 subjects in the same age range with patients, 30 males (age range 21 to 48 years) and 43 females (age range 18 to 48 years). Subjects, who formed part of the control group of a larger study of CSF and serum neuroendocrine variables in MS, were admitted to the hospital for diagnostic investigations and were found not to suffer from neurologic disease. More specifically, we included asymptomatic patients not only with positive serum treponemal tests, but also with negative CSF findings and a normal neurological and Mini Mental State Examination, as well as patients with a few nonspecific T2 lesions on brain MRI and a history atypical for MS, as well as normal neurological examination, cervical spine MRI, and CSF findings.

Written informed consent was obtained from all subjects and the study was approved by the Ethics Committee of Eginition Hospital, Athens University Medical School.

Body mass index (BMI, weight in kilograms divided by the square of height in meters) was calculated using self-reported height and weight. Blood samples were collected between 8.00 and 10.00 a.m. in all patients and controls, following an overnight fast. Serum was separated by centrifugation and kept at −30°C until estimation. Leptin is exceptionally stable in frozen serum samples, over two years at −20°C and over five freeze-thaw cycles [14]. Leptin was estimated in serum using the coated tube radioimmunoassay kit of DIAsource ImmunoAssays SA, Belgium. The manufacturer gives an analytical sensitivity of 0.1 ng/mL and intra- and interassay

Table 1: Clinical data of male and female therapy-naïve patients with clinically isolated syndrome suggestive of MS (CIS) or with relapsing-remitting MS (RRMS).

| | Males | | Females | |
|---|---|---|---|---|
| | CIS | RRMS | CIS | RRMS |
| $N$ | 21 | 14 | 32 | 22 |
| Duration, months | 1.7 ± 2.6 | 56.8 ± 47.4 | 3.9 ± 13.1 | 45.1 ± 46.8 |
| EDSS score | 1.6 ± 1.2 | 2.3 ± 1.1 | 1.4 ± 1.1 | 1.7 ± 1.1 |
| Smoking, no/yes | 10/11 | 4/10 | 18/14 | 13/9 |
| Relapse, no/yes | 7/14 | 6/8 | 13/19 | 9/13 |
| OB, no/yes | 7/14 | 3/11 | 9/23 | 5/17 |
| GEL, no/yes | 11/10 | 7/7 | 16/16 | 5/17 |
| Inactive/active | 5/16 | 4/10 | 8/24 | 4/18 |

OB: oligoclonal bands in CSF; GEL: gadolinium enhanced lesions in MRI; inactive: patients in remission without GEL in MRI; active: patients in relapse or with GEL in MRI.

sensitivities close to 5%. We calculated an intra-assay coefficient of variation of 4.8 ± 3.8% (mean ± SD, range 0.06 to 11.5%) for 38 samples with leptin concentrations from 2.72 to 38.3 ng/mL. Both control and patient sera were included in every batch, to compensate for interassay variation.

Differences in leptin levels among groups were evaluated using analysis of variance (ANOVA) with covariates age and BMI. Differences in leptin levels normalized to BMI (leptin/BMI ratio) were also evaluated as previously suggested [7], using ANOVA with age as covariate. The leptin/BMI ratio can serve as a measure of adipocyte leptin secreting activity, since BMI correlates significantly with body fat [15]. Analyses were performed separately for males and females, since leptin levels are higher in females [1, 16]. Multiple regression analyses were performed with dependent variable serum leptin levels or leptin/BMI ratio and independent variables clinical and data. Linear regression was used in searching for correlations of leptin and leptin/BMI ratio to age, BMI, and duration of illness. For this analysis, data for duration of illness, expressed in months, were log-transformed to achieve a normal distribution (Shapiro-Wilk test for normality).

## 3. Results

Table 1 summarizes the clinical data for CIS and RRMS patients, both males and females. Table 2 shows age, BMI, leptin levels, and leptin/BMI ratio in patients and controls. There were no significant differences in leptin or leptin/BMI ratio for the total group of patients (CIS + RRMS) when compared to controls, either for male or for female (Table 2). Significant differences were found when the three groups, controls, CIS, and RRMS, were compared for females. Patients with RRMS have higher values of both leptin and leptin/BMI ratio compared to controls and to female CIS. These differences were not significant for male patients.

Serum leptin levels and leptin/BMI ratios were higher in all female groups compared to all male groups. The known significant correlation between leptin and BMI was present in all groups, both male and female, with correlation coefficients ranging from 0.525 (CIS males) to 0.835 (RRMS females).

Table 2: Age, body mass index, serum leptin levels (ng/mL), and ratio leptin/BMI of controls and therapy-naïve patients with clinically isolated syndrome suggestive of MS (CIS) or relapsing-remitting MS (RRMS). Mean values ± SD. Evaluation by ANOVA with age and BMI as covariates for leptin and age as covariate for leptin/BMI ratio.

| Group | *N* | Age | BMI | Leptin | Leptin/BMI |
|---|---|---|---|---|---|
| Males | | | | | |
| Controls | 30 | 36.8 ± 8.1 | 25.7 ± 3.6 | 5.6 ± 3.5 | 0.21 ± 0.10 |
| Patients, all | 35 | 33.8 ± 6.3 | 25.4 ± 3.2 | 4.7 ± 1.6 | 0.18 ± 0.05 |
| *F/P* | | | | 1.92/.17 | 1.64/.21 |
| CIS | 21 | 34.7 ± 6.2 | 26.1 ± 3.7 | 4.8 ± 1.8 | 0.18 ± 0.06 |
| RRMS | 14 | 32.6 ± 6.3 | 24.4 ± 1.9 | 4.5 ± 1.5 | 0.18 ± 0.05 |
| *F/P* | | | | 1.26/.26 | 0.84/.44 |
| Females | | | | | |
| Controls | 43 | 33.6 ± 7.8 | 24.1 ± 3.8 | 10.9 ± 7.6 | 0.43 ± 0.25 |
| Patients, all | 54 | 32.9 ± 6.2 | 22.9 ± 4.3 | 10.6 ± 8.1 | 0.44 ± 0.25 |
| *F/P* | | | | 1.29/.26 | 0.01/.92 |
| CIS | 32 | 33.3 ± 6.1 | 23.3 ± 4.4 | 9.2 ± 8.5 | 0.36 ± 0.26 |
| RRMS | 22 | 32.3 ± 6.5 | 22.3 ± 4.3 | 12.6 ± 7.2 | 0.54 ± 0.20 |
| *F/P* | | | | 6.57/.002 | 3.54/.033 |
| Females, planned comparisons | | | | | |
| Controls versus CIS, *F/P* | | | | 0.31/.58 | 1.48/.23 |
| Controls versus RRMS, *F/P* | | | | 9.53/.003 | 2.98/.09 |
| CIS versus RRMS, *F/P* | | | | 11.70/.001 | 7.07/.009 |

Table 3: Multiple regression analyses with dependent variable ratio leptin/BMI, an index of adipocyte leptin secreting activity in therapy-naïve male and female MS patients. CIS: clinically isolated syndrome; RR: relapsing-remitting MS; duration of illness in months; OB: oligoclonal bands in CSF; GEL: gadolinium enhanced lesions in MRI; EDSS: score in the expanded disability status scale.

| | Males | | Females, all | | CIS-females | | RR-females | |
|---|---|---|---|---|---|---|---|---|
| *R* | .2551 | | .4503 | | .3881 | | .6693 | |
| *F* | 0.40 | | 2.44 | | 0.92 | | 2.60 | |
| *P* | .84 | | .047 | | .748 | | .06 | |
| Variable | Beta | *P* | Beta | *P* | Beta | *P* | Beta | *P* |
| Duration | −0.070 | .71 | 0.394 | **.007** | −0.230 | .25 | 0.671 | **.004** |
| Relapse | −0.1796 | .36 | −0.189 | .29 | −0.449 | .09 | 0.159 | .56 |
| OB | −0.014 | .94 | 0.024 | .86 | .108 | .61 | −0.054 | .78 |
| GEL | 0.230 | .23 | −0.101 | .49 | −0.096 | .65 | −0.176 | .42 |
| EDSS | 0.001 | .99 | 0.148 | .39 | 0.295 | .22 | −0.222 | .41 |

Age or smoking status had no effect on leptin or leptin/BMI ratio. No significant differences between groups were also found when patients were classified as active (patients who were in relapse or had GEL in MRI) and inactive (patients in remission without GEL in MRI). These variables were not introduced as independent variables in the following multiple regression analyses, in order to keep the number of independent variables low.

Multiple regression analyses were performed separately for male and female patients with dependent variable serum leptin levels or leptin/BMI ratio and independent variables duration of illness, relapse, oligoclonal bands in CSF, gadolinium enhancing lesions in MRI, and EDSS score. For male patients, no associations with any independent variable were found, either for leptin levels or leptin/BMI ratio (for leptin $R = .2387$, $F = .35$, and $P = .88$; for leptin/BMI ratio data are shown in Table 3). For females, no associations were found with relapse, presence of oligoclonal bands in CSF, gadolinium enhancing lesions in CSF, or EDSS score, but both leptin levels and leptin/BMI ratio were positively associated with the duration of illness (for leptin $R = .4573$, $F = 2.54$, $P = .04$, duration of illness beta = .395, and $P = .006$; for leptin/BMI ratio, see Table 3). This association though was present only for RR females, as revealed by performing multiple regressions separately for CIS and for RR patients (analytical data in Table 3).

The correlation between duration of illness and leptin/BMI ratio in female RR patients is depicted in Figure 1 ($n = 22$, $r = .4368$, and $P = .041$). The data for duration of illness were log-transformed to achieve a normal distribution. This correlation is not significant for male RR patients ($r = -.0734$, $P = .80$).

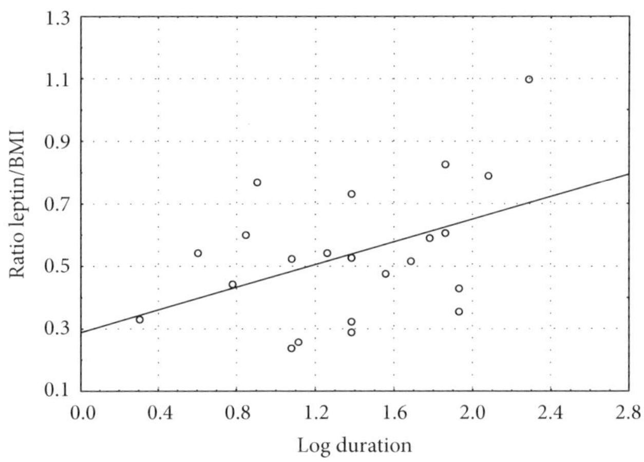


FIGURE 1: Correlation of the ratio leptin/BMI to duration of illness (in months, after logarithmic transformation) in female patients with relapsing-remitting MS ($n = 22$; $r = .4368$; $P = .04$).

## 4. Discussion

The present study evaluated serum leptin levels not only in treatment-naïve patients with RRMS, but also in patients with CIS at the early stages of disease and examined potential associations with various disease parameters. Leptin levels were increased in female patients with RRMS and correlated positively to disease duration. On the other hand, female patients with CIS had normal leptin levels. No significant changes in leptin were found in male RRMS or CIS patients.

Leptin levels were strongly correlated to gender and BMI in both MS patients and controls. The sexual dimorphism in leptin levels (higher in females) is well established in normal subjects and has also been previously observed in MS patients [10, 16]. Regarding the correlation of leptin to BMI in MS patients specifically, previous reports have been somewhat conflicting. Matarese et al. [7] reported a loss of this correlation in MS patients with low disability in relapse. Rotondi et al. [10] reported that the correlation was maintained in MS patients with low disability in remission but lost in patients with high disability in remission. Our cohort included patients with low disability both in relapse and remission. Our findings are more in agreement with the second study, but this may be due to including our patients in remission.

Increased leptin levels in RRMS patients have been previously reported in several studies [7–9]. Gender specific analyses were reported in only one of these studies, which found increased levels in both female and male patients [8]. This is in contrast with our data that showed differences restricted to female patients. It is not easy to reconcile these conflicting findings, given that male sample size and percentage of males in relapse were very similar in both studies. A possible explanation for the discrepancy may lie in the fact that Frisullo et al. [8] included patients with previous corticosteroid treatment. Corticosteroid administration has been shown to increase serum leptin levels, albeit only transiently [10, 17].

Earlier studies that found no differences in leptin levels between MS patients and controls had lower patient numbers and one of them also included subjects on immunomodulatory therapy [5, 6]. The above may partly explain discrepancies with more recent reports, including the present findings. The only recent study that reported comparable leptin levels in patients and controls investigated exclusively patients in remission [10]. This may be offered as a possible explanation for the discrepancy, since the presence of relapse has been shown to significantly affect leptin levels in some studies. Batocchi et al. [5] found that leptin levels, measured before the first clinical relapse, during the follow-up period, were significantly higher compared to baseline values. Frisullo et al. [8] reported higher serum leptin levels in female RRMS patients in remission than in female RRMS patients in relapse and female controls. Nevertheless, we did not observe significant differences in leptin levels between patients in relapse and remission. However, we did observe a borderline significant negative correlation of leptin/BMI ratio in female CIS patients.

Several studies have shown that leptin leads to increased production of proinflammatory cytokines, upregulation of costimulatory molecules, increase in Th1 type of immune response, and suppression of Treg function [18]. Several lines of evidence also suggest that it has an important role in the induction and progression of EAE, the animal model of MS. Leptin-deficient mice are resistant to EAE induction and this can be reversed by the administration of leptin [19]. Accordingly, it has been suggested that the increase in leptin levels seen in patients with active RRMS might reflect a pathogenic role [20]. If such was the case, one would expect to see increased leptin levels at the early stages of MS, in patients with CIS. However, our study found no significant differences in leptin levels between patients with CIS and controls, suggesting that the hormone may not have a pathogenic role and that higher levels observed in RRMS patients may be a secondary phenomenon induced during the course of the disease. Beyond this, the lack of significant difference in leptin levels between male patients and controls also argues strongly against a pathogenic role.

In a recent study, by our group, female RRMS patients were found to have lower BMI compared to controls [21]. Since leptin levels are secreted in proportion to energy stored in body fat, acute BMI changes have been shown to affect circulating leptin concentrations [20]. One might expect, therefore, a reduction of leptin levels in female RRMS patients. Instead, we found disproportionately increased leptin levels, suggesting a possible dysregulation of the mechanisms regulating leptin secretion to body fat in MS patients.

Several studies investigated possible correlations between leptin levels and disease parameters, such as disease duration and EDSS, with negative results [5, 6, 10]. The present study, on the other hand, found a positive correlation between leptin levels and disease duration in female patients with RRMS. This correlation was also present for leptin/BMI ratio, further suggesting that adipocyte leptin secreting activity is increased in female patients as the disease progresses. However, the lack of association with EDSS indicates that changes in leptin secretion are not directly related to accumulating central nervous system damage. It is possible that the association of leptin with disease duration was not detected in previous studies because of smaller sample sizes [5] or less stringent exclusion criteria [6, 10]. More specifically, Chatzantoni et al. [6] also included patients on immunomodulatory treatment, whereas Rotondi et al. [10] also included patients that had received past corticosteroid treatment. We designed our study to include only treatment-naïve patients, both in terms of previous corticosteroid and immunomodulatory therapy. This greatly restricted the number of RRMS patients that could be included and that affected our sample size, but it may have allowed associations with surface that would otherwise be masked by confounding factors.

Several limitations that may influence the results of the present study, beyond the relatively restricted sample size, need to be mentioned. Firstly, the control group used was not healthy volunteers but subjects investigated as in-patients for possible neurological disease with negative findings, although, unlikely, this may have influenced serum leptin in controls. Secondly, the inclusion of only treatment-naïve RRMS patients means that the sample is not representative of the entire RRMS population. However, this avoids other potentially significant confounding factors. Finally, the use of self-reported BMI is a further limitation, although this applies to both patients and controls and taking also into account the high correlation between self-reported and measured values [22], it is not expected to significantly influence results.

## 5. Conclusion

The results of the present study on treatment-naïve patients with CIS and RRMS do not indicate the involvement of leptin in the early stages of the disease. The finding of increased leptin secretion only in female patients with RRMS, but not in patients at first demyelinating episode (CIS), suggests that leptin does not have a pathogenic role from the early stages of disease. The ratio leptin/BMI increases during disease course in female MS patients in a time-dependent and disability-independent manner.

## Conflict of Interests

The authors declare that there is no conflict of interests regarding the publication of this paper.

## References

[1] R. E. Ostlund Jr., J. W. Yang, S. Klein, and R. Gingerich, "Relation between plasma leptin concentration and body fat, gender, diet, age, and metabolic covariates," *The Journal of Clinical Endocrinology & Metabolism*, vol. 81, no. 11, pp. 3909–3913, 1996.

[2] M. W. Schwartz, E. Peskind, M. Raskind, E. J. Boyko, and D. Porte Jr., "Cerebrospinal fluid leptin levels: relationship to plasma levels and to adiposity in humans," *Nature Medicine*, vol. 2, no. 5, pp. 589–593, 1996.

[3] P. M. Moraes-Vieira, Ê. J. Bassi, R. C. Araujo, and N. O. S. Câmara, "Leptin as a link between the immune system and kidney-related diseases: leading actor or just a coadjuvant?" *Obesity Reviews*, vol. 13, no. 8, pp. 733–743, 2012.

[4] V. Sanna, A. Di Giacomo, A. La Cava et al., "Leptin surge precedes onset of autoimmune encephalomyelitis and correlates with development of pathogenic T cell responses," *Journal of Clinical Investigation*, vol. 111, no. 2, pp. 241–250, 2003.

[5] A. P. Batocchi, M. Rotondi, M. Caggiula et al., "Leptin as a marker of multiple sclerosis activity in patients treated with interferon-beta," *Journal of Neuroimmunology*, vol. 139, no. 1-2, pp. 150–154, 2003.

[6] K. Chatzantoni, P. Papathanassopoulos, E. Gourzoulidou, and A. Mouzaki, "Leptin and its soluble receptor in plasma of patients suffering from remitting-relapsing multiple sclerosis (MS): in vitro effects of leptin on type-1 and type-2 cytokine secretion by peripheral blood mononuclear cells, T-cells and monocytes of MS patients," *Journal of Autoimmunity*, vol. 23, no. 2, pp. 169–177, 2004.

[7] G. Matarese, P. B. Carrieri, A. La Cava et al., "Leptin increase in multiple sclerosis associates with reduced number of $CD4^+CD25^+$ regulatory T cells," *Proceedings of the National Academy of Sciences of the United States of America*, vol. 102, no. 14, pp. 5150–5155, 2005.

[8] G. Frisullo, M. Mirabella, F. Angelucci et al., "The effect of disease activity on leptin, leptin receptor and suppressor of cytokine signalling-3 expression in relapsing-remitting multiple sclerosis," *Journal of Neuroimmunology*, vol. 192, no. 1-2, pp. 174–183, 2007.

[9] S. Emamgholipour, S. M. Eshaghi, A. Hossein-nezhad, K. Mirzaei, Z. Maghbooli, and M. A. Sahraian, "Adipocytokine profile, cytokine levels and foxp3 expression in multiple sclerosis: a possible link to susceptibility and clinical course of disease," *PLoS ONE*, vol. 8, no. 10, Article ID e76555, 2013.

[10] M. Rotondi, A. P. Batocchi, F. Coperchini et al., "Severe disability in patients with relapsing-remitting multiple sclerosis is associated with profound changes in the regulation of leptin secretion," *Neuroimmunomodulation*, vol. 20, no. 6, pp. 341–347, 2013.

[11] C. H. Polman, S. C. Reingold, G. Edan et al., "Diagnostic criteria for multiple sclerosis: 2005 Revisions to the "McDonald Criteria"," *Annals of Neurology*, vol. 58, no. 6, pp. 840–846, 2005.

[12] W. I. McDonald, A. Compston, G. Edan et al., "Recommended diagnostic criteria for multiple sclerosis: guidelines from the International Panel on the diagnosis of multiple sclerosis," *Annals of Neurology*, vol. 50, no. 1, pp. 121–127, 2001.

[13] J. F. Kurtzke, "Rating neurologic impairment in multiple sclerosis: an expanded disability status scale (EDSS)," *Neurology*, vol. 33, no. 11, pp. 1444–1452, 1983.

[14] U. Meier and A. M. Gressner, "Endocrine regulation of energy metabolism: review of pathobiochemical and clinical chemical aspects of leptin, ghrelin, adiponectin, and resistin," *Clinical Chemistry*, vol. 50, no. 9, pp. 1511–1525, 2004.

[15] D. Gallagher, M. Visser, D. Sepúlveda, R. N. Pierson, T. Harris, and S. B. Heymsfieid, "How useful is body mass index for comparison of body fatness across age, sex, and ethnic groups?" *The American Journal of Epidemiology*, vol. 143, no. 3, pp. 228–239, 1996.

[16] M. F. Saad, S. Damani, R. L. Gingerich et al., "Sexual dimorphism in plasma leptin concentration," *Journal of Clinical Endocrinology and Metabolism*, vol. 82, no. 2, pp. 579–584, 1997.

[17] H. Masuzaki, Y. Ogawa, K. Hosoda et al., "Glucocorticoid regulation of leptin synthesis and secretion in humans: elevated plasma leptin levels in Cushing's syndrome," *The Journal of Clinical Endocrinology & Metabolism*, vol. 82, no. 8, pp. 2542–2547, 1997.

[18] C. Procaccini, E. Jirillo, and G. Matarese, "Leptin as an immunomodulator," *Molecular Aspects of Medicine*, vol. 33, no. 1, pp. 35–45, 2012.

[19] G. Matarese, A. di Giacomo, V. Sanna et al., "Requirement for leptin in the induction and progression of autoimmune encephalomyelitis," *Journal of Immunology*, vol. 166, no. 10, pp. 5909–5916, 2001.

[20] G. Matarese, C. Procaccini, and V. de Rosa, "The intricate interface between immune and metabolic regulation: a role for leptin in the pathogenesis of multiple sclerosis?" *Journal of Leukocyte Biology*, vol. 84, no. 4, pp. 893–899, 2008.

[21] M. Markianos, M. E. Evangelopoulos, G. Koutsis, P. Davaki, and C. Sfagos, "Body mass index in multiple sclerosis: associations with CSF neurotransmitter metabolite levels," *ISRN Neurology*, vol. 2013, Article ID 981070, 6 pages, 2013.

[22] M. Stommel and C. A. Schoenborn, "Accuracy and usefulness of BMI measures based on self-reported weight and height: findings from the NHANES & NHIS 2001–2006," *BMC Public Health*, vol. 9, article 421, 2009.

# 11

# Pentraxin 3 Plasma Levels and Disease Activity in Systemic Lupus Erythematosus

**Roberto Assandri,[1] Marta Monari,[1] Anna Colombo,[2] Alessandra Dossi,[3] and Alessandro Montanelli[3]**

[1] *Clinical Investigation Laboratory, Humanitas Clinical and Research Center, Rozzano, Milan, Italy*
[2] *Humanitas Clinical and Research Center, Rozzano, Milan, Italy*
[3] *Clinical Investigation Laboratory, Diagnostics Department, Spedali Civili of Brescia, Brescia, Italy*

Correspondence should be addressed to Roberto Assandri; roberto.assandri@humanitas.it

Academic Editor: Ricard Cervera

SLE is an autoimmune disorder that involves polyclonal autoimmunity against multiple autoantigens. PTX3, a marker of the acute-phase inflammatory response, plays an important role in innate immunity and in modulation of the adaptive immune response. Our study tried to resolve some rather controversial aspects of the use of PTX3 as a biomarker of disease activity in SLE patients. We demonstrated that plasma PTX3 concentration of the SLE patients was significantly higher than the healthy control groups and reflected disease activity. ROC curve analysis was used to determine best cut-off point (2.8 ng/mL) with a good sensitivity and specificity. In patients with SLE, PTX3 concentrations were correlated with SLEDAI. Trend to remission (TTR) curve was created by plotting PTX3 levels and SLEDAI and we applied the curve as a model for the analysis of two patients with different follow-up. PTX3 plasma levels declined significantly and this decline occurred parallel to the clinical improvement with a complete remission of disease. In patients who experienced a clinical relapse, an increase in PTX3 levels followed the lupus flare. The proposal of PTX3 cut-off associated with TTR and monitoring of PTX3 plasma levels could be an innovative approach to follow-up of SLE patients.

## 1. Introduction

Systemic lupus erythematosus (SLE) is an autoimmune disorder with unpredictable course that involves polyclonal autoimmunity against multiple autoantigens and presents a wide spectrum of clinical manifestations (fever, skin rashes, arthralgia, and inflammation of kidney, lungs, or brain) [1]. The pathogenesis of SLE is based on combinations of genetic variants and environmental factors that promote loss-of-tolerance or tissue inflammation [2]. In fact there is growing evidence to suggest that inflammation and related molecules play a key role in the pathogenesis of SLE.

The pentraxin superfamily (PTXs), divided into long and short PTXs, can be induced by a variety of inflammation-associated stimuli [3]. Next to the classical short pentraxins C-reactive protein (CRP) and serum amyloid P component (SAP), pentraxin 3 (PTX3) is prototypic of long pentraxin family, a multifunctional protein characterized by a cyclic multimeric structure and a conserved domain [4].

An increasing number of studies have identified PTX3 as a key component in the host defence against certain infections such as fungal, bacterial, and viral ones [5, 6]. Furthermore, higher circulating PTX3 levels have been observed in cardiovascular diseases [7] and also in some autoimmune disorders, such as vasculitis [8], celiac disease (CD) [9], and SLE [3].

Despite several studies, the literature provides a contradictory description of PTX3 in SLE patients and, at the moment, it has not identified any biochemical markers that allow accurately monitoring disease activity.

Considering that SLE is characterized by chronic inflammation and immune dysfunction, PTX3 may play a role in the pathogenesis of this disease. Unlike CRP and SAP, PTX3 is produced by resident and innate immunity cells in peripheral tissues, in response to inflammatory signals [10].

However the literature provides a contradictory picture of PTX3 in SLE pathogenesis and several questions should be answered.

Our study tried to resolve some rather controversial aspects of the use of PTX as a biomarker of disease activity in SLE patients and finally proposed a model related to clinical use and follow-up.

## 2. Patients and Methods

*2.1. Subjects.* We studied 64 patients with SLE and 60 controls. We enrolled patients aged more than 18 years fulfilling the American College of Rheumatology (ACR) criteria for SLE [11]. Control subjects who did not meet the criteria for SLE or any other inflammatory disease and did not have infectious diseases were recruited.

Exclusion criteria of enrolled SLE patients were as follows: age > 50 years, pregnancy or postpartum patients, malignancy ischemic heart disease, concurrent infections, and recent trauma.

All patients subscribed written informed consent.

*2.2. Clinical Assessment.* Clinical information was obtained through a structured review of the medical records and laboratory tests. Subjects were considered to have hypertension if they took antihypertensive agents if they had a systolic blood pressure of at least 140 mmHg or a diastolic pressure of at least 90 mmHg.

The activity of SLE was measured with the SLE Disease Activity Index (SLEDAI) [11].

Antiphospholipid syndrome (APS) patients were enrolled following classification criteria established by international consensus document (2006): vascular thrombosis, one or more clinical episodes_ of arterial, venous, or small vessel thrombosis, Lupus Anticoagulant (LA) present in plasma, anticardiolipin (aCL) antibody of IgG and/or IgM isotype in serum or plasma, and anti-b2 glycoprotein-I antibody of IgG and/or IgM present in medium or high titer, on two or more occasions at least 12 weeks apart [12]. Patients with cerebrovascular accident, multi-infarct dementia, cerebral venous thrombosis, and transverse myelopathy were excluded.

Lupus nephritis was defined as present if the clinical and laboratory findings had met the ACR criteria (persistent proteinuria 0.5 mg/day or greater than 3+ by dipstick and/or cellular casts, including red blood cells, hemoglobin, granular, tubular, or mixed casts, and renal biopsy, according to the ISN/RPS 2003 classification [13]).

## 3. Methods

*3.1. Blood Samples.* Venous blood samples were collected after a minimum of 4 hours of fasting. The samples for PTX3 level analysis were stored at –75°C in small specimen containers.

*3.2. Measurement of Plasma PTX3 Concentrations.* The levels of PTX3 were measured by a sandwich ELISA kit (Hycult), on automated platform DSX (Technogenetics). Each sample was tested in duplicate with a dilution of 1 : 4 and the reported value refers to the mean of the two determinations. Both intra- and interassay coefficient of variation (CV) do not exceed 3%. The assay does not cross-react with CRP or serum amyloid A protein. Briefly, polystyrene microplates coated with a monoclonal antibody against PTX3 were incubated with serum samples for 1 hour at 37°C. For detection, biotinylated tracer polyclonal antibody specific to PTX3 was added for 1 hour and a streptavidin-peroxidase conjugate was added for 1 h. Color reaction was developed using tetramethylbenzidine and hydrogen peroxide. Optical density at 450 nm. was measured with a plate reader, and absolute values were calculated from the four-parameter logistic standard curve.

*3.3. Statistical Analysis.* Demographic characteristics were presented as the mean ± SD (median) for continuous variables and as frequencies and percentages for categorical variables. PTX3 concentrations were compared between SLE patients and healthy controls by using Wilcoxon's rank sum test.

The associations between the PTX3 level and SLEDAI or clinical characteristics CRP, ESR, anti-dsDNA antibody, C3, C4, and other laboratory parameters were examined in the SLE patients using Spearman's rank correlation analysis. Spearman's rank correlation coefficients were calculated to assess univariate associations between plasma PTX3 and continuous variables. All analyses in this study employed a significance level of $p < 0.05$ (two-sided). Cut-off value for PTX3 was selected from ROC curve analysis. Positive predictive value was calculated as (PPV = (true positive ∗ 100)/(true positive + false positive)) and negative predictive value was calculated as (NPV = (true negative ∗ 100)/(true negative + false negative)) and Youden's Index for the estimated cut-off point was calculated as sensitivity + specificity – 1.

Accuracy is measured by the area under the ROC curve.

## 4. Results

*4.1. Characteristics of Patients and Healthy Control Subjects.* Table 1 shows the baseline characteristics of the SLE patients and the control subjects.

In this study, 64 patients with SLE and 60 healthy controls were matched for age (mean ± SD 46.8 ± 15.1 years versus 41.8 ± 12.6 years, $p = 0.801$) and sex (percentage of women 87.5 versus 90%, $p = 0.92$).

In the patients' group, 15 patients had secondary form of APS and 15 patients had lupus nephritis (LN). There was no significant difference of either systolic blood pressure or diastolic blood pressure between the two groups ($p = 0.78$).

Patients with SLE had the same BMI ($p = 0.023$) as healthy control subjects and there were no significant differences with respect to smoking, history of coronary heart disease, and postmenopausal status between the two groups.

We investigated lipid profile of SLE patients and control subjects. The mean total cholesterol at diagnosis of celiac disease was 188 ± 75 mg/dL and HDL-cholesterol was 34 ± 15 mg/dL (Table 1).

Table 1: Characteristics of SLE patients and healthy controls.

| | SLE patients ($n$ = 64) | Healthy controls ($n$ = 60) | $p$ value |
|---|---|---|---|
| Clinical features | | | |
| Age (years) | 46.8 ± 15.1 | 41.8 ± 12.6 | 0.801 |
| Sex (% of women) | 87.5 | 90 | 0.84 |
| Systolic blood pressure (mmHg) | 120 ± 18 | 114 ± 12 | 0.63 |
| Diastolic blood pressure (mmHg) | 72 ± 13 | 70 ± 12 | 0.54 |
| Clinical manifestations | | | |
| Renal involvement | 23.4 | — | NA |
| Seizure | 6.2 | — | NA |
| Severe headache | 4.6 | — | NA |
| Myositis | 4.6 | — | NA |
| Arthritis | 34.3 | — | NA |
| Malar rash/alopecia | 12.5 | — | NA |
| APS | 18.4 | — | NA |
| Retinal vasculitis | 1.5 | — | NA |
| Anemia | 48.4 | — | NA |
| Lymphopenia | 40 | — | NA |
| Leukopenia | 11 | — | NA |
| Thrombocytopenia | 15.6 | — | NA |
| Laboratory parameters | | | |
| Total cholesterol (mg/dL) | 188 ± 75 | 193 ± 27 | 0.57 |
| HDL-cholesterol (mg/dL) | 48 ± 9 | 53 ± 4 | 0.54 |
| LDL-cholesterol | 95 ± 2 | 98 ± 3 | 0.91 |
| Triglycerides (mg/dL) | 49 ± 18 | 54 ± 11 | 0.54 |
| Serum iron ($\mu$g/mL) | 91 ± 14 | 98 ± 12 | <0.05 |
| Hemoglobin (g/dL) | 8 ± 2 | 9.4 ± 4 | <0.05 |
| C3 (mg/L) | 82.5 ± 32.1 | 102.5 ± 52 | <0.05 |
| C4 (mg/L) | 13.1 ± 6.7 | 31 ± 12.1 | <0.05 |
| Anti-dsDNA (IU/mL) | 814 ± 461 | 1 ± 0.2 | <0.05 |
| Serum creatinine (mg/dL) | 1.2 ± 0.9 | 0.97 ± 0.2 | <0.05 |
| Serum albumin (g/dL) | 2.8 ± 0.7 | 4.1 ± 0.4 | <0.05 |
| Inflammatory marker | | | |
| Erythrocyte sedimentation rate (mm/h) | 58 ± 40 | 10 ± 12 | <0.05 |

Both men and women with SLE had the same HDL and triglycerides in comparison to healthy control ($p = 0.54$).

Patients were at different stages of disease activity with or without major organ involvement. The frequency of SLEDAI components in these patients was as follows: renal involvement: 23.4%, seizure: 6.4%, psychosis: 1.5%, severe headache: 5.4%, myositis: 5.4%, arthritis: 33.9%, malar rash/alopecia: 13.4%, APS: 18.4%, retinal vasculitis: 1.5%, anemia: 48.9%, lymphopenia: 40%, leukopenia: 11%, and thrombocytopenia: 14.9% (see Table 1).

The mean SLEDAI in these patients was 8 ± 3.5, ranged from SLEDAI = 0 to SLEDAI = 16.

In this study, patients were divided into three groups according to SLEDAI score: inactive group (1, 18 patients, 28%: SLEDAI < 4), active group (2, 32 patients, 50%: 4 < SLEDAI < 10), and highly active group (3, 14 patients, 22%: SLEDAI > 10).

*4.2. Baseline Analysis.* Figure 1 shows the PTX3 plasma levels in SLE patients and control subjects.

In the SLE patients PTX3 plasma levels ranged from 1.18 to 95.1 ng/mL, with a mean ± SD of 14 ± 13.1 ng/mL and a median value of 5.3 ng/mL. In the control subjects, PTX3 ranged from 0.2 to 4.8 ng/mL, with a mean ± SD of 2.3 ± 1.1 ng/mL and a median value of 2.5 ng/mL. The plasma PTX3 concentration was significantly higher in the SLE patients than in the healthy controls ($p < 0.001$).

ROC curve analysis was conducted to determine a cut-off point for PTX3 plasma value between SLE patients and HS group. In the ROC curve shown PTX3 levels were plotted for

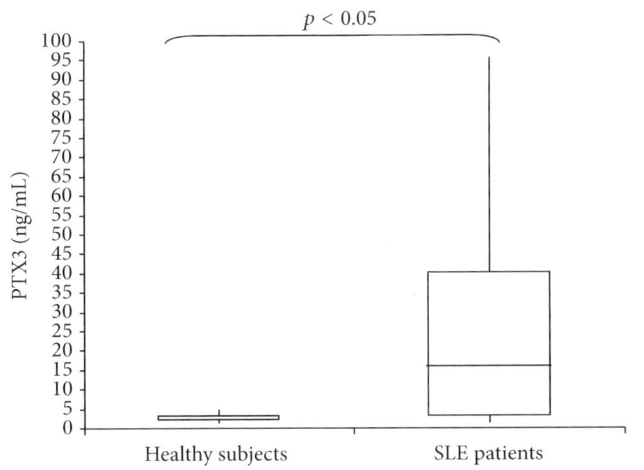


Figure 1: PTX3 plasma levels in SLE patients and healthy subjects.

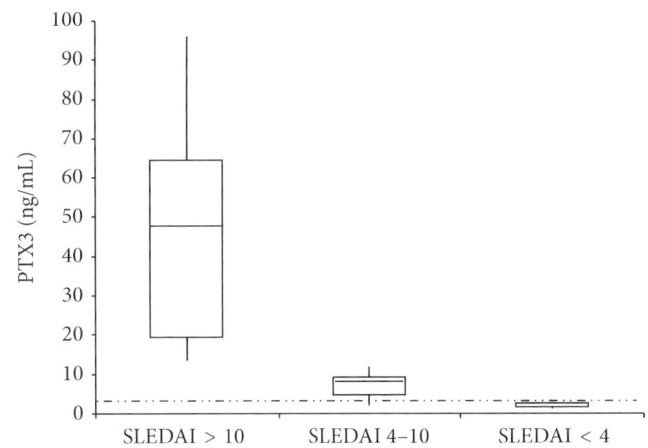


Figure 3: PTX3 plasma levels and SLEDAI patients categories. The dashed line represents cut-off value.

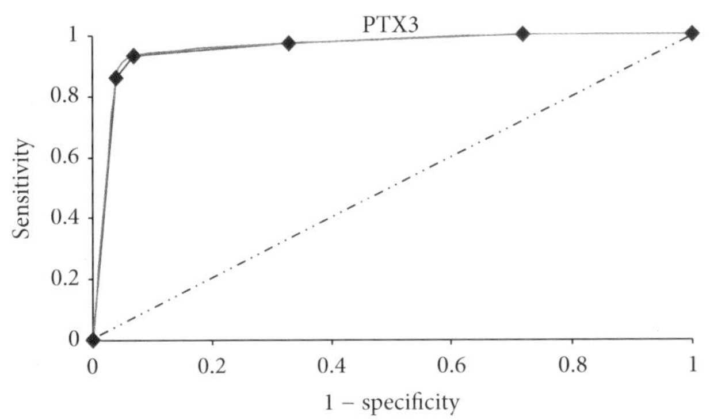


Figure 2: ROC curve analysis was used to determine PTX3 cut-off point between lupus patients and healthy controls. Example of a receiver operating characteristic curve. Solid red: ROC curve; dashed line: chance level; vertical line: (J) maximum value of Youden's Index for the ROC curve.

their ability to predict the disease activity with true positive on vertical axis (sensitivity) and false positive (1 − specificity) on horizontal axis (Figure 2).

The estimated best cut-off point for PTX3 between active SLE patients and healthy subjects was 2.8 ng/mL, characterized by a high sensitivity (100%) and high specificity (80%), with a negative predictive value of 1 (100%), positive predictive value of 0.76 (76%), and an accuracy of 0.88 (88%).

Youden's Index was determined as 0.8. (see ROC curve in Figure 2).

## 5. Plasma PTX3 Concentration in SLE Patients

Figure 3 shows the distribution of patients according to PTX3 plasma values in groups A, B, and C.

PTX3 plasma concentration in group 1 ranged from 1.18 to 2.7 ng/mL with a mean range ± SD of 1.8 ± 0.60 ng/mL. PTX3 plasma concentration in group 2 ranged from 2.7 to 11.3 ng/mL with a mean range ± SD of 9 ± 2.4 ng/mL. Finally PTX3 plasma concentration in group 3 ranged from 13.5 to 95.9 ng/mL with a mean range ± SD of 47 ± 27.6 ng/mL (see Figure 2). There was a significant difference between the 3 groups ($p < 0.001$).

When patients were divided into two groups, according to calculated diagnostic cut-off point for plasma PTX3 (2.8 ng/mL), there was significant difference between active SLEDAI score and its individual parameters in these two groups ($p = 0.001$). Distribution of patients according to PTX3 cut-off point, in three groups of inactive, moderately active, and highly active patients, shows significant difference in PTX3 plasma levels in each group.

In patients with PTX3 < 2.8 ng/mL, 28% had SLEDAI < 4. In patients with PTX3 > 2.8 ng/mL, 72% had SLEDAI > 4 (see Figure 4).

## 6. Plasma PTX3 Concentration and Disease Activity

*6.1. Complement System Fractions and CRP.* The complement system was closely linked to SLE. All patients were tested to C3 and C4 fractions.

C3 and C4 serum concentration were estimated, respectively, in 825 ± 321 mg/L and 130 ± 60 mg/L.

The proportions of patients with low levels of complement fractions (C3 fraction < 900 mg/L, C4 fraction < 160 mg/L) were, respectively, 48 (75%) and 35 (54.6%).

The PTX3 plasma concentrations were compared in SLE patients with or without normal C3 and C4 complement fractions and in healthy subjects. There was a statistical difference in PTX3 plasma concentrations between the proportions of patients with low C3 and C4 fraction levels (16.5± 11.3 ng/mL), patients with normal levels (6.5 ± 2.7 ng/mL), and HCS. According to these data we examined correlation between plasma PTX3 concentration and complements system levels. There was a significantly negative correlation between C3 and C4 fractions and PTX3 plasma levels (resp., $r = -0.34$, $p = 0.02$, and $r = -0.42$, $p = 0.002$).

CRP serum levels were estimated in the three groups mentioned above (groups 1, 2, and 3).

CRP serum levels in SLE patients were estimated in 16.1 ± 15.3 mg/L, ranged from 0.1 to 83 mg/L with a median range

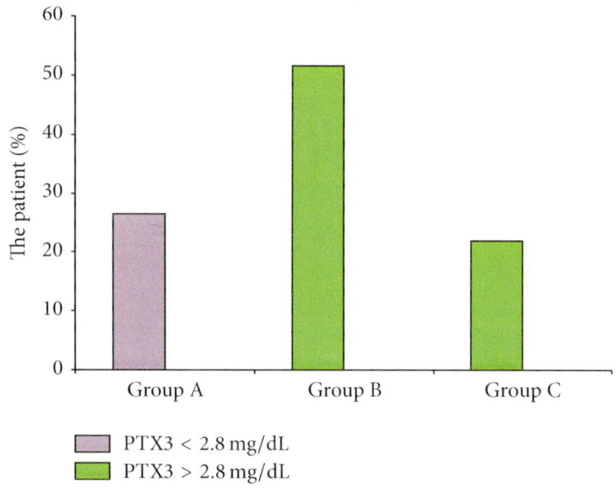


FIGURE 4: Distribution of patients according to PTX3 cut-off point in three groups of patients.

of 9.1 mg/L. In group 1 CRP serum levels ranged from 0.1 to 9 mg/L with a mean value ± SD estimated in 6 ± 3.8 ng/L. In group 2 CRP serum concentration ranged from 0.2 to 14.3 mg/L (mean value ± SD 7.2 ± 5.2 mg/L) while group 3 ranged from 8.5 to 51 mg/L (mean value ± SD 28.1 ± 12.4 mg/L).

There are statistical differences between group 1 versus group 3 and group 2 versus group 3 and HC ($p < 0.05$), but no difference appeared between group 1 and group 2 ($p = 0.62$).

In light of these data we examined correlations between CRP serum concentration and PTX3 plasma levels. No correlation appeared between CRP and PTX3 levels ($r = -0.08$, $p = 0.84$).

*6.2. Other Laboratory Biomarkers.* We examined correlations between PTX3 plasma levels and other laboratory parameters in 64 patients with SLE. PTX3 plasma concentration was negatively correlated with serum albumin ($r = -0.57$, $p = 0.01$) and hemoglobin ($r = -0.42$, $p < 0.05$). Consequently PTX3 was still significantly associated with anemia ($p = 0.020$).

However, PTX3 was not correlated to serum creatinine, ESR, white blood cell count, lymphocyte count, and platelet count. Regarding immunological parameters no correlation appeared between PTX3 concentrations and anticardiolipin (aCL) immunoglobulin isotypes G (IgG), M (IgM) and IgG, IgM anti-b2 glycoprotein-I (anti-b2GPI) or anti-dsDNA antibody titer.

There was no correlation between the PTX3 concentration and several coronary risk factors, including serum cholesterol levels (total cholesterol, HDL-cholesterol, and LDL-cholesterol). Instead PTX3 was positively correlated with triglycerides ($r = 0.39$, $p = 0.024$; see Table 2).

TABLE 2: Factors associated with plasma PTX3 levels in SLE patients.

| Variables | Correlation coefficient | $p$ value |
|---|---|---|
| Clinical features | | |
| Age (years) | 0.047 | 0.80 |
| Systolic blood pressure (mmHg) | 0.01 | 0.75 |
| Diastolic blood pressure (mmHg) | 0.10 | 0.64 |
| BMI (Kg/m$^2$) | 0.11 | 0.41 |
| Clinical manifestations | | |
| Renal involvement | 0.61 | <0.05 |
| Seizure | 0.18 | 0.71 |
| Severe headache | 0.12 | 0.27 |
| Myositis | −0.18 | 0.09 |
| Arthritis | 0.21 | 0.27 |
| Malar rash/alopecia | −0.09 | <0.05 |
| APS | 0.49 | <0.05 |
| Retinal vasculitis | 0.03 | 0.59 |
| Anemia | −0.42 | <0.05 |
| Lymphopenia | −0.13 | 0.43 |
| Leukopenia | 0.17 | 0.51 |
| Thrombocytopenia | −0.17 | 0.41 |
| Laboratory parameters | | |
| Total cholesterol (mg/dL) | 0.02 | 0.61 |
| HDL-cholesterol (mg/dL) | 0.12 | 0.51 |
| LDL-cholesterol | 0.12 | 0.42 |
| Triglycerides (mg/dL) | 0.03 | <0.05 |
| Serum iron ($\mu$g/mL) | −0.41 | <0.05 |
| Hemoglobin (g/dL) | 0.42 | <0.05 |
| C3 (mg/L) | −0.34 | 0.02 |
| C4 (mg/L) | −0.42 | 0.002 |
| Anti-dsDNA (IU/mL) | 0.14 | 0.53 |
| Serum creatinine (mg/dL) | 0.02 | 0.80 |
| Serum albumin (mg/dL) | −0.57 | <0.05 |
| AlbU (mg/dL) | 0.61 | <0.06 |
| Inflammatory marker | | |
| Erythrocyte sedimentation rate (mm/h) | 0.23 | 0.09 |
| C-reactive protein (mg/dL) | −0.08 | 0.84 |
| Fibrinogen (mg/dL) | −0.11 | 0.41 |

## 7. Medication

The median dose of prednisolone was estimated in 1.8 (0–13) mg/day, although there was significant correlation between PTX3 plasma levels and prednisolone dosage ($r = 0.49$, $p < 0.05$).

Twenty-two (36.6%) patients received cytotoxic drugs including cyclophosphamide (16.4%), azathioprine (13.5%), and mycophenolate mofetil (6.7%).

*7.1. SLEDAI, "Trend to Remission Curve," and Follow-Up of Patients.* We considered a hypothetical correlation between disease activity, CRP serum concentration, and PTX3 plasma level. Activity patients categories have been defined on the base of SLEDAI scores as mentioned above.

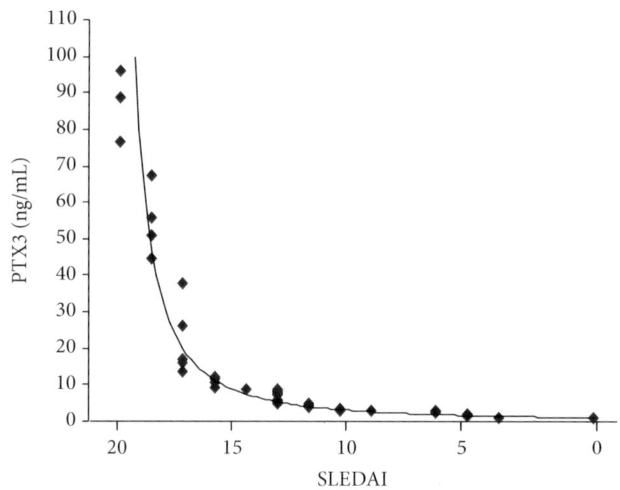


FIGURE 5: Trend to remission curve.

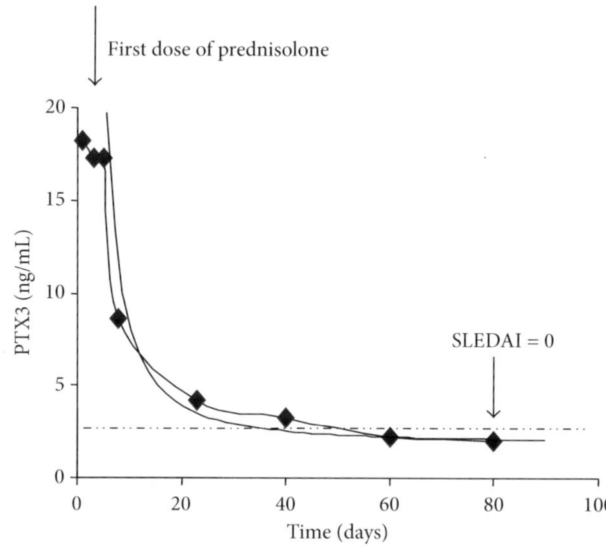


FIGURE 6: Patient 1 trend to remission. The dashed line represents the operative cut-off.

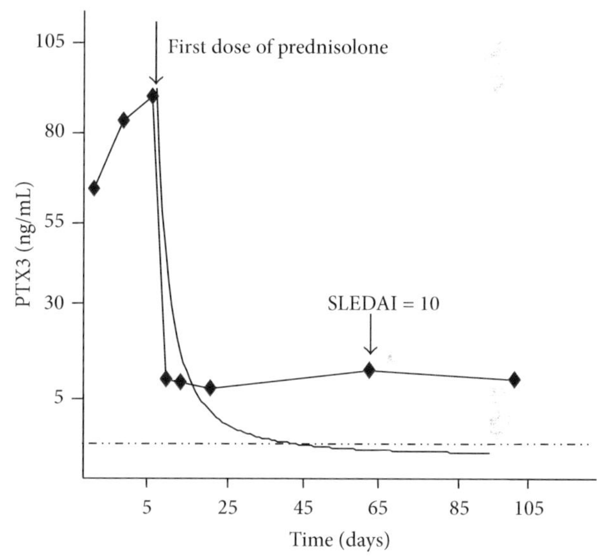


FIGURE 7: Patient 2 trend to remission curve. The dashed line represents the operative cut-off.

We evaluated a correlation between SLEDAI and PTX3 plasma levels. We noted a positive significant correlation between SLEDAI and PTX3 concentration ($r = 0.79$, $p < 0.001$).

No significant correlation appeared between SLEDAI and CRP.

According to the evidences relationship between PTX3 plasma levels and SLEDAI we tried to provide a "trend to remission curve" (TTR curve, Figure 5). In the TTR curve PTX3 levels were plotted on vertical axis and SLEDAI on horizontal axis. In this way we linked the trend of SLE activity to PTX3 plasma concentrations. After that, we applied TTR curve as a model to the analysis of 2 patients, called Patient 1 (P1, Figure 6) and Patient 2 (P2, Figure 7), with two different follow-ups.

In P1, after initiation of high-dose corticosteroid therapy, PTX3 plasma levels declined significantly (from 18.2 to 2.1 ng/mL). This decline occurred parallel to the clinical improvement.

In this patient we showed a complete remission of disease (from SLEDAI 12 to SLEDAI 0, see Figure 6). We applied the TTR curve to the disease trend and we observed a complete match between TTR curve and the Patient's trend curve.

PTX3 plasma concentration of P1 was shown in Figure 6.

In P2 who experienced a clinical relapse, an increase in PTX3 plasma levels followed the relapse (see Figure 7). We applied the TTR curve to the patient's trend and we observed no complete match between the two curves.

## 8. Relationship between PTX3 and Organ Damage in SLE Patients

Since there was a positive correlation between the PTX3 plasma concentration and the disease activity indexes, we suspected that patients with major organ damage such as APS lupus or lupus nephritis could have higher PTX3 levels. Therefore, we compared PTX3 plasma concentrations between fifteen patients with LN and other APS-SLE patients. No statistical differences appeared between the two groups. We found that the PTX3 plasma concentration of the SLE patients with APS lupus (mean 22.2 ± 20.6 ng/mL) and LN was significantly higher than mean of LES patients (mean 24.2 ± 20.3 ng/mL).

In APS-SLE patients no correlation appeared between APS-specific autoantibodies and PTX3 plasma concentration. On the other hand plasma levels PTX3 was correlated with urine albumin and spot proteinuria in patients with LN ($r = 0.62$, $p < 0.05$; $r = 0.67$, $p < 0.05$).

## 9. Discussion

Pentraxins are a family of multimeric proteins divided into short and long pentraxin, based on the primary structure:

CRP, the prototype of the short pentraxin subfamily, and PTX3, the prototypic long pentraxin.

Our study tried to resolve some rather controversial aspects of the PTX use as a biomarker of disease activity in SLE but despite several studies, the literature provides a contradictory picture of PTX3 in SLE patients and several questions should be answered.

It is now known that CRP levels, usually parallel with disease activity in inflammatory states, are almost never accompanied by elevated CRP levels [14]. Median CRP levels in patients with active RA are commonly in the range of 20–40 mg/L [14]. In contrast to this, Becker et al. and Borg et al. found median CRP levels during SLE exacerbation to be only 15 mg/L [14].

Literature provides evidences that hepatic CRP protein synthesis is inhibited by IFN$\alpha$, which could explain the lack of correlation between inflammation and CRP in SLE. In support of this evidence, it is now known that CRP are associate with SLE disease activity in patients without measurable IFN$\alpha$ and without a genetic variant of the CRP gene associated with low levels of CRP [15]. Taken together, these findings have led to the conclusion that the CRP response in lupus is less than what is expected and CRP serum concentrations were not correlated with disease activity or with any types of clinical manifestations [14]. It is a reasonable research question to check if other pentraxins can overcome this limitation of CRP use as a biomarker of systemic disease activity in SLE.

Our study emphasized the concept that CRP serum levels did not correlate with disease activity and we have demonstrated that plasma PTX3 concentration correlated with disease activity and SLEDAI.

It has been demonstrated that Toll-Like Receptor (TLR) 7 (TLR7) and TLR9 signaling play a pivotal role in SLE pathogenesis. Very recent studies revealed that estrogen receptor $\alpha$ knockout mice have impaired inflammatory responses to TLR3, TLR4, TLR7, and TLR9 ligand stimulation in Dendritic Cells (DCs) [16, 17]. Also data in mice indicate that TLR4 plays a key role in mediating autoimmunity, proinflammatory cytokine production, and other immune activation.

TLR4 is one of the best characterized and the first member of the TLR family [18].

TLR4 signaling is implicated in the innate immune responses against a wide range of microbes, including Gram-negative and Gram-positive bacteria, mycobacteria, spirochetes, yeasts, and some viruses and mammary tumor viruses [17, 18].

TLR4 is implicated in a different range of pathological processes associated with autoimmune diseases such as psoriasis, diabetic retinopathy, thrombosis, and inflammatory disorders including arthritis and atherosclerosis [18].

There is an evident role of TLR4 in SLE pathogenesis, such as the kidney damage, the induction of CD40 and autoantibodies, the suppression of regulatory T cells, and the role of proinflammatory cytokines in SLE pathogenesis [19].

In mouse-model sex hormones could directly change TLR4 responsiveness through several mechanisms. Evidences suggested that NF$\kappa$B was a focal point in the signal transduction cascades that mediate inflammatory cues from antigen receptors on T cells and B cells, 80, and from TLRs on cells of the innate immune system [20]. In addition to hypomethylation-driven activation of NF$\kappa$B-sensitive genes, other oxidation-induced alterations in transcription factor programs are implicated in SLE [21].

The corresponding PTX3 human gene is located on chromosome 3 band q 25. The proximal promoter shares numerous transcription factor binding sequences (such as NF-kB) and [20, 21] it has been demonstrated that NF-kB binding site is essential for PTX3 gene transcriptional response. Also PTX3 is produced in response to a variety of inflammatory signals mediated by TLR agonists IL-1 and tumor necrosis factor alpha (TNF-alpha) [20–22].

It was elegantly demonstrated that PTX3 was strictly necessary for NF-kB activation in intestinal reperfusion injury model and underlined a fundamental role of PTX3 in mediating tissue inflammation under sterile conditions [22].

An integrate viewpoint suggested that PTX3 responsiveness lupus is possible and it could be speculated that PTX3 may play a role as a biomarker of disease activity.

In Hollan et al. study healthy subjects showed a serum PTX3 level as 1.21 ± 0.59 ng/mL [7].

On the other hand Yamasaki reported the mean plasma PTX3 concentration around 2.00 ng/mL for healthy Japanese people [23]. These different values could be referred to the use of two different matrices (plasma and serum) during the detection of healthy control PTX3 concentration.

In Shimada et al. study the mean PTX3 plasma concentration of 53 healthy controls was 2.2 ± 1.1 ng/mL [24], which was nearly identical to that of the healthy subjects in Yamasaki et al.'s study [23].

Fazzini et al. [8] and Hollan et al. [7] reported serum concentrations PTX3 (not plasma) of 28 SLE patients and three SLE patients, respectively. The mean PTX3 serum concentration of the 28 SLE patients reported by Hollan et al. was 0.38 ± 0.50 ng/mL, which was lower than that of 1.00 ± 0.47 ng/mL in their healthy controls [7]. However, 12 of their 28 SLE subjects did not have active disease with SLEDAI at zero (SLEDAI = 0).

Our study defined PTX3 plasma value in healthy subjects (2.3 ± 1.1 ng/mL) according to other studies, the concentration of PTX3 in SLE patients at different SLEDAI stage, and most importantly an operative cut-off (2.8 ng/mL), characterized by a high sensitivity (100%) and high specificity (80%). Furthermore PTX3 concentration reflects disease activity and "trend to remission curve" is a "friendly" instrument to apply in the clinical routine and follow-up of SLE patients.

## 10. Conclusions

A SLE biomarker would be a stable molecule that is easy to sample and cheap to measure and that discriminates disease activity and flares.

According to our data we could consider PTX3 as a "single and integrate biomarker" in SLE, a multifactorial pathology with wide spectrum of clinical manifestations.

It is a new and interesting approach. Future studies are needed, but the road is drawn.

## Conflict of Interests

All authors declare no conflict of interests for this paper.

## References

[1] A. Rahman and D. A. Isenberg, "Systemic lupus erythematosus," *The New England Journal of Medicine*, vol. 358, no. 9, pp. 929–939, 2008.

[2] A. Migliorini and H.-J. Anders, "A novel pathogenetic concept-antiviral immunity in lupus nephritis," *Nature Reviews Nephrology*, vol. 8, no. 3, pp. 183–189, 2012.

[3] M. Lech, C. Römmele, O. P. Kulkarni et al., "Lack of the long pentraxin PTX3 promotes autoimmune lung disease but not glomerulonephritis in murine systemic lupus erythematosus," *PLoS ONE*, vol. 6, no. 5, Article ID e20118, 2011.

[4] L. Deban, S. Jaillon, C. Garlanda, B. Bottazzi, and A. Mantovani, "Pentraxins in innate immunity: lessons from PTX3," *Cell and Tissue Research*, vol. 343, no. 1, pp. 237–249, 2011.

[5] X. He, B. Han, X. Bai et al., "PTX3 as a potential biomarker of acute lung injury: supporting evidence from animal experimentation," *Intensive Care Medicine*, vol. 36, no. 2, pp. 356–364, 2010.

[6] X. He, B. Han, and M. Liu, "Long pentraxin 3 in pulmonary infection and acute lung injury," *American Journal of Physiology—Lung Cellular and Molecular Physiology*, vol. 292, no. 5, pp. L1039–L1049, 2007.

[7] I. Hollan, B. Bottazzi, I. Cuccovillo et al., "Increased levels of serum pentraxin 3, a novel cardiovascular biomarker, in patients with inflammatory rheumatic disease," *Arthritis Care & Research*, vol. 62, no. 3, pp. 378–385, 2010.

[8] F. Fazzini, G. Peri, A. Doni et al., "PTX3 in small-vessel vasculitides: an independent indicator of disease activity produced at sites of inflammation," *Arthritis & Rheumatism*, vol. 44, no. 12, pp. 2841–2850, 2001.

[9] R. Assandri, M. Monari, A. Colombo, and A. Montanelli, "Pentraxin 3 serum levels in celiac patients: evidences and perspectives," *Recent Patents on Food, Nutrition & Agriculture*, vol. 6, no. 2, pp. 82–92, 2015.

[10] B. Bottazzi, V. Vouret-Craviari, A. Bastone et al., "Multimer formation and ligand recognition by the long pentraxin PTX3. Similarities and differences with the short pentraxins C-reactive protein and serum amyloid P component," *The Journal of Biological Chemistry*, vol. 272, no. 52, pp. 32817–32823, 1997.

[11] D. D. Gladman and M. B. Urowitz, "The SLICC/ACR damage index: progress report and experience in the field," *Lupus*, vol. 8, no. 8, pp. 632–637, 1999.

[12] S. Miyakis, M. D. Lockshin, T. Atsumi et al., "International consensus statement on an update of the classification criteria for definite antiphospholipid syndrome (APS)," *Journal of Thrombosis and Haemostasis*, vol. 4, no. 2, pp. 295–306, 2006.

[13] J. J. Weening, V. D. D'Agati, M. M. Schwartz et al., "The classification of glomerulonephritis in systemic lupus erythematosus revisited," *Journal of the American Society of Nephrology*, vol. 15, no. 2, pp. 241–250, 2004.

[14] R. T. Keenan, C. J. Swearingen, and Y. Yazici, "Erythrocyte sedimentation rate and C-reactive protein levels are poorly correlated with clinical measures of disease activity in rheumatoid arthritis, systemic lupus erythematosus and osteoarthritis patients," *Clinical and Experimental Rheumatology*, vol. 26, no. 5, pp. 814–819, 2008.

[15] C. Mold and T. W. D. Clos, "C-reactive protein inhibits plasmacytoid dendritic cell interferon responses to autoantibody immune complexes," *Arthritis and Rheumatism*, vol. 65, no. 7, pp. 1891–1901, 2013.

[16] A. Marshak-Rothstein, "Toll-like receptors in systemic autoimmune disease," *Nature Reviews Immunology*, vol. 6, no. 11, pp. 823–835, 2006.

[17] K. A. Zarember and P. J. Godowski, "Tissue expression of human Toll-like receptors and differential regulation of Toll-like receptor mRNAs in leukocytes in response to microbes, their products, and cytokines," *Journal of Immunology*, vol. 168, no. 2, pp. 554–561, 2002.

[18] W. Jiang and G. Gilkeson, "Sex differences in monocytes and TLR4 associated immune responses; implications for systemic lupus erythematosus (SLE)," *Journal of Immunotherapy Applications*, vol. 1, no. 1, 2014.

[19] H. Qin, C. A. Wilson, S. J. Lee, X. Zhao, and E. N. Benveniste, "LPS induces CD40 gene expression through the activation of NF-κB and STAT-1α in macrophages and microglia," *Blood*, vol. 106, no. 9, pp. 3114–3122, 2005.

[20] B. Han, M. Mura, C. F. Andrade et al., "TNFα-induced long pentraxin PTX3 expression in human lung epithelial cells via JNK," *Journal of Immunology*, vol. 175, no. 12, pp. 8303–8311, 2005.

[21] D. G. Souza, A. T. Vieira, V. Pinho et al., "NF-κB plays a major role during the systemic and local acute inflammatory response following intestinal reperfusion injury," *British Journal of Pharmacology*, vol. 145, no. 2, pp. 246–254, 2005.

[22] D. G. Souza, F. A. Amaral, C. T. Fagundes et al., "The long pentraxin PTX3 is crucial for tissue inflammation after intestinal ischemia and reperfusion in mice," *The American Journal of Pathology*, vol. 174, no. 4, pp. 1309–1318, 2009.

[23] K. Yamasaki, M. Kurimura, T. Kasai, M. Sagara, T. Kodama, and K. Inoue, "Determination of physiological plasma pentraxin 3 (PTX3) levels in healthy populations," *Clinical Chemistry and Laboratory Medicine*, vol. 47, no. 4, pp. 471–477, 2009.

[24] Y. Shimada, Y. F. Asanuma, K. Yokota et al., "Pentraxin 3 is associated with disease activity but not atherosclerosis in patients with systemic lupus erythematosus," *Modern Rheumatology*, vol. 24, no. 1, pp. 78–85, 2014.

12

# A Metabolomic Perspective on Coeliac Disease

**Antonio Calabrò,[1,2] Ewa Gralka,[3] Claudio Luchinat,[3,4] Edoardo Saccenti,[5,6] and Leonardo Tenori[3,7]**

[1] *Department of Experimental and Clinical Biomedical Sciences, University of Florence, Viale Pieraccini 6, 50139 Florence, Italy*
[2] *Tuscany Referral Center for Adult Coeliac Disease, Viale Pieraccini 6, 50139 Florence, Italy*
[3] *Magnetic Resonance Center (CERM), University of Florence, Via L. Sacconi 6, 50019 Sesto Fiorentino, Italy*
[4] *Department of Chemistry, University of Florence, Via della Lastruccia 3, 50019 Sesto Fiorentino, Italy*
[5] *Biosystems Data Analysis Group, University of Amsterdam, 904 Science Park, 1098 XH Amsterdam, The Netherlands*
[6] *Laboratory of Systems and Synthetic Biology, Wageningen University and Research Center, Dreijenplein 10, 6703 HB Wageningen, The Netherlands*
[7] *FiorGen Foundation, Via L. Sacconi 6, 50019 Sesto Fiorentino, Italy*

Correspondence should be addressed to Claudio Luchinat; claudioluchinat@cerm.unifi.it

Academic Editor: Kalle Kurppa

Metabolomics is an "omic" science that is now emerging with the purpose of elaborating a comprehensive analysis of the metabolome, which is the complete set of metabolites (i.e., small molecules intermediates) in an organism, tissue, cell, or biofluid. In the past decade, metabolomics has already proved to be useful for the characterization of several pathological conditions and offers promises as a clinical tool. A metabolomics investigation of coeliac disease (CD) revealed that a metabolic fingerprint for CD can be defined, which accounts for three different but complementary components: malabsorption, energy metabolism, and alterations in gut microflora and/or intestinal permeability. In this review, we will discuss the major advancements in metabolomics of CD, in particular with respect to the role of gut microbiome and energy metabolism.

## 1. Introduction

Coeliac disease (CD, MIM 212750), first described in 1887, is a common complex chronic immune-mediated disorder with a known (gluten) environmental trigger. Recent surveys indicate that it may affect 1 in 105 subjects in the United States [1], 1 in 67 Finnish school children [2], and 1 in 230 in Italian school age children [3], with seroprevalence of about 1% in subjects of white European origin [4, 5].

Coeliac disease has a strong genetic component with multiple contributing genes: the most important and best characterized genetic risk factors are the HLA class II genes DQ2 and/or DQ8 which are located on chromosome 6p21. More than 97% of patients have at least one of the two genes: most patients (>90%) carry the DQ2 gene, while the rest expresses the DQ8 gene. HLA-DQ2 is encoded by the HLA-DQA1$^*$05 allele ($\alpha$ chain) and the HLA-DQB1$^*$02 ($\beta$ chain) [6, 7]. Common to many other autoimmune disorders, the two alleles are often present in the *cis* conformation on the DR3 haplotype [8]; HLA-DQ2 and HLA-DQ8 are necessary but not sufficient for the development of CD.

Genome wide association studies indicated 39 non-HLA loci to be predisposing to CD [9–11]. Altogether, the nonHLA loci explain only 5% of the risk for CD [6], while the HLA loci account for 35% of the risk [7].

Several of these nonHLA CD susceptibility genes are associated with other diseases/traits [6] such as type 1 diabetes [12, 13], rheumatoid arthritis [14], and systemic lupus erythematosus [15] indicating a possibly shared genetic background with other diseases [7].

The environmental trigger of coeliac disease is gluten, a protein complex formed by gliadin and glutenin, which is

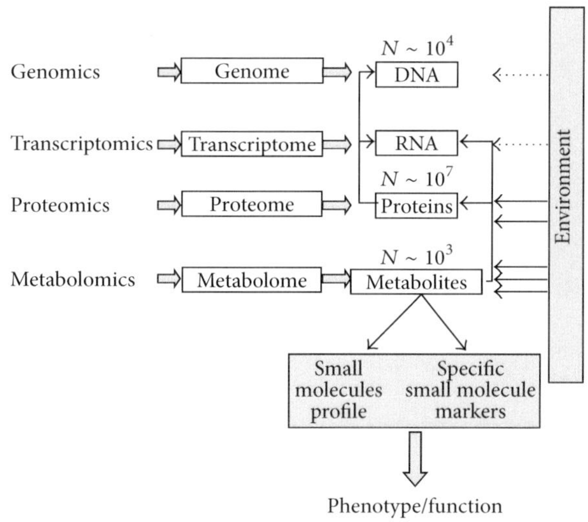


FIGURE 1: Relationships between the omics sciences.

found in wheat and related grain species like barley and rye and also in processed food where it is used to enhance food texture and as a stabilizing agent.

The active disease component is gliadin [16] with the $\alpha$-, $\beta$-, $\gamma$-, and $\omega$-fractions. These fractions are rich in proline and glutamine and resistant to enzymatic digestion; large proline/glutamine-rich peptides accumulate in the smallest intestine, triggering an abnormal innate and adaptive immune response in genetically predisposed subjects.

The response of the adaptive immune system is due to the gliadin-reactive CD4+ T cells; HLA-DQ molecules bind to these peptides which are deamidated by the intestinal brush border enzyme tissue transglutaminase; these complexes interact with the T-cell receptor on T cells leading to T-cell activation with subsequent release of proinflammatory cytokines and the production by B-cells of specific antibodies (anti-tissue transglutaminase and endomysial antibodies) [17, 18].

The role of the innate immune systems in CD is less clear [7]. Increased expression of interleukin-15 has been observed [19]; enhanced intestinal permeability has been also observed [20], induced by zonulin [21], whose release is mediated by gluten activated CXCR-3 [22, 23]. Loss of functionality in the intestinal barrier permits the passage of immunoreactive peptides and other antigens from the gut lumen to the lamina propria, with subsequent triggering of the innate immune system.

## 2. Metabolomics

The advent of high-throughput techniques led to a rapid expansion of data sets originated from the analysis of gut microbiota and currently several ongoing projects are aimed at the study and definition of the microbiome [24, 25]. In this framework, metabolomics is playing a crucial role.

Since the systematic genome sequencing of the first free-living microbe [26], we have seen the rising of genome-wide expression profiling methods, aimed to understand complex biological systems on a large scale [27]. The fast development of genomics, transcriptomics, proteomics, and the other *omics* disciplines is the consequence of this new scientific paradigm.

In this framework, metabolomics has already proved in the past decade to be a useful complement for the characterization of several physiological and pathological conditions and offers promises as a clinical tool [28]. Metabolomics is based on the analysis of the measured dynamic changes of a living organism in response to genetic modifications or physiological stimuli such as nutrients, drugs treatment, or toxic insults [29].

The metabolome, the complete collection of all metabolites contained in a biological specimen, can be considered the downstream end-product of the complex interaction of genome, transcriptome, proteome, and the environment: it can be regarded as a cascade linking genome to the phenotype [30] (Figure 1). The metabolome, consisting of low-molecular weight chemical intermediates [31], can be considered as an amplified version of gene expression. While changes in gene expression levels (and thus proteins) will have only small effects on metabolic fluxes, they must have large effects on metabolic pathways (and thus metabolites concentrations) [27]. From this point of view, the metabolite space represents the optimal level at which changes in biological systems are analyzed with optimal sensitivity [32] under conditions of negligible effects on the global phenotype [33].

Metabolomics does not rely on the measurement of a single metabolite but considers the spectrum of (possibly) all metabolites as a whole, taking a holistic approach; this offers evident advantages with respect to a targeted search of metabolites; indeed, no assumption is required on the identity of the metabolites that are or may be relevant for the biological phenomenon under investigation.

The main analytical techniques employed in metabolomics (Boxes 1 and 2) are nuclear magnetic resonance spectroscopy (NMR) and mass spectrometry (MS). Both MS and NMR methods provide information on the relative and absolute concentrations of different classes of metabolites in a single measurement (see Box 3) and can be also used

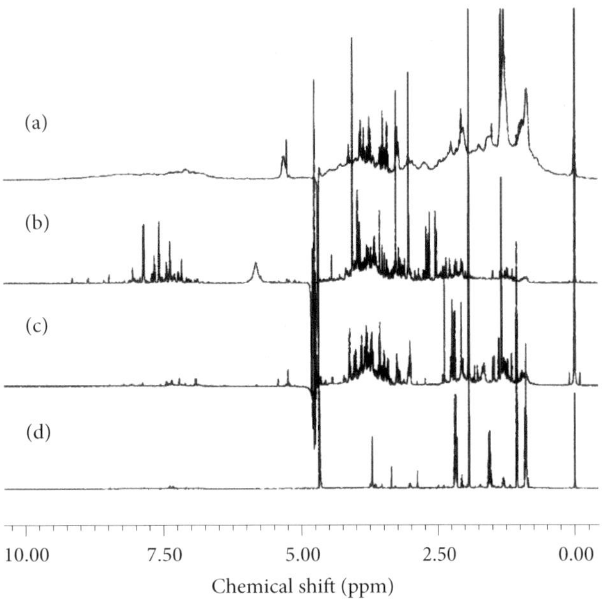


FIGURE 2: Examples of NMR profiles of (a) serum, (b) urine, (c) saliva, and (d) faecal extract.

to determine metabolite structures providing mechanistic insights.

The most common biological specimens used in metabolomics are serum/plasma and/or urines, firstly, because they can be collected with low invasiveness, and, secondly because, as they contain thousands of metabolites, they are rich in biological information at the systemic level; a number of other biofluids such as saliva [34], tissue extract [35], cerebrospinal fluid [36], bile [37], seminal fluid [38], amniotic fluid [39], synovial fluid [40], exhaled breath condensate [41, 42], and faecal extracts [43] can also be studied. Figure 2 shows typical NMR spectra of four different biofluids (Box 3).

Targeted and untargeted approaches are possible in metabolomics, the former focusing on the analysis of a subset of known compounds or class thereof (targeted MS and NMR) and the latter focusing on the whole array of metabolites within the detection limit of the technique employed (untargeted MS and NMR). Using both approaches, hundreds to thousands of metabolites are measured. Data are usually analyzed following the classical metabolomics pipeline (Box 4), and information is extracted using state-of-the-art statistical tools (Box 5).

Metabolomics has provided significant information on a wide range of pathologies, such as cancer [44], meningitis [45], neurological disorders [46], cardiovascular diseases [47], inborn errors of metabolism [48], and CD [49–51]. The first metabolomics investigation of CD revealed that a metabolic fingerprint for coeliac disease can be defined [49], which accounts for three different but complementary components: malabsorption, energy metabolism, and alterations in gut microflora and/or intestinal permeability.

In this review, we will discuss the major advancements in metabolomics of CD with respect to the role of gut microbiome and energy metabolism.

## 3. Gut Microbiota and CD

Recent studies [52–56] pointed to the possible role of intestinal microbiota (faecal and duodenal species) in the development of coeliac disease. A summary of the most relevant findings in this research area is reported in Table 1 together with the associated bacteria strains involved.

Nistal et al. [57] compared the differences between gut microorganisms in the upper small intestinal mucosa in adults and in children. A two-time higher number of microbial genera have been identified in adults compared to children, although the dominant genera were very similar: *Firmicutes*, *Proteobacteria*, *Bacteroidetes*, *Actinobacteria,* and *Fusobacteria*. Differences in the amount of bacterial communities between adult and juvenile groups can be also directly connected with the age of investigated subjects.

A comparison between healthy, diseased, and treated coeliac adults showed a lower number of *Streptococcus* spp. and *Prevotella* spp. families in untreated coeliac adults. Interestingly, similar patterns were also observed in CD children, suggesting that these bacterial populations may have been modified by changes in the intestine environment caused by active CD.

In the study by Nadal et al. [58], the bacterial species present in faeces and duodenum of children with active and treated CD were compared with a healthy control group. The ratio of harmless Gram-positive bacteria (*Lactobacillus* + *Bifidobacterium*) to potentially harmful Gram-negative (*Bacteroides*/*Prevotella* + *E. coli*) bacteria was significantly lower in CD patients than in controls, while no distinction was possible between active and inactive CD.

Sánchez et al. [59] applied denaturing gradient gel electrophoresis (DGGE) to analyze intestinal microbiota from biopsy specimens obtained from three groups of children, investigating the composition of *Bacteroides*, *Bifidobacterium*, and Lactic acid bacteria in duodenal biopsies of patients with active and treated coeliac disease. Dysbiosis in *Bacteroides* (the most abundant intestinal bacterial group) was observed, with a significant reduction in coeliac and coeliac treated patients in comparison with the control group. Moreover, it was observed that a treatment with gluten-free diet did not restore the balance of the *Bacteroides* composition. Interestingly, it was observed that the lactic acid bacteria (*Lactobacillus*) and the *Weissella* family were more abundant and diverse in treated coeliac and control patients than in patients with untreated coeliac disease. The authors suggested that some of the changes in duodenal bacterial community could be due to the inflammatory consequences of the active phase of the disease; nonetheless, the influence of different dietary habits could not be discarded.

Biopsies from treated coeliac children were analyzed in a study by di Cagno et al. [63], that also confirmed that a gluten-free diet lasting two or more years is not able to restore completely the microbiota. In addition, a higher diversity of the *Eubacteria* community was observed in the duodenum

Table 1: Most relevant findings, and associated references, for studies linking gut microbiota and CD.

| References | Type of sample | Technique | Microbiota phylum/class | Relevant findings |
|---|---|---|---|---|
| Wacklin et al. (2013) [55] | Mucosa biopsy | PCR-DGGE (real-time polymerase chain reaction, denaturing gradient gel electrophoresis), 16S rRNA sequencing | *Firmicutes Bacteroides Proteobacteria Actinobacteria* | Diversity in mucosal microbiota of celiac disease patients is associated with the symptoms of the disease. |
| Nistal et al. (2012) [57] | Duodenal biopsies | PCR (polymerase chain reaction) | *Firmicutes Proteobacteria Bacteroidetes Actinobacteria Fusobacteria* | Composition of small intestinal microbiota is similar between adults and children; there is higher number of *Streptococcus* and *Prevotella* in healthy subjects. |
| Nadal et al. (2007) [58] | Duodenal biopsy | FISH (Fluorescent in situ hybridization), Flow cytometry detection. | | In faeces and duodenum of CD children, smaller amount of harmless bacteria (*Lactobacillus* and *Bifidobacterium*) and higher number of harmful bacteria are found (*Bacteroides/Prevotella* + *E. coli*) compared to healthy children. |
| Sánchez et al. (2010) [59] | Duodenal biopsy | PCR-DGGE | *Bacteroidetes* | Reduced number of intestinal microbiota in CD children but also in treated CD children was noticed. Treatment with GFD does not restore the bacteria composition. |
| Sánchez et al. (2011) [60] | Faeces samples | PCR-DGGE | | Studies were carried out on stools of infants with high/low risk of CD and different types of milk feeding. High-risk infants have higher prevalence of *Bacteroides vulgatus*, whereas low-risk infants have higher population of *B. uniformis, B. ovatus,* and *B. plebeius* considering the subgroup of either breast-fed or formula-fed infants. |
| Cheng et al. (2013) [61] | Duodenal biopsy | qRT-PCR (quantitative real-time PCR) | *Bacilli Bacteroides Clostridium Proteobacteria* | Overall microbiota composition in the duodenal mucosa is comparable between healthy and CD children, but studied groups differ regarding bacteria subpopulation profile. |
| Sellitto et al. (2012) [51] | Faeces samples | qPCR (quantitative PCR) | *Bacteroidetes Firmicutes* | Lack of microflora maturation during first 2 years of life in infants at risk of CD. Moreover, there was observed absence of *Bacteroidetes* and abundance of *Firmicutes*. |
| Sanz et al. (2007) [54] | Faeces samples | PCR-DGGE | *Actinobacteria Firmicutes* | *Lactobacillus* and *Weissella* are more abundant and diverse in treated CD patients and control subjects than in active CD individuals. Composition of lactic bacteria and *Bifidobacterium* differs between celiac children and age-matched controls. |
| Kaufman and Rousseeuw (2009) [62] | Intestine biopsies | PCR | *Proteobacteria* | There observed no statistical differences in bacteria composition between healthy and CD children. Nevertheless, *Haemophilus* was more common in CD patients and *Neisseria polysaccharea* in control individuals. |
| di Cagno et al. (2011) [63] | Faeces sample, duodenal biopsy | RAPD (random amplification of polymorphic DNA) -PCR | *Eubacteria* | Higher number of different *Eubacteria* classes was found in duodenum of coeliac children under gluten-free diet than in healthy children. |

Table 1: Continued.

| References | Type of sample | Technique | Microbiota phylum/class | Relevant findings |
|---|---|---|---|---|
| Medina et al. (2008) [64] | Faeces sample | PBMC (peripheral blood mononuclear cell) phenotyping and flow cytometric analyses | *Actinobacteria* | Studies regarding interaction between faecal bacteria and immune system response of coeliac disease patients. It appeared that Gram-positive bacteria such as *Lactobacillus* and *Bifidobacterium* may act as inhibitors of inflammation. |

of coeliac children under a gluten-free diet with respect to healthy children. Compared to that of duodenal biopsies, the faecal bacterial population was found to be more diverse. PCR-DGGE faecal profiles of *Lactobacillus* and *Bifidobacterium* differ between treated coeliac children and healthy controls. The ratio between *Lactobacillus*/*Bifidobacterium* and *Bacteroides*/*Enterobacteria* was lower in coeliac children under treatment compared to healthy children. Some of the differences could be related to both coeliac disease and dietary variations.

Surprisingly, a study by Ou et al. [65], based on biopsies collected from the distal duodenum/proximal jejunum of 45 children, did not reveal significant differences between the microbiota in the small intestine of diseased and healthy children, although bacteria from the *Haemophilus* family were more abundant in CD patients, while *Neisseria polysaccharea* were more widespread in the control group. However, at the *genus* level, no differences between the two groups were observed. The authors commented that differences at the species level could not be excluded because complete 16 S rDNA were not sequenced. Similar results, pointing to a lack of significant differences in global composition of duodenal microbiota between healthy controls and CD patients, were obtained also by Cheng et al.; on the other hand, a subpopulation profile, containing eight genus-like bacterial groups, was found to distinguish healthy controls from CD patients [61].

The possible effect on microbiota of different types of milk feeding in early life and the link to the risk of CD development were investigated by Sánchez et al. [60]. The study was carried out on stools of breast-fed infants with different genetic risk of CD (low and high); it showed that high-risk infants had a higher prevalence of *Bacteroides vulgatus*, whereas low-risk infants had higher population of *B. uniformis*, *B. ovatus*, and *B. plebeius*. In the study group of formula-fed infants, *B. ovatus* and *B. plebeius* were increased in subjects with lower genetic risk, while *B. vulgatus* had higher prevalence in those subjects with higher genetic risk. The authors concluded that both types of milk feeding in conjunction with HLA-DQ genotype can influence the *Bacteroides* colonization, increasing the risk of coeliac disease onset. Also, the time of exposure to milk feeding was found to be relevant in prompting coeliac disease development [66].

Sellitto et al. [51] reported the impact on the intestinal tract of two different patterns of gluten introduction. A delay in gluten exposure of at least 6 to 12 months was found to have a positive effect on gluten tolerance: it caused a delay in CD autoimmunity onset in infants that were genetically susceptible to CD. Instead, the early exposure to gluten of infants at risk of coeliac disease was found to induce an immune response and led to a more frequent development of CD. Moreover, a lack of gut microflora maturation during the first 2 years of life in infants at risk of CD was also noted. The gut metabolome of the first 6 months of infant's life reflects mainly the milk diet (rich in polysaccharides and other sugars) and is very similar in all infants; once the solid food is introduced, a shift occurs and a group of short-chain fatty acids are found in faeces. By the end of the second year of life, *Bacteroides* are the main bacteria group found in the metabolome of healthy infants. Conversely, in infants with a genetic risk of celiac disease, an overall lack of bacteria of the phylum *Bacteroides* and abundance of *Firmicutes* were observed.

Recent studies [67] suggest that the colonization of gastrointestinal tract is very important in the development of autoimmune disorders and food-related disease. Furthermore, possible interaction between the intestinal bacteria and the mammalian immune system in the direct differentiation of both pro- and anti-inflammatory T-cells population has been suggested [68]. To clarify whether the gut microflora present in the faeces of CD patients is involved in the proinflammatory activity of coeliac disease, *Bifidobacterium* from healthy subjects was co-incubated together with the faecal microflora or the peripheral blood mononuclear cell culture of coeliac subjects [64]. It appeared that certain strains of *Bifidobacterium* are able to suppress and reverse the proinflammatory effect by increasing IL-10 cytokine production. These results may suggest the use of selected strains of *Bifidobacterium* as probiotics for treatment of CD.

It has been also suggested that gluten intolerance may be also triggered by environmental factors like viruses or bacteria showing molecular mimicking with gluten proteins, causing an autoimmune response that may last even after infection [69]. Several studies pointed to infections by human adenovirus [70], hepatitis C virus [71], rotaviruses [72], or *Campylobacter jejuni* [73] that could induce allergic reactions similar to that induced by gluten exposure, causing the onset of CD.

## 4. Body Composition and Energy Expenditure in CD Patients

Patients with the classic form of coeliac disease are always characterized by weight loss directly connected with malabsorption and subsequent risk of malnutrition. Often coeliac disease results in a general lack of energy and strength that can create abnormal conditions described as (chronic) fatigue. Appearance of fatigue and fatigue-related problems seems to be more frequent in nontreated coeliac patients than in patients on a gluten-free diet [74].

Body composition, resting metabolic rate (RMR), and substrate oxidation rates were investigated in [75, 76]. The results showed that untreated and treated CD patients had a lower body weight, lower levels of fat-free mass (FFM), and lower fat mass (FM) in comparison to the healthy controls. In [77], the analysis of body composition at the diagnosis time and after one year of treatment with a gluten-free diet was carried out. The analysis showed a significant increase of body weight and FM but only a slight increase of FFM after treatment with gluten-free diet. Additionally, RMR values were higher in CD patients (treated and untreated) than in controls. Moreover, untreated CD patients showed a higher npRQ (nonprotein respiratory quotient); this may indicate that untreated patients oxidize larger amounts of carbohydrate under resting metabolite conditions than treated CD and healthy subjects.

Interestingly ghrelin, one of the hormones responsible for energy balance regulation, is also changed in CD patients. Ghrelin is a 28-amino acid-peptide produced by the enteroendocrine cells of the gastric mucosa and the intestine [78]. Recent studies have shown that ghrelin is able to increase food intake, decrease fat use, and reduce energy expenditure [79]. While serum ghrelin concentration was increased in CD patients, body mass was decreased [80, 81]. Lower levels of circulating ghrelin were found in CD patients after gluten-free treatment in comparison with CD and control subjects [82]. These results suggest that low amounts of ghrelin in the blood may be partially responsible for the slight increase in body weight and FM in CD patients after treatment with a gluten-free diet.

## 5. Metabolomic Signature of CD

In many cases, the diagnosis of CD is not an easy task, mainly because CD has a variable clinical picture due to its intertwingled genetic, immunological, and environmental components. The presence of the HLA genetic factor, together with a positive biopsy and serological antibodies upon gluten-containing diet, is used to diagnose coeliac disease at any age. In order to better understand the processes underlying the activation and development of coeliac disease, it is important to examine the mechanisms from the early beginning.

To date, a limited number of metabolomics studies of coeliac disease are available, but they clearly show that metabolic differences between healthy individuals and coeliac patients exist. In the first (to our knowledge) metabolomic study on CD, Bertini et al. [49], examined adult healthy controls and coeliac patients by $^1$H NMR profiling of their serum and urine profiles before and after GFD, showing that a metabolic fingerprint for CD can be defined. This fingerprint was found to be made up by three components, one related to malabsorption, one related to energy metabolism, and the third related to alterations in gut microflora and/or intestinal permeability. Using this metabolic fingerprint, it was possible to make predictions about the coeliac status with a very good accuracy (ca. 84%). One of the most interesting findings was that the metabolic profile of CD patients reverts to normality after 12 months of a strict gluten-free diet; interestingly, a similar behavior was not found in CD patients when analyzing them from a gut microflora prospective [58, 59, 63].

The main observed differences in serum spectra between CD patients and controls were lower levels of several amino acids (asparagine, isoleucine, methionine, proline, and valine), methylamine, pyruvate, creatinine, choline, methylglutarate, lactate, lipids, and glycoproteins and higher levels of glucose and 3-hydroxybutyric acid. Notably, the best discrimination is obtained from CPMG spectra (Carr-Purcell-Meiboom-Gill spin echo sequence) [83], that is, from spectra in which signals arising from large macromolecules such as lipidic components are suppressed [49]. So, although it is known that coeliac patients usually appear to be hypocholesterolemic, lipids do not contribute significantly to the metabonomic signature of coeliac disease. A decrease in the level of pyruvate and lactate and a higher level of glucose in the blood of coeliac patients were observed, probably as a consequence of an impaired glycolysis process. Glycolysis impairment can cause a lowering of pyruvate and lactate levels and an increase of glucose levels in blood. If this metabolic way is reduced, $\beta$-oxidation is probably increased. Enhanced $\beta$-oxidation and malabsorption can then explain lower levels of lipids in serum [49]. In these conditions, the authors hypothesized an increase of the use of ketonic bodies as a source of energy in coeliac patients, consistently with the higher observed levels of 3-hydroxybutyric acid in blood and acetoacetate in urines [49].

Energy conversion from lipids and catabolism of ketonic bodies are far less efficient than that from glucids. Untreated coeliac subjects often report symptoms of fatigue. In patients on a gluten-free diet, fatigue tends to be reduced and, in fact, it has been proposed that this condition is gluten-related [74]. In [49], the authors found that in CD patients on a gluten-free diet the levels of glucose and 3-hydroxy-butyric acids revert to normality.

Further, the authors found that CD patients are characterized by higher urine levels of some metabolites related to gut microbiota: indoxyl sulfate (IS), meta-[hydroxyphenyl] propionic acid (m-HPPA), and phenylacetylglycine (PAG). M-HPPA mostly originates from gut microflora, being one of the several products of the microbially mediated breakdown of larger plant phenolic compounds such as caffeic acid and its conjugate chlorogenic acids [84]. IS is a harmful uremic toxin produced in the liver from indole through indoxyl. Indole is a subproduct of tryptophan metabolism by intestinal bacteria [85]. Modulation of PAG excretion in urine has been attributed to gut microflora, and increases of PAG have been reported in cases of drug-induced phospholipidosis; nonetheless, the contribution of mammalian and microbial sources to PAG excretion is not yet fully characterized [86]. All these findings are consistent with the hypothesis that in CD patients the gut microflora of the small bowel is altered or presents peculiar species with their own microbial metabolome.

In a following investigation [50], the same research group highlighted again the existence of a metabolic fingerprint for coeliac disease, confirming most of the previously discussed metabolites with the additional finding of higher levels of *p*-cresolsulfate in the urines of CD patients. Interestingly, *p*-cresolsulfate, a metabolite of bacterial origin, is associated with several gastric-related disease [87], including bowel cancer [88]. In the same study, the analysis of the so-called "potential coeliac patients" (i.e., subjects who have a positive antibody test but no evidence of intestinal damage) showed that the metabolic patterns of overt and potential coeliac patients are similar [50] indicating that CD-related dysmetabolism precedes the intestinal damage. Only a few serum metabolites differentiate between potential and overt CD, and none of these metabolites are related to the energy metabolism [50]. It appears that, as in overt CD patients, glycolysis is somehow impaired also in potential CD patients. Impairment of glycolysis explains both the observed lower lactate levels and the higher glucose levels in blood of potential CD patients. In urine, there are more metabolites that discriminate potential and overt CD. The key differences lie in the concentration of metabolites originating from the gut microflora (m-HPPA, IS, and PAG) which in potential coeliac subjects are similar to those of controls, suggesting a relationship between overt CD, villous atrophy, and bacterial consortia of the host [50].

The authors concluded that, although free from intestinal injury, placing potential CD subjects on a gluten-free diet could be justified because they are experiencing most of the pathological alterations experienced by overt coeliac patients [50]. Figure 3 shows the discrimination between overt CD patients and healthy controls and the statistical prediction of the potential CD patients: almost all potential CD patients are predicted as overt CD. The plot shown in Figure 3(a) was obtained using a training set composed of the serum CPMG spectra of 34 overt CD patients, 34 healthy controls, and 13 (out of the 34) CD patients after 12 months of gluten-free diet. It clearly appears that all but one patient on gluten-free diet were classified as healthy. Similarly, the plot in Figure 3(b) was built using the CPMG spectra of 61 overt CD patients, 51 healthy controls, and 29 potential CD patients. Almost all the potential CD patients fall in the CD group, underlining the affinity between the metabolic fingerprints of these two dissimilar clinical conditions.

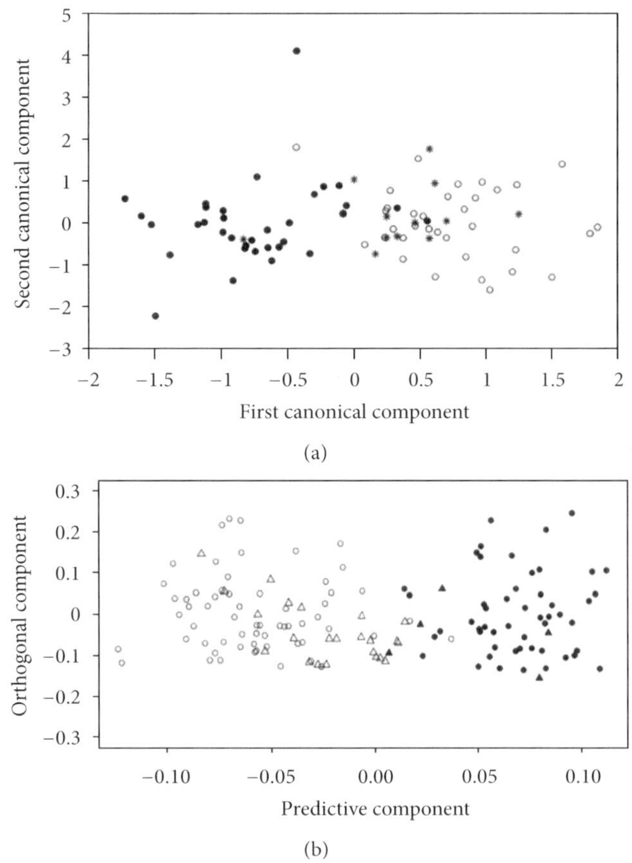


Figure 3: (a) Clustering of CMPG (Carr-Purcell-Meiboom-Gill spin echo sequence) [83] serum spectra of CD patients (filled circles) and controls (open circles). The discriminant model between the two groups was calculated using a combination of partial least square [89] and (regularized) canonical analysis [90] (PLS-RCC) and was validated using cross-validation. The CPMG spectra of 13 (out of the 34) CD patients after 12 months of gluten-free diet were then projected into the discriminant space of the model (stars) and were assigned to the CD or the healthy group applying a support vector machine [91] classifier (SVM). (b) Clustering of overt CD patients (open circles) and healthy controls (filled circles) obtained with CPMG serum spectra. The discriminant model was calculated using orthogonal partial least square [92] (OPLS) and validated using double cross-validation [93]. The CPMG spectra of 29 potential CD patients were then projected in the model (triangles) and filled or not according to the results of an SVM classifier. Adapted with permission from [49, 50]. Copyright (2009 and 2011) American Chemical Society.

Differences between the metabolic profiles of faeces and urine of CD and healthy children using a combination of $^{1}$H-NMR and GC-MS/SPME techniques were reported by di Cagno et al. [63]. The analysis allowed the identification of a group of compounds that were significantly changed in the treated coeliac children group. A set of volatile organic compounds and short fatty acids were identified using MS, whereas amino acids were identified using NMR [63]. Faecal and urine samples of treated CD children showed elevated levels of free amino acids (proline, methionine, histidine, and tryptophan) and lowered levels of some short fatty acids (butyric, isocaproic, and propanoic acids) compared to healthy children [63]. The authors suggested that these changes may be associated with intestinal and faecal bacteria modifications that could induce a nonspecific inflammation and a reduction of the absorptive surface of the intestinal mucosa; this may lead to a reduction of the absorption of amino acids which are subsequently lost with stool [63]. By combining microbiology and metabolomics, the authors showed that a gluten-free diet lasting at least two years did not completely restore the microbiota of the CD children. From that work, a broader picture seems to emerge that microbial indices (i.e., the ratio of faecal cell density of lactic acid *bacteria-Bifidobacterium* to *Bacteroides-Enterobacteria*) and the levels of some metabolites (i.e., ethyl-acetate, octyl-acetate, SCFA, and glutamine) are characteristic of CD patients [63].

## 6. Perspectives

Metabolomics is a rapidly growing discipline bringing together analytical technologies, metabolite pathways evaluation, and information technology. A major advantage is the noninvasive or minimally invasive measurement of potentially useful biomarkers from biofluids such as urine and plasma. A great deal of validation work (both at the analytical and data analysis level) has been carried out to gain full acceptance to metabolomics in routine clinical practice. Challenges for the development of metabolomics still exist, including simplified systems to present data to end-users (such as interpretation of often complex statistical models), the coordination of multiple data streams, and the implementation of quality control programs [94]. We expect that in the next few years it will be clear whether or not metabolomics will take its place as a complementary or even an alternative tool in the clinical setting.

At the present time, only few applications devoted to the investigation of coeliac disease have been presented in the literature, but a complex picture of the interaction between energy metabolism and gut microbiota seems to emerge, providing new hints on the biochemistry of the disease. In our institutions, as a logical complement to the results obtained analyzing overt coeliac and potential coeliac subjects, we are currently applying metabolomics to the biomolecular investigation of a gluten-related condition defined as gluten sensitivity [95]. This condition is still not very well characterized and its pathogenesis is caused by unknown mechanisms; we believe that metabolomics is a useful tool to expand our current limited knowledge of this condition.

Metabolomics-based approaches are expected to enable diagnosis, prognosis, and prediction of response of individuals to treatment. We can expect that metabolomics will provide more accurate and less expensive biomarkers (obtained by means of proper statistical analysis and properly validated) than presently available, which could improve diagnostic accuracy and sensitivity. However, far more research is essential to reach such a goal, and a validation of the results on an epidemiological scale is indeed needed.

*Box 1* (MS and metabolomics). The main analytical techniques used in metabolomics are nuclear magnetic resonance spectroscopy (NMR) and mass spectrometry (MS) [96]. Both MS and NMR methods provide information on a wide range of metabolites in a single measurement. Furthermore, both can be used to identify the metabolites' structures and to measure the relative and absolute concentrations of the molecules (MS has higher sensitivity but NMR is more reliable for determining concentrations) [97].

Mass spectrometry is a technique to determine extremely accurate mass of molecules in a pure sample or in a mixture. The molecules in a sample are converted to ions by an electron beam; the ions are accelerated by charged plates and then deflected by a magnetic field according to the mass-to-charge ratio of each ion. When the ions reach the detector, the mass-to-charge ratio is registered to provide a spectrum where series of peaks are shown reporting the intensity of each ion generated by the sample. MS is a destructive technique but requires a very low quantity of sample [98]. Over the last few years, its application to mammalian study increased, especially for its high sensitivity, and because it is a major technique for molecular identification [99]. As opposed to NMR, MS usually requires metabolites separation before detection, typically by using gas chromatography (GC) or liquid chromatography (LC). GC-MS is a robust technique for the analysis of volatile and semivolatile compounds suitable for chemical derivatization to increase their volatility [100]. Electron ionization (EI) in GC-MS is quite reproducible [100]. In contrast to GC-MS, LC-MS is especially suitable for the analysis of nonvolatile and/or thermally unstable metabolites. The introduction of UPLC (ultraperformance liquid chromatography) and capillary LC enabled better peak resolution and further increase in sensitivity and speed, and it is now successfully applied to metabolomics studies [101].

*Box 2* (NMR and metabolomics). NMR spectroscopy is an analytical technique that exploits the magnetic properties of certain atomic nuclei. It determines the physical and chemical properties of molecules by detecting the magnetically active nuclei. When placed in a magnetic field, an active nucleus (such as $^{1}H$ or $^{13}C$) absorbs electromagnetic radiation at a characteristic frequency and then reemits it. After absorbing electromagnetic radiation in the range of frequencies of $^{1}H$ (or $^{13}C$, or $^{31}P$,...), the sample emits all frequences of its active nuclei of that type, which constitute its $^{1}H$ (or $^{13}C$ or $^{31}P$,...) NMR spectrum. The resonance frequency and the corresponding intensity of each signal are dependent, respectively, on the chemical environment where that particular nucleus is located (i.e., molecular structure) and on the concentration of that molecule.

NMR spectroscopy is a nondestructive and highly reproducible technique and provides detailed information on the molecular structure of both pure compounds and complex mixtures [102]. In a typical biological fluid, all hydrogen-containing molecules will give a $^{1}H$-NMR spectrum as long as they are present in concentrations above the detection limit. The NMR spectrum of a biological fluid is therefore the superposition of the spectra of thousands of different small molecules (up to 2500 for urine and up to 200 for serum/plasma) present in the sample at concentrations $>1\,\mu M$ [103]. An advantage of NMR is that the biological fluid requires only a mild treatment prior to the analysis.

The main disadvantage of NMR is its relatively low sensitivity. Another disadvantage of the NMR approach is the difficult identification of all metabolites in the samples: $^{1}H$-NMR spectra of biological fluids are very complex and often additional two-dimensional NMR experiments may be needed to assign metabolites in biofluids. The development of high-resolution $^{1}H$ magic angle spinning (MAS) spectra made viable the acquisition of data on small slices of tissue without any pretreatment [104–106].

*Box 3* (biofluids and metabolomics). Most biofluids used in metabolomics can be collected noninvasively. The Human Metabolome Database (http://www.hmdb.ca/) lists 16 different biofluids investigated and up to 5000 identified or putative metabolites: amniotic fluid (17), aqueous humor (1), ascites fluid (1), bile fluid (18), blood (4297), breast milk (37), cellular cytoplasm (49), cerebrospinal fluid (436), faeces (0), lymph (1), menses (0), mucus (0), pericardial effusion (1), prostate tissue (13), saliva (70), sebum (0), semen (4), sweat (1), synovial fluid (0), tear fluid (1), urine (3873), and vaginal fluid (0). Of these, 694 have been associated with one or more diseases and pathologies.

Blood, urine, cerebrospinal fluid, and saliva are the richest in metabolites. The Human Serum Metabolome project. [107] (http://www.serummetabolome.ca/) lists 4229 *detectable* metabolites (most of them lipids) obtained by enhanced NMR, MS, and other analytical platforms. NMR was able to measure 1.2% (49/4229) of the human serum metabolome, GC 2.13% (90/4229), ESI-MS/MS (lipid mediator profiling) 2.3% (96/4229), and TLC/GC-FID-MS (general lipidomics) 79.9% (3381/4229, mostly, however, components of the complex lipid fraction) and DFI MS/MS is able to access 3.3% (139/4229) of the serum metabolome. Some of the compounds identified by NMR are urea (6 mM), glucose (5 mM), lactic acid, (1.4 mM), glutamine (0.51 mM), and glycerol (0.43 mM). The least abundant compounds were carnitine (46 $\mu$M), acetic acid (42 $\mu$M), creatine (37 $\mu$M), cysteine (34 $\mu$M), propylene glycol (22 $\mu$M), and aspartic acid (21 $\mu$M), and the lowest concentration reliably detected using NMR was 12.3 $\mu$M (for malonic acid) and 14.5 $\mu$M (for choline).

The Human Urine Metabolome project [108] (http://www.urinemetabolome.ca/) lists up to 3100 metabolites identified in urine. Human urine contains many classes of compounds excreted as waste products, including organic acids, amino acids, purines, pyrimidines, sugars, sugar alcohols, sugar acids, amines, and other compounds, at a variety of concentrations. Fresh urine is also characterized by the presence of human cells (erythrocytes, leucocytes, urothelial cells, and epithelial cells), bacteria, fungi, sperms, and noncellular components (mucus filaments, cylinders, cylindroids, pseudocylinders, and crystals, urates).

Some of the metabolites identified in saliva using NMR are [109] glucose, propionate, acetate, taurine, glycine, alanine, sucrose, dimethylamine, formate, glycine, lactate, methanol, propionate, propylene glycol, pyruvate, succinate, and taurine.

A large panel of metabolites has been also identified in cerebrospinal fluid by using NMR and GC-MS [36]. Among those obtained by NMR, there are amino acids, sugars, 2-oxoglutarate, 2-oxoisovalerate, 3-hydroxybutyrate, 3-hydroxyisovalerate, xanthine, and pyruvate.

Up to 50 metabolites were identified in faecal extracts via NMR [43]: amino acids, n-butyrate, propionate, n-caproate, 3-(4′-hydroxyphenyl) propionate, 5-aminopentanoate, glucose, 5-N-acetylneuraminate, 5-aminosalicylate, N-acetyl-5-aminosalicylate, deoxycholate, and phenylacetate, many of which are of bacterial origin.

*Box 4* (the metabolomics pipeline). The workflow of a metabolomics study is complex and each step has its own criticalities that need to be addressed. The metabolomics workflow can be summarized as follows [96, 110–112].

*Biological Question.* It includes definition of the biological/biomedical problem to be addressed.

*Study Design.* It involves power analysis and treatment design.

*Data Acquisition.* It concerns quality control strategies, experimental setting (platform specific), Sampling, and measurement design.

*Data Preprocessing.* It is a fundamental step before analysis involving alignment, baseline correction (MR), phasing, alignment, bucketing (NMR), normalization, and scaling.

*Metabolite Identification.* It includes spectral matching (MS) and peak assignment (NMR).

*Statistical Analysis.* It includes explorative (i.e., PCA and clustering), predictive (regression, PLS-DA), and univariate analysis and model optimization and validation.

*Biological Interpretation.* It involves embedding the results within the framework of existing biological knowledge.

*Box 5* (statistical analysis of metabolomic data). Metabolomic data are high dimensional in nature. Tens, hundreds, or even thousands of (un) identified metabolites (relative) concentrations are measured by means of NMR or MS platforms, usually on a limited number of samples. Biological information is retrieved from this data by means of univariate and multivariate statistical methods [27, 113, 114]. Multivariate methods make also use of covariances or correlations which reflect the extent of the relationships among the variables, in contrast to univariate methods that focus solely on the mean and variance of a *single* variable.

Commonly used univariate methods are $t$-test and ANOVA [115] together with their corresponding nonparametric versions [116] and with appropriate correction methods for multiple testing [117]. Multivariate methods are a broad category. When the interest centers on predicting or explaining one variable (either a group category like case/control or a continuous response) by the other variables, methods like multiple regression [118] or partial least squares regression and discriminant analysis (PLS-DA) [119] or its extensions like Multilevel PLS-DA [120], Orthogonal PLS-DA [121], and N-way PLS-DA [122] together with a proper optimization and validation of the models [93, 123, 124] are used. In other cases, the interest centers on providing insight into the underlying structure of the complete set of variables and other tools are used. Some examples are principal component analysis (PCA) [125], used to reduce the number of variables when there is correlation present and to explore relations between objects, or cluster analysis [62], used when objects have to be grouped to represent data structure. Hybrid methods like nearest shrunken centroids [126] or simplivariate methods [127] and machine-learning techniques like artificial neural networks [128], random forest [129], and support vector machines [91] are also used in metabolomics [27, 112, 130].

## Conflict of Interests

The authors declare that there is no conflict of interests regarding the publication of this paper.

## References


[1] J. A. Murray, C. van Dyke, M. F. Plevak, R. A. Dierkhising, A. R. Zinsmeister, and L. J. Melton III, "Trends in the identification and clinical features of celiac disease in a North American community, 1950–2001," *Clinical Gastroenterology and Hepatology*, vol. 1, no. 1, pp. 19–27, 2003.

[2] M. Mäki, K. Mustalahti, J. Kokkonen et al., "Prevalence of celiac disease among children in Finland," *The New England Journal of Medicine*, vol. 348, no. 25, pp. 2517–2524, 2003.

[3] C. Catassi, I. M. Ratsch, E. Fabiani et al., "High prevalence of undiagnosed coeliac disease in 5280 Italian students screened by antigliadin antibodies," *Acta Paediatrica*, vol. 84, no. 6, pp. 672–676, 1995.

[4] J. West, R. F. A. Logan, P. G. Hill et al., "Seroprevalence, correlates, and characteristics of undetected coeliac disease in England," *Gut*, vol. 52, no. 7, pp. 960–965, 2003.

[5] P. J. Bingley, A. J. K. Williams, A. J. Norcross et al., "Undiagnosed coeliac disease at age seven: population based prospective birth cohort study," *The British Medical Journal*, vol. 328, no. 7435, pp. 322–323, 2004.

[6] P. C. A. Dubois, G. Trynka, L. Franke et al., "Multiple common variants for celiac disease influencing immune gene expression," *Nature Genetics*, vol. 42, no. 4, pp. 295–302, 2010.

[7] G. Trynka, C. Wijmenga, and D. A. van Heel, "A genetic perspective on coeliac disease," *Trends in Molecular Medicine*, vol. 16, no. 11, pp. 537–550, 2010.

[8] P. Price, C. Witt, R. Allcock et al., "The genetic basis for the association of the 8.1 ancestral haplotype (A1, B8, DR3) with multiple immunopathological diseases," *Immunological Reviews*, vol. 167, pp. 257–274, 1999.

[9] D. A. van Heel, L. Franke, K. A. Hunt et al., "A genome-wide association study for celiac disease identifies risk variants in the region harboring IL2 and IL21," *Nature Genetics*, vol. 39, no. 7, pp. 827–829, 2007.

[10] K. A. Hunt, A. Zhernakova, G. Turner et al., "Newly identified genetic risk variants for celiac disease related to the immune response," *Nature Genetics*, vol. 40, no. 4, pp. 395–402, 2008.

[11] G. Trynka, K. A. Hunt, N. A. Bockett et al., "Dense genotyping identifies and localizes multiple common and rare variant association signals in celiac disease," *Nature Genetics*, vol. 43, no. 12, pp. 1193–1201, 2011.

[12] D. J. Smyth, V. Plagnol, N. M. Walker et al., "Shared and distinct genetic variants in type 1 diabetes and celiac disease," *The New England Journal of Medicine*, vol. 359, no. 26, pp. 2767–2777, 2008.

[13] J. C. Barrett, D. G. Clayton, P. Concannon et al., "Genome-wide association study and meta-analysis find that over 40 loci affect risk of type 1 diabetes," *Nature Genetics*, vol. 41, no. 6, pp. 703–707, 2009.

[14] A. Zhernakova, B. Z. Alizadeh, M. Bevova et al., "Novel association in chromosome 4q27 region with rheumatoid arthritis and confirmation of type 1 diabetes point to a general risk locus for autoimmune diseases," *The American Journal of Human Genetics*, vol. 81, no. 6, pp. 1284–1288, 2007.

[15] J. W. Han, H. F. Zheng, Y. Cui et al., "Genome-wide association study in a Chinese Han population identifies nine new susceptibility loci for systemic lupus erythematosus," *Nature Genetics*, vol. 41, no. 11, pp. 1234–1237, 2009.

[16] F. Koning, "Celiac disease: caught between a rock and a hard place," *Gastroenterology*, vol. 129, no. 4, pp. 1294–1301, 2005.

[17] E. M. Nilsen, F. L. Jahnsen, K. E. A. Lundin et al., "Gluten induces an intestinal cytokine response strongly dominated by interferon gamma in patients with celiac disease," *Gastroenterology*, vol. 115, no. 3, pp. 551–563, 1998.

[18] L. M. Sollid, "Coeliac disease: dissecting a complex inflammatory disorder," *Nature Reviews Immunology*, vol. 2, no. 9, pp. 647–655, 2002.

[19] J.-J. Mention, M. B. Ahmed, B. Bègue et al., "Interleukin 15: a key to disrupted intraepithelial lymphocyte homeostasis and lymphomagenesis in celiac disease," *Gastroenterology*, vol. 125, no. 3, pp. 730–745, 2003.

[20] I. Bjarnason, T. J. Peters, and N. Veall, "A persistent defect in intestinal permeability in coeliac disease demonstrated by a 51Cr-labelled EDTA absorption test," *Lancet*, vol. 1, no. 8320, pp. 323–325, 1983.

[21] A. Fasano, T. Not, W. Wang et al., "Zonulin, a newly discovered modulator of intestinal permeability, and its expression in coeliac disease," *The Lancet*, vol. 355, no. 9214, pp. 1518–1519, 2000.

[22] K. M. Lammers, R. Lu, J. Brownley et al., "Gliadin induces an increase in intestinal permeability and zonulin release by binding to the chemokine receptor CXCR3," *Gastroenterology*, vol. 135, no. 1, pp. 194–e3, 2008.

[23] A. Tripathi, K. M. Lammers, S. Goldblum et al., "Identification of human zonulin, a physiological modulator of tight junctions, as prehaptoglobin-2," *Proceedings of the National Academy of Sciences of the United States of America*, vol. 106, no. 39, pp. 16799–16804, 2009.

[24] S. Schloissnig, M. Arumugam, S. Sunagawa et al., "Genomic variation landscape of the human gut microbiome," *Nature*, vol. 493, no. 7430, pp. 45–50, 2013.

[25] H. Curtis, G. Dirk, K. Rob et al., "Structure, function and diversity of the healthy human microbiome," *Human Microbiome Project Consortium*, vol. 486, no. 7402, pp. 207–214, 2012.

[26] R. D. Fleischmann, M. D. Adams, O. White et al., "Whose-genome random sequencing and assembly of Haemophilus influenzae Rd," *Science*, vol. 269, no. 5223, pp. 496–521, 1995.

[27] M. Brown, W. B. Dunn, D. I. Ellis et al., "A metabolome pipeline: from concept to data to knowledge," *Metabolomics*, vol. 1, no. 1, pp. 39–51, 2005.

[28] C. J. Lindon, J. K. Nicholson, and E. Holmes, *The Handbook of Metabonomics and Metabolomics*, Elsevier, 2007.

[29] J. K. Nicholson, J. C. Lindon, and E. Holmes, "'Metabonomics': understanding the metabolic responses of living systems to pathophysiological stimuli via multivariate statistical analysis of biological NMR spectroscopic data," *Xenobiotica*, vol. 29, no. 11, pp. 1181–1189, 1999.

[30] O. Fiehn, "Metabolomics—the link between genotypes and phenotypes," *Plant Molecular Biology*, vol. 48, no. 1-2, pp. 155–171, 2002.

[31] S. G. Oliver, M. K. Winson, D. B. Kell, and F. Baganz, "Systematic functional analysis of the yeast genome," *Trends in Biotechnology*, vol. 16, no. 9, pp. 373–378, 1998.

[32] J. Li, O. Brazhnik, A. Kamal et al., *Metabolic Profiling—Its Role in Biomarker Discovery and Gene Function Analysis*, Kluwer Academic, 2003.

[33] L. M. Raamsdonk, B. Teusink, D. Broadhurst et al., "A functional genomics strategy that uses metabolome data to reveal the phenotype of silent mutations," *Nature Biotechnology*, vol. 19, no. 1, pp. 45–50, 2001.

[34] M. Aimetti, S. Cacciatore, A. Graziano, and L. Tenori, "Metabonomic analysis of saliva reveals generalized chronic periodontitis signature," *Metabolomics*, vol. 8, no. 3, pp. 465–474, 2012.

[35] H. Wu, A. D. Southam, A. Hines, and M. R. Viant, "High-throughput tissue extraction protocol for NMR- and MS-based metabolomics," *Analytical Biochemistry*, vol. 372, no. 2, pp. 204–212, 2008.

[36] D. S. Wishart, M. J. Lewis, J. A. Morrissey et al., "The human cerebrospinal fluid metabolome," *Journal of Chromatography B*, vol. 871, no. 2, pp. 164–173, 2008.

[37] G. A. Nagana Gowda, N. Shanaiah, A. Cooper, M. Maluccio, and D. Raftery, "Bile acids conjugation in human bile is not random: new insights from 1H-NMR spectroscopy at 800 MHz," *Lipids*, vol. 44, no. 6, pp. 527–535, 2009.

[38] A. D. Maher, O. Cloarec, P. Patki et al., "Dynamic biochemical information recovery in spontaneous human seminal fluid reactions via 1H NMR kinetic statistical total correlation spectroscopy," *Analytical Chemistry*, vol. 81, no. 1, pp. 288–295, 2009.

[39] G. Graça, I. F. Duarte, B. J. Goodfellow et al., "Metabolite profiling of human amniotic fluid by hyphenated nuclear magnetic resonance spectroscopy," *Analytical Chemistry*, vol. 80, no. 15, pp. 6085–6092, 2008.

[40] L. Lacitignola, F. P. Fanizzi, E. Francioso, and A. Crovace, "1H NMR investigation of normal and osteoarthritic synovial fluid in the horse," *Veterinary and Comparative Orthopaedics and Traumatology*, vol. 21, no. 1, pp. 85–88, 2008.

[41] P. Montuschi, D. Paris, D. Melck et al., "NMR spectroscopy metabolomic profiling of exhaled breath condensate in patients with stable and unstable cystic fibrosis," *Thorax*, vol. 67, no. 3, pp. 222–228, 2012.

[42] I. Bertini, C. Luchinat, M. Miniati, S. Monti, and L. Tenori, "Phenotyping COPD by 1H NMR of exhaled breath condensate," *Metabolomics*, 2013.

[43] G. le Gall, S. O. Noor, K. Ridgway et al., "Metabolomics of fecal extracts detects altered metabolic activity of gut microbiota in ulcerative colitis and irritable bowel syndrome," *Journal of Proteome Research*, vol. 10, no. 9, pp. 4208–4218, 2011.

[44] C. Oakman, L. Tenori, W. M. Claudino et al., "Identification of a serum-detectable metabolomic fingerprint potentially correlated with the presence of micrometastatic disease in early breast cancer patients at varying risks of disease relapse by traditional prognostic methods," *Annals of Oncology*, vol. 22, no. 6, pp. 1295–1301, 2011.

[45] M. Coen, M. O'Sullivan, W. A. Bubb, P. W. Kuchel, and T. Sorrell, "Proton nuclear magnetic resonance-based metabonomics for rapid diagnosis of meningitis and ventriculitis," *Clinical Infectious Diseases*, vol. 41, no. 11, pp. 1582–1590, 2005.

[46] T. Bartsch, K. Alfke, S. Wolff, A. Rohr, O. Jansen, and G. Deuschl, "Focal MR spectroscopy of hippocampal CA-1 lesions in transient global amnesia," *Neurology*, vol. 70, no. 13, pp. 1030–1035, 2008.

[47] P. Bernini, I. Bertini, C. Luchinat, L. Tenori, and A. Tognaccini, "The cardiovascular risk of healthy individuals studied by NMR metabonomics of plasma samples," *Journal of Proteome Research*, vol. 10, no. 11, pp. 4983–4992, 2011.

[48] S. H. Moolenaar, U. F. H. Engelke, and R. A. Wevers, "Proton nuclear magnetic resonance spectroscopy of body fluids in the field of inborn errors of metabolism," *Annals of Clinical Biochemistry*, vol. 40, part 1, pp. 16–24, 2003.

[49] I. Bertini, A. Calabró, V. de Carli et al., "The metabonomic signature of celiac disease," *Journal of Proteome Research*, vol. 8, no. 1, pp. 170–177, 2009.

[50] P. Bernini, I. Bertini, A. Calabrò et al., "Are patients with potential celiac disease really potential? The answer of metabonomics," *Journal of Proteome Research*, vol. 10, no. 2, pp. 714–721, 2011.

[51] M. Sellitto, G. Bai, G. Serena et al., "Proof of concept of microbiome-metabolome analysis and delayed gluten exposure on celiac disease autoimmunity in genetically at-risk infants," *PLoS ONE*, vol. 7, no. 3, Article ID e33387, 2012.

[52] Y. Sanz, G. D. Pama, and M. Laparra, "Unraveling the ties between celiac disease and intestinal microbiota," *International Reviews of Immunology*, vol. 30, no. 4, pp. 207–218, 2011.

[53] E. Sánchez, E. Donat, C. Ribes-Koninckx, L. Fernández-Murga, and Y. Sanz, "Duodenal-mucosal bacteria associated with celiac disease in children," *Applied and Environmental Microbiology*, vol. 79, no. 18, pp. 5472–5479, 2013.

[54] Y. Sanz, E. Sánchez, M. Marzotto, M. Calabuig, S. Torriani, and F. Dellaglio, "Differences in faecal bacterial communities in coeliac and healthy children as detected by PCR and denaturing gradient gel electrophoresis," *FEMS Immunology and Medical Microbiology*, vol. 51, no. 3, pp. 562–568, 2007.

[55] P. Wacklin, K. Kaukinen, E. Tuovinen et al., "The duodenal microbiota composition of adult celiac disease patients is associated with the clinical manifestation of the disease," *Inflammatory Bowel Diseases*, vol. 19, no. 5, pp. 934–941, 2013.

[56] M. Kalliomaki, R. Satokari, H. Lahteenoja et al., "Expression of microbiota, toll-like receptors, and their regulators in the small intestinal mucosa in celiac disease," *Journal of Pediatric Gastroenterology*, vol. 54, no. 6, pp. 727–732, 2012.

[57] E. Nistal, A. Caminero, A. R. Herrán et al., "Differences of small intestinal bacteria populations in adults and children with/without celiac disease: effect of age, gluten diet, and disease," *Inflammatory Bowel Diseases*, vol. 18, no. 4, pp. 649–656, 2012.

[58] I. Nadal, E. Donant, C. Ribes-Koninckx, M. Calabuig, and Y. Sanz, "Imbalance in the composition of the duodenal microbiota of children with coeliac disease," *Journal of Medical Microbiology*, vol. 56, no. 12, pp. 1669–1674, 2007.

[59] E. Sánchez, E. Donat, C. Ribes-Koninckx, M. Calabuig, and Y. Sanz, "Intestinal Bacteroides species associated with coeliac disease," *Journal of Clinical Pathology*, vol. 63, no. 12, pp. 1105–1111, 2010.

[60] E. Sánchez, G. de Palma, A. Capilla et al., "Influence of environmental and genetic factors linked to celiac disease risk on infant gut colonization by Bacteroides species," *Applied and Environmental Microbiology*, vol. 77, no. 15, pp. 5316–5323, 2011.

[61] J. Cheng, M. Kalliomaki, H. G. Heilig et al., "Duodenal microbiota composition and mucosal homeostasis in pediatric celiac disease," *BMC Gastroenterology*, vol. 13, article 113, 2013.

[62] L. Kaufman and P. J. Rousseeuw, *Finding Groups in Data: An Introduction to Cluster Analysis*, vol. 344, John Wiley & Sons, 2009.

[63] R. di Cagno, M. de Angelis, I. de Pasquale et al., "Duodenal and faecal microbiota of celiac children: molecular, phenotype and metabolome characterization," *BMC Microbiology*, vol. 11, article 219, 2011.

[64] M. Medina, G. de Palma, C. Ribes-Koninckx, M. Calabuig, and Y. Sanz, "Bifidobacterium strains suppress in vitro the pro-inflammatory milieu triggered by the large intestinal microbiota of coeliac patients," *Journal of Inflammation*, vol. 5, article 19, 2008.

[65] G. Ou, M. Hedberg, P. Hörstedt et al., "Proximal small intestinal microbiota and identification of rod-shaped bacteria associated with childhood celiac disease," *The American Journal of Gastroenterology*, vol. 104, no. 12, pp. 3058–3067, 2009.

[66] J. M. Norris, K. Barriga, E. J. Hoffenberg et al., "Risk of celiac disease autoimmunity and timing of gluten introduction in the diet of infants at increased risk of disease," *Journal of the American Medical Association*, vol. 293, no. 19, pp. 2343–2351, 2005.

[67] J. Kranich, K. M. Maslowski, and C. R. Mackay, "Commensal flora and the regulation of inflammatory and autoimmune responses," *Seminars in Immunology*, vol. 23, no. 2, pp. 139–145, 2011.

[68] J. L. Round and S. K. Mazmanian, "The gut microbiota shapes intestinal immune responses during health and disease," *Nature Reviews Immunology*, vol. 9, no. 5, pp. 313–323, 2009.

[69] L. Plot and H. Amital, "Infectious associations of celiac disease," *Autoimmunity Reviews*, vol. 8, no. 4, pp. 316–319, 2009.

[70] M. F. Kagnoff, R. K. Austin, and J. J. Hubert, "Possible role for a human adenovirus in the pathogenesis of celiac disease," *Journal of Experimental Medicine*, vol. 160, no. 5, pp. 1544–1557, 1984.

[71] C. Ruggeri, A. T. la Masa, S. Rudi et al., "Celiac disease and non-organ-specific autoantibodies in patients with chronic hepatitis C virus infection," *Digestive Diseases and Sciences*, vol. 53, no. 8, pp. 2151–2155, 2008.

[72] L. C. Stene, M. C. Honeyman, E. J. Hoffenberg et al., "Rotavirus infection frequency and risk of celiac disease autoimmunity in early childhood: a longitudinal study," *The American Journal of Gastroenterology*, vol. 101, no. 10, pp. 2333–2340, 2006.

[73] E. F. Verdu, M. Mauro, J. Bourgeois, and D. Armstrong, "Clinical onset of celiac disease after an episode of Campylobacter jejuni enteritis," *Canadian Journal of Gastroenterology*, vol. 21, no. 7, pp. 453–455, 2007.

[74] F. C. Jordá and J. L. Vivancos, "Fatigue as a determinant of health in patients with celiac disease," *Journal of Clinical Gastroenterology*, vol. 44, no. 6, pp. 423–427, 2009.

[75] E. Capristo, G. Addolorato, A. V. Greco et al., "Body composition and energy metabolism in celiac disease [2] (multiple letters)," *The American Journal of Gastroenterology*, vol. 93, no. 9, pp. 1596–1597, 1998.

[76] S. Bode, C. Hassager, E. Gudmand-Hoyer, and C. Christiansen, "Body composition and calcium metabolism in adult treated coeliac disease," *Gut*, vol. 32, no. 11, pp. 1342–1345, 1991.

[77] E. Capristo, G. Addolorato, G. Mingrone et al., "Changes in body composition, substrate oxidation, and resting metabolic rate in adult celiac disease patients after a 1-y gluten-free diet treatment," *The American Journal of Clinical Nutrition*, vol. 72, no. 1, pp. 76–81, 2000.

[78] M. Kojima, H. Hosoda, Y. Date, M. Nakazato, H. Matsuo, and K. Kangawa, "Ghrelin is a growth-hormone-releasing acylated peptide from stomach," *Nature*, vol. 402, no. 6762, pp. 656–660, 1999.

[79] A. M. Wren, C. J. Small, H. L. Ward et al., "The novel hypothalamic peptide ghrelin stimulates food intake and growth hormone secretion," *Endocrinology*, vol. 141, no. 11, pp. 4325–4328, 2000.

[80] A. Lanzini, P. Magni, M. L. Petroni et al., "Circulating ghrelin level is increased in coeliac disease as in functional dyspepsia and reverts to normal during gluten-free diet," *Alimentary Pharmacology and Therapeutics*, vol. 23, no. 7, pp. 907–913, 2006.

[81] M. A. Selimoglu, S. Altinkaynak, V. Ertekin, and F. Akcay, "Serum ghrelin levels in children with celiac disease," *Journal of Clinical Gastroenterology*, vol. 40, no. 3, pp. 191–194, 2006.

[82] E. Capristo, S. Farnetti, G. Mingrone et al., "Reduced plasma ghrelin concentration in celiac disease after gluten-free diet treatment," *Scandinavian Journal of Gastroenterology*, vol. 40, no. 4, pp. 430–436, 2005.

[83] S. Meiboom and D. Gill, "Modified spin-echo method for measuring nuclear relaxation times," *Review of Scientific Instruments*, vol. 29, no. 8, pp. 688–691, 1958.

[84] A. N. Phipps, J. Stewart, B. Wright, and I. D. Wilson, "Effect of diet on the urinary excretion of hippuric acid and other dietary-derived aromatics in rat. A complex interaction between diet, gut microflora and substrate specificity," *Xenobiotica*, vol. 28, no. 5, pp. 527–537, 1998.

[85] D. H. Bueschkens and M. E. Stiles, "Escherichia coli variants for gas and indole production at elevated incubation temperatures," *Applied and Environmental Microbiology*, vol. 48, no. 3, pp. 601–605, 1984.

[86] J. K. Nicholson, E. Holmes, and I. D. Wilson, "Gut microorganisms, mammalian metabolism and personalized health care," *Nature Reviews Microbiology*, vol. 3, no. 5, pp. 431–438, 2005.

[87] M. Duran, D. Ketting, P. K. de Bree, C. van der Heiden, and S. K. Wadman, "Gas chromatographic analysis of urinary volatile phenols in patients with gastro intestinal disorders and normals," *Clinica Chimica Acta*, vol. 45, no. 4, pp. 341–347, 1973.

[88] E. Bone, A. Tamm, and M. Hill, "The production of urinary phenols by gut bacteria and their possible role in the causation of large bowel cancer," *The American Journal of Clinical Nutrition*, vol. 29, no. 12, pp. 1448–1454, 1976.

[89] S. de Jong, "SIMPLS: an alternative approach to partial least squares regression," *Chemometrics and Intelligent Laboratory Systems*, vol. 18, no. 3, pp. 251–263, 1993.

[90] I. González, S. Déjean, P. Martin, and A. Baccini, "CCA: an R package to extend canonical correlation analysis," *Journal of Statistical Software*, vol. 23, no. 12, pp. 1–14, 2008.

[91] C. Cortes and V. Vapnik, "Support-vector networks," *Machine Learning*, vol. 20, no. 3, pp. 273–297, 1995.

[92] J. Trygg and S. Wold, "Orthogonal projections to latent structures (O-PLS)," *Journal of Chemometrics*, vol. 16, no. 3, pp. 119–128, 2002.

[93] E. Szymańska, E. Saccenti, A. K. Smilde, and J. A. Westerhuis, "Double-check: validation of diagnostic statistics for PLS-DA models in metabolomics studies," *Metabolomics*, vol. 8, pp. 3–16, 2012.

[94] W. M. Claudino, A. Quattrone, L. Biganzoli, M. Pestrin, I. Bertini, and A. di Leo, "Metabolomics: available results, current research projects in breast cancer, and future applications," *Journal of Clinical Oncology*, vol. 25, no. 19, pp. 2840–2846, 2007.

[95] R. Vanga and D. A. Leffler, "Gluten sensitivity: not celiac and not certain," *Gastroenterology*, vol. 145, no. 2, pp. 276–279, 2013.

[96] R. Madsen, T. Lundstedt, and J. Trygg, "Chemometrics in metabolomics—a review in human disease diagnosis," *Analytica Chimica Acta*, vol. 659, no. 1-2, pp. 23–33, 2010.

[97] J. K. Nicholson and J. C. Lindon, "Systems biology: metabonomics," *Nature*, vol. 455, no. 7216, pp. 1054–1056, 2008.

[98] R. P. Bo Zhang, "Analysis of bacterial biofilms using NMR-based metabolomics," *Future Medicinal Chemistry*, vol. 4, no. 10, pp. 1273–1306, 2012.

[99] W. Wolfram, *Metabolomics Methods and Protocols*, Humana Press Inc., 2006.

[100] Z. Wu, Z. Huang, R. Lehmann, C. Zhao, and G. Xu, "The application of chromatography-mass spectrometry: methods to metabonomics," *Chromatographia*, vol. 69, supplement 1, pp. S23–S32, 2009.

[101] I. D. Wilson, J. K. Nicholson, J. Castro-Perez et al., "High resolution "ultra performance" liquid chromatography coupled to oa-TOF mass spectrometry as a tool for differential metabolic pathway profiling in functional genomic studies," *Journal of Proteome Research*, vol. 4, no. 2, pp. 591–598, 2005.

[102] T. D. W. Claridge, *High-Resolution NMR Techniques in Organic Chemistry*, Elsevier, 2008.

[103] D. S. Wishart, D. Tzur, C. Knox et al., "HMDB: the human metabolome database," *Nucleic Acids Research*, vol. 35, no. 1, pp. D521–D526, 2007.

[104] A. M. Tomlins, P. J. D. Foxall, J. C. Lindon et al., "High resolution magic angle spinning 1H nuclear magnetic resonance analysis of intact prostatic hyperplastic and tumour tissues," *Analytical Communications*, vol. 35, no. 3, pp. 113–115, 1998.

[105] L. L. Cheng, I.-W. Chang, D. N. Louis, and R. G. Gonzalez, "Correlation of high-resolution magic angle spinning proton magnetic resonance spectroscopy with histopathology of intact human brain tumor specimens," *Cancer Research*, vol. 58, no. 9, pp. 1825–1832, 1998.

[106] S. Garrod, E. Humpfer, M. Spraul et al., "High-resolution magic angle spinning 1H NMR spectroscopic studies on intact rat renal cortex and medulla," *Magnetic Resonance in Medicine*, vol. 41, no. 6, pp. 1108–1118, 1999.

[107] N. Psychogios, D. D. Hau, J. Peng et al., "The human serum metabolome," *PLoS ONE*, vol. 6, no. 2, Article ID e16957, 2011.

[108] S. Bouatra, F. Aziat, R. Mandal et al., "The human urine metabolome," *PLoS ONE*, vol. 8, no. 9, Article ID e73076, 2013.

[109] I. Takeda, C. Stretch, P. Barnaby et al., "Understanding the human salivary metabolome," *NMR in Biomedicine*, vol. 22, no. 6, pp. 577–584, 2009.

[110] W. B. Dunn and D. I. Ellis, "Metabolomics: current analytical platforms and methodologies," *Trends in Analytical Chemistry*, vol. 24, no. 4, pp. 285–294, 2005.

[111] R. Goodacre, D. Broadhurst, A. K. Smilde et al., "Proposed minimum reporting standards for data analysis in metabolomics," *Metabolomics*, vol. 3, no. 3, pp. 231–241, 2007.

[112] M. M. W. B. Hendriks, F. A. V. Eeuwijk, R. H. Jellema et al., "Data-processing strategies for metabolomics studies," *Trends in Analytical Chemistry*, vol. 30, no. 10, pp. 1685–1698, 2011.

[113] K. H. Liland, "Multivariate methods in metabolomics—from pre-processing to dimension reduction and statistical analysis," *Trends in Analytical Chemistry*, vol. 30, no. 6, pp. 827–841, 2011.

[114] E. Saccenti, H. C. J. Hoefsloot, A. K. Smilde, J. A. Westerhuis, and M. M. W. B. Hendriks, "Reflections on univariate and multivariate analysis of metabolomics data," *Metabolomics*, 2013.

[115] R. G. Miller and B. W. Brown, *Beyond ANOVA: Basics of Applied Statistics*, Chapman & Hall/CRC, 1997.

[116] J. Fletcher, "Non-parametric tests," *The British Medical Journal*, vol. 338, 2009.

[117] D. I. Broadhurst and D. B. Kell, "Statistical strategies for avoiding false discoveries in metabolomics and related experiments," *Metabolomics*, vol. 2, no. 4, pp. 171–196, 2006.

[118] N. R. Draper and H. Smith, *Applied Regression Analysis*, Wiley Series in Probability and Statistics, 1998.

[119] S. Wold, M. Sjöström, and L. Eriksson, "PLS-regression: a basic tool of chemometrics," *Chemometrics and Intelligent Laboratory Systems*, vol. 58, no. 2, pp. 109–130, 2001.

[120] E. J. J. van Velzen, J. A. Westerhuis, J. P. M. van Duynhoven et al., "Multilevel data analysis of a crossover designed human nutritional intervention study," *Journal of Proteome Research*, vol. 7, no. 10, pp. 4483–4491, 2008.

[121] H. Stenlund, A. Gorzsás, P. Persson, B. Sundberg, and J. Trygg, "Orthogonal projections to latent structures discriminant analysis modeling on in situ FT-IR spectral imaging of liver tissue for identifying sources of variability," *Analytical Chemistry*, vol. 80, no. 18, pp. 6898–6906, 2008.

[122] R. Bro, "Multiway calibration. Multilinear PLS," *Journal of Chemometrics*, vol. 10, no. 1, pp. 47–61, 1996.

[123] J. A. Westerhuis, H. C. J. Hoefsloot, S. Smit et al., "Assessment of PLSDA cross validation," *Metabolomics*, vol. 4, no. 1, pp. 81–89, 2008.

[124] R. G. Brereton, "Consequences of sample size, variable selection, and model validation and optimisation, for predicting classification ability from analytical data," *Trends in Analytical Chemistry*, vol. 25, no. 11, pp. 1103–1111, 2006.

[125] I. T. Jolliffe, "Principal component analysis: a beginner's guide-I. Introduction and application," *Weather*, vol. 45, no. 10, pp. 375–382, 2012.

[126] R. Tibshirani, T. Hastie, B. Narasimhan, and G. Chu, "Diagnosis of multiple cancer types by shrunken centroids of gene expression," *Proceedings of the National Academy of Sciences of the United States of America*, vol. 99, no. 10, pp. 6567–6572, 2002.

[127] E. Saccenti, J. A. Westerhuis, A. K. Smilde, M. J. van der Werf, J. A. Hageman, and M. M. W. B. Hendriks, "Simplivariate models: uncovering the underlying biology in functional genomics data," *PLoS ONE*, vol. 6, no. 6, Article ID e20747, 2011.

[128] D. Lowe and D. Broomhead, "Multivariable functional interpolation and adaptive networks," *Complex Systems*, vol. 2, pp. 321–355, 1988.

[129] L. Breiman, "Random forests," *Machine Learning*, vol. 45, no. 1, pp. 5–32, 2001.

[130] M. M. W. B. Hendriks, S. Smit, W. L. M. W. Akkermans et al., "How to distinguish healthy from diseased? Classification strategy for mass spectrometry-based clinical proteomics," *Proteomics*, vol. 7, no. 20, pp. 3672–3680, 2007.

# 13

# Severe Skin Forms of Psoriasis in Black Africans: Epidemiological, Clinical, and Histological Aspects Related to 56 Cases

**Komenan Kassi,[1] Oussou Armel Mienwoley,[2,3] Mohamed Kouyate,[4] Sylvanus Koui,[4] and Kouame A. Kouassi[1]**

[1] *Department of Dermatology and Infectiology, Training and Research Unit of Medical Sciences, Félix Houphouët Boigny University (FHBU) of Abidjan-Cocody, Abidjan 21 BP 5151, Cote d'Ivoire*
[2] *Training and Research Unit of Medical Sciences, University of Bouaké, Bouaké 01 BP V18, Cote d'Ivoire*
[3] *Mother Maria Elisa Andreoli Health Center, Cocody Riviera Palmeraie, Cidex 3, Abijan-Riviera BP 51, Cote d'Ivoire*
[4] *Department of Histopathology, University Hospital of Treichville, Abidjan 01 BP V3, Cote d'Ivoire*

Correspondence should be addressed to Komenan Kassi; siskakomlo@yahoo.fr

Academic Editor: Jozélio Freire De Carvalho

*Bacground.* Psoriasis is an erythematosquamous dermatosis of chronic development. In sub-Saharan Africa, few studies have been focused on complicated forms of psoriasis. *Objective.* The aim is to describe epidemiological, clinical, and histological features of severe skin forms of psoriasis in Cote d'Ivoire. *Material and Methods.* The study was both cross-sectional and descriptive, that focused on patient admitted to the dermatology unit for complicated psoriasis, from January 1st, 1986, to December 31th, 2007. *Results.* Fifty-six patients admitted to hospital for severe skin forms of psoriasis were recorded and included in our study over 7.503 patients hospitalized during the study period. They represented 0.75% of cases. The average age was 39.6 ± 3.3 years. There were 49 male (87.5%) and 7 female patients (12.5%) with a sex ratio of 7. At socioprofessional level, 48 patients (87.5%) were from category 1. Patients' history was dominated by the psoriasis vulgaris. Physical and general signs were dominated by itching (58.9%). The three severe skin forms were observed with predominant erythrodermic psoriasis (60.7%). Fifteen patients (34.9%) were HIV positive. *Conclusion.* Severe skin forms of psoriasis are rare in our setting. But in the quarter of HIV-positive patients, they are dominated by the erythrodermic psoriasis.

## 1. Introduction

Psoriasis is an erythematosquamous dermatosis of chronic development. It is ubiquitous and seems common in the West where prevalence rate ranges from 2 to 3% in the population at large [1, 2]. The benign forms are the most numerous, around 90%, and raise an aesthetic issue. The severe forms which are life-threatening or threaten the functional prognosis account for about 10% and require an admission to hospital. Psoriasis diagnosis is clinically easy in typical forms. Yet a histological confirmation is required after a biopsy of the skin lesion. Histological images are characteristic with parakeratotic hyperkeratosis and Munro-Sabouraud's microabscesses [2]. In sub-Saharan Africa few studies have been focused on complicated forms of psoriasis [3]. The objective of this study is to describe the epidemiological, clinical, and histological aspects of psoriasis complicated forms in patients admitted to the Dermatology Unit of Treichville University Hospital.

## 2. Material and Methods

The study was cross-sectional and descriptive. It focused on all the records of patients admitted to the Dermatology Unit of Treichville University Hospital for complicated forms of psoriasis in the period covering January 1, 1986, to December 31, 2007.

In the study records of patients of all sexes and ages suffering from erythrodermic psoriasis, universal psoriasis, or pustular psoriasis confirmed by histology were included. The histological examination has been carried out in the anatomopathology labs of Treichville University Hospital on a sample of the skin lesion biopsy. The sample was stored in 10% formalin. Paraffin inclusion was performed before examining under an optical microscope.

Epidemiological, clinical, and histological data along with HIV status have been recorded in a prescribed survey form.

The socioprofessional status has been subdivided into three categories.

(i) Category I: patients with monthly pay lower than the index-linked guaranteed minimum wage in Côte d'Ivoire (35,000 FCFA, i.e. 53,8 Euros).

(ii) Category II: medium ranking civil servants of Ivorian public civil service with an average wage of 137 Euros [3].

(iii) Category III: patients with more than 300 Euros as monthly wage.

Data analysis has been performed with the software Epi info 6.04 and has consisted in calculating the rates.

## 3. Results

We selected 56 records of patients suffering from complicated forms of psoriasis out of a total of 7503 hospitalization records during the 22-year study period representing 2.5 cases per year. Cumulative incidence of complicated forms of psoriasis was 0.7%. There were 49 male (87.5%) and 7 female patients (12.5%) which equals a sex ratio of 7. Average age was 39.6±3.3 years with extremes of 4 and 77 years. There were 3 children (5.3%) and 53 adults (94.7%). From the adults, 38 patients (67%) were between 30 and 50 years old. At socioeconomic level, patients earning a monthly income less than 53.8 Euros accounted for 85.7% of cases. Our patients' history was dominated by psoriasis vulgaris in 21 cases (37.5%) followed by medication use in 18 cases (32.1%), tobacco in 14 cases (25%), alcohol in 14 cases (25%), combination of tobacco and alcohol in 8 cases (14.3%), stress in 3 cases (5.3%), and other variables in 7 cases (12.5%). Benzathine-penicillin and non steroidal topical remedies were the most used medecine in respectivily 22% of cases. Three severe forms have been observed. There were erythrodermic psoriasis in 34 cases (60.7%), universal psoriasis in 21 cases (37.5%), and generalized pustular psoriasis in 1 case (1.8%). Physical and general signs were dominated by itching in 33 cases (58.9%) (Table 2). Ungual impairments were observed in 33 patients (58.9%) and were dominated by "thimble-like" aspect in 13 cases (39.4%) followed bysubungual hyperkeratosis and pachyonychia in 4 cases (12.1%), onycholysis in 2 cases (6.1%), and others in 9 cases (27.3%). Patients were screened for HIV infection in 43 cases (76.8%). Fifteen patients (34.9%) were HIV positive with 9 cases of erythrodermic psoriasis and 6 cases of universal psoriasis. Histology involved 11 patients (19.6%). At the epidermic level, hyperkeratosis and agranulosis were observed in all the slides. Munro-Sabouraud abscesses were objectified in 8 slides (72.7%) (Table 1). Histological changes of the dermis were dominated by a lymphocytic infiltrate objectified in all the slides and a hyperpapillomatosis in 9 cases (81.8%) (Table 2).

Table 1: Histological epidermal changes in 11 severe psoriasis cases.

| Epidermal changes | Number ($n$) | Percentage ($n$/11) |
|---|---|---|
| Hyperkeratosis | 11 | 100.0 |
| Parakeratosis | 8 | 72.7 |
| Parakeratosis and orthokeratosis | 3 | 27.3 |
| Microabscesses | 8 | 72.7 |
| Agranulosis | 11 | 100.0 |
| Thinning of the dermal papilla roof | 10 | 90.9 |
| Interpapillary bud changes | | |
| Acanthosis | 10 | 90.9 |
| Elongation | 8 | 72.7 |
| Club aspect | 7 | 63.6 |
| Exocytosis | 8 | 72.7 |
| Polynuclear and mononuclear neutrophils | 7 | 63.6 |
| Mononuclear | 1 | 9.1 |
| Spongiosis | 4 | 36.4 |
| Minimal | 3 | 27.3 |
| Moderate | 1 | 9.1 |

Table 2: Histological dermal changes in 11 severe psoriasis cases.

| Dermal changes | Number ($n$) | Percentage ($n$/11) |
|---|---|---|
| Hyperpapillomatosis | 9 | 81.8 |
| Turgidity of dermal papilla | 4 | 36.4 |
| Presence of dilated capillaries | 7 | 63.6 |
| Superficial dermal infiltrate | 11 | 100.0 |
| Lymphocytes | 11 | 100.0 |
| Polynuclear | 10 | 90.9 |
| Neutrophil | 8 | 72.7 |
| Eosinophil | 1 | 9.1 |
| Neutrophil and eosinophil | 1 | 9.1 |
| Histiocytes | 10 | 90.9 |
| Plasmacytes | 8 | 72.7 |

## 4. Discussion

The severe psoriasis is rarely seen in the Dermatology Unit of Treichville University Hospital. This rareness has been reported by Kundakci et al. [4] in the Turkish in 2002 with an incidence of 0.07%. Our data is relatively low compared to those raised by Jalal et al. [5] in 2005 in Morocco and Lapeyre et al. [6] in 2007 in France with, respectively, 13 and 4.5 cases per year. This observation should confirm this disease rareness in blacks and particularly in West Africans [3, 7, 8]. Our study has pointed out a clear male predominance with 7 as sex ratio. This male predominance has been reported by many authors [5, 9, 10]. This marked difference observed in our study may be due to the delay in caring for the initially benign skin disorders in male patients for they show little concern for their physical look. Adults accounted for 94.7% and children 5.3%. They were adults of average age (39.6 ± 3.3 years old). This observation is in line with many authors' data [4, 5, 11]. Yet, Fortune et al. [12] in 2010 in Saudi Arabia have observed the severe psoriasis in adults of 22 to 26 years old. Kundakci et al. [4] reported the rareness of the disease in children (≤10 years old; 5.7%).

In our study, the severe psoriasis observed in adults may provide a proof of a late start of the (type II) disease in relation to non pustular clinical forms [1]. More than four-fifths of patients suffering from severe psoriasis were from category I. Public health facilities are visited by poor income patients in most cases due to the social rates charged whereas middle and high income patients would favor private health facilities. Moreover, we should not systematically reject the psychological impact of the bad living condition of category I patients on psoriasis beginning and/or worsening. According to Griffiths and Richards [11], psoriasis is a complex disease combining biological, psychological, and social contributors. Patients have different medical histories. Tobacco intoxication accounted for 25%. Alcohol consumption along with tobacco-alcohol combination accounted for 14.3% of cases. Dereure and Guilhou [8] mentioned tobacco and alcohol to be the psoriasis exogenous risks. Jalal et al. [5] found 8.9% of tobacco intoxication in patients suffering from severe psoriasis. In 2007, in Spain, Huerta et al. [13] reported that tobacco was an independent psoriasis risk factor. In 2008, Kirby et al. [10] observed link between psoriasis severity and weekly alcohol consumption. More than one-third of the patients suffering from severe psoriasis in our study have already been diagnosed with psoriasis vulgaris. The switch from psoriasis vulgaris to severe psoriasis is well known. Jalal et al. [5] in their series have reported a history of psoriasis vulgaris in 89.4% of cases. This precession of the severe psoriasis by the psoriasis vulgaris is caused by some contributors including drugs. Many authors have reported drug involvement in worsening or leading to psoriasis outbreak [2, 5, 6, 13]. Bérard et al. [2] have observed that mechanisms with which environment contributors such as drugs worsen or lead to outbreak are well known. Jalal et al. [5] reported an incidence of 12.5% of patients suffering from severe psoriasis triggered by the use of drug. Lapeyre et al. [6] observed that the erythrodermic psoriasis may be sparked by the introduction of new drugs. Huerta et al. [13] stated that antibiotics' use might cause an existing psoriasis to exacerbate.

The stress may be another contributor likely to lead to psoriasis outbreak or worsen an existing one according to some authors [2, 9, 11, 14]. In our study, 5.3% of patients have pointed out stress presence. However, Huerta et al. [13] stated that there was no connection between psoriasis occurrence risk and stress histories. The three severe skin forms of psoriasis have been observed in our study and are the erythrodermic psoriasis (60.7%), the universal psoriasis (37.5%), and pustular psoriasis (1.8%). Jalal et al. [5] and Lapeyre et al. [6] have reported the three severe skin forms of the psoriasis in their series at the following respective rates: erythrodermic psoriasis (54.4% and 14.2%), universal psoriasis (19.4% and 67.8%), and pustular psoriasis (19.4% and 18.0%). Kundakci et al. [4] reported the pustular psoriasis only with 17 cases. Fatani et al. [9] observed the erythrodermic psoriasis (57.9%) and the pustular psoriasis (42.1%). Our study pointed out rareness of the pustular psoriasis while this clinical form seems to be more common in the Maghreb, in Europe, and in the Middle East. This observation may suggest that there is a difference in the genetic factors associated with the onset of psoriasis between Caucasian and black African patients [8]. Severe skin forms of the psoriasis were accompanied with physical and general signs. Our study provided that there were itching (58.7%), oedema of lower limbs (28.6%), and hyperthermia (26.8%). Fatani et al. [9] have reported itching in 43% of cases. Globe et al. [15] have shown that itching was the most important sign and the most severe in the course of psoriasis. For patients included in this study, itching would cause an important deterioration of the quality of life. Jalal et al. [5] have found hyperthermia in 3% of patients. These physical and general signs are mostly observed in erythrodermic forms of psoriasis. The important impairment of the skin barrier may be the cause of biochemical disorders, thermoregulation changes, and hydroelectrolytic and protein disorders. More than half of our patients (58.9%) had ungual impairments dominated by "thimble-like aspect" (39.4%). Kundakci et al. [4] reported the ungual impairments in 16.4% of cases with "thimble-like aspect" dominating (79.6%). Mak et al. [14] asserted that almost half of the patients suffering from psoriasis had ungual impairment dominated by the "thimble-like aspect." For some authors, HIV infection is a contributing factor to the occurrence of severe and extensive forms of psoriasis [8, 14, 16, 17]. According to most of these authors, there was no change in the incidence of psoriasis patients associated with HIV in comparison to the general population. But, in our series, 15 patients in 43 detected were HIV positive, that is, 34.9% of cases. The prevalence of patients suffering from severe psoriasis associated with HIV seemed high, in 28.8% of cases, yet the study does not allow checking whether severe psoriasis erupted before or after the HIV infection. This limit does not help to assess involvement of HIV infection in occurrence of severe forms of psoriasis. This prevalence observed in our study was lower than in the study conducted in eastern Africa where it was 41.6% of cases (in a population of 61 HIV-positive patients diagnosed for complicated psoriasis) [18]. However, it was higher than in Caucasians. In fact, a study in 2000 on HIV-positive patients showed a prevalence of 2.5% of cases compared to the general population in San Francisco [19]. Another study in Berlin on 700 patients infected by HIV reported a prevalence of 5% of cases, 3 times higher compared to the general population [16]. This high rate of HIV associated with severe forms of psoriasis in our setting could be explained by the high rate of HIV/AIDS incidence and prevalence in sub-Saharan Africa (the most infected region worldwide), in particular in Côte d'Ivoire.

## 5. Conclusion

Although they are scarce, severe forms of psoriasis are a concern to practitioners for being more often life-threatening because of the biological disorders and infectious complications they involve. Incidence of these severe cases of psoriasis in HIV-positive patients requires systematic HIV testing.

## Conflict of Interests

The authors declare that there is no conflict of interests regarding this paper.

## References


[1] E. Christophers, "Psoriasis—epidemiology and clinical spectrum," *Clinical and Experimental Dermatology*, vol. 26, no. 4, pp. 314–320, 2001.

[2] F. Bérard, I. Guillot, N. Saad, and J. F. Nicolas, "Comment comprendre le psoriasis," *La Revue Du Praticien*, vol. 54, no. 1, pp. 28–34, 2004.

[3] R. O. Leder and E. M. Farber, "The variable incidence of psoriasis in sub-saharan Africa," *International Journal of Dermatology*, vol. 36, no. 12, pp. 911–919, 1997.

[4] N. Kundakci, Ü. Türsen, M. O. A. Babiker, and E. Gürgey, "The evaluation of the sociodemographic and clinical features of Turkish psoriasis patients," *International Journal of Dermatology*, vol. 41, no. 4, pp. 220–224, 2002.

[5] O. Jalal, S. Houass, K. Laissaoui, O. Hocar, S. Charioui, and S. Amal, "Formes graves de psoriasis: 160 cas," *Annales de Dermatologie et de Vénéréologie*, vol. 132, no. 2, pp. 126–128, 2005.

[6] H. Lapeyre, M. F. Hellot, and P. Jolly Motifs, "d'hospitalisation des maladies attaints de psoriasis," *Annales de Dermatologie et de Vénéréologie*, vol. 134, pp. 433–436, 2007.

[7] M. R. Namazi, "Why is psoriasis uncommon in Africans? the influence of dietary factors on the expression of psoriasis," *International Journal of Dermatology*, vol. 43, no. 5, pp. 391–392, 2004.

[8] O. Dereure and J.-J. Guilhou, "Epidémiologie et génétique du psoriasis.," *Annales De Dermatologie Et De Vénéréologie*, vol. 130, no. 8-9, pp. 829–836, 2003.

[9] M. I. Fatani, M. M. Abdulghani, and K. A. Al-Afif, "Psoriasis in the eastern Saudi Arabia," *Saudi Medical Journal*, vol. 23, no. 2, pp. 213–217, 2002.

[10] B. Kirby, H. L. Richards, D. L. Mason, D. G. Fortune, C. J. Main, and C. E. M. Griffiths, "Alcohol consumption and psychological distress in patients with psoriasis," *British Journal of Dermatology*, vol. 158, no. 1, pp. 138–140, 2008.

[11] C. E. M. Griffiths and H. L. Richards, "Psychological influences in psoriasis," *Clinical and Experimental Dermatology*, vol. 26, pp. 338–342, 2001.

[12] D. G. Fortune, H. L. Richards, and C. E. M. Griffiths, "Psychologic factors in psoriasis: consequences, mechanisms, and interventions," *Dermatologic Clinics*, vol. 23, no. 4, pp. 681–694, 2005.

[13] C. Huerta, E. Rivero, and L. A. García Rodríguez, "Incidence and risk factors for psoriasis in the general population," *Archives of Dermatology*, vol. 143, no. 12, pp. 1559–1565, 2007.

[14] R. K. H. Mak, C. Hundhausen, and F. O. Nestle, "Progress in understanding the immunopathogenesis of psoriasis," *Actas Dermo-Sifiliograficas*, vol. 100, no. 2, pp. 2–13, 2009.

[15] D. Globe, M. S. Bayliss, and D. J. Harrison, "The impact of itch symptoms in psoriasis: results from physician interviews and patient focus groups," *Health and Quality of Life Outcomes*, vol. 7, article 62, 2009.

[16] L. Leal, M. Ribera, and E. Daudén, "Psoriasis and hiv infection," *Actas Dermo-Sifiliograficas*, vol. 99, no. 10, pp. 753–763, 2008.

[17] I. Mamkin, A. Mamkin, and S. V. Ramanan, "HIV-associated psoriasis," *Lancet Infectious Diseases*, vol. 7, no. 7, p. 496, 2007.

[18] D. D. Odraogo and B. O. Mayer, "Le rhumatisme psoriasique en Afrique sub-saharienne," *Revue De Rhumatologie*, vol. 78, no. 5, pp. 412–415, 2011.

[19] M. L. Obush, T. A. Maurer, and B. Becker, "Berger TG. psoariasis and human immunodeficiency virus infection," *Journal of the American Academy of Dermatology*, vol. 27, pp. 667–671, 1992.

# 14

# Social Support and Self-Reported Stress Levels in a Predominantly African American Sample of Women with Systemic Lupus Erythematosus

**Edith Marie Williams,[1] Jiajia Zhang,[2] Judith Anderson,[3] Larisa Bruner,[2] and Laurene Tumiel-Berhalter[3]**

[1]*Department of Public Health Sciences, Medical University of South Carolina, 135 Cannon Street, Suite 303, Charleston, SC 29425, USA*
[2]*University of South Carolina, Columbia, SC 29208, USA*
[3]*State University of New York at Buffalo, Buffalo, NY 14215, USA*

Correspondence should be addressed to Edith Marie Williams; willi425@mailbox.sc.edu

Academic Editor: Ricard Cervera

Lupus patients should avoid stress because physical or emotional stress can affect overall physical health. It has been suggested that social support has a positive influence on health status, but there is a lack of information in the literature on the association between the two among lupus patients. The current study investigated the association between social support and self-reported stress and coping status among African American women with lupus using data collected from two linked cross-sectional surveys. No social support differences in groups of high and low stress/coping were revealed; a duplicate study with a larger sample size is required.

## 1. Introduction

Stress can be a physical, mental, and/or emotional response to life's changes and demands. Stress can have immediate and chronic effects. The stress response is the set of physical and emotional changes the human body makes in response to a threat or stress [1]. Stress has been linked to chronic disease because if it occurs too often or lasts too long, the immune system can be weakened, making it harder to fight off disease and/or worsening existent health problems. Thus, stress is a particularly important issue for lupus patients, since lupus is an autoimmune disease wherein the immune system is already dysfunctionally attacking the body's own cells. Lupus patients are advised to avoid stress and to try to lead lives that are close to normal because physical or emotional stress can trigger an exacerbation and affect overall physical health [2–4]. It has been suggested that social support or the extent to which resources in the social environment meet an individual's interpersonal needs has a positive influence on health status. Social support has gained much research attention due to its believed beneficial effects on the psychosocial and physical well-being of lupus patients [5–10].

Some researchers have examined both stress and social support and their effects on the mental and physical health of SLE patients, but not their relation to each other. Dobkin and associates [11] assessed daily hassles, social support, psychologic distress, and quality of life in 44 women with SLE, using standardized instruments, and found that high stress (assessed by hassles severity) and poor social support were the strongest predictors of patients' perceived global physical health and psychologic distress. Other variables investigated included SLE disease activity and damage, age, disease duration, education, and ethnicity [11].

In addition to life stress and social support, Kozora et al. [12] examined coping styles in relation to psychological processes in SLE and Rheumatoid Arthritis (RA) patients. Investigators measured depression, mood, disease activity, perceived health, and cognitive ability and found that increased depressive symptoms and distressed mood state in

SLE patients were related to use of disengaging and emotional coping styles [12]. Dobkin and colleagues [13] assessed psychological distress, social support, stress, coping, and health-related quality of life. They observed that better physical health was predicted by more emotion-oriented coping in patients in a more active disease state, suggesting that this style of coping may be more adaptive in situations that are considered uncontrollable (e.g., SLE flare) [13]. McCracken and associates [14] investigated the relations of coping with psychological adjustment and functional status in 46 adults with SLE and found that seeking social support was a significant predictor of adjustment, although neither perceived nor tangible social support was measured in relation to coping [14].

While the effects of stress and social support on disease activity in lupus patients have been well-documented, there is lack of information in the literature on the association between social support and stress levels among lupus patients. Therefore, the objective of this study was to determine if there is a link between social support and self-reported stress and coping status among African American women with lupus.

## 2. Patients and Methods

In brief, this paper reflects the analysis stress/coping and social support data, collected from two linked cross-sectional surveys. Cases analyzed for the current study were participants in the Buffalo Lupus Project and Breakfast with a Buddy Biomarkers of Lupus Study. The Buffalo Lupus Project, a partnership between the Toxic Waste Lupus Coalition and the University at Buffalo, was formed to count the number of people in the Buffalo community who had lupus and other autoimmune diseases and also to uncover any common factors that may elucidate the complex causes of lupus and other autoimmune diseases. At its onset, the Buffalo Lupus Project consisted of a registry and survey. The survey component of the Buffalo Lupus Project focused on the east side of the city of Buffalo, NY, which is predominantly African American. These areas were targeted due to citizens' concern about high rates of autoimmune disease in the area that they believed may be related to the presence of a toxic waste site there. Trained interviewers completed surveys with 66 patients with SLE, 52 of whom were African American women. Survey topics included demographics, diagnosis, health care utilization, residential history, residential history exposure, occupational history, occupational history exposure, smoking history, family health history, and social support.

Upon completion of the survey, each participant was invited to participate in the Breakfast with a Buddy Biomarkers of Lupus Study, which was developed to investigate the relationship between inflammation and heart disease in African American women with lupus. Participation in the study included a fasting blood draw, carotid ultrasound, physical measurements, and a short questionnaire assessing traditional cardiovascular risk factors, including stress/coping status.

Currently, 317 residents with lupus and other autoimmune diseases have registered with the Buffalo Lupus Project. Out of the 317 current registrants, 194 have reported being diagnosed with SLE, and, of those SLE cases, 92 were eligible to participate in the Buffalo Lupus Project survey due to having ever lived or currently living in zip codes 14211 or 14215. Sixty-six SLE cases completed the survey and all were invited to participate in the biomarkers study; 44 consented, corresponding to a 67 percent response rate. Responses to the social support variables from the Buffalo Lupus Project survey were merged with the Breakfast with a Buddy Biomarkers of Lupus Study database, and those cases who had participated in both projects and responded to both social support and stress questions were selected out for analysis. Forty-three cases had available values for both stress and social support inquiries. After exclusion of those cases with "Do not know/Not applicable" (DK/NA) responses for the dichotomized stress/coping variable, 41 cases were included in analysis.

Stress and coping status was measured as self-reported perceived level of stress and ability to cope, using a question, adapted from the American Heart Association (AHA) Coronary Risk Assessment Questionnaire [15], which asked the participants to describe how they currently coped with stress in their life using a five-item scale (seldom feeling stress, coping very well; sometimes stressed, coping fairly well; often stressed, having trouble coping at times; heavily stressed, often having trouble coping; or excessively stressed, or unable to cope). Responses were dichotomized for analysis. Specifically, "seldom" and "sometimes" responses were coded as no/low stress, and "often," "heavily," and "excessively" responses were codes as yes/high stress. Social support was assessed by six questions, adapted from the Social Support Questionnaire 6 and Medical Outcomes Study Short Form Health Survey (SF-36) [6, 16–21]. Five themes were evaluated: perception of having a support system and individuals/groups comprising it, proximity and number of perceived close friends and family members, perception of having someone there to take over tasks and chores if sick, membership and attendance at faith based and other types of meetings, and frequency of get-togethers and conversations with friends, relatives, and neighbors.

Participants were asked how many close friends or relatives they saw at least one time per month (none through 5 or more), how many times in a typical week participants talk on the phone (more than once per week, once per week, and less than once per week), and how often patients get together with friends or relatives (more than once per week, less than once per month, once per week, never or almost never, and 1–3 times per month). Participants were also asked if they had a support system, if they lived with someone they considered to be a close friend or relative, and if they belonged to any clubs and/or organizations. Confounding variables assessed included age, highest level of education attained, annual household income, smoking status, and race.

The stress/coping variable was cross-tabulated with each of the six social support variables investigated, using SPSS, and percentages were calculated. Statistical tests were conducted based on the Fisher exact test and $t$-test due to the

TABLE 1: Demographic characteristics of SLE cases in the Buffalo Lupus Project and Breakfast with a Buddy Biomarkers of Lupus Study ($N = 41$).

| | Total (41) | Low stress (28) | High stress (13) | *P* value |
|---|---|---|---|---|
| Age, years, mean (SD) | | 52 (13.11) | 49 (5.48) | 0.3084 |
| Education, *n* (%) | | | | 0.3523 |
| <Grade 12 | 2 (4.9) | 2 (7.1) | 0 (0) | |
| High school grad | 11 (26.8) | 7 (25.0) | 4 (30.8) | |
| Some college | 19 (46.3) | 11 (39.3) | 8 (61.5) | |
| College graduate | 9 (22.0) | 8 (28.6) | 1 (7.7) | |
| Annual household income, *n* (%) | | | | 0.5815 |
| Under $10,000 | 7 (17.1) | 4 (14.3) | 3 (23.1) | |
| $10,000–29,999 | 15 (36.6) | 9 (32.1) | 6 (46.2) | |
| $30,000–49,999 | 8 (19.5) | 7 (25.0) | 1 (7.7) | |
| Over $50,000 | 8 (19.5) | 5 (17.9) | 3 (23.1) | |
| Smoking status, *n* (%) | | | | 0.6666 |
| Never | 17 (41.5) | 13 (46.4) | 4 (30.8) | |
| Past (quit) | 18 (43.9) | 11 (39.3) | 7 (53.9) | |
| Current | 6 (14.6) | 4 (14.3) | 2 (15.4) | |
| Race, *n* (%) | | | | 0.5698 |
| African American | 36 (87.8) | 26 (92.9) | 10 (76.9) | |
| White | 5 (12.2) | 2 (7.1) | 3 (23.1) | |

*N*: total number of participants, *n*: number of participants in each cell, %: percent, and SD: standard deviation.

small sample size by assuming the independence among the high and low stress group.

## 3. Results

Approximately 88 percent of participants were African American and the remaining 12 percent were Caucasian. The mean age of participants was 50.8 years. Less than ten percent of participants completed less than 12 years of school. Approximately 77 percent of participants graduated from high school, and 17 percent attained a college degree or higher. Table 1 shows that 28 participants were classified as "no/low stress." The remaining 13 participants were classified as "yes/high stress." When divided into categories of low and high stress, those reporting higher levels of stress were slightly younger than those in the "no/low stress" category (mean age of 49 years compared with 52 years). There were more White participants in the "yes/high stress category" than there were in the "no/low stress category." Conversely, there were more Black participants in the "no/low stress category" than there were in the "yes/high stress category." In both categories, the majority of participants reported attending some college or attaining a college degree or higher. In the "yes/high stress category," the majority of respondents reported annual household incomes below $30,000.00. Conversely, in the "no/low stress category," the most respondents reported annual household incomes at or above $30,000.00. In both stress categories, few participants reported being current smokers (less than 16 percent).

Table 2 shows that most of the SLE patients in the current study (97.6 percent) had a support system that was comprised of both immediate family members and unrelated sources of support. While the majority of participants in both stress categories reported their family, children, siblings, other family members, and friends to be part of their support systems, more participants in the "yes/high stress" category reported their spouse and a spiritual leader to be part of their support system compared to participants classified as "no/low stress" ($P = 0.02$). Additionally, approximately half of participants in the "no/low stress" category reported coworkers to be a part of their support system, while less than a quarter of participants in the "yes/high stress" category (23.1 percent) reported coworkers to be a part of their support system. More than half of participants reported living with someone they considered a close friend or relative, and the majority of participants reported belonging to at least one club or organization (73 percent).

Few differences were observed between the two stress categories with respect to the six social support variables investigated (Table 3). In both categories, the majority of participants reported having four or more close friends and/or relatives they see at least once per month (68 percent of no/low stress group and 69 percent of yes/high stress group) and talking on the phone with family, friends, and/or neighbors more than once per week (86 percent of no/low stress group and 92 percent of yes/high stress group). The largest number of participants in both of the stress/coping categories reported getting together with friends and/or relatives one to three times per month or once per week or more. However, a smaller percentage of participants in the "no/low stress" category reported getting together with friends and/or relatives one to three times per month when compared with participants in the "yes/high stress" category (32 percent of the no/low stress group and 54 percent of

Table 2: Social support characteristics of SLE cases in the Buffalo Lupus Project and Breakfast with a Buddy Biomarkers of Lupus Study ($N = 41$).

| Social support parameters | Total (41) | Low stress (28) | High stress (13) | P value |
|---|---|---|---|---|
| Having support system, n (%) | 40 (97.6) | 27 (96.4) | 13 (100) | 1 |
| Family | 38 (92.7) | 25 (89.3) | 13 (100) | 0.5390 |
| Spouse | 23 (56.1) | 12 (42.9) | 11 (84.6) | 0.0181* |
| Children | 35 (85.4) | 23 (82.1) | 12 (92.3) | 0.6448 |
| Siblings | 29 (70.7) | 19 (67.9) | 10 (76.9) | 0.7186 |
| Other family members | 30 (73.2) | 20 (71.4) | 10 (76.9) | 1 |
| Coworkers | 16 (39.0) | 13 (46.4) | 3 (23.1) | 0.1874 |
| Friends | 35 (85.4) | 23 (82.1) | 12 (92.3) | 0.6448 |
| Spiritual leader | 31 (75.6) | 19 (67.9) | 12 (92.3) | 0.1286 |
| Support group | 9 (22.0) | 5 (17.9) | 4 (30.8) | 0.4288 |
| Living with someone considered close friend and/or relative, n (%) | 25 (61.0) | 17 (60.7) | 8 (61.5) | 1 |
| Belonging to clubs/organizations, n (%) | 30 (73.2) | 19 (67.9) | 11 (84.6) | 0.4507 |

N: total number of participants, n: number of participants in each cell, %: percent, and SD: standard deviation.
* indicates statistical significance.

Table 3: Social support characteristics of SLE cases in categories of high and low stress ($N = 41$).

| Characteristics | Total (41) | Low stress (28) | High stress (13) | P value |
|---|---|---|---|---|
| Number of close friends/relatives seen at least once per month, n (%) | | | | 1 |
| None | 3 (7.3) | 2 (7.1) | 1 (7.7) | |
| 1–3 | 10 (24.4) | 7 (24.9) | 3 (23.1) | |
| 4 or more | 28 (68.3) | 19 (67.9) | 9 (69.3) | |
| Number of times of talk on the phone with family/friends/neighbors in a typical week, n (%) | | | | 1 |
| More than once | 36 (87.8) | 24 (85.7) | 12 (92.3) | |
| Once per week | 5 (12.2) | 4 (14.3) | 1 (7.7) | |
| How often patients get together with friends/relatives, n (%) | | | | 0.6453 |
| Once per week or more | 18 (43.9) | 14 (50.0) | 4 (30.8) | |
| 1–3 times per month | 16 (39.0) | 9 (32.1) | 7 (53.8) | |
| Less than once/month | 3 (7.3) | 2 (7.1) | 1 (7.7) | |
| Never/almost never | 3 (7.3) | 2 (7.1) | 1 (7.7) | |
| Having support system, n (%) | | | | 1 |
| Yes | 40 (97.6) | 27 (96.4) | 13 (100) | |
| No | 1 (2.4) | 1 (3.6) | 0 (0) | |
| Living with close friend/relative, n (%) | | | | 1 |
| Yes | 25 (61.0) | 17 (60.7) | 8 (61.5) | |
| No | 15 (36.6) | 10 (35.7) | 5 (38.5) | |
| Belonging to any clubs/organizations, n (%) | | | | 0.2307 |
| Yes | 30 (73.2) | 19 (67.9) | 11 (84.6) | |
| No | 10 (24.4) | 9 (32.1) | 1 (7.7) | |

N: total number of participants, n: number of participants in each cell, %: percent, and SD: standard deviation.

the yes/high stress group), and a smaller percentage of participants in the "yes/high stress" category reported getting together with friends and/or relatives once per week or more when compared with participants in the "no/low stress" category (31 percent of the yes/high stress group and 50 percent of the no/low stress group). In both categories, the majority of participants perceived themselves to have a support system (96 percent of no/low stress group and 100 percent of yes/high stress group) and live with someone they consider a close friend and/or relative (61 percent of no/low stress group and 62 percent of yes/high stress group). The same trend was observed with respect to club/organization membership. In both categories, the majority of participants reported belonging to a club or organization, although a smaller percentage of participants in the "no/low stress" category reported this trend when compared with participants in the "yes/high stress" category (68 percent of no/low stress group and 85 percent of yes/high stress group).

## 4. Discussion

The current study did not observe social support differences in groups of high and low stress/coping from a predominantly African American sample of middle-aged women with SLE. A key finding indicates that most SLE patients in the current study had social support.

There are a variety of reasons where a link between higher levels of social support and lower levels of stress was not observed. There may, in fact, not be a relationship between the two factors. However, statistical tests were not conducted due to small overall sample size and inability to compare such small groups as independent samples when divided into groups of high and low stress. It will require a duplicate study with a larger sample size to determine if findings are reproducible and statistically valid. It is more likely that the homogeneity of the study sample made it impossible to observe existent trends. In addition to very little variability with regard to social support, there was very little variability in the sample with regard to race and education. However, the slight differences in age, race, and/or income (proxy marker of SES) between the two stress categories could have masked the effects of social support. It is also possible that the way social support and stress/coping were assessed was not comprehensive enough and, therefore, did not truly measure what the present study aimed to measure. Other studies of stress and coping in SLE populations used entire scales, such as the Daily Stress Inventory and Daily Hassles Questionnaire [4, 22–26], whereas the current study assessed stress and coping using one question, although the question incorporates response choices reminiscent of such validated scales. The scales used may not have been appropriate since participants usually want to report what they think the interviewer wants to hear. Misclassification may have occurred due to such response bias. Since other studies have not examined stress and social support in relation to one another, present results could not be compared to those of other investigators. It was assumed, however, that a positive relationship between stress and social support would be observed, similar to the positive relationships between social support and physical well-being of lupus patients observed by other researchers [5–10].

It cannot be ignored, however, that social support is one of the most important factors in predicting the physical health and well-being of everyone, ranging from childhood to older adults. The absence of social support shows some disadvantage among the impacted individuals. In most cases, it can predict the deterioration of physical and mental health among the victims. The initial social support given is also a determining factor in successfully overcoming life stress. Studies in the general population have observed that the presence of social support significantly predicts the individual's ability to cope with stress. Knowing that they are valued by others is an important psychological factor in helping them to forget the negative aspects of their lives and think more positively about their environment. Not only does social support help improve a person's well-being, it affects the immune system as well. Thus, it is also a major factor in preventing negative symptoms such as depression and anxiety from developing [27]. While the present study did not observe differences in an SLE cohort, broken into groups of high and low stress with respect to amount of social support perceived, it is an area that should be explored further. Health status and disease activity in patients with SLE and other chronic diseases are strongly associated with social support, which suggests that enhanced social support in medical care might improve SLE outcome.

## Conflict of Interests

The authors have no conflict of interests or financial ties to disclose.

## Acknowledgments

This work was supported by the following Grants: DAMD17-02-1-0252, 1 P20 CA96256-01A1, 1 R03 CA103475-01, and R01 ES11368.

## References

[1] I. Healthwise, "Stress management: topic overview," *WebMD*, 2006.

[2] M. H. Liang, A. J. Partridge, L. H. Daltroy, K. V. Straaton, S. R. Galper, and H. R. Holman, "Strategies for reducing excess morbidity and mortality in blacks with systemic lupus erythematosus," *Arthritis & Rheumatism*, vol. 34, no. 9, pp. 1187–1196, 1991.

[3] O. Bricou, O. Taïeb, T. Baubet, B. Gal, L. Guillevin, and M.-R. Moro, "Stress and coping strategies in systemic lupus erythematosus," *Presse Medicale*, vol. 33, no. 18, pp. 1284–1292, 2004.

[4] M. I. Peralta-Ramírez, J. Jiménez-Alonso, J. F. Godoy-García et al., "The effects of daily stress and stressful life events on the clinical symptomatology of patients with lupus erythematosus," *Psychosomatic Medicine*, vol. 66, no. 5, pp. 788–794, 2004.

[5] E. W. Karlson, L. H. Daltroy, R. A. Lew et al., "The relationship of socioeconomic status, race, and modifiable risk factors to outcomes in patients with systemic lupus erythematosus," *Arthritis & Rheumatism*, vol. 40, no. 1, pp. 47–56, 1997.

[6] D. da Costa, A. E. Clarke, P. L. Dobkin et al., "The relationship between health status, social support and satisfaction with medical care among patients with systemic lupus erythematosus," *International Journal for Quality in Health Care*, vol. 11, no. 3, pp. 201–207, 1999.

[7] N. Sutcliffe, A. E. Clarke, C. Gordon, V. Farewell, and D. A. Isenberg, "The association of socio-economic status, race, psychosocial factors and outcome in patients with systemic lupus erythematosus," *Rheumatology*, vol. 38, no. 11, pp. 1130–1137, 1999.

[8] J. Thumboo, K.-Y. Fong, S.-P. Chan et al., "A prospective study of factors affecting quality of life in systemic lupus erythematosus," *Journal of Rheumatology*, vol. 27, no. 6, pp. 1414–1420, 2000.

[9] S.-C. Bae, H. Hashimoto, E. W. Karlson, M. H. Liang, and L. H. Daltroy, "Variable effects of social support by race, economic status, and disease activity in systemic lupus erythematosus," *Journal of Rheumatology*, vol. 28, no. 6, pp. 1245–1251, 2001.

[10] G. S. Alarcón, J. Calvo-Alén, G. McGwin Jr. et al., "Systemic lupus erythematosus in a multiethnic cohort: LUMINA XXXV. Predictive factors of high disease activity over time," *Annals of the Rheumatic Diseases*, vol. 65, no. 9, pp. 1168–1174, 2006.

[11] P. L. Dobkin, P. R. Fortin, L. Joseph, J. M. Esdaile, D. S. Danoff, and A. E. Clarke, "Psychosocial contributors to mental and physical health in patients with systemic lupus erythematosus," *Arthritis Care & Research*, vol. 11, no. 1, pp. 23–31, 1998.

[12] E. Kozora, M. C. Ellison, J. A. Waxmonsky, F. S. Wamboldt, and T. L. Patterson, "Major life stress, coping styles, and social support in relation to psychological distress in patients with systemic lupus erythematosus," *Lupus*, vol. 14, no. 5, pp. 363–372, 2005.

[13] P. L. Dobkin, D. Da Costa, M. Dritsa et al., "Quality of life in systemic lupus erythematosus patients during more and less active disease states: Differential contributors to mental and physical health," *Arthritis Care & Research*, vol. 12, no. 6, pp. 401–410, 1999.

[14] L. M. McCracken, E. M. Semenchuk, and V. L. Goetsch, "Cross-sectional and longitudinal analyses of coping responses and health status in persons with systemic lupus erythematosus," *Behavioral Medicine*, vol. 20, no. 4, pp. 179–187, 1995.

[15] A. H. Association, "Search your heart: our faith-based program for heart health and stroke prevention," Coronary Risk Assessment Questionaire, Channing Bete Company, South Deerfield, Mass, USA, 2003.

[16] I. G. Sarason, B. R. Sarason, E. N. Shearin, and G. R. Pierce, "A brief measure of social support: practical and theoretical implications," *Journal of Social and Personal Relationships*, vol. 4, no. 4, pp. 497–510, 1987.

[17] G. D. Zimet, N. W. Dahlem, S. G. Zimet, and G. K. Farley, "The multidimensional scale of perceived social support," *Journal of Personality Assessment*, vol. 52, no. 1, pp. 30–41, 1988.

[18] J. E. Ware Jr. and C. D. Sherbourne, "The MOS 36-item short-form health survey (SF-36). I. Conceptual framework and item selection," *Medical Care*, vol. 30, no. 6, pp. 473–483, 1992.

[19] C. A. McHorney, J. E. Ware Jr., and A. E. Raczek, "The MOS 36-Item Short-Form Health Survey (SF-36): II. Psychometric and clinical tests of validity in measuring physical and mental health constructs," *Medical Care*, vol. 31, no. 3, pp. 247–263, 1993.

[20] J. E. Ware Jr., M. M. Kosinski, and S. D. Keller, "A 12-item short-form health survey: construction of scales and preliminary tests of reliability and validity," *Medical Care*, vol. 34, no. 3, pp. 220–233, 1996.

[21] S. Swindells, J. Mohr, J. C. Justis et al., "Quality of life in patients with human immunodeficiency virus infection: impact of social support, coping style and hopelessness," *International Journal of STD & AIDS*, vol. 10, no. 6, pp. 383–391, 1999.

[22] D. P. Mueller, D. W. Edwards, and R. M. Yarvis, "Stressful life events and psychiatric symptomatology: change or undesirability?" *Journal of Health and Social Behavior*, vol. 18, no. 3, pp. 307–317, 1977.

[23] B. S. Dohrenwend, L. Krasnoff, A. R. Askenasy, and B. P. Dohrenwend, "Exemplification of a method for scaling life events: the Peri Life Events Scale," *Journal of Health and Social Behavior*, vol. 19, no. 2, pp. 205–229, 1978.

[24] P. J. Brantley, C. D. Waggoner, G. N. Jones, and N. B. Rappaport, "A daily stress inventory: development, reliability, and validity," *Journal of Behavioral Medicine*, vol. 10, no. 1, pp. 61–73, 1987.

[25] P. J. Brantley, T. B. Cocke, G. N. Jones, and A. J. Goreczny, "The Daily Stress Inventory: validity and effect of repeated administration," *Journal of Psychopathology and Behavioral Assessment*, vol. 10, no. 1, pp. 75–81, 1988.

[26] R. T. Rowlison and R. D. Felner, "Major life events, hassles, and adaptation in adolescence: confounding in the conceptualization and measurement of life stress and adjustment revisited," *Journal of Personality and Social Psychology*, vol. 55, no. 3, pp. 432–444, 1988.

[27] A. W. Clark, "Personal and social resources as correlates of coping behaviour among the aged," *Psychological Reports*, vol. 51, no. 2, pp. 577–578, 1982.

other disorders [47, 52]. After an ADEM event occurs, the clinical manifestations and neuroimaging findings can fluctuate during the next 3 months and are considered to be part of the same event, rather than separate events. The occurrence of a second event characterized by clinical encephalopathy plus polyfocal neurological deficits at least 3 months after the first episode irrespective of steroid treatment is characterized as multiphasic disseminated encephalomyelitis (MDEM) [5]. Relapsing disease that follows ADEM beyond a second encephalopathic event currently suggests a chronic disorder that often predates the diagnosis of MS or NMO [53, 54]. Some studies have suggested that 18% to 29% of patients with ADEM as their first demyelinating attack progress to MS [47, 55]. However, in a recent prospective study following the definitions proposed by the International Pediatric Multiple Sclerosis Study Group (IPMSSG) on children with ADEM, only 6% developed MS in a 9-year followup [53].

Typical MRI characteristics of ADEM are large, usually at least 2 cm, hyperintense asymmetric lesions, disseminated and confluent, involving white matter, cortex, and the deep grey nuclei with gadolinium enhancement. Recently Callen et al. [56] proposed several MRI findings to better differentiate ADEM from MS. Most patients with ADEM show (a) a diffuse bilateral pattern, (b) absence of black holes, and (c) fewer than two periventricular lesions (sensitivity 81%, specificity 95%). As a consequence, the diagnosis of ADEM is based only on the combination of clinical and neuroimaging findings and exclusion of disorders that resemble this entity.

In children younger than 12 years with features of ADEM to include encephalopathy and polyfocal neurological deficits, application of the revised 2010 MS McDonald criteria for dissemination in space and time on initial MRI is considered inappropriate, and continued follow-up of clinical and MRI findings is needed to confirm a diagnosis of MS [5].

*4.5. Neuromyelitis Optica (NMO).* Neuromyelitis optica (NMO) is an uncommon inflammatory demyelinating disorder characterized by severe acute transverse myelitis (TM) with simultaneous or sequential unilateral or bilateral optic neuritis (ON). Usually reported in adults and rarely in children, NMO has been considered an exceptional manifestation of multiple sclerosis (MS). However, the discovery of a highly specific aquaporin-4 (AQP4) autoantibody (AQP4-IgG) has demonstrated that NMO is a distinct pathophysiological disorder [57].

Over the last five years a better understanding of pediatric NMO has emerged. A median age of onset of 10–14 years and strong female predominance have been observed [54, 57–59]. Pediatric NMO spectrum can either be monophasic or manifest clinical relapses of ON or TM. Relapsing attacks of ON and TM separated in time are more common, and up to 80% of this group of patients is AQP4-IgG seropositive. Relapsing NMO tends to progress more slowly in children than in adults [60], and clinical relapses of NMO can resemble features of ADEM to include the presence of encephalopathy and large hemispheric lesions on MRI [54, 61].

Diagnostic workup for NMO includes brain and spinal cord MRI and serum AQP4-IgG testing which is 99% specific and 60%–70% sensitive even in pediatric patients [62]. Forty-two percent of children with features of NMO may display serologic (76%) or clinical evidence of systemic lupus erythematosus, Sjogren syndrome, or other autoimmune diseases [58].

Standard CSF analysis during an NMO attack may show pleocytosis with significant number of neutrophils and eosinophils and/or elevation of proteins; oligoclonal bands are generally absent [57, 60, 61].

Current diagnostic criteria are summarized in List 1. Features that suggest NMO or an NMO-spectrum disorder include (1) presence of longitudinally T2-hyperintense spinal cord lesions extending for greater than 3 vertebral segments, (2) optic neuritis, which may have a greater risk of residual deficit compared to ON associated with MS, and (3) brainstem symptoms to include intractable nausea/vomiting, vertigo, hearing loss, facial weakness, trigeminal neuralgia, diplopia, ptosis, and nystagmus [5].

*4.6. Pediatric Multiple Sclerosis.* According to international consensus clinical criteria, pediatric MS is defined by multiple episodes of demyelination of the CNS separated by time and space as specified in adults, eliminating any lower age limit [4, 5]. Therefore, pediatric MS can be diagnosed in patients younger than 18 years with two episodes of CNS demyelination separated by more than 30 days and involving more than one area of the CNS. The consensus is that clinical and radiological criteria of dissemination in time and space must be met [5, 43]. In children aged 12 years and older presenting with an acute event, some typical findings on a baseline MRI may facilitate establishing an early diagnosis when the observed changes are consistent with dissemination in space and time [5, 43].

A high sensitivity (84%) and specificity (93%) of T1 hypointense lesions and T2 periventricular lesions have been recently confirmed and validated as strong early predictors of MS diagnosis in children with acquired demyelinating syndrome (ADS) [63]. As noted earlier, most children with a single demyelinating attack of the CNS will not have recurrences, and only the assessments of clinical investigations, such as neuroimaging, analyses of the CSF, and other laboratory tests, can provide more accurate information regarding which children are at higher risk for developing MS among those who have a single monophasic event. The objective demonstration of dissemination of lesions in both space and time, based on either clinical findings alone or a combination of clinical and MRI findings, remains the core requirement for establishing the diagnosis of MS (List 1).

Most patients with pediatric MS present with a relapsing-remitting course and have much higher relapse rates compared to adults. Gorman et al. [64] have reported that the annualized relapse rate in the pediatric group was significantly higher than that in the adult-onset group (1.13 versus 0.40; $P < 0.001$). This higher rate of early relapses in pediatric MS may be related to different immune activation or levels of cells and cytokines in the CNS. However, the result may have been influenced by referral, since large tertiary referral centers may see patients with a more aggressive disease course. Further prospective studies of early relapse rate in children from first attack are required. Adolescents generally have a second clinical attack within 12 months after the first event, whereas the younger children have a greater time interval between the first and second attacks [7]. Most pediatric patients have complete recovery after their first attacks. A higher risk of experiencing permanent disability seems to be linked to the increased relapse rate within the first 2 years of the disease in pediatric patients [1, 7]. In general, disease progression is slower in pediatric MS, recovery after a clinical exacerbation is shorter in children compared to adults, and a lower proportion of children are classified with progressive forms of the disease [1, 7].

*4.7. Cognitive Impairment.* Available data suggest that approximately one-third of children and adolescents with MS experience cognitive impairment, defined as having at least one-third of completed test scores falling 1 standard deviation or more below published normative data. Areas of cognitive deficit can vary but often include attention and speeded processing, visuomotor functions, memory, and language [47, 65, 66]. Receptive language and verbal fluency are often more affected in pediatric compared with adult MS patients in whom the aspects of language are usually preserved. Interestingly, cognitive impairment was identified in 65 (35%) of 187 children with multiple sclerosis and 8 of 44 (18%) with clinically isolated syndrome in the largest sample studied to date [65]. The most frequent areas involved were fine motor coordination (54%), visuomotor integration (50%) and speeded information processing (35%). This relatively increased proportion of impairment in pediatric MS patients compared to CIS is consistent with the observation that cognitive impairments in children with multiple sclerosis progress over time [67]. Furthermore, the striking difference of cognitive impairment in the early disease course between children and adults with MS may be due to the effects of the inflammatory demyelinating process on the ongoing myelination in the developing brain and neuronal networks [47, 65].

Cognitive dysfunction is a major feature of pediatric multiple sclerosis that can occur at the earliest stages of the disease, interfering with the child's present and future academic performance. In addition, fatigue, depression, and reduced quality of life are important issues in pediatric demyelinating disorders and may occur at a rate up to three times that of controls [66, 67]. Depression or anxiety is present in 50% of children and adolescents with multiple sclerosis, thus interfering with their quality of daily life [65, 66]. Periodic neuropsychological and psychiatric assessment along with the development of interventions for cognitive decline, fatigue, and depression is warranted as part of routine care [68].

## 5. Differential Diagnosis

The diagnosis of pediatric MS is a clinical one, requiring the presence of recurrent episodes of CNS demyelination with supportive ancillary paraclinical data in the absence of another plausible diagnosis. Neuroimaging and CSF analysis features help to establish the diagnosis of pediatric MS. Accordingly, before giving a patient a diagnosis of MS, clinicians should rule out other disorders that may display similar symptoms to include vascular, inflammatory, infectious, metabolic, and neurodegenerative disorders. In a prospective cohort of 332 children meeting clinical criteria for ADS, 20 (6%) were ultimately diagnosed with nondemyelinating disorders [69]. Clinical and paraclinical findings that suggest an alternative diagnosis to initial presentation of MS include fever, encephalopathy, progressive clinical course, involvement of the peripheral nervous system or other organ systems, increased leukocyte count or ESR, markedly elevated pleocytosis or proteinorraquia, and the absence of CSF oligoclonal bands [70]. The combination of peripheral neuropathy and CNS demyelination argue against MS and favor other entities such as leukodystrophies or mitochondrial diseases.

This group of disorders usually exhibits progressive neurologic deterioration in absence of a clear relapsing-remitting disease.

CNS vasculitis is a challenging differential diagnosis of ADS with occasional overlapping features to include optic neuritis, transverse myelitis, and polyfocal supratentorial and infratentorial neurologic deficits [69, 71]. Persistent headache, rarely observed in MS or children with CIS, was present in 4 of the 5 patients with childhood primary angiitis of the CNS in the O'Mahony et al.'s study [69]. Seizures were observed in 4 of the 5 children with childhood primary angiitis compared to only 3 of more than 301 children with CNS demyelination. Focal seizures in the absence of persistent neurological deficits may be associated with CNS malignancy.

The evolution of disease by neuroimaging can help to confirm or exclude an MS diagnosis. White matter abnormalities on MRI in pediatric patients have a wide range of differential diagnoses (List 2). These entities should more often be considered in the younger child or when the presentation is atypical [70].

*List 2: Diagnostic Categories to Exclude in Pediatric Multiple Sclerosis*

*Vascular/Inflammatory Disease*

(i) CNS vasculitis/childhood primary CNS angiitis,

(ii) Stroke,

(iii) CADASIL,

(iv) Autoimmune disease: systemic lupus erythematous, antiphospholipid antibody syndrome, neurosarcoidosis, Sjogren's syndrome,

(v) Migraine.

*Metabolic/Nutritional*

(i) Mitochondrial encephalopathy,

(ii) Leukodystrophies,

(iii) B12 or folate deficiency.

*CNS Infection*

(i) Neuroborreliosis,

(ii) Herpes simplex encephalitis,

(iii) Influenza ANE,

(iv) Viral encephalitis.

*Malignancy*

(i) Lymphoma,

(ii) Astrocytoma.

Regarding neuroimaging, persistent lesion enhancement and edema or increasing size of lesions over time are considered "red flags" for an underlying malignant condition. Leptomeningeal enhancement uncommon in MS may point to either childhood primary angiitis of the CNS or an inflammatory disorder with meningeal infiltration as neurosarcoidosis [69]). Alternatively, clinical and imaging involvement of basal ganglia is not common in MS and may suggest other diagnosis such as mitochondrial disease, infectious encephalitis, or histiocytosis [69, 70]. A correct and timely diagnosis is vital to lead the children and their families to the appropriate treatment and reduce the potential long-term disability [70].

## 6. Diagnostic Tools

In patients with demyelinating events, evaluation by neuroimaging, analysis of the CSF, visual testing including the visual evoked potentials (VEP), and ocular coherence tomography (OCT) are important diagnostic tools.

*6.1. Neuroimaging (Brain MRI).* Currently, MRI is the most important diagnostic tool for evaluating MS in both children and adults, as it has invaluable utility in the recognition of other disorders that may resemble ADEM or MS. MRI findings in MS consist of plaques of demyelination particularly visible on T2-weighted sequences and typically located in the deep white matter, corpus callosum, periventricular zone, and brainstem. T1 sequences may demonstrate "black holes" or hypointense lesions that represent complete tissue loss resulting from a previous inflammatory event (Figures 1(a)–1(f)). Enhancement of active areas of inflammation and blood-brain barrier compromise can be displayed with T1 gadolinium contrast sequences. Tumefactive T2-bright lesions can be seen in up to 0.3 cases per 100.000 per year. Characteristic features that can help to distinguish demyelination from a malignant process include preferential enhancement of the lesional rim facing the lateral ventricles [72, 73].

Retrospective data suggest that children at MS onset have a higher number of total hyperintense T2 lesions in the posterior fossa and overall more gadolinium-enhancing lesions than adults do. In addition, compared to adults, pediatric MS patients tend to have greater resolution of the initial T2 lesion burden on follow-up MRI, suggesting better recovery of demyelination in children [74].

Current diagnostic criteria for MS admit MRI evidence of new lesions over time to substitute for clinical relapses. The most recent revision of the McDonald criteria specifically outlines the applicability for the use of the revised criteria in children and permits the diagnosis of pediatric MS at a first clinical event [43]. According to these criteria, dissemination in space (DIS) can be fulfilled with one or more lesions in at least two of four CNS areas (periventricular, juxtacortical, infratentorial, or spinal cord). Additionally, DIT can also be fulfilled in patients with typical acute demyelinating syndrome with a single MRI study that demonstrates simultaneous presence of asymptomatic gadolinium-enhancing and nonenhancing lesions [5, 43].

In the prospective cohort study by Sadaka et al. [75], the 2010 revised McDonald criteria demonstrated high sensitivity (100%), specificity (86%), positive predictive value (76%), and negative predictive value (100%) for children older than 12 years with non-ADEM presentations. In younger children, these criteria are of less predictive value and not appropriate for application in the context of ADEM-like presentations.

The emerging emphasis on the MRI features in the diagnosis of MS in younger children can be challenging, given the higher incidence of ADEM in this age group and often equivalent imaging features between ADEM and MS in this population with large confluent, ill-defined lesions early in the disease course. This particular phenotype contributes considerably to misdiagnosis of a significant number of patients [76].

*6.2. Cerebrospinal Fluid (CSF) Analysis.* CSF provides valuable information about the inflammatory process of the CNS. Its analysis, which includes cellular profiles, oligoclonal bands, and IgG Index, has been used to define and differentiate MS from other disorders. The profile of the CSF in pediatric MS may vary depending on the child's age. Compared to adolescents, children younger than 10 years of age tend to show more neutrophils in the CSF, and the CSF cellular profile in children tends to disappear in repeated analyses, on average 19 months after the initial examination [77]. The absence of neutrophils in the CSF at the onset of the disease may be a predictive factor of a second and early neurological episode. These observations suggest that the age of the patient exerts a modifying effect on the CSF cellular profile at the beginning of the disorder, which leads to activation of the innate immune system in the early stages or to an immature immune response [77].

CSF cell count and protein are normal in as many as 60% of pediatric patients with MS; the other patients show a discrete increase in the number of white blood cells or proteins [1, 78]. The percentage of pediatric patients with MS who also have oligoclonal bands has been reported to be up to 92%, providing that the spinal fluid is analyzed using isoelectric focusing assays [79, 80]. In some cases, the oligoclonal bands initially can be negative and detected only later in the course of the disease. It has been reported that positive oligoclonal bands may be found in 29% of patients with ADEM [78]. Mikaeloff et al., [55] in a study with 72 children presenting with a first demyelinating event, found

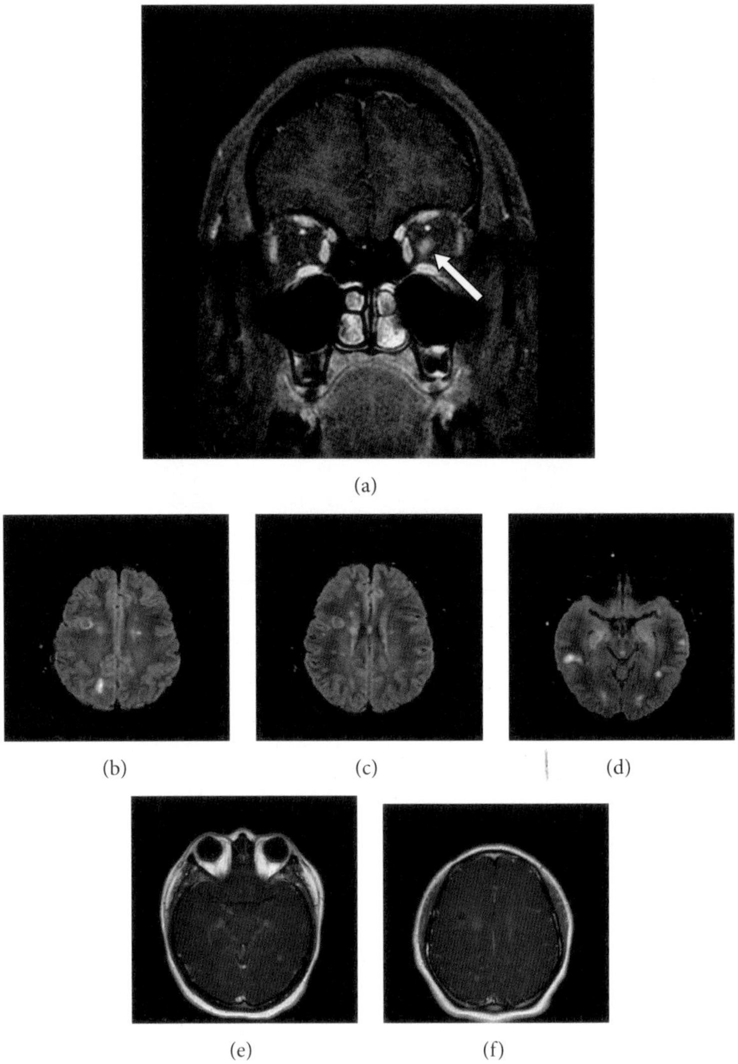

FIGURE 1: (a) Coronal T1 gadolinium enhanced sequence demonstrating left optic neuritis with enhancement and enlargement of the left optic nerve (arrow). (b) and (c) Axial FLAIR demonstrating typical well-circumscribed ovoid lesions in the juxtacortical and periventricular regions consistent with 2010 McDonald criteria for dissemination in space. (d) and (e) Axial FLAIR and gadolinium enhanced sequences with corresponding asymptomatic enhancing and nonenhancing lesions consistent with 2010 McDonald criteria for dissemination in time. (f) Axial T1 sequence with hypointense lesion associated with acute demyelination and axonal injury.

that 94% of children with positive oligoclonal bands went on to develop MS. Moreover, only 40% of patients with definitive diagnosis of MS had oligoclonal bands. These results suggest that oligoclonal bands have low sensitivity but high specificity for the development of MS.

*6.3. Visual Evaluation.* Visual deficit may go unnoticed in children with MS. Although ON may be a presenting symptom, a significant number of patients may have subclinical abnormalities of the visual pathway [81]. In fact, the visual pathways frequently are affected in MS, even in patients without visual disturbances. The visual evoked potential has diagnostic utility in pediatric MS, revealing a second focus of demyelination before a second clinical attack occurs [81]. Ocular coherence tomography (OCT), which permits *in vivo* characterization of the tissue structures with higher resolution by quantifying the thickness of the retinal nerve fiber layer containing nonmyelinated axons as well as the macular volume, has been proposed as a useful tool to evaluate patients with demyelinating disorders [82, 83]. The determination of the total macular volume has been suggested as a marker for neuronal loss in patients with MS. Similarly, a correlation between reduction of retinal nerve fiber layer thickness and both brain atrophy (by MRI) and level of disability (by Kurtzke's EDSS score) also has been reported [84, 85]. In children with MS, this tool provides a sensitive demonstration of optic atrophy and, together with the ophthalmological assessment to include visual evoked potentials, provides objective evidence of a previous inflammatory insult to the optic nerve. A recent study on OCT in children reported a significant retinal atrophy in the pediatric population with demyelinating disorders including optic neuritis, MS, and ADEM. Retinal atrophy was found to be more marked in patients with a previous episode of ON [86].

## 7. Treatment

*7.1. Acute Treatment.* Acute relapses of pediatric MS are usually treated with IV methyl prednisolone 20–30 mg/kg (maximum 1 g daily) for 3–5 days followed by oral taper. Available data in adults do not support the need for a corticosteroid taper after completion of pulse corticosteroid therapy. Pediatric patients with recurrent symptoms after discontinuation of intravenous corticosteroids may raise the possible need for an oral taper [87]. If there is an incomplete response or in case of a severe attack, intravenous immune globulin (IVIG) at 0.4 g/kg/day for 5 days or plasmapheresis should be considered.

*7.2. Preventive Therapy.* To date, there have been no randomized control trials of any DMT in the pediatric population, and the use of these treatments is mainly based on several adult clinical trials and small retrospective, observational studies. First-line therapies include intramuscular interferon (IFN)-b1a (300 mcg once a week), subcutaneous IFN b-1a (22 or 44 mcg 3 times a week), subcutaneous IFN-b1 b (0.25 mg every other day), or glatiramer acetate (20 mg/day) [88, 89].

Gradual titration of the interferon dosing over four to six weeks is common practice in children. In published studies, the majority of patients were escalated to full dose, unadjusted for age or body weight. Disease control is not always achieved immediately. Adherence to medication and time to effective dosing should be evaluated if relapses continue. If disease activity continues after 6–12 months of treatment, a change in therapies may be considered. Although there is no evidence-based guidelines as to when to switch therapies, working definitions of breakthrough disease in need of treatment modification from the IPMSSG suggest the following: (1) minimum time of full dose therapy of 6 months and (2) full medication adherence and one of the following: (a) increase or no reduction in the relapse rate or new T2 or enhancing lesion on MRI as compared to previous treatment or (b) ≥2 confirmed MRI or clinical relapses within a 12-month period [90].

Refractory disease may be considered if there are further relapses or silent progression of disease on MRI. There are several new immunomodulatory agents for refractory pediatric MS. These therapies include monoclonal antibody therapy (e.g., natalizumab, daclizumab), chemotherapeutic agents (e.g., cyclophosphamide, mitoxantrone), and oral medications with novel mechanisms of action (e.g., fingolimod, teriflunomide, and dimethyl fumarate (BG-12)). Among this group, only natalizumab, mitoxantrone, fingolimod, and teriflunomide have been approved by the FDA for use in adults with MS.

*7.3. Challenges regarding Current and Future MS Therapies.* Available data suggest that about 40% of pediatric MS patients discontinue treatment owing to intolerance, toxicity, persisting relapses, or nonadherence, supporting a need for developing new therapies in this population. Only well-designed clinical trials and long-term safety monitoring may allow the pediatric patients to benefit from the advances in MS standard of care.

Recent legislation in the United States and Europe has now mandated pediatric studies for new biological products. In Europe, a pediatric investigation plan (PIP) must be submitted to the European Medicines Agency (EMA). Similarly, the Pediatric Research Equity Act (PREA) in the United States requires pediatric studies for any new active molecule, new dosage form, or new route of administration.

A full or partial waiver is possible if the treated condition does not occur in the pediatric population or if studies are not feasible or appropriate or safe for the age group. Additionally, the Best Pharmaceuticals Act for Children (BPCA) in the United States allows for voluntary pediatric drug assessments via written requests issued by the FDA, with the incentive of eligibility of an additional 6 months of market exclusivity [91].

A meeting report on Clinical Trial Summit from the Steering Committee of the International Pediatric MS Study Group (IPMSSG) has been recently published [91]. The academic leaders established guidelines for outcome measures, including clinical, cognitive, and MRI, to be considered in the pediatric MS clinical drug trials. Despite the growing arsenal of therapies that offers substantial promise for pediatric patients, there are some immediate and long-term health risks, and only well-designed, multicenter trials with long-term followup will properly assess accompanying hazards and safety.

## 8. Conclusions

The diagnosis of pediatric MS needs to be considered in those patients in whom optic nerve, sensory, motor, brainstem, and/or cerebellar disturbance are the presenting symptoms. A comprehensive history aided by clinical, neuroimaging, and laboratory clues can help to assure a prompt diagnosis and the exclusion of other neurological disorders. In younger patients, however, a polyfocal presentation with associated encephalopathy may be difficult to distinguish from ADEM. As in adult-onset MS, the MRI features of pediatric MS involve the presence of multiple lesions, mostly in the white matter and typically observed in the periventricular area of the corpus callosum and spinal cord. Children often show more infratentorial lesions, predominantly in the pons, and can have large and tumefactive lesions with perilesional edema. The most recent revision of the McDonald criteria specifically underscores its applicability in diagnosing MS in children older than 12 years and in facilitating the diagnosis at a first clinical attack, providing the criteria for dissemination in space and time are met.

During the last 10 years, new insights regarding the pathology and immunobiology, clinical features, and neuroimaging have increased the ability to better understand pediatric MS. For example, different studies have identified the potential roles of EBV and low vitamin D in the pathogenesis of MS. However, information about the nature of the immune mechanisms involved in pediatric MS and the interactions of risk factors with genetic susceptibility is limited. On the horizon, identification of biomarkers with the promise to predict disease onset and monitor disease course, severity, and response to treatment has led to a renewed and increased interest and may provide important information for the best management of patients.

## References

[1] P. Duquette, T. J. Murray, J. Pleines et al., "Multiple sclerosis in childhood: clinical profile in 125 patients," *Journal of Pediatrics*, vol. 111, no. 3, pp. 359–363, 1987.

[2] A. Ghezzi, V. Deplano, J. Faroni et al., "Multiple sclerosis in childhood: clinical features of 149 cases," *Multiple Sclerosis*, vol. 3, no. 1, pp. 43–46, 1997.

[3] M. Ruggieri, P. Iannetti, A. Polizzi, L. Pavone, and L. M. Grimaldi, "Multiple sclerosis in children under 10 years of age," *Neurological Sciences*, vol. 25, no. 4, pp. S326–S335, 2004.

[4] L. B. Krupp, B. Banwell, and S. Tenembaum, "International Pediatric MS Study Group, Consensus definitions proposed for pediatric multiple sclerosis and related disorders," *Neurology*, vol. 68, no. 16, supplement 2, pp. S7–S12, 2007.

[5] L. B. Krupp, M. Tardieu, M. P. Amato et al., "International Pediatric Multiple Sclerosis Study Group criteria for pediatric multiple sclerosis and immune-mediated central nervous system demyelinating disorders: revisions to the 2007 definitions," *Multiple Sclerosis Journal*, vol. 19, no. 10, pp. 1261–1267, 2013.

[6] O. Deryck, P. Ketelaer, and B. Dubois, "Clinical characteristics and long term prognosis in early onset multiple sclerosis," *Journal of Neurology*, vol. 253, no. 6, pp. 720–723, 2006.

[7] C. Renoux, S. Vukusic, Y. Mikaeloff et al., "Natural history of multiple sclerosis with childhood onset," *New England Journal of Medicine*, vol. 356, no. 25, pp. 2603–2613, 2007.

[8] A. Langer-Gould, J. L. Zhang, J. Chung, Y. Yeung, E. Waubant, and J. Yao, "Incidence of acquired CNS demyelinating syndromes in a multiethnic cohort of children," *Neurology*, vol. 77, no. 12, pp. 1143–1148, 2011.

[9] B. Banwell, J. Kennedy, D. Sadovnick et al., "Incidence of acquired demyelination of the CNS in Canadian children," *Neurology*, vol. 72, no. 3, pp. 232–239, 2009.

[10] I. A. Ketelslegers, C. E. Catsman-Berrevoets, R. F. Neuteboom et al., "Incidence of acquired demyelinating syndromes of the CNS in Dutch children: a nationwide study," *Journal of Neurology*, vol. 259, no. 9, pp. 1929–1935, 2012.

[11] J. Kennedy, P. O'Connor, A. D. Sadovnick, M. Perara, I. Yee, and B. Banwell, "Age at onset of multiple sclerosis may be influenced by place of residence during childhood rather than ancestry," *Neuroepidemiology*, vol. 26, no. 3, pp. 162–167, 2006.

[12] B. Banwell, A. Ghezzi, A. Bar-Or, Y. Mikaeloff, and M. Tardieu, "Multiple sclerosis in children: clinical diagnosis, therapeutic strategies, and future directions," *Lancet Neurology*, vol. 6, no. 10, pp. 887–902, 2007.

[13] T. Chitnis, B. Glanz, S. Jaffin, and B. Healy, "Demographics of pediatric-onset multiple sclerosis in an MS center population from the Northeastern United States," *Multiple Sclerosis*, vol. 15, no. 5, pp. 627–631, 2009.

[14] E. A. Yeh, T. Chitnis, L. Krupp et al., "Pediatric multiple sclerosis," *Nature Reviews Neurology*, vol. 5, no. 11, pp. 621–631, 2009.

[15] T. Chitnis, L. Krupp, A. Yeh et al., "Pediatric Multiple Sclerosis," *Neurologic Clinics*, vol. 29, no. 2, pp. 481–505, 2011.

[16] B. K. Mehta, "New hypotheses on sunlight and the geographic variability of multiple sclerosis prevalence," *Journal of the Neurological Sciences*, vol. 292, no. 1-2, pp. 5–10, 2010.

[17] E. M. Mowry, "Vitamin D: evidence for its role as a prognostic factor in multiple sclerosis," *Journal of the Neurological Sciences*, vol. 311, no. 1-2, pp. 19–22, 2011.

[18] S. Chen, G. P. Sims, X. C. Xiao, Y. G. Yue, S. Chen, and P. E. Lipsky, "Modulatory effects of 1,25-dihydroxyvitamin D3 on human B cell differentiation," *Journal of Immunology*, vol. 179, no. 3, pp. 1634–1647, 2007.

[19] S. Simpson Jr., B. Taylor, L. Blizzard et al., "Higher 25-hydroxyvitamin D is associated with lower relapse risk in multiple sclerosis," *Annals of Neurology*, vol. 68, no. 2, pp. 193–203, 2010.

[20] E. M. Mowry, L. B. Krupp, M. Milazzo et al., "Vitamin D status is associated with relapse rate in pediatric-onset multiple sclerosis," *Annals of Neurology*, vol. 67, no. 5, pp. 618–624, 2010.

[21] E. M. Mowry, E. Waubant, C. E. McCulloch et al., "Vitamin D status predicts new brain magnetic resonance imaging activity in multiple sclerosis," *Annals of Neurology Journal*, vol. 72, no. 2, pp. 234–240, 2012.

[22] A. Ascherio, K. L. Munger, E. T. Lennette et al., "Epstein-Barr virus antibodies and risk of multiple sclerosis: a prospective study," *Journal of the American Medical Association*, vol. 286, no. 24, pp. 3083–3088, 2001.

[23] S. Alotaibi, J. Kennedy, R. Tellier, D. Stephens, and B. Banwell, "Epstein-Barr virus in pediatric multiple sclerosis," *Journal of the American Medical Association*, vol. 291, no. 15, pp. 1875–1879, 2004.

[24] B. Banwell, L. Krupp, J. Kennedy et al., "Clinical features and viral serologies in children with multiple sclerosis: a multinational observational study," *Lancet Neurology*, vol. 6, no. 9, pp. 773–781, 2007.

[25] D. Pohl, B. Krone, K. Rostasy et al., "High seroprevalence of Epstein-Barr virus in children with multiple sclerosis," *Neurology*, vol. 67, no. 11, pp. 2063–2065, 2006.

[26] E. Waubant, E. M. Mowry, L. Krupp et al., "Common viruses associated with lower pediatric multiple sclerosis risk," *Neurology*, vol. 76, no. 23, pp. 1989–1995, 2011.

[27] D. Pohl, "Epstein-Barr virus and multiple sclerosis," *Journal of the Neurological Sciences*, vol. 286, no. 1-2, pp. 62–64, 2009.

[28] Y. Mikaeloff, G. Caridade, M. Rossier, S. Suissa, and M. Tardieu, "Hepatitis B vaccination and the risk of childhood-onset multiple sclerosis," *Archives of Pediatrics and Adolescent Medicine*, vol. 161, no. 12, pp. 1176–1182, 2007.

[29] Y. Mikaeloff, G. Caridade, S. Assi, M. Tardieu, and S. Suissa, "Hepatitis B vaccine and risk of relapse after a first childhood episode of CNS inflammatory demyelination," *Brain*, vol. 130, part 4, pp. 1105–1110, 2007.

[30] Y. Mikaeloff, G. Caridade, S. Suissa, and M. Tardieu, "Hepatitis B vaccine and the risk of CNS inflammatory demyelination in childhood," *Neurology*, vol. 72, no. 10, pp. 873–880, 2009.

[31] Y. Mikaeloff, G. Caridade, M. Tardieu, and S. Suissa, "Parental smoking at home and the risk of childhood-onset multiple sclerosis in children," *Brain*, vol. 130, part 10, pp. 2589–2595, 2007.

[32] D. A. Dyment, G. C. Ebers, and A. D. Sadovnick, "Genetics of multiple sclerosis," *Lancet Neurology*, vol. 3, no. 2, pp. 104–110, 2004.

[33] P. L. de Jager, X. Jia, J. Wang et al., "Meta-analysis of genome scans and replication identify CD6, IRF8 and TNFRSF1A as new multiple sclerosis susceptibility loci," *Nature Genetics*, vol. 41, no. 7, pp. 776–782, 2009.

[34] T. Derfuss, C. Linington, R. Hohlfeld, and E. Meinl, "Axo-glial antigens as targets in multiple sclerosis: implications for axonal and grey matter injury," *Journal of Molecular Medicine*, vol. 88, no. 8, pp. 753–761, 2010.

[35] P. K. Stys, G. W. Zamponi, J. van Minnen, and J. J. Geurts, "Will the real multiple sclerosis please stand up?" *Nature Reviews Neuroscience*, vol. 13, no. 7, pp. 507–514, 2012.

[36] K. Rostasy, E. Withut, D. Pohl et al., "Tau, phospho-tau, and S-100B in the cerebrospinal fluid of children with multiple sclerosis," *Journal of Child Neurology*, vol. 20, no. 10, pp. 822–825, 2005.

[37] T. Derfuss, K. Parikh, S. Velhin et al., "Contactin-2/TAG-1-directed autoimmunity is identified in multiple sclerosis patients and mediates gray matter pathology in animals," *Proceedings of the National Academy of Sciences of the United States of America*, vol. 106, no. 20, pp. 8302–8307, 2009.

[38] E. K. Mathey, T. Derfuss, M. K. Storch et al., "Neurofascin as a novel target for autoantibody-mediated axonal injury," *Journal of Experimental Medicine*, vol. 204, no. 10, pp. 2363–2372, 2007.

[39] E. Meinl, T. Derfuss, M. Krumbholz, A. K. Pröbstel, and R. Hohlfeld, "Humoral autoimmunity in multiple sclerosis," *Journal of the Neurological Sciences*, vol. 306, no. 1-2, pp. 180–182, 2011.

[40] A. S. Dhaunchak, C. Becker, H. Schulman et al., "Implication of perturbed axoglial apparatus in early pediatric multiple sclerosis," *Annals of Neurology*, vol. 71, no. 5, pp. 601–613, 2012.

[41] J. M. Van Noort, M. Bsibsi, W. H. Gerritsen et al., "αB-crystallin is a target for adaptive immune responses and a trigger of innate responses in preactive multiple sclerosis lesions," *Journal of Neuropathology and Experimental Neurology*, vol. 69, no. 7, pp. 694–703, 2010.

[42] J. L. Bennett and G. P. Owens, "Cerebrospinal fluid proteomics: a new window for understanding human demyelinating disorders?" *Annals of Neurology*, vol. 71, no. 5, pp. 587–588, 2012.

[43] C. H. Polman, S. C. Reingold, B. Banwell et al., "Diagnostic criteria for multiple sclerosis: 2010 revisions to the McDonald criteria," *Annals of Neurology*, vol. 69, no. 2, pp. 292–302, 2011.

[44] R. F. Neuteboom, M. Boon, C. E. Catsman Berrevoets et al., "Prognostic factors after a first attack of inflammatory CNS demyelination in children," *Neurology*, vol. 71, no. 13, pp. 967–973, 2008.

[45] M. Wilejto, M. Shroff, J. R. Buncic, J. Kennedy, C. Goia, and B. Banwell, "The clinical features, MRI findings, and outcome of optic neuritis in children," *Neurology*, vol. 67, no. 2, pp. 258–262, 2006.

[46] L. H. Verhey, H. M. Branson, M. M. Shroff et al., "MRI parameters for prediction of multiple sclerosis diagnosis in children with acute CNS demyelination: a prospective national cohort study," *The Lancet Neurology*, vol. 10, no. 12, pp. 1065–1073, 2011.

[47] S. Bigi and B. Banwell, "Pediatric multiple sclerosis," *Journal of Child Neurology*, vol. 27, no. 11, pp. 1378–1383, 2012.

[48] G. Alper and L. Wang, "Demyelinating optic neuritis in children," *Journal of Child Neurology*, vol. 24, no. 1, pp. 45–48, 2009.

[49] R. Miyazawa, Y. Ikeuchi, T. Tomomasa, H. Ushiku, T. Ogawa, and A. Morikawa, "Determinants of prognosis of acute transverse myelitis in children," *Pediatrics International*, vol. 45, no. 5, pp. 512–516, 2003.

[50] A. T. Borchers and M. E. Gershwin, "Transverse myelitis," *Autoimmunity Reviews*, vol. 11, no. 3, pp. 231–248, 2012.

[51] F. S. Pidcock, C. Krishnan, T. O. Crawford, C. F. Salorio, M. Trovato, and D. A. Kerr, "Acute transverse myelitis in childhood: center-based analysis of 47 cases," *Neurology*, vol. 68, no. 18, pp. 1474–1480, 2007.

[52] D. Pohl and S. Tenembaum, "Treatment of acute disseminated encephalomyelitis," *Current Treatment Options in Neurology*, vol. 14, no. 3, pp. 264–275, 2012.

[53] S. Mar, J. Lenox, T. Benzinger, S. Brown, and M. Noetzel, "Long-term prognosis of pediatric patients with relapsing acute disseminated encephalomyelitis," *Journal of Child Neurology*, vol. 25, no. 6, pp. 681–688, 2010.

[54] T. E. Lotze, J. L. Northrop, G. J. Hutton, B. Ross, J. S. Schiffman, and J. V. Hunter, "Spectrum of pediatric neuromyelitis optica," *Pediatrics*, vol. 122, no. 5, pp. e1039–e1047, 2008.

[55] Y. Mikaeloff, S. Suissa, L. Vallée et al., "First episode of acute CNS inflammatory demyelination in childhood: prognostic factors for multiple sclerosis and disability," *Journal of Pediatrics*, vol. 144, no. 2, pp. 246–252, 2004.

[56] D. J. A. Callen, M. M. Shroff, H. M. Branson et al., "Role of MRI in the differentiation of ADEM from MS in children," *Neurology*, vol. 72, no. 11, pp. 968–973, 2009.

[57] D. M. Wingerchuk, "Neuromyelitis optica spectrum disorders," *CONTINUUM Lifelong Learning in Neurology*, vol. 16, no. 5, pp. 105–121, 2010.

[58] A. McKeon, V. A. Lennon, T. Lotze et al., "CNS aquaporin-4 autoimmunity in children," *Neurology*, vol. 71, no. 2, pp. 93–100, 2008.

[59] J. A. Peña, M. E. Ravelo, E. Mora-La Cruz, and C. Montiel-Nava, "NMO in pediatric patients: brain involvement and clinical expression," *Arquivos de Neuro-Psiquiatria*, vol. 69, no. 1, pp. 34–38, 2011.

[60] M. J. Morrow and D. Wingerchuk, "Neuromyelitis optica," *Journal of Neuro-Ophthalmology*, vol. 32, no. 2, pp. 154–166, 2012.

[61] J. M. Tillema and A. McKeon, "The spectrum of neuromyelitis optica (NMO) in childhood," *Journal of Child Neurology*, vol. 27, no. 11, pp. 1437–1447, 2012.

[62] B. Banwell, S. Tenembaum, V. A. Lennon et al., "Neuromyelitis optica-IgG in childhood inflammatory demyelinating CNS disorders," *Neurology*, vol. 70, no. 5, pp. 344–352, 2008.

[63] L. H. Verhey, E. D. van Pelt-Gravesteijnc, A. Ketelslegersc et al., "Validation of MRI predictors of multiple sclerosis diagnosis in children with acute CNS demyelination," *Multiple Sclerosis and Related Disorders*, vol. 2, no. 3, pp. 193–199, 2013.

[64] M. P. Gorman, B. C. Healy, M. Polgar-Turcsanyi, and T. Chitnis, "Increased relapse rate in pediatric-onset compared with adult-onset multiple sclerosis," *Archives of Neurology*, vol. 66, no. 1, pp. 54–59, 2009.

[65] L. Julian, D. Serafin, L. Charvet et al., "Cognitive impairment occurs in children and adolescents with multiple sclerosis: results from a United States network," *Journal of Child Neurology*, vol. 28, no. 1, pp. 102–107, 2013.

[66] W. S. MacAllister, J. R. Boyd, N. J. Holland, M. C. Milazzo, and L. B. Krupp, "The psychosocial consequences of pediatric multiple sclerosis," *Neurology*, vol. 68, no. 16, supplement 2, pp. S66–S69, 2007.

[67] W. S. MacAllister, C. Christodoulou, M. Milazzo, and L. B. Krupp, "Longitudinal neuropsychological assessment in pediatric multiple sclerosis," *Developmental Neuropsychology*, vol. 32, no. 2, pp. 625–644, 2007.

[68] B. I. Glanz, B. C. Healy, L. E. Hviid, T. Chitnis, and H. L. Weiner, "Cognitive deterioration in patients with early multiple sclerosis: a 5-year study," *Journal of Neurology, Neurosurgery and Psychiatry*, vol. 83, no. 1, pp. 38–43, 2012.

[69] J. O'Mahony, A. Bar-Or, D. L. Arnold, A. D. Sadovnick, R. A. Marrie, and B. Banwell, "Masquerades of acquired demyelination in children: experiences of a national demyelinating disease program," *Journal of Child Neurology*, vol. 28, no. 2, pp. 184–197, 2013.

[70] J. S. Hahn, D. Pohl, M. Rensel, and S. Rao, "Differential diagnosis and evaluation in pediatric multiple sclerosis," *Neurology*, vol. 68, no. 16, supplement 2, pp. S13–S22, 2007.

[71] M. Twilt and S. M. Benseler, "CNS vasculitis in children," *Multiple Sclerosis and Related Disorders*, vol. 2, no. 3, pp. 162–171, 2013.

[72] L. C. McAdam, S. I. Blaser, and B. L. Banwell, "Pediatric tumefactive demyelination: case series and review of the literature," *Pediatric Neurology*, vol. 26, no. 1, pp. 18–25, 2002.

[73] D. Riva, L. Chiapparini, B. Pollo, M. R. Balestrini, M. Massimino, and N. Milani, "A case of pediatric tumefactive demyelinating lesion misdiagnosed and treated as glioblastoma," *Journal of Child Neurology*, vol. 23, no. 8, pp. 944–947, 2008.

[74] E. Waubant, D. Chabas, D. T. Okuda et al., "Difference in disease burden and activity in pediatric patients on brain magnetic resonance imaging at time of multiple sclerosis onset vs adults," *Archives of Neurology*, vol. 66, no. 8, pp. 967–971, 2009.

[75] Y. Sadaka, L. H. Verhey, M. M. Shroff et al., "2010 McDonald criteria for diagnosing pediatric multiple sclerosis," *Annals of Neurology*, vol. 72, no. 2, pp. 211–223, 2012.

[76] D. Chabas, T. Castillo-Trivino, E. M. Mowry, J. B. Strober, O. A. Glenn, and E. Waubant, "Vanishing MS T2-bright lesions before puberty: a distinct MRI phenotype?" *Neurology*, vol. 71, no. 14, pp. 1090–1093, 2008.

[77] D. Chabas, J. Ness, A. Belman et al., "Younger children with MS have a distinct CSF inflammatory profile at disease onset," *Neurology*, vol. 74, no. 5, pp. 399–405, 2010.

[78] R. C. Dale, C. de Sousa, W. K. Chong, T. C. S. Cox, B. Harding, and B. G. R. Neville, "Acute disseminated encephalomyelitis, multiphasic disseminated encephalomyelitis and multiple sclerosis in children," *Brain*, vol. 123, no. 12, pp. 2407–2422, 2000.

[79] A. Ghezzi, C. Pozzilli, M. Liguori et al., "Prospective study of multiple sclerosis with early onset," *Multiple Sclerosis*, vol. 8, no. 2, pp. 115–118, 2002.

[80] D. Pohl, K. Rostasy, H. Reiber, and F. Hanefeld, "CSF characteristics in early-onset multiple sclerosis," *Neurology*, vol. 63, no. 10, pp. 1966–1967, 2004.

[81] D. Pohl, K. Rostasy, S. Treiber-Held, K. Brockmann, J. Gärtner, and F. Hanefeld, "Pediatric multiple sclerosis: detection of clinically silent lesions by multimodal evoked potentials," *Journal of Pediatrics*, vol. 149, no. 1, pp. 125–127, 2006.

[82] F. Costello, S. Coupland, W. Hodge et al., "Quantifying axonal loss after optic neuritis with optical coherence tomography," *Annals of Neurology*, vol. 59, no. 6, pp. 963–969, 2006.

[83] E. Frohman, F. Costello, R. Zivadinov et al., "Optical coherence tomography in multiple sclerosis," *Lancet Neurology*, vol. 5, no. 10, pp. 853–863, 2006.

[84] E. Gordon-Lipkin, B. Chodkowski, D. S. Reich et al., "Retinal nerve fiber layer is associated with brain atrophy in multiple sclerosis," *Neurology*, vol. 69, no. 16, pp. 1603–1609, 2007.

[85] A. P. D. Henderson, S. A. Trip, P. G. Schlottmann et al., "An investigation of the retinal nerve fibre layer in progressive multiple sclerosis using optical coherence tomography," *Brain*, vol. 131, part 1, pp. 277–287, 2008.

[86] E. A. Yeh, B. Weinstock-Guttman, N. Lincoff et al., "Retinal nerve fiber thickness in inflammatory demyelinating diseases of childhood onset," *Multiple Sclerosis*, vol. 15, no. 7, pp. 802–810, 2009.

[87] E. A. Yeh, "Management of children with multiple sclerosis," *Pediatric Drugs*, vol. 14, no. 3, pp. 165–177, 2012.

[88] A. Ghezzi, M. P. Amato, M. Capobianco et al., "Disease-modifying drugs in childhood-juvenile multiple sclerosis: results of an Italian co-operative study," *Multiple Sclerosis*, vol. 11, no. 4, pp. 420–424, 2005.

[89] E. A. Yeh, "Current therapeutic options in pediatric multiple sclerosis," *Current Treatment Options in Neurology*, vol. 13, no. 6, pp. 544–559, 2011.

[90] T. Chitnis, S. Tenembaum, B. Banwell et al., "Consensus statement: evaluation of new and existing therapeutics for pediatric multiple sclerosis," *Multiple Sclerosis*, vol. 18, no. 1, pp. 116–127, 2012.

[91] T. Chitnis, M. Tardieu, M. P. Amato et al., "International Pediatric MS Study Group Clinical Trials Summit: meeting report," *Neurology*, vol. 80, no. 12, pp. 1161–1168, 2013.

# Prevalence of Thyroid Autoimmunity in Children with Celiac Disease Compared to Healthy 12-Year Olds

**Maria van der Pals,[1] Anneli Ivarsson,[2] Fredrik Norström,[2] Lotta Högberg,[3,4] Johan Svensson,[1] and Annelie Carlsson[1]**

[1] *Department of Pediatrics, Clinical Sciences, Skåne University Hospital, Lund University, 205 02 Lund, Sweden*
[2] *Department of Public Health and Clinical Medicine, Epidemiology and Global Health, Umeå University, 905 85 Umeå, Sweden*
[3] *Division of Pediatrics, Department of Clinical and Experimental Medicine, Faculty of Health Sciences, Linköping University, 581 85 Linköping, Sweden*
[4] *Department of Pediatrics in Norrköping, County Council of Östergötland, 603 79 Norrköping, Sweden*

Correspondence should be addressed to Maria van der Pals; maria.vanderpals@med.lu.se

Academic Editor: Alina Popp

*Objectives.* Studies have suggested a correlation between untreated celiac disease and risk for other autoimmune diseases. We investigated the prevalence of thyroid autoimmunity in 12-year-old children (i) with symptomatic celiac disease diagnosed and treated with a gluten-free diet, (ii) with screening-detected untreated celiac disease, and (iii) without celiac disease. *Methods.* Blood samples from 12632 children were collected. All celiac disease cases, previously diagnosed and newly screening-detected, were identified. Per case, 4 referents were matched. Blood samples were analyzed for autoantibodies against thyroid peroxidase (TPOAb). The cut-off value for TPO positivity was set to 100 U/mL. *Results.* Altogether, 335 celiac disease cases were found. In the entire celiac disease group, 7.2% (24/335) had elevated titers of TPOAb compared to 2.8% (48/1695) of the referents. Among the previously diagnosed celiac disease cases, 7.5% (7/93, OR 2.8, 95% CI 1.2–6.4) was TPOAb positive and among screening-detected cases, 7.0% (17/242, OR 2.6, 95% CI 1.5–4.6) was TPOAb positive. *Conclusion.* Children with celiac disease showed a higher prevalence of thyroid autoimmunity. We could not confirm the hypothesis that untreated celiac disease is associated with increased risk of developing thyroid autoimmunity. Early initiation of celiac disease treatment might not lower the risk for other autoimmune diseases.

## 1. Introduction

Celiac disease is one of the most common chronic diseases in childhood, affecting approximately 0.5–3% of the population in the Western world [1–3]. It is characterized by an autoimmune response triggered by gluten and possibly other environmental cofactors, leading to small-intestinal mucosal injury [4]. This in turn leads to malabsorption with a variable clinical expression ranging from no symptoms to severe malnutrition. The disease can have its onset at any age throughout life [5, 6]. The human leukocyte antigen HLA DQ2 or DQ8 haplotype is carried by all celiac disease cases, and the prevalence in the general population has been assumed to be about 30% [7, 8]. The presence of HLA DQ2 and/or DQ8 is necessary but not sufficient for development of the disease. Studies of identical twins and siblings suggest the HLA contribution to be less than 50%, with the remaining part being explained by a combination of non-HLA genes and environmental factors [9].

Autoimmune conditions including thyroid diseases such as Hashimoto thyroiditis and Grave's disease are associated with celiac disease [10–13] with a reported prevalence up to 10 times that in the general population [14–17]. Some studies have suggested that untreated celiac disease and thus also gluten exposure, with subsequent inflammation and mucosal injury, increase the risk for developing other autoimmune diseases such as thyroid diseases and insulin dependent diabetes mellitus. Ventura et al. showed that patients with celiac disease had a high prevalence of both insulin dependent diabetes mellitus autoantibodies and thyroid-related serum autoantibodies. Moreover, these autoantibodies were supposed to be gluten-dependent, because they disappeared during treatment with a gluten-free diet [12, 18].

These findings raise questions as to whether abnormal immune responses, at the level of the gut mucosa when exposed to environmental antigens, play a role in systemic autoimmune disease or if these associations instead reflect an underlying joint genetic predisposition. If the duration of gluten exposure is positively correlated to development of autoimmune disease, and if early detection and initiated treatment of the disease reduces the risk for development of autoimmune disease, this would point in the direction of a general celiac disease screening at as early an age as possible.

The aim of our study was to investigate the prevalence of thyroid autoimmunity in 12-year-old children with celiac disease compared to sex-matched referents and to investigate if early introduction of a gluten-free diet in children with celiac disease reduces the risk for developing autoimmune thyroid disease. The hypothesis is that previously diagnosed cases with a consequentially reduced exposure (after the time of the diagnosis) can be expected to display a lower incidence of TPOAbs than screening-detected cases (with ongoing exposure).

## 2. Materials and Methods

*2.1. A Population-Based Celiac Disease Screening Study.* A two-phased population-based cross-sectional multicenter screening study for celiac disease in 12-year olds was performed in 2005-2006 and 2009-2010 representing two birth cohorts (children born in 1993 and 1997, resp.) [3, 19]. The study was entitled the ETICS study (Exploring the Iceberg of Celiacs in Sweden) and was part of the PreventCD European project [3, 20]. Both screening efforts covered the same geographical areas and followed a similar protocol, including collaboration with school health services. Families gave their signed informed consent before being enrolled. The study was approved by the Regional Ethical Review Board of Umeå University, Umeå, Sweden.

In total, 12632 children (69% of those invited) participated, with similar sex ratios in both birth cohorts (48% and 49% girls in the 1993 and 1997 groups, resp.). Details of the celiac disease screening strategy and descriptions of both cohorts have been published previously [3, 19]. In brief, blood samples from all participating children were analyzed for antihuman tissue transglutaminase and if borderline values were obtained also for endomysial antibodies (both of isotype IgA). Children with values above a predefined cut-off were referred to the closest pediatric clinic for a small intestinal biopsy, which represents the gold standard for diagnosis [21, 22]. Criteria for diagnosis were Marsh 3a–c enteropathy or the combination of Marsh 1-2 enteropathy, HLA-DQ2/DQ8 haplotype, and symptoms and/or signs compatible with celiac disease [22].Genotyping for HLA alleles encoding for HLA-DQ2/DQ8 was performed by oligonucleotide probe hybridization and was verified in all screening-detected cases. For those who reported clinically detected celiac disease, diagnosis was confirmed by review of histology and serological markers from the National Swedish Childhood Celiac Disease Register [23] and/or medical records.

*2.2. A Nested Case-Referent Study on Thyroid Autoimmunity.* A case-referent design nested within the ETICS study was used to evaluate the risk of thyroid autoimmunity related to treated (i.e., the previously diagnosed celiac disease cases) and untreated celiac disease, respectively. The mean age at diagnosis among the previously diagnosed celiac disease cases was 4.7 and the median was 2.75 years. They had thus been on a gluten-free diet for approximately 7 to 9 years since the screening was performed at 12 years of age. The total number of celiac disease cases from both screening efforts, including previously diagnosed cases and newly screening-detected cases, together formed our celiac disease case group. This cohort was used as a basis for screening of thyroid autoimmunity, defined as significant titers of TPOAb. The blood samples drawn for the TPOAbs were taken at 12 years of age, that is, at the time of the screening. Autoantibodies of IgG type directed against thyroid peroxidase (TPOAb) that were measured in blood samples were used as an indicator of thyroid autoimmunity and expressed as arbitrary units per milliliter (U/mL). The cut-off value for TPO positivity was set to 100 U/mL (Varelisa TPO Antibodies, Phadia GmbH, Freiburg, Germany).

Four referents were selected for each celiac disease case. Referents, matched for sex, were randomly selected from all cohort members free of celiac disease at the time of diagnosis. In this paper we included cases with a confirmed celiac disease diagnosis, obtained either through the ETICS screening ($n = 242$) or ahead of the screening ($n = 93$). We therefore excluded 90 children, either because of incorrect information about the existing celiac disease diagnosis ($n = 36$ children) or because of no biopsy verifying a celiac disease diagnosis ($n = 54$ children). This resulted in 213 cases and 1150 referents from the first phase (a rate of 5.4 referents per case) and 122 cases and 545 referents from the second phase (a rate of 4.5 referents per case) for the analyses in this paper.

*2.3. Statistical Analysis.* The relation between celiac disease and TPOAb positivity was analyzed with logistic regression using the nonceliac disease children as the reference group. Results are presented as odds ratios (OR) with 95% confidence intervals (CI). Microsoft Access was used for data handling and Stata 10 for statistical analysis (StataCorp LP, College Station, TX). Statistical significance was accepted at $P < 0.05$ corresponding to a CI not including 1.

## 3. Results

*3.1. Study Population Characteristics.* In total, among the 12632 children, we identified 335 celiac disease cases whereof 93 had previously diagnosed celiac disease and 242 were detected within the study (Figure 1). Details regarding the prevalence of celiac disease have been published elsewhere, but in short, the screening procedure revealed a total celiac disease prevalence of 29/1 000 in the 1993 cohort, including

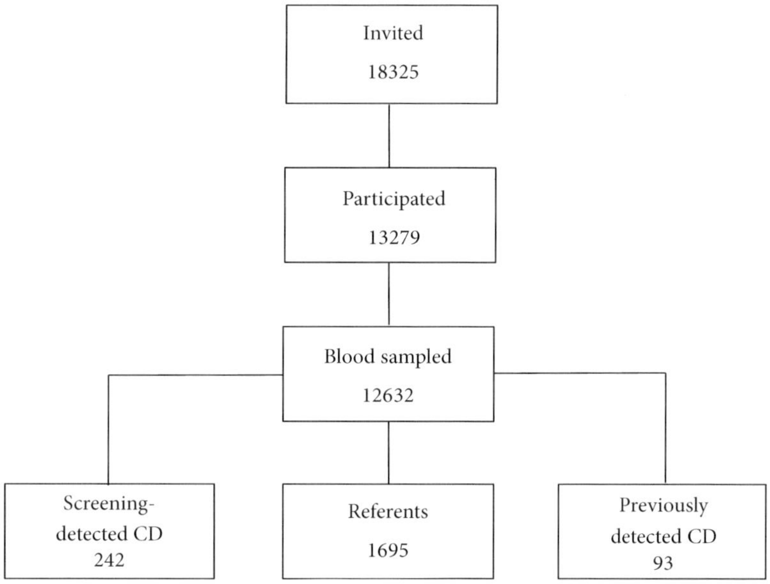


FIGURE 1: Flowchart depicting the screening procedure. Cross-sectional screenings performed in 12-year olds across Sweden to investigate the total prevalence of celiac disease (CD), including both clinically- and screening-detected cases. Numbers of children are given in the boxes.

TABLE 1: Risk for thyroid peroxidase antibody (TPO) positivity in 12-year olds when comparing treated and untreated celiac disease (CD) cases with non-CD children through a case-referent study nested within the ETICS[1] study.

| Groups | TPO[2] Positive ($n$ = 72) | | Negative ($n$ = 1958) | | OR[3] | 95% CI[3] |
|---|---|---|---|---|---|---|
| | $n$ | %[4] | $n$ | % | | |
| Non-CD[5] | 48 | 2.8 | 1647 | 97.2 | 1.0 | — |
| Previously diagnosed CD | 7 | 7.5 | 86 | 92.5 | 2.8 | 1.2–6.4 |
| Screening-detected CD | 17 | 7.0 | 225 | 93.0 | 2.6 | 1.5–4.6 |

[1] Exploring the Iceberg of celiacs in Sweden (ETICS).
[2] The thyroid peroxidase (TPO) cut-off used was 100 U/mL.
[3] Logistic regression was used to estimate odds ratio (OR) with 95% confidence interval (CI).
[4] Row percentages.
[5] Children not diagnosed with celiac disease (CD).

both previously and screening-detected cases, and 22/1 000 in the 1997 cohort [3, 19]. The proportions of children with previously diagnosed celiac disease and those with screening-detected disease were similar in the cohorts. The mean age at diagnosis among the previously diagnosed children was 4.7 years (SD 4.0) and the median was 2.75 years.

*3.2. Thyroid Autoimmunity.* In the celiac disease group, 7.2% (24/335) had elevated titers of TPOAb compared to 2.8% (48/1695) of the referents. Among the previously diagnosed celiac disease cases 7.5% (7/93, OR 2.8, 95% CI 1.2–6.4) was TPOAb positive and among the screening-detected cases 7.0% (17/242, OR 2.6, 95% CI 1.5–4.6) was TPOAb positive (Table 1).

## 4. Discussion

This study demonstrates an increased prevalence of thyroid autoimmunity among 12-year-old children with celiac disease compared to healthy controls. We found the prevalence of thyroid autoimmunity to be almost three times higher than in the age- and sex-matched control group of children without celiac disease. We did not find any difference in the prevalence of thyroid autoantibodies in the group of children with previously diagnosed celiac disease compared to the screening-detected cases. Our previous pilot screening studies, performed on the same birth cohorts, showed that 2.5-year olds have approximately the same prevalence of undiagnosed celiac disease as found in the ETICS study [24]. This supports the theory that not all cases detected through screening are of recent onset and these may constitute a group of children who have had untreated celiac disease since early childhood [24, 25]. The previously diagnosed cases had already been treated for several years with a gluten-free diet. The mean age at diagnosis among the previously diagnosed celiac disease cases was 4.7 years (SD 4.0) and the median age was 2.75 years; they had thus been on a gluten-free diet for approximately 9 years since the screening was performed at 12 years of age. Adherence to a gluten-free diet among children is generally good [26–28]. In our cohort, 83 out of the 93 previously diagnosed cases had normal tTG at the time of the screening as a measure of very good compliance and only 10 out of 93 had slightly raised tTG (range 4.1 to 29.95) above normal. According to our study results, a gluten-free diet does not seem to be protective against the development of thyroid autoimmunity.

The results are in accordance with those of Sategna Guidetti et al. who observed that many celiac patients developed autoimmune disorders despite strict adherence to a gluten-free diet [29]. Viljamaa et al. also investigated the prevalence of autoimmune disease associated with celiac disease among both adults and children. They found that the duration of gluten exposure did not seem to be of crucial importance regarding development of autoimmune diseases. One-third of the patients in their study developed associated autoimmune diseases despite being on a gluten-free diet [16]. In fact, in the latter study the development of autoimmune disease decreased with duration of gluten exposure. One can hypothesize that these patients, who were diagnosed with celiac disease at a later age, might be generally less susceptible to developing autoimmune diseases. This is also supported by Cosnes et al. who showed that a late diagnosis of celiac disease was associated with a decreased risk of autoimmunity [26]. The above-mentioned findings might support a common genetic susceptibility to the autoimmune conditions. It is important to bear in mind that autoimmune diseases develop at different ages; for example, type 1 diabetes mellitus often develops during childhood, while development of autoimmune thyroiditis increases with increasing age and has its peak incidence in the fifth decade of life [30, 31]. It is thus important to analyze the incidence of autoimmune diseases in relation to both age and compliance with a gluten-free diet. Cosnes et al. found that the risk of development of an autoimmune disease in celiac patients was increased in patients with a family history of autoimmune disease when celiac disease was diagnosed early in childhood or adolescence compared to adulthood [26]. The fact that family history was a strong contributing factor to the development of autoimmune disease also favors a linkage disequilibrium between the genes responsible for celiac disease and those responsible for the coexpressed autoimmune disease [32].

Contrary to the abovementioned findings, Ventura et al. showed that patients with celiac disease had a high prevalence of both insulin dependent diabetes mellitus autoantibodies and thyroid-related serum autoantibodies. These autoantibodies were supposed to be gluten-dependent, since they disappeared during treatment with a gluten-free diet [12]. They also observed that the prevalence of autoimmune disorders in children in whom celiac disease was diagnosed before the age of two years, and who were treated with a gluten-free diet, was comparable to that of controls [18]. In our study, the distribution of TPO positivity at 12 years of age among the previously diagnosed celiac disease cases was equal among those diagnosed before 2 years of age and after 2 years of age. It was also equally distributed regardless of the degree of mucosal damage in the entire celiac disease cohort.

Sategna Guidetti et al. hypothesized that gluten ingestion plays a central role in modifying the immunological response early in life [29]. As mentioned above, we could not verify this theory in our study since we did not find any difference in the prevalence of TPOAb among the screening-detected, and thus untreated, celiac disease cases and the previously diagnosed celiac disease cases. However, some of the previously diagnosed cases in our study were diagnosed at a later age than before the age of two. If the hypothesis of Sategna Guidetti et al. is true and this is a crucial age, the opportunity to modify the immunological response might have disappeared after that age.

The present trial was based on a nationwide, contemporary study on celiac disease in 12632 children/almost 13000 children. Yet, it has some limitations that merit consideration. First, celiac disease was defined pathologically as Marsh 1–3c. The inclusion of Marsh 1 in the diagnosis is currently an unsettled issue in the scientific community. We chose to include Marsh 1 in accordance with previous publications [3, 19] and research showing that patients with low-grade inflammation still benefit from a gluten-free diet [33]. Second, albeit the screening study included 12632 children, power nevertheless constitutes a limitation of the current study, as diagnosis of concomitant celiac disease and elevated TPOAb was relatively rare in our cohorts. Thus, the lack of a significant difference in TPOAb between the screening-detected and previously detected CD cases could possibly be due to a lack of power. The third limitation of the present study is that we only analyzed TPO markers as an indicator of autoimmune disease. We did not investigate how many of the children developed clinical autoimmune thyroiditis, defined as TPOAb positivity in combination with goiter and/or hypothyroidism. Although the clinical significance of these antibodies in celiac disease is still unclear, there is probably a higher propensity for thyroid autoimmunity in children with positive TPO markers. In most cases the immune response to the target cells progressively destroys the endocrine gland, and hypofunction is the main clinical manifestation [34]. The presence of TPOAb in serum is an independent risk factor for the development of hypothyroidism in patients with subclinical hypothyroidism [35, 36]. The Whickham study demonstrated that the presence of antithyroid microsomal (TPO is the antigen involved in the "microsomal" response) antibodies, or elevated serum TSH alone, was associated with a significant increased risk of developing hypothyroidism at 20 years of age [36]. A longitudinal followup would, therefore, seem necessary in patients with positive autoimmune thyroid serology but who are currently euthyroid.

## 5. Conclusion

Thus far, we can conclude that having celiac disease as a 12-year old increases the risk of also having thyroid autoimmunity almost threefold compared to healthy children. Our findings do not support a general screening for celiac disease on the basis of trying to protect against thyroid disease through earlier diagnosis of celiac disease and initiation of treatment with a gluten-free diet.

## Abbreviations

tTG: Transglutaminase
EMA: Endomysial antibodies
TPOAb: Thyroid peroxidase antibodies
OR: Odds ratio
SD: Standard deviation
CI: Confidence interval.

## Conflict of Interests

The authors declare no conflict of interests.

## Acknowledgments

The study was funded by the Swedish Research Council (Grants 521-2004-7093 and 521-2007-2953), the Swedish Research Council for Environment, Agricultural Sciences and Spatial Planning (Grants 222-2004-1918 and 222-2007-1394), and the Swedish Council for Working Life and Social Research (Grant 2005-0802). In addition, a minor contribution was made by Skane County Council. The study was part of the European Union-supported Project FP6-2005-FOOD-4B-36383-PREVENTCD. Phadia (Freiburg, Germany) and Eurospital SpA (Trieste, Italy) contributed with analyses of coded serum samples. The authors thank all participating children and their families and all personnel working with the study including research nurses, laboratory personnel, administrative staff, and collaborators within the school health services and pediatric departments. We thank Anna Myleus for carefully reading the paper and for her valuable contributions to its content. The authors also thank Associate Professor Hans Stenlund for his contribution during the planning of the study and interpretation of results. The study was performed in cooperation with the county councils of Västerbotten, Stockholm, Östergötland, Kronoberg, and Skåne. It was undertaken within the Centre for Global Health at Umeå University, with support from FAS, the Swedish Council for Working Life and Social Research.

## References

[1] P. H. Green and C. Cellier, "Medical progress: celiac disease," *New England Journal of Medicine*, vol. 357, no. 17, pp. 1731–1743, 2007.

[2] K. Mustalahti, C. Catassi, A. Reunanen et al., "The prevalence of celiac disease in Europe: results of a centralized, international mass screening project," *Annals of Medicine*, vol. 42, no. 8, pp. 587–595, 2010.

[3] A. Myléus, A. Ivarsson, C. Webb et al., "Celiac disease revealed in 3% of Swedish 12-year-olds born during an epidemic," *Journal of Pediatric Gastroenterology and Nutrition*, vol. 49, no. 2, pp. 170–176, 2009.

[4] P. H. Green and B. Jabri, "Coeliac disease," *The Lancet*, vol. 362, no. 9381, pp. 383–391, 2003.

[5] E. Lionetti and C. Catassi, "New clues in celiac disease epidemiology, pathogenesis, clinical manifestations, and treatment," *International Reviews of Immunology*, vol. 30, no. 4, pp. 219–231, 2011.

[6] S. Zawahir, A. Safta, and A. Fasano, "Pediatric celiac disease," *Current Opinion in Pediatrics*, vol. 21, no. 5, pp. 655–660, 2009.

[7] L. M. Sollid and E. Thorsby, "HLA susceptibility genes in celiac disease: genetic mapping and role in pathogenesis," *Gastroenterology*, vol. 105, no. 3, pp. 910–922, 1993.

[8] F. Bao, P. H. Green, and G. Bhagat, "An update on celiac disease histopathology and the road ahead," *Archives of Pathology & Laboratory Medicine*, vol. 136, no. 7, pp. 735–745, 2012.

[9] L. Greco, R. Romino, I. Coto et al., "The first large population based twin study of coeliac disease," *Gut*, vol. 50, no. 5, pp. 624–628, 2002.

[10] C. E. Counsell, A. Taha, and W. S. J. Ruddell, "Coeliac disease and autoimmune thyroid disease," *Gut*, vol. 35, no. 6, pp. 844–846, 1994.

[11] C. Sategna-Guidetti, M. Bruno, E. Mazza et al., "Autoimmune thyroid diseases and coeliac disease," *European Journal of Gastroenterology and Hepatology*, vol. 10, no. 11, pp. 927–931, 1998.

[12] A. Ventura, E. Neri, C. Ughi, A. Leopaldi, A. Città, and T. Not, "Gluten-dependent diabetes-related and thyroid-related autoantibodies in patients with celiac disease," *Journal of Pediatrics*, vol. 137, no. 2, pp. 263–265, 2000.

[13] D. Larizza, V. Calcaterra, C. De Giacomo et al., "Celiac disease in children with autoimmune thyroid disease," *Journal of Pediatrics*, vol. 139, no. 5, pp. 738–740, 2001.

[14] F. Norstrom, O. Sandstrom, L. Lindholm, and A. Ivarsson, "A gluten-free diet effectively reduces symptoms and health care consumption in a Swedish celiac disease population," *BMC Gastroenterology*, vol. 12, p. 125, 2012.

[15] G. Guariso, S. Conte, F. Presotto et al., "Clinical, subclinical and potential autoimmune diseases in an Italian population of children with coeliac disease," *Alimentary Pharmacology and Therapeutics*, vol. 26, no. 10, pp. 1409–1417, 2007.

[16] M. Viljamaa, K. Kaukinen, H. Huhtala, S. Kyrönpalo, M. Rasmussen, and P. Collin, "Coeliac disease, autoimmune diseases and gluten exposure," *Scandinavian Journal of Gastroenterology*, vol. 40, no. 4, pp. 437–443, 2005.

[17] L. C. Chin, M. K. Jones, and J. G. C. Kingham, "Celiac disease and autoimmune thyroid disease," *Clinical Medicine and Research*, vol. 5, no. 3, pp. 184–192, 2007.

[18] A. Ventura, G. Magazzu, and L. Greco, "Duration of exposure to gluten and risk for autoimmune disorders in patients with celiac disease," *Gastroenterology*, vol. 117, no. 2, pp. 297–303, 1999.

[19] A. Ivarsson, A. Myleus, F. Norstrom et al., "Reduced prevalence of childhood celiac disease: an effect of changes in infant feeding?" *The Journal of Pediatrics*, vol. 131, no. 3, pp. e687–e694, 2013.

[20] C. E. Hogen Esch, A. Rosén, R. Auricchio et al., "The PreventCD Study design: towards new strategies for the prevention of coeliac disease," *European Journal of Gastroenterology and Hepatology*, vol. 22, no. 12, pp. 1424–1430, 2010.

[21] A. Di Sabatino and G. R. Corazza, "Coeliac disease," *The Lancet*, vol. 373, no. 9673, pp. 1480–1493, 2009.

[22] C. Webb, B. Halvarsson, F. Norström et al., "Accuracy in celiac disease diagnostics by controlling the small-bowel biopsy process," *Journal of Pediatric Gastroenterology and Nutrition*, vol. 52, no. 5, pp. 549–553, 2011.

[23] A. Ivarsson, L. Högberg, and L. Stenhammar, "The Swedish childhood coeliac disease working group after 20 years: history and future," *Acta Paediatrica*, vol. 99, no. 9, pp. 1429–1431, 2010.

[24] A. K. Carlsson, I. E. M. Axelsson, S. K. Borulf, A. C. A. Bredberg, and S. Ivarsson, "Serological screening for celiac disease in healthy 2.5-year-old children in Sweden," *Pediatrics*, vol. 107, no. 1, pp. 42–45, 2001.

[25] A. Carlsson, D. Agardh, S. Borulf, E. Grodzinsky, I. Axelsson, and S. Ivarsson, "Prevalence of celiac disease: before and after a national change in feeding recommendations," *Scandinavian Journal of Gastroenterology*, vol. 41, no. 5, pp. 553–558, 2006.

[26] J. Cosnes, C. Cellier, S. Viola et al., "Incidence of autoimmune diseases in celiac disease: protective effect of the gluten-free diet," *Clinical Gastroenterology and Hepatology*, vol. 6, no. 7, pp. 753–758, 2008.

[27] E. J. van Koppen, J. J. Schweizer, C. G. D. S. Csizmadia et al., "Long-term health and quality-of-life consequences of mass screening for childhood celiac disease: a 10-year follow-up study," *Pediatrics*, vol. 123, no. 4, pp. e582–e588, 2009.

[28] E. G. Hopman, S. Le Cessie, B. M. von Blomberg, and M. L. Mearin, "Nutritional management of the gluten-free diet in young people with celiac disease in The Netherlands," *Journal of Pediatric Gastroenterology and Nutrition*, vol. 43, no. 1, pp. 102–108, 2006.

[29] C. Sategna Guidetti, E. Solerio, N. Scaglione, G. Aimo, and G. Mengozzi, "Duration of gluten exposure in adult coeliac disease does not correlate with the risk for autoimmune disorders," *Gut*, vol. 49, no. 4, pp. 502–505, 2001.

[30] A. Green, "The EURODIAB studies on childhood diabetes 1988–1999," *Diabetologia*, vol. 44, supplement 3, pp. B1–B2, 2001.

[31] M. P. Vanderpump and W. M. Tunbridge, "Epidemiology and prevention of clinical and subclinical hypothyroidism," *Thyroid*, vol. 12, no. 10, pp. 839–847, 2002.

[32] A. Fasano, "Systemic autoimmune disorders in celiac disease," *Current Opinion in Gastroenterology*, vol. 22, no. 6, pp. 674–679, 2006.

[33] K. Kurppa, P. Collin, M. Viljamaa et al., "Diagnosing mild enteropathy celiac disease: a randomized, controlled clinical study," *Gastroenterology*, vol. 136, no. 3, pp. 816–823, 2009.

[34] J. R. Baker Jr., "Autoimmune endocrine disease," *Journal of the American Medical Association*, vol. 278, no. 22, pp. 1931–1937, 1997.

[35] G. Huber, J. Staub, C. Meier et al., "Prospective study of the spontaneous course of subclinical hypothyroidism: prognostic value of thyrotropin, thyroid reserve, and thyroid antibodies," *Journal of Clinical Endocrinology and Metabolism*, vol. 87, no. 7, pp. 3221–3226, 2002.

[36] M. P. Vanderpump, W. M. Tunbridge, J. M. French et al., "The incidence of thyroid disorders in the community: a twenty-year follow-up of the Whickham Survey," *Clinical Endocrinology*, vol. 43, no. 1, pp. 55–68, 1995.

17

# Silent Burdens in Disease: Fatigue and Depression in SLE

**R. Fonseca,[1] M. Bernardes,[2] G. Terroso,[2] M. de Sousa,[3] and M. Figueiredo-Braga[1]**

[1] *Department of Clinical Neurosciences and Mental Health, Faculty of Medicine, University of Porto, 4200-319 Porto, Portugal*
[2] *Rheumatology Department, São João Hospital, 4200-319 Porto, Portugal*
[3] *IBMC/GABBA, University of Porto, 4150-180 Porto, Portugal*

Correspondence should be addressed to M. Figueiredo-Braga; mmfb@med.up.pt

Academic Editor: Juan-Manuel Anaya

At a time when health is being recognized as more than just avoiding death, age and comorbidity are becoming increasingly important aspects of chronic disease. Systemic Lupus Erythematous (SLE) is probably one of the best paradigms of modern chronic disease, sitting at the crossroads of numerous somatic health problems, immune activation, depression, pain, and fatigue. One hundred forty-eight female participants were enrolled in the present study: 50 diagnosed with SLE, 45 with major depressive disorder (MDD), and 53 age-matched controls. Statistically significant lower scores in quality-of-life dimensions related to physical impairment were found in SLE. Patients with MDD presented significant levels of pain, reduced physical summary component (PSC), and general health scores different from healthy controls. Fatigue was reported in 90% of women with SLE and 77.8% of the MDD patients in contrast with 39.6% in the control group. Significant correlations were seen among fatigue severity, age, and educational level in SLE. From our own previous work and more recent work on the association of immune activation and depression, unexplained fatigue in SLE may signify an early sign of immune activation flare-up. The search for cytokine markers should perhaps be extended to fatigue in SLE.

## 1. Introduction

The more recent analysis of the Global Burden of Disease has identified mental disorders and musculoskeletal diseases as some of the major contributors to Years Lived in Disability (YLD) [1]. One consequence of this study that has particularly interested us has led to the question of how such global findings can be reflected in the care of the individual patient and the understanding of the complexity of comorbidity in chronic disease. Although fatigue, anxiety, and depression crosstalk with the clinical presentation and progression of Systemic Lupus Erythematosus (SLE), clinicians generally pay more attention to the somatic health problems posed by illness [2]. This can be explained in part by present-day medical education's emphasis on the biological, genomic, and statistically significant dimensions of disease.

Studies of SLE patients have shown, however, the impact of individual elements such as anxiety and depression on the course of disease as experienced by individual patients and how, collectively, such elements have an impact on health care costs [3].

SLE is also a particularly good example of how progress in the dissection of genes and molecules involved in autoimmunity continues to be disappointingly reflected in helping the individual patient [4]. In addition, SLE as a chronic inflammatory autoimmune disease with multisystem involvement, secondary to the production of autoantibodies and to the production of Type 1 interferon by innate immune cells [5, 6], represents a singularly revealing model of the crossroads that individual clinicians or clinical teams must face to deal adequately with an individual patient.

Presently, clinical evaluation of disease relies mostly upon objective criteria, contemplating clinical features whose significance may nevertheless escape the patient. Particular symptoms such as pain and fatigue can, on the contrary, be experienced and reported exclusively by the patient, escaping regular clinical assessment. We would like to identify such individual burdens as silent burdens of disease.

TABLE 1: Sociodemographic characterization.

| | Total $n = 148$ | SLE (1) $n = 50$ | Depression (2) $n = 45$ | Controls (3) $n = 53$ | $P$ | Post hoc analysis |
|---|---|---|---|---|---|---|
| Age (years)[a] | 44.5 (11.6) | 44.1 (10.1) | 41.7 (13.7) | 47.2 (11.8) | 0.108[c] | |
| Education (years)[a] | 10.7 (4.8) | 9.1 (3.9) | 13.0 (4.2) | 10.9 (5.4) | 0.001[c] | 2 > 1, 3 |
| Marital status[b] | | | | | | |
| Single | 26 (17.6) | 8 (16.0) | 10 (22.2) | 8 (15.1) | | |
| Married | 101 (68.2) | 38 (76.0) | 25 (55.6) | 38 (71.7) | | |
| Divorced | 15 (10.1) | 2 (4.0) | 9 (20.0) | 4 (7.5) | 0.254[d] | |
| Widow | 4 (2.7) | 1 (2.0) | 1 (2.2) | 2 (3.6) | | |
| Common-law marriage | 2 (1.4) | 1 (2.0) | 0 (0.0) | 1 (1.9) | | |
| Employment status[b] | | | | | | |
| Active | 86 (58.1) | 15 (30.0) | 27 (60.0) | 44 (83.0) | 0.000[d] | |
| Nonactive | 62 (41.9) | 35 (70.0) | 18 (40.0) | 9 (17.0) | | |

[a]Mean (standard deviation), [b]$n$ (%), [c]ANOVA, [d]Chi-square test.

Eventually, the disrupted immunological tolerance seen in SLE patients results in immune complex deposition that ends in permanent damage, most frequently affecting the musculoskeletal, cutaneous, renal, central nervous, and gastrointestinal systems [7]. The diversity of the resulting clinical manifestations led to the establishment of consensual, valuable, sensitive, and specific diagnostic criteria: the American College of Rheumatology (ACR) Criteria for Classification of Systemic Lupus Erythematosus. Although not formally contemplated in these criteria, fatigue is the most common symptom in SLE, affecting 67% to 90% of the patients, even in mild disease presentations [8–10]. Patients often describe their fatigue as debilitating, causing a severe impact on personal, family, and social functioning [10]. Resulting from a complex interplay of biological, behavioral, and psychological factors, fatigue appears to have a privileged association with depressive symptoms, independently of genetic background [11]. Indeed, fatigue cannot be seen as a purely physical sign, as it is also a common symptom in depressive disorder [12].

Anxiety and depression are highly prevalent among patients with lupus, thought to represent central nervous system involvement [13] or immune dysfunction manifestation [14, 15], or denoting the emotional burden of the disease [16, 17]. Recently, a link has been established among neurotransmitter dysfunction, immune activation (lymphocyte abnormalities and cytokine expression), and major depression [18, 19]. In this paper, we consider fatigue and depression as examples of silent burdens of disease, in a cross-sectional study of three groups of participants: patients with SLE, patients with major depressive disorder, and age- and sex-matched controls.

The principal objective of the work was twofold: to highlight the importance of single patient derived symptoms over the course of the disease and to stress the importance of SLE as a modern model chronic disease as important as cancer, if not more so. This importance is derived from the multiple effects resulting from the challenge of crosstalk between the immunological system and other systems, in the absence of infection.

## 2. Study Participants and Methods

One hundred forty-eight female participants were enrolled in the present study, 50 of whom were patients diagnosed with SLE, recruited from the rheumatology outpatient clinic of the São João Hospital, EPE. All SLE patients fulfilled the ACR diagnostic criteria. Only adult patients (>18 years old) without diagnosed psychiatric comorbidities were selected. All patients attended routine visits at the hospital and completed regular clinic and laboratorial assessments.

Patients with lupus were compared to one group of 53 healthy age-matched subjects and a group of 45 patients with major depressive disorder (MDD), followed by one of the authors (mmfb) in her private psychiatric clinic. Psychiatric patients were diagnosed by a psychiatrist according to the Diagnostic and Statistical Manual of Mental Disorders (DSM-IV-TR) [20]. The study was submitted and approved by the Ethical Committee of the São João Hospital (EPE). Participants received oral and written information about the study's goals, methods, expected benefits, and discomfort, after which they gave their oral and written informed consent. The confidentiality and privacy of the collected data were guaranteed during the data collection and analysis stages according to the Declaration of Helsinki.

The sociodemographic characterization of the populations studied is shown in Table 1.

## 3. Data Collection

Following a cross-sectional approach, psychosocial data were collected between September 2012 and June 2013. A first contact established the willingness of the patients to participate. After a first verbal consent was obtained, written informed consent was mailed and retrieved from all participants before the study began. Recruited patients and controls were subsequently interviewed by phone by a trained interviewer (RF). The literature corroborates phone interviews as valid and precise tools for psychological data collection [21–25].

Participants' sociodemographic data included age, educational level, employment status (active/nonactive), and marital status. Laboratorial and SLE standardized clinical evaluation were obtained exclusively in the SLE patients through the clinical records.

## 4. Instruments

*4.1. Psychosocial Evaluation.* Psychological variables were obtained through a battery test: the Fatigue Severity Scale (FSS), the Hospital Anxiety and Depression Scale (HADS), the Pittsburgh Sleep Quality Index (PSQI), and the Short Form-36 Health Survey (SF-36v2).

Self-reported fatigue was evaluated through the short version of the FSS [26]. This unidimensional nine-item Likert scale was designed to assess fatigue in chronic medical and rheumatologic conditions and is recommended as the instrument of choice for research purposes in studies involving patients diagnosed with SLE [27]. The Portuguese version of the FSS used in the present work has been validated for SLE patients [28].

The FSS demonstrates good internal consistency (Cronbach's $\alpha = 0.89$ in SLE patients), test-retest reliability (0.84), and construct and discriminative validity and is sensitive to change. Each question is scored from 1 to 7, and a final score is obtained from the mean of all scored items. Higher scores reveal increasing severity of fatigue. Presence of clinical levels of fatigue was defined by a FSS score >3, as proposed by Krupp and collaborators [26]. The use of FSS assessment in an SLE population by telephone interview has been established [29].

The Hospital Anxiety and Depression Scale (HADS) [30] is used to assess depressive and anxiety symptoms. This questionnaire contains 14 items, scored from 0 to 3, to achieve a total of 0 to 21. It is divided into two sets of seven questions aiming to detect, respectively, depressive and anxiety states. Scores exceeding 8 points indicate possible mood disorder, and 10 points delimit pathological situations. This instrument does not contain items focused in physical indicators of psychological distress or somatic complaints, which improves its sensitivity to anxiety and depression in physically ill individuals. Factor analysis confirmed the bidimensionality of the scale and the correlation between the anxiety and depression subscales. Both subscales showed suitable internal consistency (Mean Cronbach's alpha = 0.83 for HADS-A and 0.82 for HADS-D) [31]. Telephone-administered mode has been described for the HADS, maintaining similar psychometric properties [32].

Participants were also screened for sleep quality through the Pittsburgh Sleep Quality Index (PSQI). A weighted global score of 0 to 21, reflecting a four-week time interval, is yielded from the seven components subjectively evaluated: sleep latency, sleep disturbances, sleep duration, sleep quality, sleep efficiency, use of sleep medications, and daytime dysfunction. This instrument has good psychometric properties, with high homogeneity, reliability (Cronbach's alpha = 0.83), and validity [33, 34]. Poor sleepers are identified by a PSQI score >5 [33]. When used in a telephone interview, the PSQI presented an adequate internal consistency and proved to be a reliable mode for sleep quality assessment [35, 36].

The Short-Form 36 Health Survey Version 2.0 (SF-36v2) was elected to assess health-related quality of life (HRQoL) [37]. This scale comprises 36 self-rated questions, reproducing eight domains: physical functioning (PF), role limitations due to physical problems (RP), bodily pain (BP), general health (GH), vitality (VT), social functioning (SF), role limitations due to emotional problems (RE), and mental health (MH). These domains can be individually evaluated or summarized in the physical (PSC) and mental (MSC) summary components. A gradual score ranging from 0 to 100 in each area reflects enhanced quality of life. The SF-36 can be either self-administered or administered by a trained interviewer, either in person or by telephone [38, 39]. The SF-36-v2 is the most widely used questionnaire to assess quality-of-life-related outcomes in SLE patients, providing the additional possibility of comparing the obtained results with those of other healthy or patient populations [40].The Cronbach's alpha for studies enrolling SLE patients was recently computed from the available literature (Cronbach's $\alpha = 0.71$–$0.95$) [41].

*4.2. Clinical SLE Indexes.* Disease activity was estimated with the Systemic Lupus Erythematosus Disease Activity Index (SLEDAI) [42]. This physician-rated instrument reports 16 clinical and eight laboratorial descriptors appraised during the previous 10 or 30 days. The SLEDAI score retrieved during the last (most recent) patient visit was used. Patients were grouped into four categories, according to SLEDAI total score, representing increasing activity of the disease: no activity (0), mild activity (1–5), moderate activity (6–10), high activity (11–19), and very high activity (20) [43]. A score of 6 or more was considered as clinically active disease.

The Systemic Lupus International Collaborating Clinics/American College of Rheumatology (SLICC/ACR) damage index [44] was used to compile irreversible impairment in all SLE patients. This index reflects accumulated damage continuously present in a six-month period and targets 12 distinct organs/systems.

*4.3. Laboratory Evaluation.* Laboratorial evaluation included in the patient's clinical records was used to determine immune activation, inflammatory status, antibody profile, and vitamin D quantifications. Immune activation was determined by autoantibodies detection: antidouble stranded DNA, nucleosome, Smith, Sjogren Syndrome A, Sjogren Syndrome B, histones, cardiolipin (IgG and IgM isotypes), $\beta 2$-glycoprotein I (IgG and IgM isotypes), antiribonucleoproteins, and Ribosomal P substance. The C-Reactive Protein (CRP), inactive C1, C1q, C3c, C4, and CH50 complement fractions and Erythrocyte Sedimentation Rate (ESR) determinations were also considered. Blood and serological measurements were performed according to standardized methods in the hospital's laboratory, and standardized cutoff levels were established. Only two laboratory tests correlate with fatigue: CH50 and anti-ds-DNA determinations (data not shown).

Table 2: Fatigue assessment.

| | Total $n = 148$ | SLE (1) $n = 50$ | Depression (2) $n = 45$ | Controls (3) $n = 53$ | $P$ | Post hoc analysis |
|---|---|---|---|---|---|---|
| FSS global score[a,b] | 4.3 (1.7)<br>1.0–7.0 | 5.2 (1.3)<br>1.6–7.0 | 4.5 (1.4)<br>1.7–7.0 | 3.2 (1.8)<br>1.0–10.4 | 0.000[d] | 2, 1 > 3 |
| Fatigue severity level[c] | | | | | | |
| Nonclinical | 36 (24.3) | 5 (10.0) | 6 (13.3) | 25 (47.2) | | |
| Clinical | 101 (68.2) | 45 (90.0) | 35 (77.8) | 21 (39.6) | 0.000[e] | |
| Missing | 11 (7.4) | | 4 (8.9) | 7 (13.2) | | |

[a]Mean (standard deviation); [b]minimum–maximum; [c]$n$ (%); [d]ANOVA; [e]Chi-square test.

Table 3: Correlations (Pearson) between fatigue and psychosocial and anthropometric characteristics, quality of life, and sleep quality.

| | SLE (1) $n = 50$ | Depression (2) $n = 45$ | Controls (3) $n = 53$ |
|---|---|---|---|
| Age (years) | 0.489** | −0.061 | 0.243 |
| Education (years) | −0.476** | −0.043 | −0.294 |
| HADS | | | |
| Anxiety | 0.542** | 0.202 | 0.397** |
| Depression | 0.576** | 0.402* | 0.410** |
| SF-36 | | | |
| PSC | −0.717** | −0.351* | −0.466** |
| Physical functioning | −0.648** | −0.103 | −0.318* |
| Role limitations due to physical health problems | −0.699** | −0.393* | −0.302* |
| Social functioning | −0.354* | −0.389* | −0.226 |
| Mental health | −0.464** | −0.416** | −0.435** |
| Role limitations due to emotional problems | −0.315* | −0.249 | −0.274 |
| Vitality | −0.677** | −0.323* | −0.660** |
| Bodily pain | −0.563** | −0.450** | −0.287 |
| General health | −0.617** | −0.418** | −0.580** |
| PSQI global score | 0.401** | 0.334* | 0.425** |
| BMI (kg/m$^2$) | 0.135 | −0.82 | −0.301* |

*$P < 0.05$, **$P < 0.01$; PSC: Physical summary component; BMI: body mass index.

*4.4. Statistical Analysis.* Statistical analysis was performed using the Statistical Package for Social Science 18.0 (SPSS).

A descriptive analysis of the obtained results was performed, and the data were expressed as frequencies (%), minimums, maximums, means, and standard deviations.

Analysis of variance (ANOVA) was used to investigate differences between groups, and Pearson Chi-square test was conducted for categorical variables. Post-hoc Tukey test was performed to provide a stratified comparison between groups, when necessary. For correlation analysis, the Spearman's coefficient was computed. Confidence intervals of 95% and a significance level of 0.05 were adopted.

## 5. Results

*5.1. Fatigue Assessment: Significant Associations with Age, Psychological Suffering, and Educational Level (Tables 1, 2, and 3).* The sociodemographic characterization of the three groups showed that all participants presented similar age, with a mean value of 44.5 years and similar marital status. Regarding employment status and education, however, lower scores were observed in the SLE group, with statistical significance when compared to depressed and control women (Table 1).

Fatigue was not an exclusive burden of SLE. It was reported in 90% of women with SLE and 77.8% of the female MDD patients, in contrast with 39.6% in the control group.

The global score of FSS revealed similar fatigue severity in SLE and MDD patients ($5.2 \pm 1.3$ and $4.5 \pm 1.4$, resp.), which is significantly higher than the scores found in the control group ($3.2 \pm 1.8$, $P = 0.0001$) (Table 2).

The result of the search for significant correlations between fatigue and markers of psychological suffering is detailed as a correlational analysis in Table 3.

Significant correlations were detected between fatigue severity, age, and education exclusively in patients with SLE. Higher fatigue was associated with older age, possibly reflecting the cumulative physical impairment of disease and aging.

TABLE 4: Anthropometric characterization, health-related behaviors, and sleep quality.

| | Total $n = 148$ | SLE (1) $n = 50$ | Depression (2) $n = 45$ | Controls (3) $n = 53$ | $P$ | Post hoc analysis |
|---|---|---|---|---|---|---|
| BMI ($kg/m^2$)[a] | 24.9 (5.5) | 24.8 (4.1) | 25.7 (7.8) | 24.3 (4.0) | 0.466[c] | |
| BMI categories[b] | | | | | | |
| Underweight | 7 (4.7) | 1 (2.0) | 3 (6.7) | 3 (5.7) | | |
| Normal range | 85 ( 57.4) | 31 (62.0) | 24 (53.3) | 30 (56.6) | | |
| Preobesity | 32 (21.6) | 13 (26.0) | 8 (17.8) | 11 (20.8) | 0.701[d] | |
| Obesity | 18 (12.2) | 5 (10.0) | 8 (17.8) | 5 (9.4) | | |
| Missing | 6 (4.1) | 0 (0.0) | 2 (4.4) | 4 (7.5) | | |
| Smoking habits[b] | | | | | | |
| Smokers | 34 (23.0) | 10 (20.0) | 18 (40.0) | 6 (11.3) | 0.003[d] | |
| Nonsmokers | 114 (77.0) | 40 (80.0) | 27 (60.0) | 47 (88.7) | | |
| Alcohol consumption[b] | | | | | | |
| Yes | 13 (8.8) | 3 (6.0) | 2 (4.4) | 8 (15.1) | 0.124[d] | |
| No | 135 (91.2) | 47 (94.0) | 43 (95.6) | 45 (84.9) | | |
| Physical activity[b] | | | | | | |
| Yes | 63 (42.6) | 18 (36.0) | 18 (40.0) | 27 (50.9) | 0.283[d] | |
| No | 85 (57.4) | 32 (64.0) | 27 (60.0) | 26 (49.1) | | |
| Sleep | | | | | | |
| PSQI global score[a] | 10.3 (3.8) | 10.9 (4.0) | 11.3 (3.7) | 9.0 (3.4) | 0.007[c] | 2, 1 > 3 |
| Quality of sleep[b] | | | | | | |
| Good sleepers | 16 (10.8) | 3 (6.0) | 3 (6.7) | 10 (18.9) | | |
| Poor sleepers | 126 (85.1) | 46 (92.0) | 39 (86.7) | 41 (77.4) | 0.140[d] | |
| Missing | 6 (4.1) | 1 (2.0) | 3 (6.7) | 2 (3.8) | | |

[a]Mean (standard deviation), [b]$n$ (%), [c]ANOVA, [d]Chi-square test; BMI: body mass index.

Lower education was seen to be related to higher fatigue scores.

Significant correlations between anxiety and fatigue were detected in SLE and control population ($r = 0.542$ and $r = 0.397$, resp.).

Mental health scores, vitality, and depressive symptoms presented significant associations with fatigue severity, regardless of participant group (Table 3).

In the SLE group of women, education correlated significantly with anxiety (HADS-A: $r = 0.313$, $P = 0.027$), depressive symptoms (HADS D $r = 0.452$, $P = 0.001$), and bodily pain ($r = 0.527$, $P < 0.005$).

*5.2. Weight, Sleep, and Physical Activity (Table 4).* In order to clarify classically reported associations among fatigue, excessive weight, sleep abnormalities, and physical activity, participants were subjected to anthropometric, sleep quality, and health-related behavior evaluations.

In our study, disturbed sleep quality affected the three groups, although higher global PSQI scores ($P = 0.007$), representing poorer sleep quality, were detected in SLE and MDD patients.

The presence of obesity and preobesity was equally distributed across the studied sample, and BMI scores were similar in all the groups. Evaluation of health-related behaviors revealed that physical activity and alcohol consumption were similar in the three groups. Smoking habits, on the contrary, were more prevalent in psychiatric patients (Table 4).

*5.3. Fatigue and Quality-of-Life Dimensions: Physical Summary Components, Pain, and General Health (Table 5).* Fatigue has been extensively associated with poorer health-related quality of life in SLE patients. Accordingly, we detected statistically significant lower scores in quality-of-life dimensions related to physical impairment in SLE patients; results in physical summary components, bodily pain and general health were statistically significantly different in the SLE group when compared to the MDD group and control subjects. MDD patients, however, presented significant levels of pain, reduced PSC, and general health scores different from healthy controls.

Other dimensions expressed in mental summary components (social functioning, mental health, and role limitations due to emotional problems), while showing significant impairment in SLE patients, presented lower scores in the MDD group when compared to the control population (Table 5).

*5.4. Fatigue, Anxiety, and Depression (Table 6).* Loss of energy or exhaustion can characterize fatigue and also be regarded as a depressive symptom. In the present study, measures of depression were obtained using HADS depression subscale in the three groups of participants, and they revealed

Table 5: Health-related quality of life.

| | Total $n = 148$ | SLE (1) $n = 50$ | Depression (2) $n = 45$ | Controls (3) $n = 53$ | $P$ | Post hoc analysis |
|---|---|---|---|---|---|---|
| SF-36 | | | | | | |
| Physical functioning[a] | 71.8 (26.7) | 55.8 (30.5) | 75.9 (22.2) | 84.3 (16.7) | 0.000[b] | 1 < 2, 3 |
| Role limitations due to physical health problems[a] | 62.5 (30.8) | 44.5 (32.6) | 59.8 (23.5) | 81.3 (22.4) | 0.000[b] | 1 < 2 < 3 |
| Social functioning[a] | 63.0 (28.6) | 61.5 (31.0) | 46.6 (22.5) | 78.1 (22.5) | 0.000[b] | 2 < 1 < 3 |
| Mental health[a] | 56.8 (22.1) | 55.8 (20.2) | 43.0 (17.5) | 69.3 (20.2) | 0.000[b] | 2 < 1 < 3 |
| Role limitations due to emotional problems[a] | 70.1 (27.9) | 68.7 (29.0) | 52.4 (22.9) | 86.5 (20.5) | 0.000[b] | 2 < 1 < 3 |
| Vitality[a] | 45.6 (22.9) | 34.9 (23.1) | 39.4 (16.8) | 70.0 (18.8) | 0.000[b] | 1, 2 < 3 |
| Bodily pain[a] | 60.7 (31.6) | 43.7 (34.6) | 64.5 (26.1) | 73.7 (25.5) | 0.000[b] | 1 < 2, 3 |
| General health[a] | 49.8 (23.7) | 31.3 (18.5) | 56.2 (21.2) | 61.9 (19.2) | 0.000[b] | 1 < 2, 3 |
| PSC[a] | 0.0 (1.0) | −0.8 (0.9) | 0.4 (0.7) | 0.5 (0.6) | 0.000[b] | 1 < 2, 3 |
| MSC[a] | 0.0 (1.0) | 0.1 (0.9) | −0.8 (0.8) | 0.6 (0.8) | 0.000[b] | 2 < 3 < 1 |

[a]Mean (standard deviation); [b]ANOVA; PSC: physical summary component; MSC: mental summary component.

Table 6: Depression and anxiety symptoms.

| | Total $n = 148$ | SLE (1) $n = 50$ | Depression (2) $n = 45$ | Controls (3) $n = 53$ | $P$ | Post hoc analysis |
|---|---|---|---|---|---|---|
| HADS-D[a] | 6.4 (4.5) | 6.7 (5.0) | 8.4 (4.0) | 4.5 (3.5) | 0.000[b] | 2, 1 > 3 |
| HADS-A[a] | 8.8 (4.6) | 8.5 (4.8) | 11.4 (3.7) | 6.8 (4.1) | 0.000[b] | 2 > 1, 3 |

[a]Mean (standard deviation); [b]ANOVA.

Table 7: Correlation (Pearson) between fatigue and disease-related markers in SLE patients.

| | FSS |
|---|---|
| SLEDAI | –100 |
| SLICC | 0.043 |

the occurrence of similar depressive symptoms in SLE patients and MDD patients (6.7 ± 5.0 and 8.4 ± 4.0, resp.), which are significantly higher than in the normal population. Anxiety presented higher scores in MDD patients (11.4±3.7), which are statistically significantly different from the SLE and control groups.

*5.5. Lack of Correlations between Clinical SLE Evaluation and Severity of Fatigue (Table 7).* Clinical indexes used to assess disease activity and damage in SLE patients did not present significant associations with fatigue severity, failing to translate subjective patients' complaints into clinical standardized evaluation.

## 6. Discussion

The spectacular progress in our understanding of the molecular and genetic basis of disease is transforming clinical practice and the nature of patient-physician interaction. Indeed, distracted by the panoply of biological markers at his/her disposal, the clinician may miss subjective symptoms of relevance to the development of disease. Fatigue, anxiety, and depression fall in the category of subjective symptoms that may escape the attention of clinicians *and* patients. Because of their impact in the course of a chronic disease such as SLE, such symptoms will become of increasing clinical and social value as the concept of health itself changes. As emphasized by others, "health is about more than avoiding death" [1].

As shown by the results of the present study, some correlations of fatigue, for example, with sleep quality were common to all groups examined, namely, SLE, MDD, and the control group. A correlation of fatigue with anxiety was also seen within the control group.

The presence of obesity and BMI scores was similar in all groups just as alcohol consumption and physical activity. Smoking habits were more prevalent in the psychiatric group.

We would like to highlight two observations made exclusively in SLE: the correlation with age and education and the correlation with depression (not exclusively seen in SLE).

*6.1. Fatigue and Depression.* In a recent analysis of fatigue in monozygotic and dizygotic twins, chronic fatigue and psychological distress were strongly associated without evidence of genetic covariation, implying, according to the authors, that the "association is environmental" [11]. In an earlier large analysis of a World Health Organization longitudinal study of fatigue and depression, Skapinakis et al. concluded that unexplained fatigue and depression might act as independent factors of each other [45].

However, Palagini et al., in a review based on the search of SLE and depression as key-words in several major databases, concluded that to date, the relationship between depression and SLE disease activity appears controversial, stressing the need for identification of SLE-specific biomarkers of depression. Methodological limitations are present in the available literature, and the standardization of methodologies should be considered a high priority in SLE research [46].

In the present cross-sectional study, we confirmed the existence of a link between fatigue and depression in the patients studied. From our own previous work [14] and more recent work on the association of immune activation and depression, unexplained fatigue may signify an early alert signal of a flare-up of immune activation [18, 19], and the search for cytokine markers in SLE [47] should perhaps be extended to fatigue in SLE.

*6.2. Fatigue and Education Level.* Comparison of educational levels can be done only between the SLE and control groups. The link between education level and fatigue strengthens the point made by others about the importance of the role of health professionals, including nurses, in explaining the disease to patients [48]. Patients with lower education levels challenge clinicians and other health professionals' ability to gather and share important information. Reduced educational achievement may affect a patient's ability to understand, and, in addition, to seek appropriate clarification of doubts regarding the disease, the treatment, or its expected outcomes [49]. Lack of knowledge can comprehensibly add more anxiety and suffering to the difficulty of living with a disease with uncertain evolution and unpredictable flares.

## 7. Conclusion

Giving the attention that fatigue and depression may deserve as silent burdens of disease in SLE, we may be preventing a deleterious progression of a disease and, thus, diminishing the costs recently estimated in Sweden, where a total of 339 patients with the mean age of 55 years were analyzed. The mean Health Related Quality of Life (HRQoL) measured through the five-item EQ-5D instrument was 0.64, and total costs were estimated at €22,594 (direct costs €7,818; indirect costs €14,776). Disease activity, fatigue, and corticosteroid doses had a statistically significant impact on costs and HRQoL. This study demonstrates that Swedish patients with SLE have low HRQoL and incur high societal costs that are both associated with and most likely driven by disease activity, fatigue, and corticosteroid use [3].

The objective measure of costs has, like molecular and genetic progress, become a carefully "listened to" burden of health care and chronic disease.

We wish to conclude by returning to our starting reference to the Global Burden of Disease study, referencing one of their interpretations: *"Prevalences of the most common causes of YLDs such as mental and behavioural disorders and musculoskeletal disorders have not decreased. Health systems will need to address the needs of the rising numbers of individuals with a range of disorders that largely cause disability but not mortality"*—such as SLE [1].

The health system will work well proportionally to the attention and time clinicians can give to one patient. We hope this study of SLE as a model of all modern chronic diseases, with all its limitations as a cross-sectional study and its small numbers, will nevertheless help clinicians and patients to become aware of the importance of the weight of their silent burden in the global burden of modern disease, where *"health is about more than avoiding death"* [1].

Identifying silent burdens in SLE is essential at all times to the care and follow-up of disease progression.

## Conflict of Interests

The authors declare that there is no conflict of interests regarding the publication of this paper.

## References

[1] T. Vos, A. D. Flaxman, M. Naghavi et al., "Years lived with disability (YLDs) for 1160 sequelae of 289 diseases and injuries 1990–2010: a systematic analysis for the Global Burden of Disease Study 2010," *The Lancet*, vol. 380, no. 9859, pp. 2163–2196, 2012.

[2] M. M. Gerrits, H. W. van Marwijk, P. van Oppen, H. van der Horst, and B. W. Penninx, "The role of somatic health problems in the recognition of depressive and anxiety disorders by general practitioners," *Journal of Affective Disorders*, vol. 151, no. 3, pp. 1025–1032, 2013.

[3] C. Bexelius, K. Wachtmeister, P. Skare, L. Jonsson, and R. Vollenhoven, "Drivers of cost and health-related quality of life in patients with systemic lupus erythematosus (SLE): a Swedish nationwide study based on patient reports," *Lupus*, vol. 22, no. 8, pp. 793–801, 2013.

[4] E. A. Frangou, G. K. Bertsias, and D. T. Boumpas, "Gene expression and regulation in systemic lupus erythematosus," *European Journal of Clinical Investigation*, vol. 43, no. 10, pp. 1084–1096, 2013.

[5] M. Wahren-Herlenius and T. Dorner, "Immunopathogenic mechanisms of systemic autoimmune disease," *The Lancet*, vol. 382, no. 9894, pp. 819–831, 2013.

[6] E. S. Kellner, P. Y. Lee, Y. Li et al., "Endogenous type-I interferon activity is not associated with depression or fatigue in systemic lupus erythematosus," *Journal of Neuroimmunology*, vol. 223, no. 1-2, pp. 13–19, 2010.

[7] R. Cervera, M. A. Khamashta, J. Font et al., "Systemic lupus erythematosus: clinical and immunologic patterns of disease expression in a cohort of 1,000 patients. The European Working Party on Systemic Lupus Erythematosus," *Medicine*, vol. 72, no. 2, pp. 113–124, 1993.

[8] S. Cleanthous, M. Tyagi, D. A. Isenberg, and S. P. Newman, "What do we know about self-reported fatigue in systemic lupus erythematosus?" *Lupus*, vol. 21, no. 5, pp. 465–476, 2012.

[9] C. M. Tench, I. McCurdie, P. D. White, and D. P. D'Cruz, "The prevalence and associations of fatigue in systemic lupus erythematosus," *Rheumatology*, vol. 39, no. 11, pp. 1249–1254, 2000.

[10] C. Gordon, D. Isenberg, K. Lerstrom et al., "The substantial burden of systemic lupus erythematosus on the productivity and careers of patients: a European patient-driven online survey," *Rheumatology*, 2013.

[11] P. Roy-Byrne, N. Afari, S. Ashton, M. Fischer, J. Goldberg, and D. Buchwald, "Chronic fatigue and anxiety/depression: a twin study," *British Journal of Psychiatry*, vol. 180, no. 1, pp. 29–34, 2002.

[12] L. M. Arnold, "Understanding fatigue in major depressive disorder and other medical disorders," *Psychosomatics*, vol. 49, no. 3, pp. 185–190, 2008.

[13] "ACR Ad Hoc Committee on Neuropsychiatric Lupus Nomenclature, The American College of Rheumatology nomenclature and case definitions for neuropsychiatric lupus syndromes," *Arthritis and Rheumatism*, vol. 42, no. 4, pp. 599–608, 1999.

[14] M. Figueiredo-Braga, F. Mota-Garcia, J.-E. O'Connor et al., "Cytokines and Anxiety in Systemic Lupus Erythematosus (SLE) patients not receiving antidepressant medication: a little-explored frontier and some of its brief history," *Annals of the New York Academy of Sciences*, vol. 1173, pp. 286–291, 2009.

[15] M. Figueiredo-Braga, *Depression and Immunity: Lessons From a Study of Patients with Systemic Lupus Erythematosus*, University of Porto, Porto, Portugal, 2009.

[16] F. G. Nery, E. F. Borba, V. S. T. Viana et al., "Prevalence of depressive and anxiety disorders in systemic lupus erythematosus and their association with anti-ribosomal P antibodies," *Progress in Neuro-Psychopharmacology and Biological Psychiatry*, vol. 32, no. 3, pp. 695–700, 2008.

[17] E. A. Bachen, M. A. Chesney, and L. A. Criswell, "Prevalence of mood and anxiety disorders in women with systemic lupus erythematosus," *Arthritis Care and Research*, vol. 61, no. 6, pp. 822–829, 2009.

[18] R. Dantzer, "Cytokine, sickness behavior, and depression," *Neurologic Clinics*, vol. 24, no. 3, pp. 441–460, 2006.

[19] M. Maes, M. Berk, L. Goehler et al., "Depression and sickness behavior are Janus-faced responses to shared inflammatory pathways," *BMC Medicine*, vol. 10, no. 1, article 66, 2012.

[20] American Psychiatric Association, *Diagnostic and Statistical Manual of Mental Disorders: DSM-IV-TR*, American Psychiatric Pub, 2000.

[21] P. Carrete, F. Augustovski, N. Gimpel et al., "Validation of a telephone-administered Geriatric Depression Scale in a hispanic elderly population," *Journal of General Internal Medicine*, vol. 16, no. 7, pp. 446–450, 2001.

[22] L. S. Cook, J. L. White, G. C. E. Stuart, and A. M. Magliocco, "The reliability of telephone interviews compared with in-person interviews using memory aids," *Annals of Epidemiology*, vol. 13, no. 7, pp. 495–501, 2003.

[23] J. Siemiatycki, "A comparison of mail, telephone, and home interview strategies for household health surveys," *American Journal of Public Health*, vol. 69, no. 3, pp. 238–245, 1979.

[24] P. Rohde, P. M. Lewinsohn, and J. R. Seeley, "Comparability of telephone and face-to-face interviews in assessing axis I and II disorders," *American Journal of Psychiatry*, vol. 154, no. 11, pp. 1593–1598, 1997.

[25] B. B. Cohen and D. C. Vinson, "Retrospective self-report of alcohol consumption: test-retest reliability by telephone," *Alcoholism*, vol. 19, no. 5, pp. 1156–1161, 1995.

[26] L. B. Krupp, N. G. LaRocca, J. Muir-Nash, and A. D. Steinberg, "The fatigue severity scale. Application to patients with multiple sclerosis and systemic lupus erythematosus," *Archives of Neurology*, vol. 46, no. 10, pp. 1121–1123, 1989.

[27] "Ad Hoc Committee on Systemic Lupus Erythematosus Response Criteria for Fatigue, Measurement of fatigue in systemic lupus erythematosus: a systematic review," *Arthritis Care & Research*, vol. 57, no. 8, pp. 1348–1357, 2007.

[28] M. G. Pereira and S. Duarte, "Fadiga intensa em doentes com lúpus eritematoso sistémico: estudo das características psicométricas da escala da intensidade da fadiga," *Psicologia, Saúde&Doenças*, vol. 11, no. 1, pp. 121–136, 2010.

[29] J. S. Austin, R. S. Maisiak, D. M. Macrina, and L. W. Heck, "Health outcome improvements in patients with systemic lupus erythematosus using two telephone counseling interventions," *Arthritis Care and Research*, vol. 9, no. 5, pp. 391–399, 1996.

[30] A. S. Zigmond and R. P. Snaith, "The hospital anxiety and depression scale," *Acta Psychiatrica Scandinavica*, vol. 67, no. 6, pp. 361–370, 1983.

[31] I. Bjelland, A. A. Dahl, T. T. Haug, and D. Neckelmann, "The validity of the Hospital Anxiety and Depression Scale. An updated literature review," *Journal of Psychosomatic Research*, vol. 52, no. 2, pp. 69–77, 2002.

[32] L. Wettergren, E. Mattsson, and L. von Essen, "Mode of administration only has a small effect on data quality and self-reported health status and emotional distress among Swedish adolescents and young adults," *Journal of Clinical Nursing*, vol. 20, no. 11-12, pp. 1568–1577, 2011.

[33] D. J. Buysse, C. F. Reynolds III, T. H. Monk, S. R. Berman, and D. J. Kupfer, "The Pittsburgh Sleep Quality Index: a new instrument for psychiatric practice and research," *Psychiatry Research*, vol. 28, no. 2, pp. 193–213, 1989.

[34] J. S. Carpenter and M. A. Andrykowski, "Psychometric evaluation of the Pittsburgh Sleep Quality Index," *Journal of Psychosomatic Research*, vol. 45, no. 1, pp. 5–13, 1998.

[35] T. H. Monk, D. J. Buysse, B. D. Billy et al., "Shiftworkers report worse sleep than day workers, even in retirement," *Journal of Sleep Research*, vol. 22, no. 2, pp. 201–208, 2013.

[36] P. A. Palmieri, K. J. Chipman, D. Canetti, R. J. Johnson, and S. E. Hobfoll, "Prevalence and correlates of sleep problems in adult Israeli Jews exposed to actual or threatened terrorist or rocket attacks," *Journal of Clinical Sleep Medicine*, vol. 6, no. 6, pp. 557–564, 2010.

[37] J. E. Ware Jr. and C. D. Sherbourne, "The MOS 36-item short-form health survey (SF-36). I. Conceptual framework and item selection," *Medical Care*, vol. 30, no. 6, pp. 473–483, 1992.

[38] C. A. McHorney, M. Kosinski, and J. E. Ware Jr., "Comparisons of the costs and quality of norms for the SF-36 health survey collected by mail versus telephone interview: results from a national survey," *Medical Care*, vol. 32, no. 6, pp. 551–567, 1994.

[39] E. K. Watson, D. W. Firman, P. D. Baade, and I. Ring, "Telephone administration of the SF-36 health survey: validation studies and population norms for adults in Queensland," *Australian and New Zealand Journal of Public Health*, vol. 20, no. 4, pp. 359–363, 1996.

[40] K. McElhone, J. Abbott, and L.-S. Teh, "A review of health related quality of life in systemic lupus erythematosus," *Lupus*, vol. 15, no. 10, pp. 633–643, 2006.

[41] M. Castelino, J. Abbott, K. McElhone, and L. S. Teh, "Comparison of the psychometric properties of health-related quality of life measures used in adults with systemic lupus erythematosus: a review of the literature," *Rheumatology*, vol. 52, no. 4, pp. 684–696, 2013.

[42] C. Bombardier, D. D. Gladman, M. B. Urowitz, D. Caron, and C. H. C. Chi Hsing Chang, "Derivation of the SLEDAI. A disease activity index for lupus patients. The Committee on Prognosis Studies in SLE," *Arthritis and Rheumatism*, vol. 35, no. 6, pp. 630–640, 1992.

[43] M. Petri, M. Genovese, E. Engle, and M. Hochberg, "Definition, incidence, and clinical description of flare in systemic lupus erythematosus: a prospective cohort study," *Arthritis and Rheumatism*, vol. 34, no. 8, pp. 937–944, 1991.

[44] D. Gladman, E. Ginzler, C. Goldsmith et al., "The development and initial validation of the systemic lupus international collaborating clinics/American college of rheumatology damage index for systemic lupus erythematosus," *Arthritis and Rheumatism*, vol. 39, no. 3, pp. 363–369, 1996.

[45] P. Skapinakis, G. Lewis, and V. Mavreas, "Temporal relations between unexplained fatigue and depression: longitudinal data from an international study in primary care," *Psychosomatic Medicine*, vol. 66, no. 3, pp. 330–335, 2004.

[46] L. Palagini, M. Mosca, C. Tani, A. Gemignani, M. Mauri, and S. Bombardieri, "Depression and systemic lupus erythematosus: a systematic review," *Lupus*, vol. 22, no. 5, pp. 409–416, 2013.

[47] A. da Silva, E. T. Dos Reis-Neto, N. da Silva, and E. Sato, "The effect of acute physical exercise on cytokine levels in patients with systemic lupus erythematosus," *Lupus*, vol. 22, no. 14, pp. 1479–1483, 2013.

[48] K. Beusterien, J. Bell, J. Grinspan, T. Utset, H. Kan, and S. Narayanan, "Physician-patient interactions and outcomes in systemic lupus erythematosus (SLE): a conceptual model," *Lupus*, vol. 22, no. 10, pp. 1038–1045, 2013.

[49] J. G. Schwartzberg, A. Cowett, J. VanGeest, and M. S. Wolf, "Communication techniques for patients with low health literacy: a survey of physicians, nurses, and pharmacists," *American Journal of Health Behavior*, vol. 31, no. 1, pp. s96–s104, 2007.

# 18

# Nail Involvement in Patients with Psoriatic Arthritis

**O. Zargari,[1] E. Kazemnezhad Leyli,[2] and S. Z. Azimi[3]**

[1]*Department of Dermatology, Skin Research Center, Shahid Beheshti University of Medical Sciences, Tehran, Iran*
[2]*Department of Biostatistics, Guilan University of Medical Sciences, Rasht, Iran*
[3]*Department of Dermatology, Skin Research Center, Guilan University of Medical Sciences, Rasht, Iran*

Correspondence should be addressed to S. Z. Azimi; sz.azimi@yahoo.com

Academic Editor: Ricard Cervera

*Background.* Psoriatic arthritis (PsA) results in an increased burden of psoriasis and impairs both quality of life and an individual's functional capacity. The relationship between nail involvement and PsA in psoriasis is not fully characterized. *Aim.* To evaluate the frequency and characteristics of nail involvement in psoriatic patients and to assess the relationship with joint involvement. *Methods.* A total of 197 patients with moderate-to-severe psoriasis were consecutively invited to participate in this cross-sectional study. The patients are divided into two groups: those with and those without psoriatic arthritis. *Results.* 69.5% of psoriatic (137 out of 197) patients had nail involvement. The most common nail abnormality was onycholysis, followed by pitting and oil droplet changes. Nail involvement was more common in patients with psoriatic arthritis (82.1% versus 57.8%, p=0.001). *Conclusion.* Nail involvement is commonly associated with PsA. Onycholysis, splinter hemorrhage, and oil drop were significantly more common in the PsA group as opposed to patients with just skin findings. In general, psoriatic patients with arthritis had more severe disease.

## 1. Introduction

Psoriasis is a chronic inflammatory disease affecting up to 3% of the general population. It has a substantial negative impact on health-related quality of life (HRQOL), especially when it involves visible areas of the body such as the face, hands, and nails [1]. Psoriatic arthritis (PsA) has been defined as inflammatory arthritis, usually seronegative, associated with psoriasis [1]. The exact prevalence of PsA is unknown but up to 30% of patients with psoriasis develop psoriatic arthritis [2, 3].

A substantial number of psoriatic patients have nail involvement, varying from 10% to 80%, with an estimated lifetime incidence of 80–90% [4–6].

Nail involvement may be considered an indicator for patients at risk for future psoriatic joint damage [7, 8]; however, this relationship has not been proven [9]. The aim of this study was to assess the overall prevalence of nail involvement in patients with moderate-to-severe psoriasis and to achieve more details on the possible relationship between nail psoriasis and PsA.

## 2. Materials and Methods

*2.1. Patients.* This cross-sectional study was conducted from January 2017 to December 2017. During this period, all eligible patients with moderate-to-severe psoriasis who attended to our psoriasis clinic and were candidates for systemic therapy were enrolled in the study. Moderate-to-severe psoriasis was defined as body surface area (BSA) >10% or psoriasis area and severity index (PASI) >10 [10]. The study was approved by the Shahid Beheshti institutional board committee. Informed consent was obtained from each subject.

A detailed history was recorded for all subjects, including gender, age, age at the time of onset of the disease, phenotype of psoriasis, disease duration, extent, and severity of the disease. We diagnosed psoriasis according to the clinical findings, and if necessary, a skin biopsy was performed. All patients underwent dermatological examination by a dermatologist (O.Z.). The following nail changes were recorded: pitting, crumbling, onycholysis, oil drop, subungual hyperkeratosis, and splinter hemorrhage.

Psoriasis skin severity was assessed by using psoriasis area and severity index (PASI) at the time of the physical examination. Mycological investigations were performed in patients with nail changes suspicious for fungal infection such as onychorrhexis, hyperkeratosis, thickening, or crumbling. Nail clippings and subungual scrapings were collected. One part of nail specimens was exposed to direct microscopic examination with 10% potassium hydroxide aqueous solution and the other part was cultured on Sabouraud's dextrose agar medium with cycloheximide. Also, other causes of nail changes, like congenital and traumatic dystrophy were excluded from the study. Isolated nail psoriasis patients were not included in the study.

On the basis of musculoskeletal findings, patients with arthralgia or other joint symptoms were referred to a rheumatologist. The diagnosis of psoriatic arthritis was established in accordance with the Classification Criteria for Psoriatic Arthritis (CASPAR).

*2.2. Statistical Analysis.* Statistical analysis was performed using software SPSS 18.0 (SPSS Inc., IBM Corporation, Armonk, New York). Categorical variables were expressed as frequencies and percentages and analyzed by Chi-square test or Fisher's exact test. Normality of variables was verified by Kolmogorov-Smirnov test. Continuous variables were given as means (SD) or medians (range). Student t-test was used for continuous variables with normal distribution. For continuous variables with an abnormal distribution, the Mann–Whitney test was performed. Statistical significance was considered at a level of 5% ($p<0.05$) for all tests.

## 3. Results

In total, 197 patients participated in the study. There was a slight female preponderance in our sample with 54 % (n = 107) female patients and 46% (n = 90) male patients.

The mean duration of the disease was 15 years (SD: 11 years; ranging from one month to 46 years) and the mean age of disease onset was 30 ±17 years. The subjects were divided into two groups: those with and those without psoriatic arthritis. In the study population, 95 patients (48%) had psoriatic arthritis. Of these, 56 patients were women and 39 patients were men (Table 1).

We found no significant difference between the two groups in terms of age, gender, the presence of comorbidities, alcohol intake and smoking. However, patients with PsA had lower median age of onset [26.91 ± 16.65 versus 31.87 ± 17.06 years, p=0.04] and longer disease duration [17.24 ± 10.79 versus 13.06 ± 10.42, p=0.006]. Also, the frequency of facial involvement was higher in those with PsA (74.7% versus 54.9%, p=0.001). In general, patients with PsA had more severe psoriasis reflected by higher median PASI scores [20.05 ± 11.54 versus 15.37 ± 8.97, p=0.016]. Also, positive family history for psoriasis was more often reported in those with PsA (49.5% versus 34.3%, p=0.03).

Overall, methotrexate was the most used medication among patients (88.3%). Patients in PsA group had a higher rate for the history of using different systemic treatments.

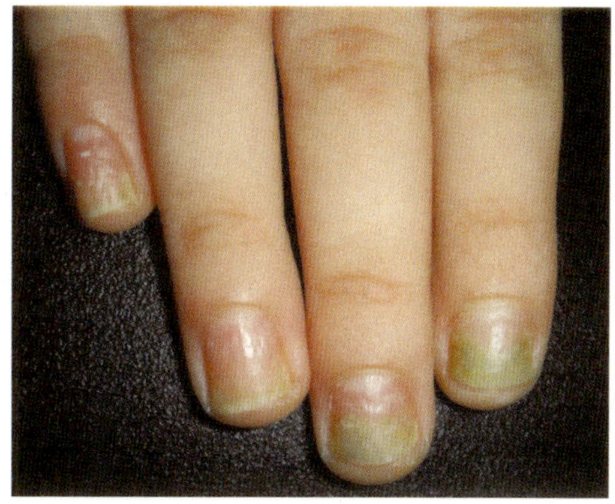

FIGURE 1: Pitting and onycholysis in a psoriatic patient.

Prevalence of plaque-type psoriasis was significantly higher in patients with PsA (Table 2).

Nail involvement was present in 69.5% (137 out of 197) of patients. The most common nail abnormality was onycholysis, followed by pitting and oil drop (68.4%, 34.7%, and 30.5%, respectively). Nail changes were more common in patients with PsA (82.1% vs. 57.8%, p=0.001). Prevalence of onycholysis, splinter hemorrhage, and oil drop were significantly higher in PsA patients in comparison with patients without psoriatic arthritis (Table 3). Figure 1, illustrates pitting and onycholysis in a patient.

## 4. Discussion

The prevalence of nail changes in psoriatic patients reportedly presents great variety in the literature. Nail involvement in psoriasis usually is divided into two major groups: (a) signs of involvement of nail matrix including pitting, leukonychia, red spots of the lunula, transverse grooves (Beau's lines), and crumbling of the nail plate and (b) signs of involvement of the nail bed which present as oil-drop discoloration, splinter hemorrhages, subungual hyperkeratosis, and onycholysis [5].

The most common psoriasic nail features were dissimilar in different studies. In a report by Kyriakou et al., oil droplet changes were the most common finding [11]. In another study, by Kaur et al. nail pitting was the most common finding [12]. On the other hand, there are reports showing that subungual hyperkeratosis is the most common feature [13]. Our study was in concordance with Grover's paper [14] that the most common nail finding was onycholysis, which was present in 54.8% of our patients (108 out or 197) and significantly was more prevalent in the PsA group.

Pits can be seen in normal individuals as well as those with chronic eczema, alopecia areata, and lichen planus. Therefore, seeking other psoriatic nail features would be helpful for the identification of psoriatic nail pitting. Also, it is suggested that pits in patients with nail psoriasis are typically deeper than those observed in association with other dermatological conditions [10, 15].

Forty-eight percent of our patients had PsA. This figure is slightly higher than previous studies, which suggest a prevalence of around 30% [16, 17]. The higher rate of PsA in

Table 1: Demographic and clinical characteristics of patients.

| | All patients (N= 197) | Patients without PsA (N=102) | Patients with PsA (N=95) | P Value |
|---|---|---|---|---|
| **Age** (Year, mean ±SD) | 44.56 ± 14.73 | 44.93 ± 16.06 | 44.16 ± 13.24 | 0.71 |
| **Sex** | | | | |
| Male | 90 (45.7%) | 51 (50%) | 39 (41.1%) | 0.21 |
| Female | 107 (54.3%) | 51 (50%) | 56 (58.9%) | |
| **Age at onset** (Year, mean ±SD) | 29.48 ± 17.00 | 31.87 ± 17.06 | 26.91 ± 16.65 | **0.04** |
| **Duration of psoriasis** (Year, mean ±SD) | 15.08 ± 10.78 | 13.06 ± 10.42 | 17.24 ± 10.79 | **0.006** |
| **Positive family history** | 82 (41.6%) | 35 (34.3%) | 47 (49.5%) | **0.03** |
| **BMI,** ($kg/m^2$; mean ± SD) | 28.97 ± 6.33 | 28.11± 6.05 | 29.95 ± 6.52 | **0.05** |
| **PASI** | 17.67 ± 10.53 | 15.37 ± 8.97 | 20.05 ± 11.54 | **0.01** |
| **Nail involvement** | 137 (69.5%) | 59 (57.8%) | 78 (82.1%) | **0.001** |
| **Face involvement** | 127 (64.5%) | 56 (54.9%) | 71 (74.7%) | **0.004** |
| **Genital involvement** | 126 (64%) | 59 (57.8%) | 67 (70.5%) | 0.06 |
| **Smoking** | 32 (16.2%) | 19 (18.6%) | 13 (13.7%) | 0.35 |
| **Alcohol** | 26 (13.2%) | 14 (13.7%) | 12 (12.6%) | 0.82 |
| **Comorbidities** | | | | |
| **DM** | 36 (18.3%) | 17 (16.7%) | 19 (20%) | 0.54 |
| **HTN** | 36 (18.3%) | 17 (16.7%) | 19 (20%) | 0.54 |
| **CVD** | 11 (5.6%) | 6 (5.9%) | 5 (5.3%) | 0.85 |
| **HLP** | 37 (18.8%) | 20 (19.6%) | 17 (17.9%) | 0.76 |
| **Prior Treatments** | | | | |
| **Methotrexate** | 174 (88.3%) | 85 (83.3%) | 89 (93.7%) | **0.024** |
| **Acitretin** | 122 (61.9%) | 62 (60.8%) | 60 (63.2%) | 0.73 |
| **CyA** | 73 (37.1%) | 27 (26.5%) | 46 (48.4%) | **0.001** |
| **Phototherapy** | 36 (18.3%) | 13 (12.7%) | 23 (24.2%) | **0.04** |
| **Systemic steroids** | 21 (10.7%) | 7 (6.9%) | 14 (14.7%) | 0.07 |
| **Biologics** | 64 (32.5%) | 18 (17.6%) | 46 (48.4%) | **0.001** |

BMI: body mass index, PASI: psoriasis and area severity index, DM: diabetes mellitus, HTN: hypertension, CVD: cardio vascular disease, HLP: hyperlipidemia, and CyA: cyclosporine A.

TABLE 2: Psoriasis phenotypes in the groups studied.

| Type of Psoriasis | All patients (N= 197) | Patients without PsA (N=102) | Patients with PsA (N=95) | P Value |
|---|---|---|---|---|
| **Chronic plaque** | 181 (91.9%) | 90 (88.2%) | 91 (95.8%) | **0.05** |
| **Pustular** | 2 (1%) | 1 (1%) | 1 (1.1%) | 0.96 |
| **Palmoplantar** | 33 (16.8%) | 19 (18.6%) | 14 (14.7%) | 0.53 |
| **Flexural** | 13 (6.6%) | 8 (7.8%) | 5 (5.8%) | 0.46 |
| **Guttate** | 32 (16.2%) | 13 (12.7%) | 19 (20%) | 0.16 |
| **Erythrodermic** | 5 (2.5%) | 2 (2%) | 3 (3.2%) | 0.59 |

TABLE 3: Morphologic features of nail changes.

| Nail Features | All patients (N= 197) | Patients without PsA (N=102) | Patients with PsA (N=95) | P Value |
|---|---|---|---|---|
| **Pitting** | | | | 0.34 |
| **Yes** | 62 (31.5%) | 29 (28.4%) | 33 (34.7%) | |
| **No** | 135 (68.5%) | 73 (71.6%) | 62 (65.3%) | |
| **Total Dystrophy** | | | | 0.71 |
| **Yes** | 3 (1.5%) | 0 (0) | 3 (3.2%) | |
| **No** | 194 (98.5%) | 102 (100%) | 92 (96.8%) | |
| **Onycholysis** | | | | **0.001** |
| **Yes** | 108 (54.8%) | 43 (42.2%) | 65 (68.4%) | |
| **No** | 89 (45.2%) | 59 (57.8%) | 30 (31.6%) | |
| **Oil Drop** | | | | **0.013** |
| **Yes** | 45 (22.8%) | 16 (15.7%) | 29 (30.5%) | |
| **No** | 152 (77.2%) | 86 (84.3%) | 66 (69.5%) | |
| **Subungual hyperkeratosis** | | | | 0.69 |
| **Yes** | 19 (9.6%) | 9 (8.8%) | 10 (10.5%) | |
| **No** | 178 (90.4%) | 93 (91.2%) | 85 (89.5%) | |
| **Splinter hemorrhage** | | | | **0.05** |
| **Yes** | 12 (6.1%) | 3 (2.9%) | 9 (9.5%) | |
| **No** | 185 (93.9%) | 99 (97.1%) | 86 (90.5%) | |
| **Longitudinal ridging** | | | | 0.28 |
| **Yes** | 4 (2%) | 1 (1%) | 3 (3.2%) | |
| **No** | 193 (98%) | 101 (99%) | 92 (96.8%) | |

our patients is probably due to the selection of relatively more severe cases in this study.

Our study revealed that the prevalence of nail changes is higher in PsA, than has been suggested by some previous observations [18, 19]. We found that onycholysis, oil drop, and splinter hemorrhage, in particular, were significantly more prevalent in PsA patients. Fonseca et al. found no statistical difference in NAPSI (Nail Psoriasis Severity Index) values among patients with or without psoriatic arthritis [20]. Perhaps, the type of nail involvement is more important than the severity of nail changes in terms of correlation with PsA.

The pathophysiology of nail dystrophy has been postulated to be more closely associated with joint symptoms than with skin symptoms [21]. However, there is still no clear explanation for this association and some believe that this association is limited only to distal interphalangeal (DIP) joints [22]. The suggested theories are (a) having a common (and yet unknown) autoantigen in both nail apparatus and synovial membrane, (b) anatomic connection between nail structures and DIP joints, and (c) the common role of trauma (Koebner phenomenon) in both nail and arthropathic psoriasis [20, 23, 24].

In this study, patients with PsA had more severe psoriasis and an earlier age of onset and longer duration than those without PsA. Also, they had a higher rate of facial involvement. To our knowledge, this association has not been reported previously and further studies are needed to corroborate this association.

We excluded all psoriatic patients with onychomycosis from the study after positive direct examination, KOH smear and/or fungal culture. However, onychomycosis may present with clinical features similar to nail psoriasis. In addition, it is anticipated that the prevalence of onychomycosis is about 4.6 to 30% of psoriatic patients with nail involvement [25, 26].

Our study had certain limitations. One of them was lack of information about the subtypes of PsA. Also, we have not recorded the severity of nail involvements. Furthermore, previous medications may have interfered with the degree of nail changes in our patients.

## 5. Conclusion

In summary, we have shown that there is an association between nail involvement and PsA and this association is most significant for onycholysis. Also, patients with PsA have a higher probability of positive family history for psoriasis, earlier onset, longer duration, more severe psoriasis and a higher rate of facial involvement. It should be kept in mind that while there is a strong association between PsA and nail changes, every psoriasis patient should be asked about joint symptoms even if they have no nail changes.

## Disclosure

Earlier version of this work was presented at "5th World Psoriasis & Psoriatic Arthritis Conference, Stockholm, Sweden, 2018".

## Conflicts of Interest

The authors have no conflicts of interest to disclose.

## Acknowledgments

The authors are grateful to Professor A. Menter and Professor S. Feldman for their review of the manuscript and insightful suggestions.

## References

[1] K. M. Klaassen, P. C. van de Kerkhof, and M. C. Pasch, "Nail Psoriasis, the unknown burden of disease," *Journal of the European Academy of Dermatology and Venereology*, 2014.

[2] T. C. Namey, "Seronegative Polyarthritis. Verna Wright and John H. Moll. Amsterdam and New York, North Holland Press, 1976, 488 Pages. Price: $65.50.," *Arthritis & Rheumatism*, vol. 21, no. 3, pp. 398-399, 1978.

[3] P. J. Mease, D. D. Gladman, K. A. Papp et al., "Prevalence of rheumatologist-diagnosed psoriatic arthritis in patients with psoriasis in European/North American dermatology clinics," *Journal of the American Academy of Dermatology*, vol. 69, no. 5, pp. 729–735, 2013.

[4] D. D. Gladman, C. Antoni, P. Mease, D. O. Clegg, and O. Nash, "Psoriatic arthritis: epidemiology, clinical features, course, and outcome," *Annals of the Rheumatic Diseases*, vol. 64, no. 2, pp. ii14–ii17, 2005.

[5] K. Reich, "Approach to managing patients with nail psoriasis," *Journal of the European Academy of Dermatology and Venereology*, vol. 23, supplement 1, pp. 15–21, 2009.

[6] M. C. Pasch, "Nail Psoriasis: A Review of Treatment Options," *Drugs*, vol. 76, no. 6, pp. 675–705, 2016.

[7] K. M. G. Klaassen, P. C. M. Van De Kerkhof, and M. C. Pasch, "Nail psoriasis: A questionnaire-based survey," *British Journal of Dermatology*, vol. 169, no. 2, pp. 314–319, 2013.

[8] A. Langenbruch, M. A. Radtke, M. Krensel, A. Jacobi, K. Reich, and M. Augustin, "Nail involvement as a predictor of concomitant psoriatic arthritis in patients with psoriasis," *British Journal of Dermatology*, vol. 171, no. 5, pp. 1123–1128, 2014.

[9] D. McGonagle, Z. Ash, L. Dickie, M. McDermott, and S. Z. Aydin, "The early phase of psoriatic arthritis," *Annals of the Rheumatic Diseases*, vol. 70, no. 1, pp. i71–i76, 2011.

[10] U. Mrowietz, K. Kragballe, K. Reich et al., "Definition of treatment goals for moderate to severe psoriasis: A European consensus," *Archives of Dermatological Research*, vol. 303, no. 1, pp. 1–10, 2011.

[11] A. Kyriakou, A. Patsatsi, and D. Sotiriadis, "Detailed analysis of specific nail psoriasis features and their correlations with clinical parameters: a cross-sectional study," *Dermatology*, vol. 223, no. 3, pp. 222–229, 2011.

[12] I. Kaur, A. Saraswat, and B. Kumar, "Nail changes in psoriasis: A study of 167 patients," *International Journal of Dermatology*, vol. 40, no. 9, pp. 601–603, 2001.

[13] J. Salomon, J. C. Szepietowski, and A. Proniewicz, "Psoriatic Nails: A Prospective Clinical Study," *Journal of Cutaneous Medicine and Surgery*, vol. 7, no. 4, pp. 317–321, 2003.

[14] C. Grover, B. S. N. Reddy, and K. U. Chaturvedi, "Diagnosis of nail psoriasis: Importance of biopsy and histopathology," *British Journal of Dermatology*, vol. 153, no. 6, pp. 1153–1158, 2005.

[15] R. Baran, R. Dawber, D. de Berker, E. Haneke, and A. Tosti, *Baran and Dawber's Diseases of the Nails and their Management*, Blackwell Science Ltd, Oxford, UK, 2001.

[16] H. Zachariae, "Prevalence of joint disease in patients with psoriasis: implications for therapy," *American Journal of Clinical Dermatology*, vol. 4, no. 7, pp. 441–447, 2003.

[17] V. Chandran, C. T. Schentag, and D. D. Gladman, "Sensitivity of the classification of psoriatic arthritis criteria in early psoriatic arthritis," *Arthritis & Rheumatism*, vol. 57, no. 8, pp. 1560–1563, 2007.

[18] V. Brazzelli, A. Carugno, A. Alborghetti et al., "Prevalence, severity and clinical features of psoriasis in fingernails and toenails in adult patients: Italian experience," *Journal of the European Academy of Dermatology and Venereology*, vol. 26, no. 11, pp. 1354–1359, 2012.

[19] F. Lavaroni Kokelj, P. Pauluzzi, and G. Trevisan, "The nail in psoriatic arthritis. Acta Derm Venereol Suppl (Stockh," in *Lavaroni G*, pp. 186-113, 186, 113, 1994.

[20] G. P. Fonseca, G. Seidel, B. Werner, and H. L. Staub, "Comparative microscopic analysis of nail clippings from patients with cutaneous psoriasis and psoriatic arthritis," *Anais Brasileiros de Dermatologia*, vol. 92, no. 1, pp. 21–25, 2017.

[21] D. McGonagle, M. Benjamin, and A. L. Tan, "The pathogenesis of psoriatic arthritis and associated nail disease: not autoimmune after all?" *Current Opinion in Rheumatology*, vol. 21, no. 4, pp. 340–347, 2009.

[22] K. M. Wittkowski, C. Leonardi, A. Gottlieb et al., "Clinical Symptoms of Skin, Nails, and Joints Manifest Independently in Patients with Concomitant Psoriasis and Psoriatic Arthritis," *PLoS ONE*, vol. 6, no. 6, p. e20279, 2011.

[23] D. McGonagle, "Enthesitis: an autoinflammatory lesion linking nail and joint involvement in psoriatic disease," *Journal of the European Academy of Dermatology and Venereology*, vol. 23, no. 1, pp. 9–13, 2009.

[24] H. Maejima, T. Taniguchi, A. Watarai, and K. Katsuoka, "Evaluation of nail disease in psoriatic arthritis by using a modified nail psoriasis severity score index," *International Journal of Dermatology*, vol. 49, no. 8, pp. 901–906, 2010.

[25] K. R. R. Schons, M. D. O. Beck, A. A. C. Beber, and O. A. Monticielo, "Nail involvement in adult patients with plaque-type psoriasis: Prevalence and clinical features," *Anais Brasileiros de Dermatologia*, vol. 90, no. 3, pp. 314–319, 2015.

[26] V. Natarajan, A. Nath, D. Thappa, R. Singh, and S. Verma, "Coexistence of onychomycosis in psoriatic nails: A descriptive study," *Indian Journal of Dermatology, Venereology and Leprology*, vol. 76, no. 6, p. 723, 2010.

# 19

# Exploring T Cell Reactivity to Gliadin in Young Children with Newly Diagnosed Celiac Disease

**Edwin Liu,[1] Kristen McDaniel,[1] Stephanie Case,[1] Liping Yu,[1] Bernd Gerhartz,[2] Nils Ostermann,[2] Gabriela Fankhauser,[2] Valerie Hungerford,[2] Chao Zou,[2] Marcel Luyten,[2] Katherine J. Seidl,[2] and Aaron W. Michels[1]**

[1] *Barbara Davis Center for Childhood Diabetes, School of Medicine, University of Colorado Denver, Mail Stop A140, 1775 Aurora Court, Aurora, CO 80045, USA*
[2] *Novartis Institutes for Biomedical Research, 4002 Basel, Switzerland*

Correspondence should be addressed to Aaron W. Michels; aaron.michels@ucdenver.edu

Academic Editor: Raffaella Nenna

Class II major histocompatibility molecules confer disease risk in Celiac disease (CD) by presenting gliadin peptides to CD4 T cells in the small intestine. Deamidation of gliadin peptides by tissue transglutaminase creates immunogenic peptides presented by HLA-DQ2 and DQ8 molecules to activate proinflammatory CD4 T cells. Detecting gliadin specific T cell responses from the peripheral blood has been challenging due to low circulating frequencies and heterogeneity in response to gliadin epitopes. We investigated the peripheral T cell responses to alpha and gamma gliadin epitopes in young children with newly diagnosed and untreated CD. Using peptide/MHC recombinant protein constructs, we are able to robustly stimulate CD4 T cell clones previously derived from intestinal biopsies of CD patients. These recombinant proteins and a panel of $\alpha$- and $\gamma$-gliadin peptides were used to assess T cell responses from the peripheral blood. Proliferation assays using peripheral blood mononuclear cells revealed more CD4 T cell responses to $\alpha$-gliadin than $\gamma$-gliadin peptides with a single deamidated $\alpha$-gliadin peptide able to identify 60% of CD children. We conclude that it is possible to detect T cell responses without a gluten challenge or in vitro stimulus other than antigen, when measuring proliferative responses.

## 1. Introduction

Celiac disease (CD) is a T cell mediated enteropathy triggered by the ingestion of dietary gluten resulting in villous atrophy and crypt hyperplasia in the small intestine [1]. Specific human leukocyte antigen (HLA) genes are involved in the disease process with restriction primarily limited to HLA-DQ2 (DQA∗05:01, DQB∗02:01 and DQA∗02:01, DQB∗02:02) and DQ8 (DQA∗03:01, DQB∗3:02) [2]. HLA genes encode class II major histocompatibility molecules (MHC), which present antigens to CD4 T cells. There has been remarkable progress in the understanding of the pathogenesis and epitopes involved in the disease process [3–6]. Gliadin, one of the two principle protein components of gluten, contains a number of well-studied T cell epitopes. Deamidation of gliadin peptides by tissue transglutaminase (TTG) type 2 converts glutamine into glutamic acid, resulting in immunogenic T cell epitopes [7].

Despite the current understanding of T cell—peptide—MHC interaction, simple and reliable T cell assays from the peripheral blood to monitor CD activity have been difficult to develop. Peripheral blood biomarkers for CD are hindered by variables such as the type of assay, use of the proper antigen, low circulating frequencies of T cells, and the timing of gluten exposure when the assay is performed. For example, it has been reported that, to obtain sufficient T cells for study without in vitro expansion, CD blood donors on a gluten-free diet need to undergo short-term gluten challenge, to detect IFN-$\gamma$ T cell responses by enzyme linked immunospot (ELISPOT) assays [8, 9]. However, both gluten-free and gluten-exposed CD patients can have measurable T cell proliferative responses with response rates more frequent in gluten-exposed patients [10]. Comprehensive epitope mapping studies have identified four immunodominant DQ2 epitopes in treated CD adults (gluten-free diet) followed by a gluten challenge [11]. Such an unbiased epitope mapping project has not been undertaken for children with CD, even though there are several well-studied epitopes in the literature.

In this study, we investigated the peripheral T cell responses to alpha and gamma gliadin epitopes in young children with newly diagnosed and untreated CD. The selected epitopes are known to stimulate T cell clones derived from adult CD patient intestinal biopsies [12, 13]. Recombinant DQ2 and DQ8 proteins with α-gliadin epitopes were created to test T cell clone stimulation without the use of antigen presenting cells, as part of an effort to develop a T cell stimulation assay feasible for large scale, consistent, and rapid assessment of CD activity. We explored the utility of peptide/MHC complexes first in stimulating T cell clones and then peripheral blood mononuclear cells (PBMCs) of newly diagnosed CD children prior to treatment with a gluten-free diet to produce inflammatory cytokines. Subsequently, proliferation assays utilizing a panel of previously described DQ2 and DQ8 peptides on the same CD children provide insight into the possible degenerate nature of α-gliadin peptide binding motifs for HLA-DQ2.

## 2. Methods

*2.1. Subjects and Samples.* Subjects were recruited from the Children's Hospital Colorado, and written informed consent was obtained after the nature and possible consequences of the study were explained to individuals. The clinical investigation in this study was conducted in accordance with the Declaration of Helsinki principles, and study approval was provided by the Colorado Multiple Institutional Review Board. Peripheral blood was obtained for T cell assays, TTG antibodies, and HLA genotyping. TTG antibodies were measured from the serum by radioimmunoassay as previously described [14]. HLA-DRB, DQA, and DQB genotyping were performed using linear arrays of immobilized sequence-specific oligonucleotides similar to previously described methodology [15].

*2.2. Expression and Purification of Recombinant Protein.* The extracellular domains of the HLA-DQ8 α chain (residue 24–204) and β chain (residue 33–221) were coexpressed in S2 drosophila cells (ExpreS2ion Biotechnologies, Denmark). Double deamidated α-gliadin (QQYPSGEGSFQPSQENPQ) was covalently attached to the N-terminus of β chain with a Factor *X* cleavage site (GGGGSIEGRGSGGGS) between the peptide and the β chain. To stabilize the heterodimer, Fos and Jun leucine zippers were attached to the C-terminus of α chain and β chain via a thrombin cleavage sequence (SSADLVPRGS). Deamidated α-gliadin/DQ8 was extracted from the medium using anti-FLAG M2 (Sigma Aldrich) affinity chromatography. The recombinant protein was purified by Superdex 200 column in buffer containing 10 mMTris, pH 8.0, and 150 mM NaCl. For the α-I-gliadin/DQ2 construct, the extracellular domains of HLA-DQ2 α chain (residue 24–206) and β chain (residue 33–221) were used, expressed in S2 drosophila cells, and purified in a similar manner to the DQ8 recombinant protein construct. The amino acid sequence of α-I gliadin, QLQPFPQPELPY, was covalently attached to the N-terminus of the β chain via TEV cleavage site (GGGGENLYFQGGSGGGS). To stabilize the heterodimer, Fos and Jun leucine zippers were attached via PreScission cleavage site (SSADLEVLFQGP) to the C-termini of α chain and β chain, respectively. The final proteins were confirmed by LC-MS. Diagrams of the two recombinant protein constructs are depicted in Figure 1(a).

*2.3. Generation of T Cell Receptor Hybridomas.* T cell receptor (TCR) hybridomas, containing the TCR from a DQ2 and DQ8 restricted T cell clone responding to α-gliadin peptides, were created as previously described [16]. The sequences for the αβ TCR clones in Figure 2 were a kind gift from Ludvig Sollid. The sequences for the αβ TCR clones in the supplemental Figures (see supplementary material available online at http://dx.doi.org/10.1155/2014/927190) were derived from published information on gene usage [13]. Briefly, a single TCR sequence, α and β chains linked by the PTV1.2A sequence, was cloned into MSCV-based retroviral vectors carrying green fluorescent protein (GFP) (pMIGII) [17], followed by production of replication-incompetent retroviruses encoding TCR sequences. The 5KC hybridoma line lacking TCR α and β chains was used to reconstitute TCRs [18]. The transduced 5KC hybridomas were sorted by GFP expression and TCR expression was confirmed by staining with anti-mouse TCRβ antibody (clone H57-597, BD Biosciences). Alternatively, the expression of plasmids in the pMSCVpuro retroviral vector (Clontech) was transfected to AmphoPack-293 or GP2-293 (VSV-G envelope) packaging cells (Clontech) to produce retrovirus and mouse 5KC cells were spin-infected with retroviral supernatants and cultured with puromycin. TCR expression was confirmed in isolated single clones by staining with anti-mouse CD3 (clone 145-2C11; BD Biosciences) or mouse TCRβ antibody (clone H57-597; BD Biosciences).

*2.4. Cytokine Stimulation Assays.* Peripheral blood mononuclear cells (PBMCs) were isolated from whole blood using Ficoll-Paque and resuspended at a density of $10^6$/mL in IMDM-C media (IMDM supplemented with 5% heat inactivated human AB serum, 100 μg/mL Pen-Strep, 100 μM MEM NEAA, and 50 μM 2-mercaptoethanol). $2 \times 10^5$ PBMCs or T cell hybridomas in 200 μL of media were added to a 96-well tissue culture plate coated with 1 μg/well of recombinant protein and cultured at 37°C in 5% $CO_2$ overnight. Secreted cytokine was measured in the supernatant by electrochemiluminescence assay (Meso Scale Discovery) for human IFN-γ, IL-2, and by ELISA for IL-17 (R&D Systems). PBMCs in culture without protein (background) were a negative control, while anti-CD3 stimulation (OKT3, eBioscience) was a positive control. DQ antibody SPV-L3 (Abcam, Cambridge, UK), 1a3 (Leinco, St. Louis, MO, USA), or HB-144 (ATCC, Manassas, VA, USA) was added at either 10 μg/mL or at

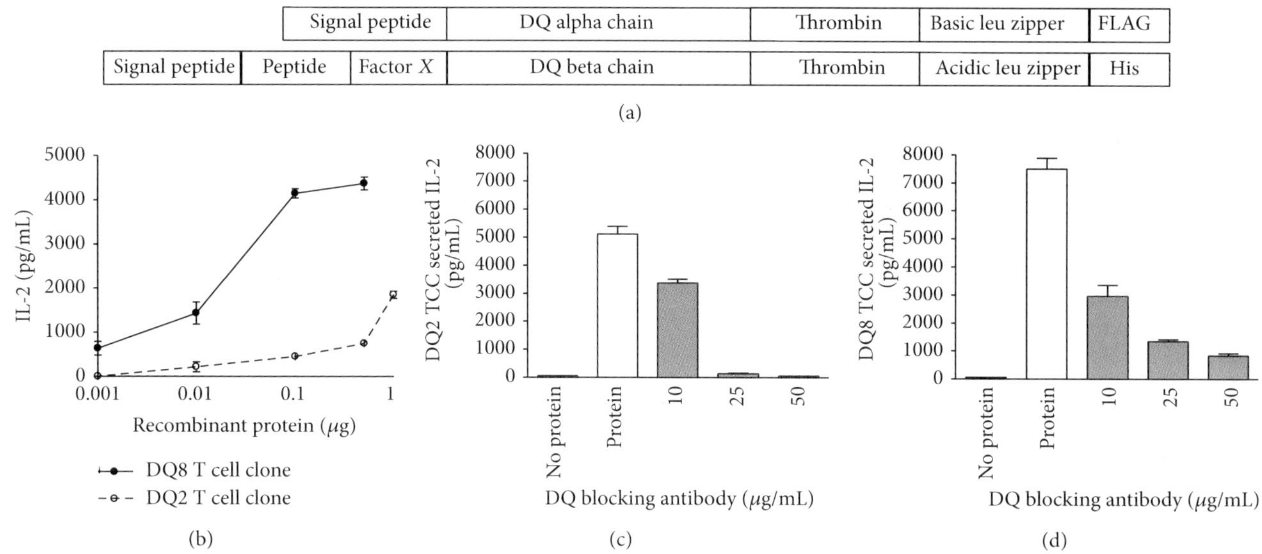


FIGURE 1: Recombinant DQ8 and DQ2 proteins with gliadin epitopes stimulate T cell clones. (a) Diagrams of the constructs used to produce recombinant protein for deamidated $\alpha$-gliadin p1E, p9E/DQ8, and $\alpha$-I gliadin/DQ2. The amino acid sequence of the $\alpha$-gliadin peptide in DQ8 is QQYPSG**E**GSFQPSQ**E**NPQ and the $\alpha$-I gliadin peptide (QLQPFPQP**E**LPY) with DQ2. Thrombin, TEV, and PreScission are protease cleavage sites incorporated into the protein constructs. (b) T cell clones restricted to either DQ8 or DQ2 produce IL-2 in response to the deamidated $\alpha$-gliadin/DQ8 or $\alpha$-I gliadin/DQ2 recombinant protein, respectively. (c) The DQ2 and (d) DQ8 T cell responses can be blocked in a dose dependent manner with a monoclonal DQ antibody.

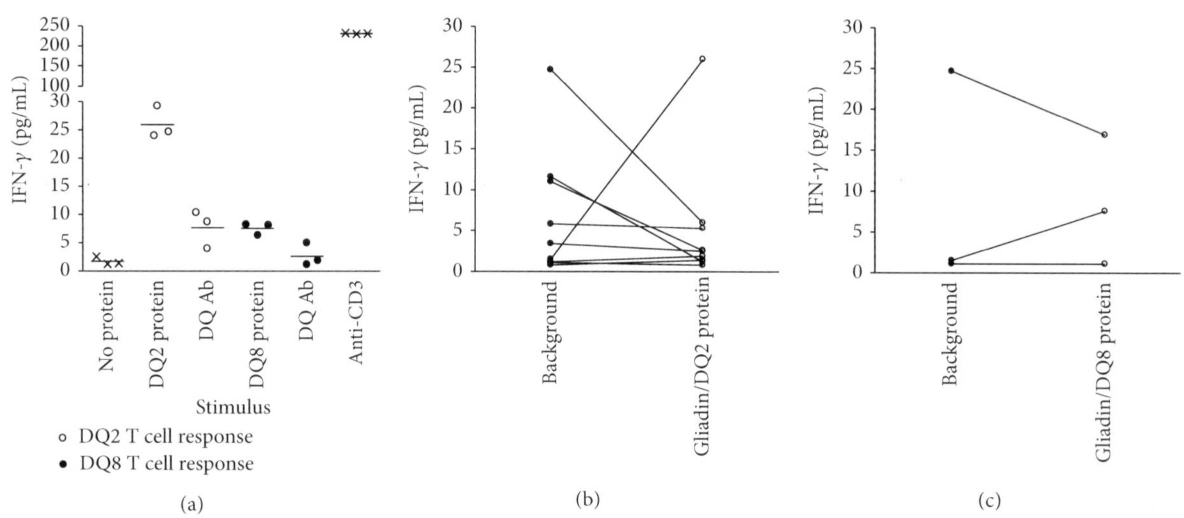


FIGURE 2: Recombinant peptide/MHC protein stimulates IFN-$\gamma$ production from bulk unfractionated PBMCs. (a) Stimulation of PBMCs from a single subject in triplicate having both HLA-DQ8 and DQ2 alleles showing response to the recombinant proteins greater than background. The IFN-$\gamma$ response is DQ restricted as it can be blocked with a monoclonal DQ antibody. An anti-CD3 monoclonal antibody is used to stimulate T cells as a positive control. The $\alpha$-gliadin p1E, p9E peptide (QQYPSG**E**GSFQPSQ**E**NPQ) is present in the DQ8 recombinant protein, while $\alpha$-I gliadin (QLQPFPQP**E**LPY) is present in the DQ2 protein. (b) Summative stimulation data from nine subjects all with HLA-DQ2 (DQA∗05:01, DQB∗02:01). (c) Data from three subjects having the HLA-DQ8 (DQA∗03:01, DQB∗03:02) allele.

varying concentrations for blocking experiments. All study subjects had cytokine stimulation assays performed.

*2.5. CFSE Proliferation Assay.* Isolated and unfractionated PBMCs were suspended at a density of $10^6$/mL in CFSE labeling buffer (1% BSA in PBS). Cells were labeled with 1 $\mu$M CFSE (eBioscience) for 10 minutes at 37°C. Labeling was quenched by adding chilled IMDM-C media at 5 times the volume at 0°C; cells were then incubated on ice for 5 minutes. Labeled cells were washed in PBS with 1% human AB serum, resuspended in media, and plated into a 24-well tissue culture plate at $10^6$ cells/well in 1 mL of media. Peptides (Genemed Synthesis Inc.) were HPLC purified (>95%), dissolved in PBS at a neutral pH, and used at a concentration of 10 $\mu$M. Pentacel vaccine (Sanofi Pasteur) was added at 2 $\mu$L per well as a positive control. After seven days of incubation

Table 1: Clinical characteristics, TTG antibody levels, histology, and HLA genotype of study participants.

| Case | Age (yrs) | Sex | TTG Ab level* | Histology marsh score | HLA DQ and DR alleles | | | | | |
|---|---|---|---|---|---|---|---|---|---|---|
| | | | | | DRB1 | DQA1 | DQB1 | DRB2 | DQA2 | DQB2 |
| 1 | 4 | F | 0.145 | 2 | 0404 | 0301 | 0302 | 0301 | 0501 | 0201 |
| 2 | 5 | F | 0.130 | 0 | 0403 | 0301 | 0302 | 0301 | 0501 | 0201 |
| 3 | 5 | M | 0.064 | 1 | 0301 | 0501 | 0201 | 1602 | 0501 | 0301 |
| 4 | 5 | M | 0.178 | 3b | 0301 | 0501 | 0201 | 0301 | 0501 | 0201 |
| 5 | 4 | F | 1.127 | 3c | 0301 | 0501 | 0201 | 0801 | 0401 | 0402 |
| 6 | 7 | F | 0.877 | No biopsy | 0701 | 0201 | 0202 | 1104 | 0501 | 0301 |
| 7 | 7 | F | 0.608 | 3c | 0301 | 0501 | 0201 | 1301 | 0103 | 0603 |
| 8 | 7 | M | 0.755 | 3b | 0301 | 0501 | 0201 | 0701 | 0201 | 0202 |
| 9 | 7 | F | 0.461 | 3b | 0301 | 0501 | 0201 | 1501 | 0102 | 0602 |
| 10 | 12 | F | 0.624 | 3b | 0701 | 0201 | 0202 | 1101 | 0501 | 0301 |
| 11 | 13 | M | 0.511 | 3b | 0403 | 0301 | 0302 | 0701 | 0201 | 0202 |
| 12 | 9 | F | 0.169 | 3b | 0301 | 0501 | 0201 | 0301 | 0501 | 0201 |

*TTG Ab ≥ 0.05 is elevated.

at 37°C in 5% $CO_2$, nonadherent cells were harvested and stained for FACS analysis using antibodies to CD4 (RPA-T4, BD Bioscience) and CD8 (RPA-T8, BD Bioscience). FACS analysis was done using a Becton-Dickenson FACS Caliber. Ten of the 12 study participants gave adequate numbers of PBMCs to perform CFSE proliferation assays.

*2.6. Statistical Analysis.* The percentage of $CD4^+CFSE^{lo}$ after proliferation to a given stimulus was compared with a paired Student's $t$-test as conditions were matched in the same subject. Response rates between $\alpha$-gliadin and $\gamma$-gliadin peptides were compared with a two-sided Fisher's exact text. For all statistical tests, a two-tailed $P$ value of $<0.05$ is considered significant. Analyses were performed using GraphPad Prism 4.0 software (La Jolla, CA).

## 3. Results

*3.1. Subjects.* Subjects with new-onset Celiac disease ($n = 12$) were recruited from the Children's Hospital Colorado Celiac Disease Center clinics. The study protocol was approved by the Institutional Review Board and written informed consent was obtained from all study participants. The Celiac subjects were young children and adolescents, with a mean age of 7.1 years, known to be TTG antibody positive and not on a gluten-free diet prior to having a small intestine biopsy. At the visit for intestinal biopsy, 11/12 (92%) patients had a biopsy and blood was collected for TTG antibody levels, HLA genotyping, and immune assays. Demographic and clinical characteristics are presented in Table 1. All of the subjects had positive TTG antibody levels and the majority 8/12 (75%) had stage 3 Marsh scores on histologic examination of a small intestine biopsy. HLA typing revealed that 9/12 (75%) subjects had the high risk HLA-DQ2 (DQA1∗05:01, DQB1∗02:01) allele and 3/12 (25%) had HLA-DQ8 (DQA1∗03:01, DQB1∗03:02) in addition to DQ2.

*3.2. T Cell Hybridomas Respond Robustly to Recombinant Peptide/MHC Protein.* We produced recombinant peptide/MHC protein to known $\alpha$-gliadin epitopes presented by HLA-DQ2 or DQ8 (Figure 1(a)). The two recombinant proteins, $\alpha$-I gliadin/DQ2 and deamidated $\alpha$-gliadin p1E, p9E/DQ8, are bioactive and able to robustly stimulate T cell hybridomas created from CD4 T cells cloned from small intestine lesions of adult CD subjects [12, 13]. The responses of these T cell hybridomas, measured by secreted IL-2, are dose dependent and required minimal amounts of protein (less than 1 $\mu$g/well) for stimulation (Figure 1(b), supplemental Figure 1(a)). The T cell responses are restricted to DQ2 or DQ8, depending on the class II molecule of the recombinant protein, as a DQ monoclonal antibody added in culture was able to abrogate IL-2 secretion (Figures 1(c) and 1(d) and supplemental Figures 1(b) and 1(c)).

*3.3. Detection of IFN-$\gamma$ Responses to Recombinant Peptide/MHC Proteins.* Having recombinant $\alpha$-gliadin/DQ proteins able to robustly stimulate T cell hybridomas, we evaluated the ability of the recombinant proteins to stimulate T cell responses from the peripheral blood of newly diagnosed CD subjects. We measured secreted cytokine responses (IFN-$\gamma$, IL-2, and IL-17) after culturing bulk unfractionated PBMCs in the presence of the $\alpha$-I gliadin/DQ2 or $\alpha$-gliadin p1E, p9E/DQ8 recombinant protein. Figure 2(a) depicts IFN-$\gamma$ responses to an individual having both the DQ2 (DQA1∗05:01, DQB1∗02:01) and DQ8 (DQA1∗03:01, DQB1∗03:02) alleles, which are identical to that of the recombinant proteins. There are responses to the protein greater than that of background alone and the responses are blocked by a DQ monoclonal antibody, suggesting that the measured responses are due to reactivity to the $\alpha$-gliadin/DQ proteins. The cumulative data from subjects having corresponding HLA alleles to that of the recombinant protein, however, failed to identify T cell reactivity above background responses (Figures 2(b) and 2(c)). The measured IL-2 and IL-17 responses were not greater than background in any of the subjects (data not shown).

*3.4. Proliferation of CD4 T Cells to the $\alpha$- and $\gamma$-Gliadin Peptides.* We next examined T cell responses to eleven known $\alpha$- and $\gamma$-gliadin epitopes [12, 19, 20], in contrast to recombinant peptide/MHC protein, previously identified from CD patients. CD4 T cell proliferation was assessed from the

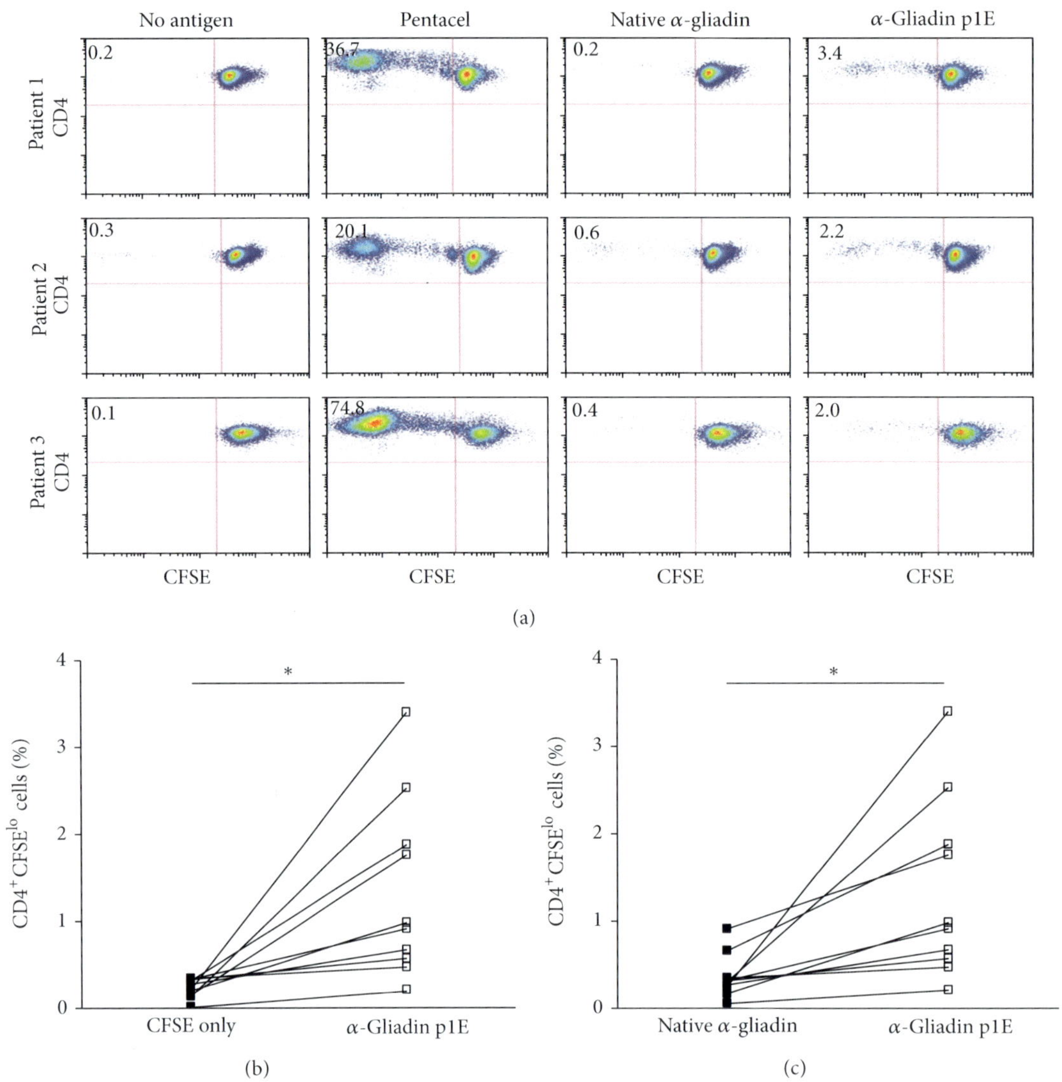


FIGURE 3: Proliferation of unfractionated PBMCs with α-gliadin peptides. (a) Representative data from three newly diagnosed Celiac subjects with 7-day CFSE proliferation assays. CD4 T cells proliferate in response to the α-gliadin p1E deamidated peptide without the in vitro addition of cytokines. (b) Summary data of proliferative responses comparing CFSE only (no antigen background) to the α-gliadin p1E peptide. (c) Proliferation of native α-gliadin to the α-gliadin p1E deamidated peptide. $^*P < 0.01$ using a paired $t$-test. Pentacel (positive control) is a childhood vaccine containing immunogens directed against diphtheria, tetanus, pertussis, poliomyelitis, and *Haemophilus influenzae* type b.

peripheral blood of newly diagnosed CD subjects. Figure 3 shows the proliferation results after bulk unfractionated PBMCs were labeled with CFSE and cultured for 7 days in the presence of a single gliadin peptide without the addition of any in vitro stimulus, that is, no IL-2, anti-CD3, or anti-CD28. Of the individuals having CFSE proliferation assays performed, there were robust responses to the α-gliadin$_{228-240}$ peptide (SGQGSFQPSQQNP), especially with a deamidated glutamate residue at the pocket 1 position. In all of the subjects, the single deamidated peptide (SG**E**GSFQPSQQNP) resulted in significantly more proliferation as measured by $CD4^+CFSE^{lo}$ cells compared to background (no antigen in culture) and the native α-gliadin peptide (Figures 3(b) and 3(c)). Interestingly, none of the subject's PBMC proliferated in response to the double deamidated α-gliadin peptide (α-gliadin p1E, p9E) and few responded (3/10) to the α-I-gliadin peptide, which are the peptides in the DQ8 and DQ2 recombinant protein, respectively (Table 2). Evaluating proliferative responses with a stimulation index ($CD4^+CFSE^{lo}$ condition/$CD4^+CFSE^{lo}$ background) greater than 3 revealed 12/60 (20%) responses to α-gliadin peptides compared to 3/50 (6%) of γ-gliadin peptides ($P = 0.049$). Overall, there were more proliferative responses to α-gliadin peptides compared to γ-gliadin in young children with newly diagnosed CD (Figure 4). In those children responding to two or more peptides, all three were HLA-DQ2/2 homozygotes (Table 3). Interestingly, the HLA-DQ2/2 children responded to epitopes which have been previously reported in the literature to be

TABLE 2: Proliferative responses to $\alpha$- and $\gamma$-gliadin epitopes.

| Epitope | Amino acid sequence* | Proliferation response** |
|---|---|---|
| Native $\alpha$-gliadin | SGQGSFQPSQQNP | 1/10 (10%) |
| $\alpha$-Gliadin p1E | SG**E**GSFQPSQQNP | 6/10 (60%) |
| $\alpha$-Gliadin p9E | SGQGSFQPSQ**E**NP | 2/10 (20%) |
| $\alpha$-Gliadin p1E, p9E | SG**E**GSFQPSQ**E**NP | 0/10 (0%) |
| $\alpha$-I-Gliadin | QLQPFPQP**E**LPY | 3/10 (30%) |
| $\alpha$-II-Gliadin | PQP**E**LPYPQPQL | 0/10 (0%) |
| Native $\gamma$-gliadin | FPQQPQQPYPQQPQQ | 0/10 (0%) |
| $\gamma$-Gliadin p1E | FP**E**QPQQPYPQQPQQ | 1/10 (10%) |
| $\gamma$-Gliadin p9E | FPQQPQQPYP**E**QPQQ | 0/10 (0%) |
| $\gamma$-Gliadin p1E, p9E | FP**E**QPQQPYP**E**QPQQ | 2/10 (20%) |
| $\gamma$-I-Gliadin | PEQPQQSFP**E**QERP | 0/10 (0%) |

*Glutamic acid (E) residues in bold are formed by tissue transglutaminase mediated deamidation. Underlined residues form the MHC class II peptide binding register.
**A stimulation index $\geq 3$ is considered a response.

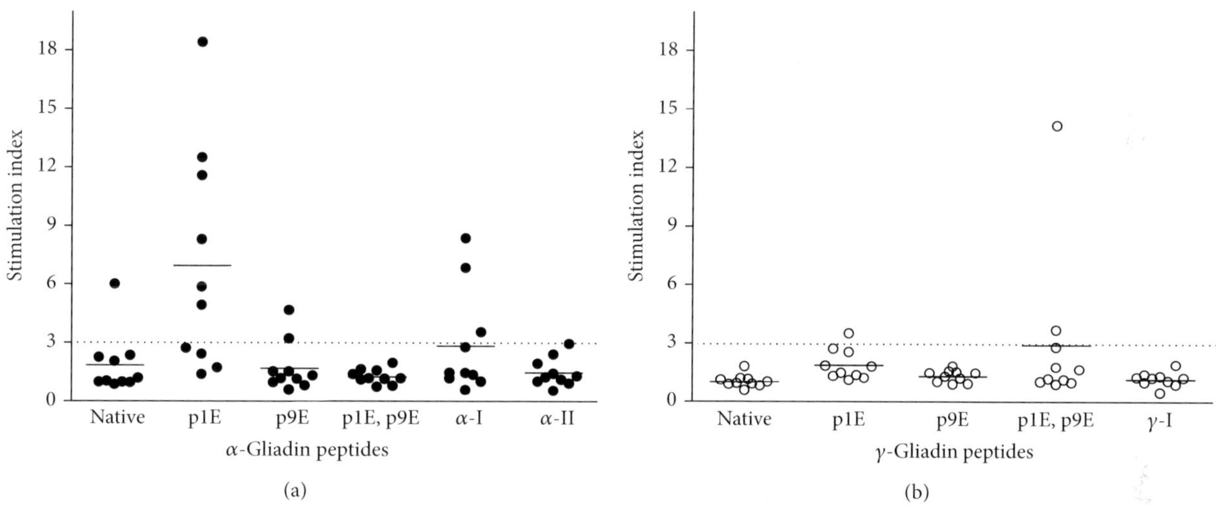


FIGURE 4: Proliferation of PBMCs from newly diagnosed Celiac patients to $\alpha$- and $\gamma$-gliadin peptides.(a) Proliferative responses to $\alpha$-gliadin and (b) $\gamma$-gliadin epitopes. Celiac subjects proliferate more in response to $\alpha$-gliadin peptides compared to $\gamma$-gliadin, especially the peptide deamidated at pocket 1 in which 6/10 subjects responded. Overall, there are 12/60 responses to $\alpha$-gliadin peptides compared to 3/50 for $\gamma$-gliadin ($P = 0.049$ with a Fisher's exact test). Dotted line is at a stimulation index ($CD4^+CFSE^{lo}$ cells at background/peptide condition) of 3, above which a responder is considered.

DQ8 restricted, suggesting that certain $\alpha$-gliadin peptides may be presented by either DQ8 or DQ2, particularly after selective deamidation.

## 4. Discussion

In the present study, we investigated peripheral T cell responses from young children with newly diagnosed CD prior to treatment with a gluten-free diet for two purposes: (1) develop a consistent and rapid assay to monitor peripheral T cell responses and (2) assess T cell responses to a panel of $\alpha$- and $\gamma$-gliadin epitopes. To develop a consistent and rapid assay using limited PBMCs, $\alpha$-gliadin/DQ2 and DQ8 recombinant protein constructs were produced which have the ability to robustly stimulate six different T cell clones derived from adult CD patients, suggesting the utility of this approach with polyclonal T cells from the peripheral blood. However, stimulation of PBMCs from young untreated children with CD did not uniformly elicit T cell responses. There are several possible reasons for the inability to detect reactivity with these protein constructs including the possibility that CD donors lack T cells that recognize a single DQ2 or DQ8 $\alpha$-gliadin epitope. Interestingly, the double deamidated $\alpha$-gliadin epitope covalently linked to recombinant DQ8 protein failed to elicit proliferative T cell responses in our study population, while three individuals with proliferative responses to $\alpha$-I gliadin did not produce IFN-$\gamma$ above background levels when stimulated with the recombinant $\alpha$-I gliadin/DQ2 protein. As these epitopes were identified from adult CD patients, our data supports the heterogeneity of T cell responses in CD and that children

Table 3: Overview of the T cell responses to tested DQ2 and DQ8 gliadin epitopes.

| Epitopes | | $\alpha$-gliadin | | | | | | $\gamma$-gliadin | | | | |
|---|---|---|---|---|---|---|---|---|---|---|---|---|
| | | DQ8 epitopes | | | | DQ2 epitopes | | | DQ8 epitopes | | | |
| Case | HLA-DQ genotype | Native | p1E | p9E | p1E, p9E | $\alpha$-I | $\alpha$-II | $\gamma$-I | Native | p1E | p9E | p1E, p9E |
| 2 | 2/8 | | ■ | | | | | | | | | |
| 3 | 2/7 | | ■ | | | | | | | | | |
| 4 | 2/2 | | ■ | | | ■ | | | | | | |
| 6 | 2/7 | | | | | | | | | | | |
| 7 | 2/6 | | | | | | | | | | | |
| 8 | 2/2 | ■ | ■ | ■ | | ■ | | | | | | ■ |
| 9 | 2/6 | | | | | | | | | | | |
| 10 | 2/7 | | ■ | | | | | | | | | |
| 11 | 2/8 | | | | | | | | | | | |
| 12 | 2/2 | | ■ | ■ | | ■ | | | | ■ | | ■ |

Peripheral T cell responses as measured by $CD4^{+}CFSE^{lo}$ proliferated cells for each individual with correlation to HLA-DQ genotype. Black boxes represent a response to the peptide with the SI $\geq 3$. Gliadin epitopes are denoted as previously reported in the literature to be presented by HLA-DQ2 ($\alpha$-I gliadin$_{57-68}$ QLQPFPQPELPY, $\alpha$-II gliadin$_{62-73}$ PQPELPYPQPQL, and $\gamma$-1 gliadin$_{139-152}$ PEQPQQSFPEQERP) or HLA-DQ8 ($\alpha$-gliadin$_{228-240}$ SGQGSFQPSQQNP and $\gamma$-gliadin$_{65-79}$ FPQQPQQPYPQQPQQ with and without deamidation at p1 and p9). Three of the new-onset CD children responding to two or more peptides have the DQ2/2 genotype.

may respond to different epitopes than adults [21]. Second, the donor's T cells may already be maximally stimulated as our patient population had not yet started a gluten-free diet. This is in agreement with studies reporting the need for a short-term gluten challenge in adult CD patients already on a gluten-free diet to elicit robust peripheral T cell responses [8, 9]. However, peripheral T cell responses can exist at disease onset and disappear with a gluten-free diet. Finally, it is possible that measuring secreted IFN-$\gamma$ may not be the best way to detect responses, and other methods for detecting antigen specific T cell responses to gliadin may be necessary, such as using gliadin/DQ2 fluorescent tetramers [22].

In addition to evaluating peptide/MHC recombinant protein to elicit T cell responses, we utilized proliferation assays with bulk unfractionated PBMCs to assess peptide reactivity. Stimulation of PBMCs from newly diagnosed and untreated CD children is better detected using proliferation assays rather than measurement of secreted cytokine. In our panel of DQ2 and DQ8 restricted antigens, we found that 6/10 children responded to at least one of the peptides tested, and the remainder did not respond to any tested peptide. It is notable that a peptide traditionally considered to be a DQ8 epitope, $\alpha$-gliadin p1E $^{228}$SG**E**GSFQPSQQNP$^{240}$, showed the greatest ability to stimulate T cells in 60% of children, even though only two children expressed the HLA-DQ8 allele (all of the children had at least one DQ2 allele). Furthermore, there were three subjects that had responses to two or more peptides and all three were DQ2/DQ2 homozygotes (Table 3). The peptide binding grooves of HLA-DQ2 and DQ8 share structural similarity with both molecules capable of anchoring peptides with acidic side chains (glutamic and aspartic acid) at pockets 1 and 9 [23]. With tissue transglutaminase present to deamidate gliadin peptides, it is plausible to hypothesize that certain deamidated epitopes have the potential to be presented by both the DQ2 and DQ8 molecules [24, 25]. There is precedence for this concept as both HLA-DR1 and DR4 class II molecules are capable of presenting the hemagglutinin peptide, HA$_{306-318}$, to T cells [26, 27].

In summary, T cell reactivity in young children with newly diagnosed and untreated CD is heterogeneous but favors reactivity to $\alpha$-gliadin epitopes more than $\gamma$-gliadin. It is unlikely that a single gliadin epitope will elicit T cell responses in all individuals and a short-term gluten challenge may be necessary to detect ample T cell reactivity in the peripheral circulation. However, it is possible to detect T cell responses without a gluten challenge or in vitro stimulus other than antigen, when measuring proliferative responses. A more comprehensive screening of gliadin epitopes in young children with newly diagnosed CD is necessary to identify peripheral blood T cell reactivity, followed by repeat assessments over time to correlate responses to disease activity and treatment with a gluten-free diet. Monitoring peripheral T cell responses to gliadin epitopes present at disease onset, which can disappear with a gluten-free diet, has clinical utility in identifying cases of refractory CD or in assessing the effectiveness of emerging therapies for CD treatment.

## Conflict of Interests

The authors E. Liu, K. McDaniel, S. Case, L. Yu, and A. W. Michels have no conflict of interests regarding the publication of this paper. The authors B. Gerhartz, N. Ostermann, G. Fankhauser, V. Hungerford, C. Zou, M. Luyten, and K. J. Seidl are all employees at Novartis and may own Novartis stock.

## Acknowledgments

This work was supported by Grants from the National Institute of Diabetes and Digestive Kidney Diseases (R01 DK032083 and K08 DK095995) and the Celiac Disease Center at the Children's Hospital Colorado. The authors would like to thank Ludvig Sollid for providing DNA constructs of the T cell receptor from gliadin responsive T cell clones.

## References


[1] P. H. R. Green and C. Cellier, "Medical progress: celiac disease," *The New England Journal of Medicine*, vol. 357, no. 17, pp. 1731–1743, 2007.

[2] L.-E. Fallang, E. Bergseng, K. Hotta, A. Berg-Larsen, C.-Y. Kim, and L. M. Sollid, "Differences in the risk of celiac disease associated with HLA-DQ2.5 or HLA-DQ2.2 are related to sustained gluten antigen presentation," *Nature Immunology*, vol. 10, no. 10, pp. 1096–1101, 2009.

[3] L. Shan, Ø. Molberg, I. Parrot et al., "Structural basis for gluten intolerance in Celiac Sprue," *Science*, vol. 297, no. 5590, pp. 2275–2279, 2002.

[4] M. F. Kagnoff, "Celiac disease: pathogenesis of a model immunogenetic disease," *Journal of Clinical Investigation*, vol. 117, no. 1, pp. 41–49, 2007.

[5] V. Abadie, L. M. Sollid, L. B. Barreiro, and B. Jabri, "Integration of genetic and immunological insights into a model of celiac disease pathogenesis," *Annual Review of Immunology*, vol. 29, pp. 493–525, 2011.

[6] S. Guandalini and M. Setty, "Celiac disease," *Current Opinion in Gastroenterology*, vol. 24, no. 6, pp. 707–712, 2008.

[7] Ø. Molberg, S. N. Mcadam, R. Körner et al., "Tissue transglutaminase selectively modifies gliadin peptides that are recognized by gut-derived T cells in celiac disease," *Nature Medicine*, vol. 4, no. 6, pp. 713–717, 1998.

[8] R. P. Anderson, P. Degano, A. J. Godkin, D. P. Jewell, and A. V. S. Hill, "In vivo antigen challenge in celiac disease identifies a single transglutaminase-modified peptide as the dominant A-gliadin T-cell epitope," *Nature Medicine*, vol. 6, no. 3, pp. 337–342, 2000.

[9] R. P. Anderson, D. A. van Heel, J. A. Tye-Din et al., "T cells in peripheral blood after gluten challenge in coeliac disease," *Gut*, vol. 54, no. 9, pp. 1217–1223, 2005.

[10] J. O'Keeffe, K. Mills, J. Jackson, and C. Feighery, "T cell proliferation, MHC class II restriction and cytokine products of gliadin-stimulated peripheral blood mononuclear cells (PBMC)," *Clinical and Experimental Immunology*, vol. 117, no. 2, pp. 269–276, 1999.

[11] J. A. Tye-Din, J. A. Stewart, J. A. Dromey et al., "Comprehensive, quantitative mapping of T cell epitopes in gluten in celiac disease," *Science Translational Medicine*, vol. 2, no. 41, Article ID 41ra51, 2010.

[12] S. Tollefsen, H. Arentz-Hansen, B. Fleckenstein et al., "HLA-DQ2 and -DQ8 signatures of gluten T cell epitopes in celiac disease," *Journal of Clinical Investigation*, vol. 116, no. 8, pp. 2226–2236, 2006.

[13] S. E. Broughton, J. Petersen, A. Theodossis et al., "Biased T cell receptor usage directed against human leukocyte antigen DQ8-restricted gliadin peptides is associated with celiac disease," *Immunity*, vol. 37, no. 4, pp. 611–621, 2012.

[14] M. Li, L. Yu, C. Tiberti et al., "A report on the international transglutaminase autoantibody workshop for celiac disease," *American Journal of Gastroenterology*, vol. 104, no. 1, pp. 154–163, 2009.

[15] T. L. Bugawan and H. A. Erlich, "Rapid typing of HLA-DQB1 DNA polymorphism using nonradioactive oligonucleotide probes and amplified DNA," *Immunogenetics*, vol. 33, no. 3, pp. 163–170, 1991.

[16] A. W. Michels, D. A. Ostrov, L. Zhang et al., "Structure-based selection of small molecules to alter allele-specific MHC class II antigen presentation," *Journal of Immunology*, vol. 187, no. 11, pp. 5921–5930, 2011.

[17] J. Holst, A. L. Szymczak-Workman, K. M. Vignali, A. R. Burton, C. J. Workman, and D. A. Vignali, "Generation of T-cell receptor retrogenic mice," *Nature Protocols*, vol. 1, no. 1, pp. 406–417, 2006.

[18] J. P. Scott-Browne, J. White, J. W. Kappler, L. Gapin, and P. Marrack, "Germline-encoded amino acids in the $\alpha$B T-cell receptor control thymic selection," *Nature*, vol. 458, no. 7241, pp. 1043–1046, 2009.

[19] H. Sjöström, K. E. A. Lundin, Ø. Molberg et al., "Identification of a gliadin T-cell epitope in coeliac disease: general importance of gliadin deamidation for intestinal T-cell recognition," *Scandinavian Journal of Immunology*, vol. 48, no. 2, pp. 111–115, 1998.

[20] H. Arentz-Hansen, R. Körner, Ø. Molberg et al., "The intestinal T cell response to $\alpha$-gliadin in adult celiac disease is focused on a single deamidated glutamine targeted by tissue transglutaminase," *The Journal of Experimental Medicine*, vol. 191, no. 4, pp. 603–612, 2000.

[21] W. Vader, Y. Kooy, P. van Veelen et al., "The Gluten response in children with celiac disease is directed toward multiple gliadin and glutenin peptides," *Gastroenterology*, vol. 122, no. 7, pp. 1729–1737, 2002.

[22] H. Quarsten, S. N. McAdam, T. Jensen et al., "Staining of celiac disease-relevant T cells by peptide-DQ2 multimers," *Journal of Immunology*, vol. 167, no. 9, pp. 4861–4868, 2001.

[23] E. Y. Jones, L. Fugger, J. L. Strominger, and C. Siebold, "MHC class II proteins and disease: a structural perspective," *Nature Reviews Immunology*, vol. 6, no. 4, pp. 271–282, 2006.

[24] K. N. Henderson, J. A. Tye-Din, H. H. Reid et al., "A structural and immunological basis for the role of human leukocyte antigen DQ8 in celiac disease," *Immunity*, vol. 27, no. 1, pp. 23–34, 2007.

[25] K. N. Henderson, H. H. Reid, N. A. Borg et al., "The production and crystallization of the human leukocyte antigen class II molecules HLA-DQ2 and HLA-DQ8 complexed with deamidated gliadin peptides implicated in coeliac disease," *Acta Crystallographica Section F*, vol. 63, part 12, pp. 1021–1025, 2007.

[26] J. V. Brawley and P. Concannon, "Complementarity-determining region 1 sequence requirements drive limited V$\alpha$ usage in response to influenza hemagglutinin 307-319 peptide," *Journal of Immunology*, vol. 168, no. 8, pp. 3894–3901, 2002.

[27] J. Hennecke and D. C. Wiley, "Structure of a complex of the human $\alpha/\beta$ T cell receptor (TCR) HA1.7, Influenza hemagglutinin peptide, and major histocompatibility complex class II molecule, HLA-DR4 (DRA*0101 and DRBI*0401): insight into TCR cross-restriction and alloreactivity," *The Journal of Experimental Medicine*, vol. 195, no. 5, pp. 571–581, 2002.

# 20

# Differential Immunotoxicity Induced by Two Different Windows of Developmental Trichloroethylene Exposure

**Kathleen M. Gilbert, William Woodruff, and Sarah J. Blossom**

*University of Arkansas for Medical Sciences, Arkansas Children's Hospital Research Institute, 13 Children's Way, Little Rock, AR 72202, USA*

Correspondence should be addressed to Kathleen M. Gilbert; gilbertkathleenm@uams.edu

Academic Editor: Aristo Vojdani

Developmental exposure to environmental toxicants may induce immune system alterations that contribute to adult stage autoimmune disease. We have shown that continuous exposure of MRL+/+ mice to trichloroethylene (TCE) from gestational day (GD) 0 to postnatal day (PND) 49 alters several aspects of $CD4^+$ T cell function. This window of exposure corresponds to conception-adolescence/young adulthood in humans. More narrowly defining the window of TCE developmental exposure causes immunotoxicity that would establish the stage at which avoidance and/or intervention would be most effective. The current study divided continuous TCE exposure into two separate windows, namely, gestation only (GD0 to birth (PND0)) and early-life only (PND0-PND49). The mice were examined for specific alterations in $CD4^+$ T cell function at PND49. One potentially long-lasting effect of developmental exposure, alterations in retrotransposon expression indicative of epigenetic alterations, was found in peripheral $CD4^+$ T cells from both sets of developmentally exposed mice. Interestingly, certain other effects, such as alterations in thymus cellularity, were only found in mice exposed to TCE during gestation. In contrast, expansion of memory/activation cell subset of peripheral $CD4^+$ T cells were only found in mice exposed to TCE during early life. Different windows of developmental TCE exposure can have different functional consequences.

## 1. Introduction

The chlorinated hydrocarbon and industrial solvent trichloroethylene (TCE) is a widespread environmental contaminant. As noted in a 2011 IRIS report, the EPA has concluded that "there is substantial potential for environmental exposure to TCE as its improper disposal has resulted in the widespread contamination of groundwater and soil" [1]. Contact with TCE may be elevated for people living near waste facilities, where TCE is released, residents of some urban or industrialized areas, or individuals using TCE-containing products. Regardless of whether TCE exposure is oral, dermal, or inhalation-based, the chemical is rabidly absorbed and distributed. Based on the likelihood of exposure together with likely negative health impact TCE is consistently ranked 16th out of 275 chemicals on the CERCLA list of hazardous chemicals.

One of the predominant human health effects associated with TCE exposure is immunotoxicity, most notably the development of autoimmunity and other types of hypersensitivity diseases. Chronic TCE exposure in adults (both occupational and environmental) has been linked to a variety of autoimmune diseases including systemic lupus erythematosus, scleroderma, hepatitis, and diabetes [2–10]. In addition, there are many cases in recent years of a TCE-induced hypersensitivity disorder that targets the skin and liver [11, 12]. Alterations in $CD4^+$ T cells are often found to be an effect biomarker in patients suffering from TCE-induced immunotoxicity [2, 13–15].

Most studies of TCE-induced autoimmunity or hypersensitivity in humans have focused on adult exposure to the higher concentrations of TCE that are most commonly found in the workplace. The type of low-level TCE exposure people may experience through drinking water contamination is generally thought to be risk-free. However, there is evidence that the developing immune system is especially sensitive to even low-level immunotoxicants. A recent review compared early versus adult exposure to several immunosuppressive toxins including lead and tributyltin in animal models [16]. In all cases, sensitivity was greater if exposure occurred during development. In fact, immune suppression in developmentally-exposed offspring often occurred at doses that were ineffective in adults. Developmental sensitivity to toxicants has also been found in humans [17, 18]. This includes evidence that adult onset autoimmune disease can be triggered by pre- and early postnatal toxicant exposure [19, 20].

Developmental exposure to TCE in humans is not uncommon; one study showed that 100% of breast milk samples from 4 US urban areas had detectable levels of TCE [21]. Gestational and early life TCE exposure has primarily been examined for its neurotoxicity [22]. However, children continuously exposed for 3–19 years beginning *in utero* to a water supply contaminated with solvents [with TCE being the predominant toxicant (267 ppb)] had altered ratios of T cell subsets and increased levels of autoantibodies [2].

We have studied a direct cause and effect relationship between TCE exposure and immunotoxicity in a mouse model. Adult exposure to TCE primarily altered effector $CD4^+$ T cells, with little effect on $CD8^+$ T cells, B cells, or $T_{reg}$ cells. The effects of TCE on $CD4^+$ T cells were seen after only 4 weeks and included expansion of activated/memory ($CD44^{hi}$ $CD62L^{lo}$) $CD4^+$ T cells and altered cytokine production [23–25]. Adult TCE exposure seemed to have minimal effect on thymus cellularity. After chronic adult exposure (26–32 weeks) the TCE-induced alterations in $CD4^+$ T cells led to T cell-mediated liver inflammation identical to that seen in idiopathic autoimmune hepatitis (AIH) in humans [24, 26].

We have also examined mice following continuous TCE exposure beginning *in utero* and then encompassing lactation as well as an additional 4 weeks of direct exposure. This continuous exposure to TCE at concentrations lower than that used for adult exposure altered thymocyte cellularity and modified the phenotype and function of peripheral $CD4^+$ T cells [27].

Although informative, studies of continuous toxicant exposure do not reveal which windows of exposure have the most impact on the developing immune system. For example, it has been shown that early gestational exposure to certain toxicants such as lead are not as likely to suppress Th1 function as late gestational exposure [28]. This suggests that within the developmental period there exists particular windows of relative susceptibility and resistance [29]. Thus, knowing more about the functional outcomes of particular developmental windows of TCE exposure is needed to accurately estimate risk and to plan interventions. This study was designed to compare central and peripheral immune system alterations in mice exposed to TCE during two crucial windows of immune development and toxicant sensitivity, namely, gestation [GD0 to birth (PND0)] and early life (PND0 to PND49).

## 2. Materials and Methods

*2.1. Mice and TCE Exposure.* Developmental exposure to TCE has been described [30]. Basically, breeding pairs of 8-week-old MRL+/+ mice (Jackson Laboratories, Bar Harbor, ME) were established. In one experiment immediately following detection of pregnancy, GD0, the females were divided (following stratified randomization) into 3 groups and given water with 0, 0.01, or 0.1 mg/mL TCE. Controls were given water containing only 1% Alkamuls EL-620, the reagent used to solubilize the TCE. All the drinking water was Ultrapure unchlorinated to assure that chlorination by-products do not confound the results. The TCE-containing drinking water was changed 3 times/week to offset degradation of TCE. Maternal exposure to TCE-containing drinking water ended at birth in this experiment. The female pups that underwent the gestation only exposure to TCE were examined at PND49. As observed previously maternal toxicity was not noted at the level of body weight, mating index, fertility index, sex ratio of litters, gestational length, and food and water consumption.

In the second experiment, the female breeders were not exposed to TCE during pregnancy, but were given TCE-containing drinking water immediately after giving birth. Thus, the pups were exposed to TCE from PND0 to PND21 via lactation. Once the female pups were weaned at PND21 they were exposed to TCE directly in their drinking water for the duration of the experiment. The female pups from this early life exposure were sacrificed at PND49.

Both female breeders and resulting pups in both experiments were weighed weekly and water consumption was monitored. All studies were approved by the Animal Care and Use Committee at the University of Arkansas for Medical Sciences.

When the female pups were sacrificed at PND49 pooled spleen cell suspensions and thymus cell suspensions from paired mice from each litter ($n$ = 5–7 litters/treatment group) were examined by flow cytometry. In addition, $CD4^+$ T cells were isolated from the pooled spleen cell suspensions and stimulated with immobilized anti-CD3 antibody and anti-CD28 antibody for 24 hours as described [25]. Culture supernatants were then collected for cytokine evaluation, and the activated $CD4^+$ T cells were frozen for subsequent qRT-PCR analysis. In addition, adherent macrophages isolated from pooled peritoneal exudates from 2-3 mice/litter were incubated for 20 hours in medium alone or in the presence of LPS (1 $\mu$g/mL) and IFN-$\gamma$ (100 units/mL). Approximately 80% of adherent peritoneal exudate cells (PEC), regardless of treatment group, expressed the transmembrane protein F4/80, a marker of mature macrophages (data not shown). Culture supernatants from the peritoneal macrophages were then collected for cytokine evaluation. RLT Lysis Buffer (Qiagen Sciences, Germantown, MD) was then added directly to the remaining adherent cells before freezing for subsequent qRT-PCR analysis.

*2.2. qRT-PCR.* Fluorescence-based quantitative reverse transcriptase polymerase chain reaction (qRT-PCR) was conducted using RNA isolated from activated $CD4^+$ T cells,

Table 1: Primer sequences used for qRT-PCR.

| Gene | | Primer sequences 5′ to 3′ | Tm (°C) |
|---|---|---|---|
| *Aire* | Sense | AGATCGCGGTGGCCATAG | 57.4 |
| | Antisense | TCGTGGTCGGCTAGAGCAT | 58.4 |
| *Bax* | Sense | TTGCTGATGGCAACTTCAACTGGG | 60.2 |
| | Antisense | TGTCCAGCCCATGATGGTTCTGAT | 60.4 |
| *Bim* | Sense | CTGTGTAATGTGCCCTACTGTTTC | 55.8 |
| | Antisense | GGAAGAGAACCAGCCACTACC | 57.3 |
| *CD70* | Sense | TGCTGGTGGTGTTTATTACTGTG | 55.4 |
| | Antisense | CTCTGGTCCGTGTGTGAAGG | 57.7 |
| *Cdkn1a* | Sense | AATCCTGGTGATGTCCGACCTGTT | 60.2 |
| | Antisense | GTGACGAAGTCAAAGTTCCACCGT | 59.4 |
| *Dnmt1* | Sense | TGATAAGGAGGACAAGGAGAATGC | 56.4 |
| | Antisense | CACCGCCAAGTTAGGACACC | 58.3 |
| *Dnmt3a* | Sense | CAGCACCATTCCTGGTCATGCAAA | 60.2 |
| | Antisense | TCCTGTGTGGTAGGCACCTGAAAT | 60.2 |
| *Fas* | Sense | CGCCCGCTGTTTTCCC | 57.6 |
| | Antisense | GCAAGCACCAGAGGCAGG | 59.4 |
| *FasL* | Sense | GGCTGGGTGCCATGCA | 59.4 |
| | Antisense | GGCACTGCTGTCTACCCAGAA | 59.2 |
| *IAP* | Sense | GCACCCTCAAAGCCTATCTTAT | 54.6 |
| | Antisense | TCCCTTGGTCAGTCTGGATTT | 55.8 |
| *Ifng* | Sense | AGCTCATCCGAGTGGTCCAC | 59.1 |
| | Antisense | AGCAGCGACTCCTTTTCCG | 57.8 |
| *Il2* | Sense | CCCAAGCAGGCCACAGAATTGAAA | 60.2 |
| | Antisense | AGTCAAATCCAGAACATGCCGCAG | 59.9 |
| *Il4* | Sense | AGCCATATCCACGGATGCGACAAA | 60.8 |
| | Antisense | AATATGCGAAGCACCTTGGAAGCC | 60.0 |
| *Il6* | Sense | AGAGGAGACTTCACAGAGGATACC | 57.1 |
| | Antisense | CATTTCCACGATTTCCCAGAGAAC | 56.1 |
| *Muerv* | Sense | TGGTGGTCGAGATGGAGGTTA | 57.5 |
| | Antisense | CCGTGAATGGTGGTTTTAGCA | 55.8 |

peritoneal macrophages or thymocytes. The details for conducting qRT-PCR, including quality control and reference gene selection, have been described previously [31]. The primers used are described in Table 1.

*2.3. Phenotypic Analysis of Spleen and Thymus Cells.* The phenotypic analysis of 30,000 events per sample was carried out using a CyFlow ML (Partec GmbH, Munster, Germany) as described previously using monoclonal antibodies from BD Biosciences or eBioscience [32], and the data were presented as mean percentage ± standard error. Fluorescence Minus One controls and isotype Ig controls were included.

*2.4. Cytokine Analysis.* The culture supernatants from the activated $CD4^+$ T cells or peritoneal macrophages were examined using READY-SET-GO ELISA kits for mouse IL-2, IL-6, or TNF-$\alpha$ from eBioscience, San Diego, CA.

*2.5. Statistics.* The data are presented as means and standard deviations. Assays were conducted using samples from 5–7 individual litters per treatment group. Comparisons between values obtained from controls and different treatment were made using a Student's $t$-test. The threshold for statistical significance was set at $\alpha = 0.05$.

## 3. Results

*3.1. Gross Changes Induced by TCE Exposure.* Two windows of TCE developmental exposure were examined in female MRL+/+ mice. The mice were either exposed to TCE during gestation (GD0-PND0) or during early life (PND0-PND49). All of the mice were assessed at 7 weeks of age (PND49) for a variety of immune parameters. TCE was added at 0.01 or 0.1 mg/mL to the drinking water of the dams and/or the pups. Based on water consumption, the resulting TCE exposures were described in Figure 1. Many of the alterations in $CD4^+$ T

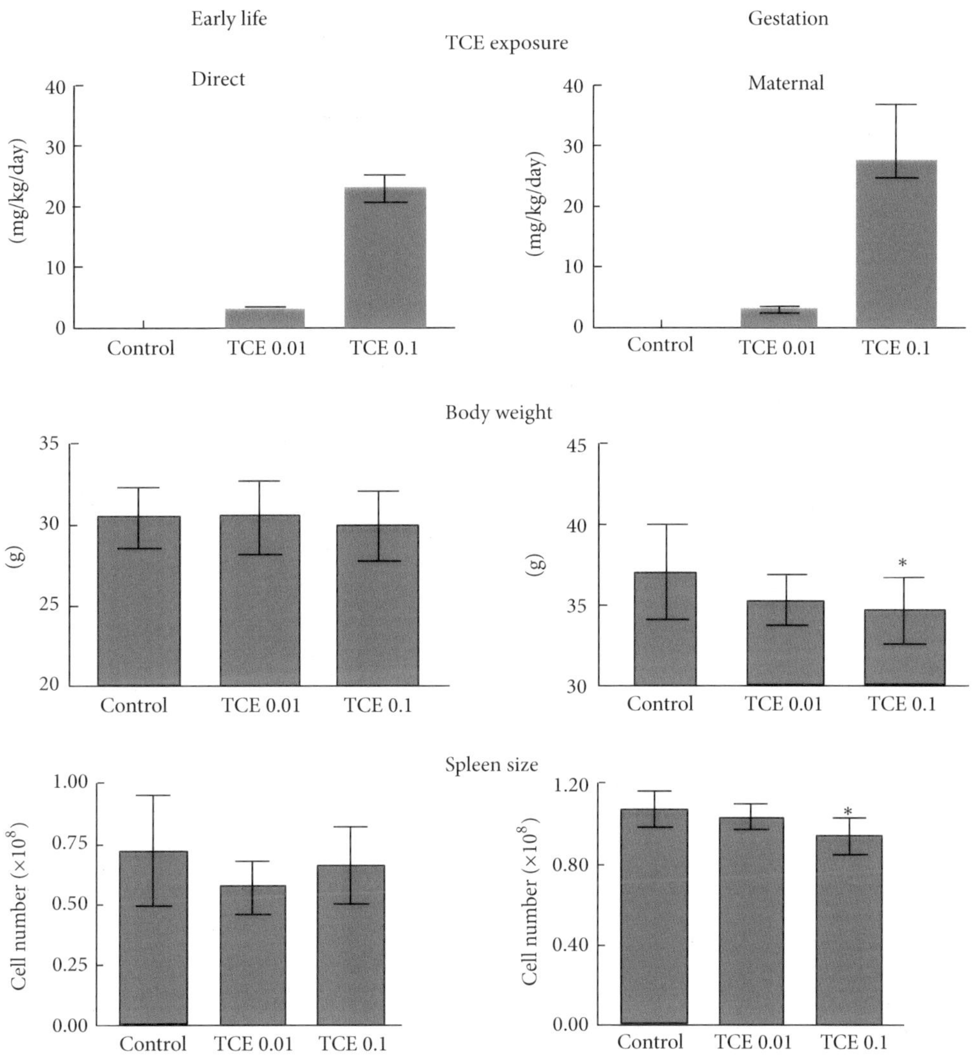


FIGURE 1: Characteristics of two windows of developmental TCE exposure. Female mice were exposed to TCE (0.01 or 0.1 mg/mL) during gestation only, or during early life only (lactation and 4 weeks of direct exposure). All of the developmentally-exposed mice were examined at PND49. For the gestation only exposure, maternal TCE ingestion based on water consumption was presented. For the early life exposure direct TCE ingestion of the pups postweaning based on water consumption was presented. Body weight and spleen cell numbers (mean ± SD) were determined at PND49. *Significantly different ($\alpha < 0.05$) compared to control values.

cells associated with adult-only direct exposure to TCE were found after 4 weeks [23, 25, 33]. Thus, the PND49 end point can be used to test how the effects of gestational or early life exposure compared to the effects of a direct 4-week adult-only exposure.

Similar to adult exposure to TCE, the early life exposure in the current study did not alter the weight of the female pups at PND49 (Figure 1). In contrast, female pups exposed to the highest concentration of TCE during gestation were significantly smaller than controls. Spleen cell numbers in the same mice were also lower than those of controls. Spleen cell numbers were not altered in mice exposed to TCE during early life only. Thus, TCE exposure during gestation rather than early life, did induce some gross changes in body weight and spleen size.

*3.2. Developmental TCE Exposure and Changes in Macrophage Function.* Potential TCE-induced alterations in peripheral immune function were examined. These included spleen cellularity and functional activity of key cellular components of chronic inflammation, namely, macrophages and $CD4^+$ T cells. IL-6 is a pleiotropic cytokine that has proinflammatory, anti-inflammatory and growth factor properties. Adult exposure to TCE has been shown to suppress macrophage production of IL-6 [34]. In the current study early life exposure to TCE at 0.1 mg/mL similarly inhibited IL-6 production at both the protein and gene expression level (Figure 2). In contrast, gestational exposure to TCE did not suppress IL-6 production by peritoneal macrophages.

*3.3. Developmental TCE Exposure and Changes in $CD4^+$ T Cell Gene Expression.* Early-occurring changes in peripheral

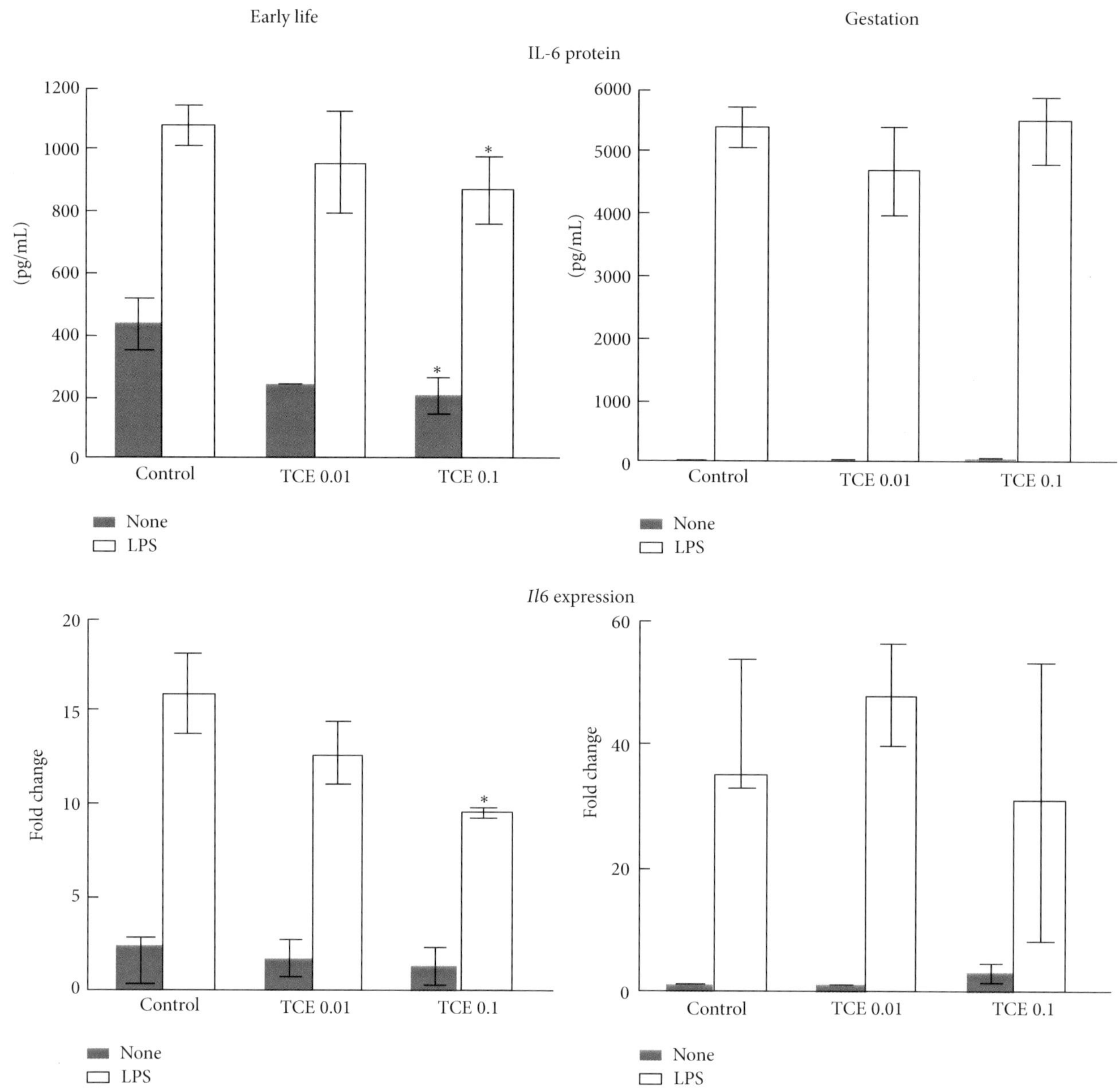


FIGURE 2: TCE inhibited IL-6 production and *Il6* expression in macrophages. Peritoneal macrophages were incubated with LPS and IFN-$\gamma$ following isolation from untreated control mice or from mice exposed to TCE (0.01 or 0.1 mg/mL) during gestation only or during early life only. Culture supernatants were examined for IL-6 (mean ± SD). *Il6* gene expression was examined in the same peritoneal macrophages. The data represents the mean ± SD. *Significantly different ($\alpha < 0.05$) compared to control values.

$CD4^+$ T cells have been observed following adult and continuous exposure to TCE. These include expansion of the activation/memory subset of peripheral $CD4^+$ T cells and increases in the production of T cell-derived cytokines [24]. These potential alterations were assessed in the current study. TCE did not alter the percentages of total splenic $CD4^+$ T cells, $CD8^+$ T cells, or B cells, regardless of concentration or window of exposure (data not shown). However, similar to both adult and continuous TCE exposure, early life exposure to TCE at 0.01 or 0.1 mg/mL did increase the percentage of $CD44^{hi}$ $CD62L^{lo}$ $CD4^+$ T cells, the population of $CD4^+$ T cells considered to represent a memory/activated $CD4^+$ T cell phenotype (Figure 3). Gestational exposure did not increase the percentage of activated/memory $CD4^+$ T cells in the periphery at PND49.

Splenic $CD4^+$ T cells isolated from control and TCE-treated mice were activated *in vitro* prior to an examination of gene expression.Compared to baseline gene expression in unstimulated $CD4^+$ T cells, activation *in vitro* increased expression of almost all genes in all $CD4^+$ T cells (data not shown). To simplify comparison the gene expression of *in vitro* stimulated $CD4^+$ T cells from TCE-treated mice was compared to that of similarly activated $CD4^+$ T cells from control mice. This comparison yielded some subtle but

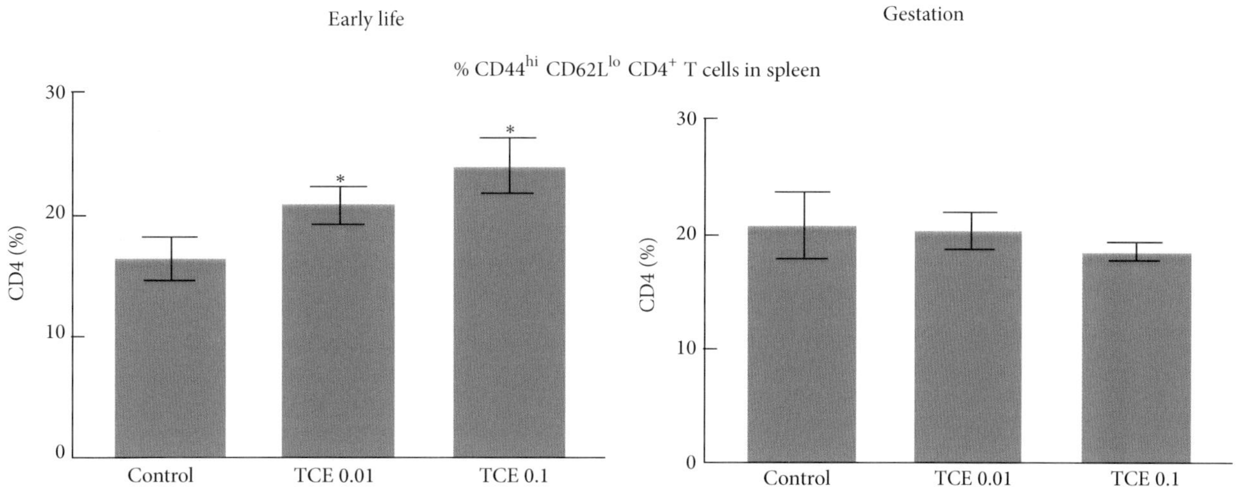


FIGURE 3: TCE enhanced the percentage of memory/activated $CD4^+$ T cells following early life exposure. Spleen cell suspensions from PND49 mice that had been exposed to TCE during gestation only or during early life only were examined by flow cytometry to determine the percentage of $CD4^+$ T cells that expressed high levels of CD44 and low levels of CD62L. *Significantly different ($\alpha < 0.05$) compared to control values.

significant differences. As observed previously following adult exposure early life exposure to TCE increased expression of *Ifng* and *Il2* but had little effect on *Il4* (Table 2). Gestational exposure, unlike early life exposure, did not increase the expression of these cytokine genes in activated peripheral $CD4^+$ T cells. Thus, once again, early life exposure, unlike gestational exposure, mirrored what has been observed in adult and continuous TCE exposure.

Although $CD4^+$ T cells from the two windows of developmental TCE exposure differed in their expression of cytokine genes, they demonstrated remarkably similar expression profiles for *Iap* and *Muerv*. These two genes encode for retrotransposons Intracisternal A particle and murine endogenous retrovirus. The expression of these two retrotransposons is kept in check by epigenetic processes, predominantly DNA methylation [35]. Events that cause global DNA hypomethylation tend to increase expression of *Iap* and *Muerv*, while DNA hypermethylation tends to suppress baseline expression of the retrotransposons. In this study both gestational and early life exposure to the lower concentration of TCE inhibited expression of Iap and MuERV in peripheral $CD4^+$ T cells.

DNA methylation is regulated by DNA methyltransferases, a family of enzymes that catalyze the transfer of a methyl group to DNA. This family encompasses *Dnmt1* that is thought to participate in maintenance DNA methylation, and *Dnmt3a*, involved in *de novo* DNA methylation in response to external stimuli [36]. At PND49, neither TCE exposure appreciably altered expression of *Dnmt1* or *Dnmt3a* in $CD4^+$ T cells. Thus, the downregulation of *Iap* and *Muerv* in $CD4^+$ T cells from mice developmentally exposed to TCE, regardless of gestation or early life, could not be explained by an increase in the expression of *Dnmt1* or *Dnmt3a*.

*3.4. Developmental TCE Exposure and Changes in $CD4^+$ T Cell Function.* In addition to gene expression, cytokine production was examined as a potential marker of TCE-induced alterations in $CD4^+$ T cell function. Early life exposure to TCE, similar to adult exposure, increased the production of certain cytokines including IL-2 by $CD4^+$ T cells (Figure 4). Gestational exposure alone was not sufficient to increase cytokine production in the peripheral $CD4^+$ T cells.

*3.5. Developmental TCE Exposure and Thymus Cellularity.* The effects of developmental TCE exposure on central immune function were also examined. The number of total thymocytes was not altered by TCE exposure during gestation or early life (data not shown). However, the composition of thymic subsets was altered in one set of the TCE-exposed mice. Exposure to the lower concentration of TCE during gestation increased the percentage of thymic single positive $CD4^+$ T cells (Figure 5). The same mice also demonstrated an increase in the percentage of double negative population 1 (DN1) thymocytes as well as a decrease in percentage of DN4 thymocytes. Unlike gestational exposure early life exposure to TCE did not change the percentages of the different thymocyte subsets measured. Thus, in terms of thymocyte cellularity early life exposure generated results that resembled that of adult exposure, while gestational exposure generated results that most resembled that of previously documented continuous exposure [27]. The thymocytes were then incubated for 18 hours to promote gene expression. Interestingly, neither gestational nor early life exposure to TCE altered *Iap* expression in the thymus, unlike peripheral $CD4^+$ T cells (Figure 6). This decreases the likelihood that the altered thymus cellularity of the gestationally exposed mice could be attributed to global changes in DNA methylation.

*3.6. Developmental TCE Exposure and Thymus Gene Expression.* The expression of genes that regulate thymic apoptosis and development were examined in an attempt to explain

TABLE 2: Gene expression in CD4$^+$ T cells from mice exposed to TCE during gestation or early life.

| | Control | Early life TCE 0.01 | TCE0.1 | Control | Gestation TCE 0.01 | TCE 0.1 |
|---|---|---|---|---|---|---|
| *Iap* | 1.0 ± 0.17 | **0.12 ± 0.02** | 0.42 ± 0.36 | 1.00 ± 0.1 | **0.43 ± 0.05** | **0.72 ± 0.19** |
| *Muerv* | 0.95 ± 0.26 | **0.6 ± 0.11** | 0.76 ± 0.23 | 1.0 ± 0.15 | **0.44 ± 0.04** | 0.95 ± 0.26 |
| *Il2* | 1.0 ± 0.1 | **1.49 ± 0.2** | **1.31 ± 0.1** | 0.91 ± 0.1 | 0.97 ± 0.29 | **0.66 ± 0.1** |
| *Il4* | 1.0 ± 0.17 | 1.1 ± 0.35 | 1.4 ± 0.34 | 1.1 ± 0.43 | 1.47 ± 0.75 | 1.44 ± 0.93 |
| *Cdknla* | 1.0 ± 0.03 | 0.9 ± 0.07 | 0.92 ± 0.07 | 1.05 ± 0.38 | 1.62 ± 0.64 | 1.41 ± 1.1 |
| *Ifng* | 0.91 ± 0.16 | 0.95 ± 0.11 | **1.31 + 0.22** | 1.32 ± 1.0 | 1.0 ± 0.81 | 1.42 ± 1.11 |
| *Dnmtl* | 1.0 ± 0.24 | 1.05 ± 0.12 | 0.89 ± 0.22 | 1.11 ± 0.51 | 1.58 ± 0.36 | 1.73 ± 0.71 |
| *Dnmt3a* | 0.98 ± 0.02 | 1.08 ± 0.07 | 1.09 ± 0.07 | 0.98 ± 0.51 | 1.12 ± 0.35 | 1.2 ± 0.87 |

Gene expression was examined in splenic CD4$^+$ T cells incubated with anti-CD3 and anti-CD28 Abs for 24 hours following isolation from untreated control mice or from mice exposed to TCE during gestation only, or during early life only. The data represents the mean ± SD. *Significantly different ($\alpha < 0.05$) compared to control values.
The bolded text represents values that are significantly different from control values ($\alpha < 0.05$).

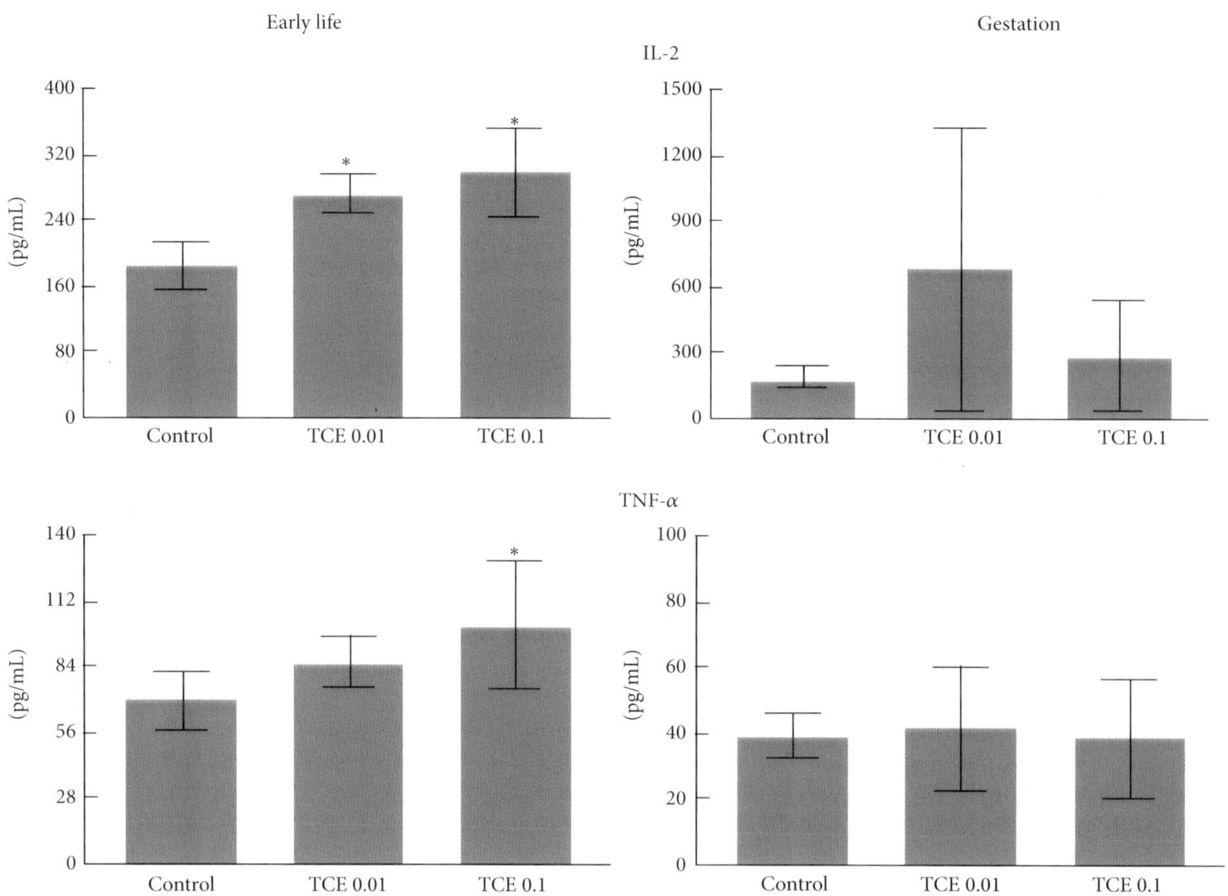


FIGURE 4: TCE altered cytokines in CD4$^+$ T cells from mice exposed to TCE during early life. Cytokine levels in culture supernatants from CD4$^+$ T cells prepared as described in Figure 4 were examined. *Significantly different ($\alpha < 0.05$) compared to control values.

the altered cellularity in the thymi of mice gestationally exposed to the lower concentration of TCE. In line with the unaltered *Iap* expression in the thymi of mice gestationally exposed to TCE, the expression of enzymes that regulate DNA methylation, namely, *Dnmtl* and *Dnmt3a*, were also unaltered by TCE in the thymus (Table 3). Deficiencies in thymic expression of the gene for the proapoptotic protein Bim or its downstream protein Bax can cause a defect in the negative selection process [37]. Neither of these genes was altered by TCE exposure in the thymus. Survivin, a protein originally described as an inhibitor of apoptosis, has more recently been shown to be required for maturation of DN thymocytes to DP thymocytes [38]. Even though gestational TCE exposure did seem to block an early stage

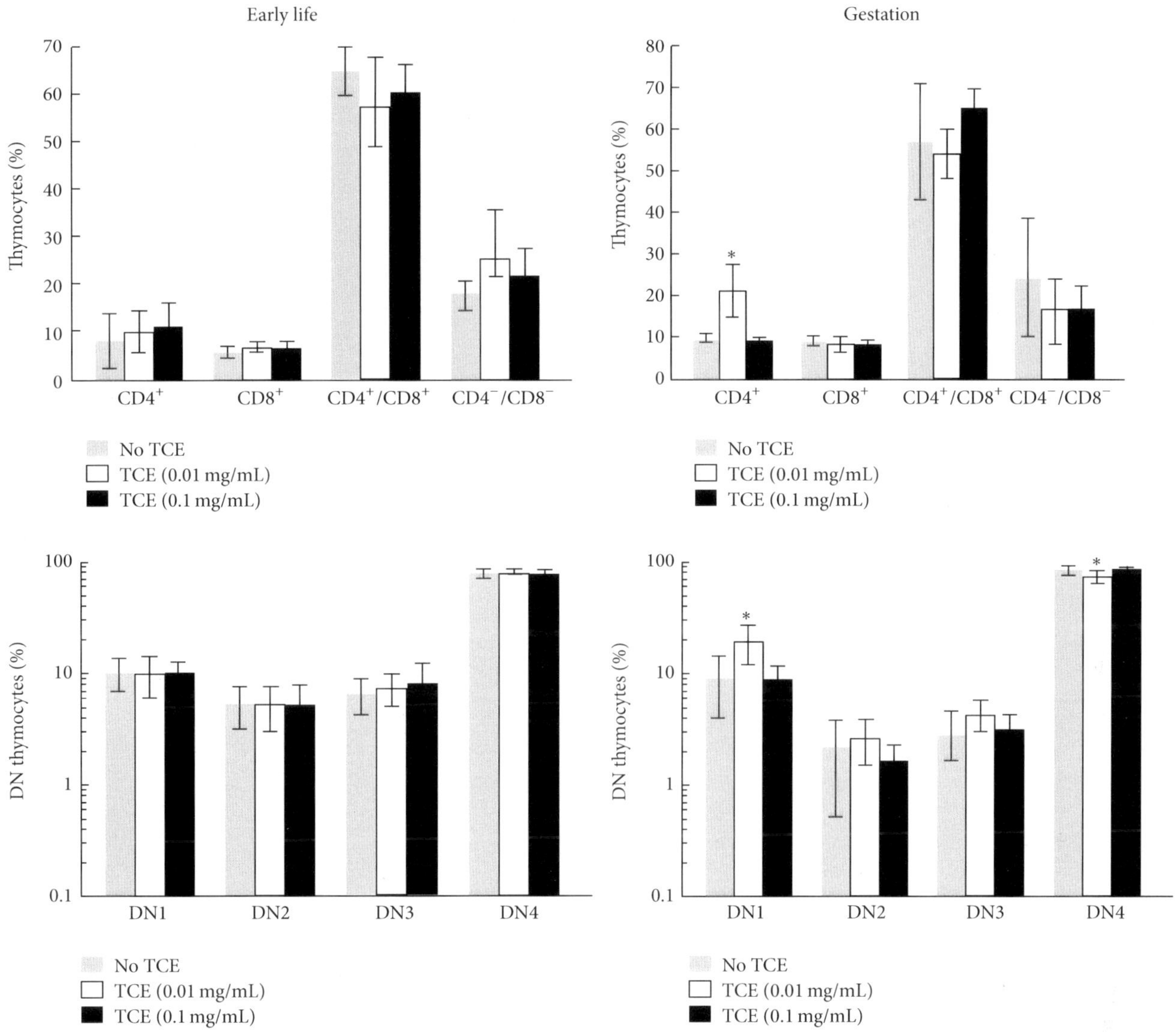


FIGURE 5: TCE altered thymus cellularity in mice exposed to TCE during gestation. Thymocyte suspensions from PND49 mice that had been exposed to TCE during gestation only or during early life only were incubated for 18 hours and then examined by flow cytometry to determine the percentage of single positive, double negative, and double positive cells. In addition, after gating on the double negative cell population, the cells were stained with anti-CD44 and anti-CD25 Abs and labeled as DN1 ($CD44^+CD25^-$), DN2 ($CD44^+CD25^+$), DN3 ($CD44^-CD25^+$), and DN4 ($CD44^-CD25^-$). *Significantly different ($\alpha < 0.05$) compared to control values.

of DN thymocyte differentiation, it did not alter expression of *Survivin*. Gestational exposure to TCE did not alter expression of *Fas*. However, both concentrations of TCE did suppress expression of *Fasl*, the gene that encodes for the ligand for *Fas*, and an important mediator of activation-induced apoptosis. Thus, the increase in SP $CD4^+$ thymocytes and DN1 thymocytes may be attributable to a decrease in apoptosis mediated by a TCE-induced decrease in the expression of *Fasl*. However, since the altered cellularity was only found in thymi of mice gestationally exposed to 0.01 mg/mL TCE, while the decrease in *Fasl* was found in mice exposed to either concentration of TCE, the role of *Fasl* in the altered cellularity needs to be clarified.

## 4. Discussion

The concordance rate for developing an autoimmune disease in identical twins demonstrates the involvement of an ill-defined genetic susceptibility [39]. To mimic this requirement "autoimmune-prone", MRL+/+ mice were used in our studies. Late in life, MRL+/+ mice can spontaneously develop a relatively mild lupus-like disease, as well as other autoimmune disorders such as Sjogren's syndrome and T cell-infiltrating pancreatitis [40, 41]. Young female MRL+/+ mice, with their propensity for autoimmunity but absence of overt disease, make a good model to test the immunostimulatory capacity of developmental TCE exposure. Others have similarly used

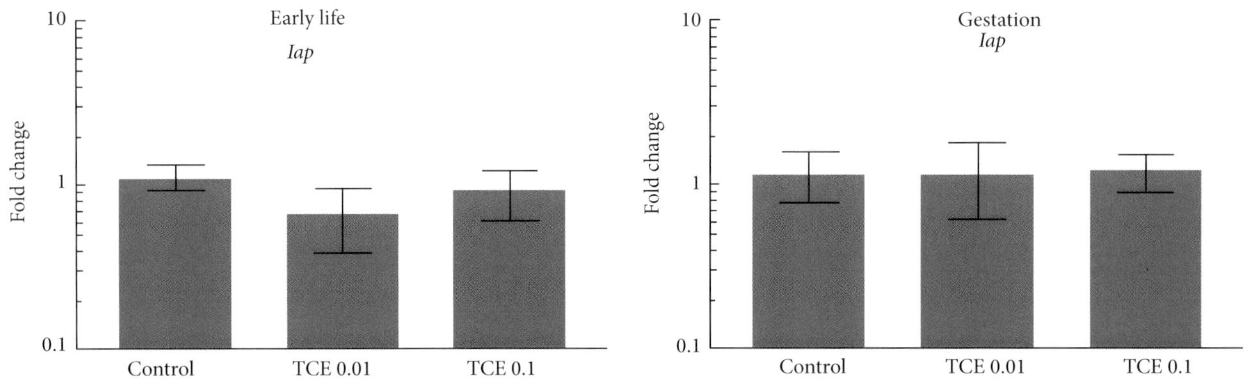


Figure 6: TCE did not inhibit *Iap* in thymocytes from either window of developmental TCE exposure. Gene expression was examined in thymocytes incubated for 18 hours following isolation from untreated control mice or from mice exposed to TCE during gestation only, or during early life only. The data represents the mean ± SD. *Significantly different ($\alpha < 0.05$) compared to control values.

Table 3: Gene expression in thymi of mice exposed to TCE during gestation.

| | | Gestation | |
|---|---|---|---|
| | Control | TCE 0.01 | TCE 0.1 |
| *Bax* | 1.04 ± 0.14 | 0.78 ± 0.24 | 1.06 ± 0.75 |
| *Bim* | 1.02 ± 0.15 | 0.82 ± 0.3 | 0.87 ± 0.21 |
| *Dnmt1* | 1.0 ± 0.3 | 1.16 ± 0.5 | 1.03 ± 0.25 |
| *Dnmt3a* | 1.14 ± 0.56 | 1.17 ± 0.46 | 0.93 ± 0.26 |
| *Survivin* | 1.3 ± 0.97 | 0.53 ± 0.47 | 0.68 ± 0.42 |
| *Aire* | 1.1 ± 0.58 | 0.71 ± 0.09 | 0.76 ± 0.51 |
| *Fas* | 0.96 ± 0.49 | 0.83 ± 0.46 | 0.78 ± 0.28 |
| *Fasl* | 1.06 ± 0.42 | **0.4 ± 0.25** | **0.45 ± 0.28** |

Gene expression was examined in thymocytes incubated for 18 hours following isolation from untreated control mice or from mice exposed to TCE during gestation only.
The data represents the mean ± SD. *Significantly different ($\alpha < 0.05$) compared to control values.
The bolded text represents values that are significantly different from control values ($\alpha < 0.05$).

"autoimmune-prone" mouse strains to test the developmental immunotoxicity of chemicals such as dioxin, bisphenol A, and mercury [42–44].

The exposure associated with the highest TCE concentration of 0.01 mg/mL (10 ppm) is considerably lower than acceptable human occupational exposure. The EPA's Maximum Contaminant Level for public drinking water is 5 ppb, but TCE has been found at levels up to 1.4 ppm [45] In humans exposed to TCE-contaminated water the amount ingested is only a fraction of the TCE absorbed via inhalation and dermal contact [46]. Since TCE exposure in the mice will be limited to ingestion it could be argued that mouse exposure to 10 ppm is within the range of possible human environmental exposure.

For essentially all of the parameters tested the early life exposure to TCE induced immune system changes similar to adult exposure, albeit at much lower concentrations. On the other hand, the results obtained from gestational only exposure to TCE were similar to those documented after continuous exposure to TCE. Gestational exposure to TCE caused alterations in thymic cellularity and effects on body weight and spleen size. In contrast, gestational TCE exposure had little effect on peripheral $CD4^+$ T cells, at least the parameters measured at PND 49. Unlike gestational exposure, early life exposure to TCE had no effect on thymic cellularity but was able to increase the percentage of activated/memory $CD4^+$ T cells in association with increased production of cytokines. This implies that exposure to TCE even as early as PND0 had more of an impact on deployed peripheral $CD4^+$ T cells than on the thymus. It is possible that lactational exposure to TCE at the concentrations used was not sufficient to impact the still-developing thymus, and that the effects observed following early life exposure were primarily attributable to the direct TCE exposure begun at PND21. An additional study of lactational only exposure to TCE is needed to resolve this question. Immune development in mice correlates well with immune development in humans, albeit with different kinetics [47]. One difference is that the perinatal immune system in mice is even more immature than that of humans. This means that the immune maturation that occurs during human gestation is commensurate with that found in mice at weaning at PND21. Thus, lactation only exposure in mice would correspond with late gestation in humans.

Taken together, it would seem that the individuals most susceptible to the most wide-ranging effects of TCE on the central and peripheral immune system are those exposed to the chemical during gestation as well as early life. Such a scenario in humans could occur when contaminated drinking water for both mother and child results in indirect TCE exposure during gestation and lactation and then direct exposure after weaning. However, it should be noted that, although the two different windows of TCE developmental exposure had distinct effects on peripheral and central T cells, both windows of exposure inhibited expression of retrotransposons in peripheral $CD4^+$ T cells. This implies that both gestation and early life are times during which epigenetic changes can be induced. Whether these changes manifest themselves in functional alterations that promote

TCE-induced hypersensitivity later in life needs to be determined. Epigenetic processes can regulate several aspects of normal $CD4^+$ T cell function including Th1/Th2 differentiation [48], cytokine production [49], and maintenance of Treg cells [50]. There are also several pieces of evidence that epigenetic processes regulate the activity of self-reactive $CD4^+$ T cells that mediate autoimmune disease [51–53]. In view of the connection between epigenetic alterations and $CD4^+$ T cell autoreactivity, the need to further investigate the capacity of TCE to induce these alterations becomes even more important.

How TCE impacts $CD4^+$ T cells is still being defined. Earlier studies showed that the $CD4^+$ T cell-altering effects of TCE were most likely mediated by its primary oxidative metabolite trichloroacetaldehyde hydrate (TCAH) [32, 33]. As an aldehyde TCAH can form a functionally active chemical interaction known as a Schiff base with amines on the surface of the $CD4^+$ T cells [54]. The possibility that TCAH forms a Schiff base with a costimulator receptor such as CD28, and thus provides bystander costimulation for antigen-activated $CD4^+$ T cells is being investigated. How this mechanism would impact thymocytes during development is unclear. In adults, TCE metabolism to TCAH is primarily mediated by cytochrome P450 2E1 (CYP2E1), and to a lesser extent by CYP1A1, and occurs primarily in the liver. However, since CYP1A1, unlike CYP2E1, can be detected in GD7 in the thymus [55], it is possible that CYP1A1 generates TCAH in the thymus of mice developmentally exposed to TCE.

Characterizing TCE-induced developmental immunotoxicity may be part of an important big picture. Immune dysfunction in the form of hypersensitivity disorders are among the most common medical conditions affecting children in the USA. Many of these appear to be increasing. For example, more children are being diagnosed with type I diabetes [56], childhood Graves' disease [57], and lupus nephritis [58] than ever before. Similarly, the CDC reports that the prevalence of food allergies increased from 3.4% in 1997–1999 to 5.1% in 2009–2011 [59]. The prevalence of skin allergies also increased from 7.4% in 1997–1999 to 12.5% 2009–2011. It is possible that the increase in childhood hypersensitivity is linked to increased exposure to environmental chemicals with potential developmental toxicity. More than 85,000 synthetic chemicals have been developed in the past 75 years, and only about 20% of the 3,000 most widely used chemicals have ever been tested for general developmental toxicity let alone developmental immunotoxicity [60]. As part of NHANES 2003-2004, it was found that after adjusting for covariates levels of many chemicals in pregnant women were increased compared to nonpregnant women [61]. Certain polychlorinated biphenyls, organochlorine pesticides, polycyclic aromatic hydrocarbons and many other chemicals were detected in 99-100% of pregnant women. Some of these chemicals cross the placenta and mediate developmental immunotoxicity. Developmental immunotoxicity is based on the premise that during the maturation of the immune system toxicant exposure results in a qualitative or quantitative difference in the effect or a greater persistence of effect. This increased sensitivity may be attributed to (i) a greater chemical exposure per pound of body weight, (ii) immature metabolic systems unable efficiently clear toxicants, (iii) developing immune system that is easily disrupted, and (iv) more time to develop chemical-induced immune-mediated diseases. Studying developmental immunotoxicity of chemicals such as TCE with proinflammatory effects may provide important clues to the etiology of idiopathic autoimmune disease.

## 5. Conclusion

Early life exposure to TCE induced changes in peripheral $CD4^+$ T cell commensurate with those found in mice exposed to TCE as an adult. Gestational TCE exposure induced changes in central immune function similar to that observed following continuous exposure. However, the two windows of exposure did have one effect in common, namely, the down-regulation of retrotransposon expression in $CD4^+$ T cells. Since the effects induced by the two developmental windows of TCE exposure were associated with TCE concentrations lower than those effective in adult, exposure the differential responses are functionally important.

## Conflict of Interests

There is no conflict of interests regarding the publication of this paper.

## Acknowledgments

The authors would like to gratefully acknowledge the excellent technical assistance of Brannon Broadfoot, Kirk West, and Rachel Lee and the support of the UAMS Translational Research Institute (National Institutes of Health UL1RR029884). This work was supported by Grants from the Arkansas Biosciences Institute, the National Institutes of Health (1R01ES017286; 1R01ES021484, R21ES017311), and the Organic Compounds Property Contamination class action settlement (CV 1992-002603).

## References

[1] US EPA, *Toxicological Review of Trichloroethylene. In Suppot of Summay Information on the integrated Risk Information System (IRIS)*, US Environmental Protection Agency, Washington, DC, USA, 2011.

[2] V. S. Byers, A. S. Levin, D. M. Ozonoff, and R. W. Baldwin, "Association between clinical symptoms and lymphocyte abnormalities in a population with chronic domestic exposure to industrial solvent-contaminated domestic water supply and a high incidence of leukaemia," *Cancer Immunology Immunotherapy*, vol. 27, no. 1, pp. 77–81, 1988.

[3] S. Yanez Diaz, M. Moran, P. Unamuno, and M. Armijo, "Silica and trichloroethylene-induced progressive systemic sclerosis," *Dermatology*, vol. 184, no. 2, pp. 98–102, 1992.

[4] B. L. Hansen and H. Isager, "A scleroderma-resembling disease-exposure to trichloroethylene and trichloroethane, is there a causal connection?" *Ugeskrift for Laeger*, vol. 150, no. 13, pp. 805–808, 1988.

[5] E. M. Saihan, J. L. Burton, and K. W. Heaton, "A new syndrome with pigmentation, scleroderma, gynaecomastia, Raynaud's phenomenon and peripheral neuropathy," *British Journal of Dermatology*, vol. 99, no. 4, pp. 437–440, 1978.

[6] H. Flindt-Hansen and H. Isager, "Scleroderma after occupational exposure to trichloroethylene and trichlorethane," *Toxicology Letters*, vol. 95, pp. 173–181, 1987.

[7] L. Czirjak, E. Pocs, and G. Szegedi, "Localized scleroderma after exposure to organic solvents," *Dermatology*, vol. 189, no. 4, pp. 399–401, 1994.

[8] J. E. Lockey, C. R. Kelly, and G. W. Cannon, "Progressive systemic sclerosis associated with exposure to trichloroethylene," *Journal of Occupational Medicine*, vol. 29, no. 6, pp. 493–496, 1987.

[9] R. Dubrow and D. M. Gute, "Cause-specific mortality among Rhode Island jewelry workers," *American Journal of Industrial Medicine*, vol. 12, no. 5, pp. 579–593, 1987.

[10] G. L. Gist and J. R. Burg, "Trichloroethylene-a review of the literature in view of the results of the trichloroethylene subregistry," *Toxicology and Industrial Health*, vol. 11, no. 3, pp. 253–307, 1995.

[11] G. R. Bond, "Hepatitis, rash and eosinophilia following trichloroethylene exposure: a case report and speculation on mechanistic similarity to halothane induced hepatitis," *Journal of Toxicology*, vol. 34, no. 4, pp. 461–466, 1996.

[12] X. Xu, R. Yang, N. Wu et al., "Severe hypersensitivity dermatitis and liver dysfunction induced by occupational exposure to trichloroethylene," *Industrial Health*, vol. 47, no. 2, pp. 107–112, 2009.

[13] J. Yi, Y. X. Teng, D. Zang et al., "Analysis of subgroups of lymphocyte in peripheral blood among dermatitis medicamentosa-like of trichloroethylene patients and healthy exposed workers," *Zhonghua Yu Fang Yi Xue Za Zhi*, vol. 45, pp. 1017–1021, 2011.

[14] K. H. Kilburn and R. H. Warshaw, "Prevalence of symptoms of systemic lupus erythematosus (SLE) and of fluorescent antinuclear antibodies associated with chronic exposure to trichloroethylene and other chemicals in well water," *Environmental Research*, vol. 57, no. 1, pp. 1–9, 1992.

[15] I. Iavicoli, A. Marinaccio, and G. Carelli, "Effects of occupational trichloroethylene exposure on cytokine levels in workers," *Journal of Occupational and Environmental Medicine*, vol. 47, no. 5, pp. 453–457, 2005.

[16] R. W. Luebke, D. H. Chen, R. Dietert, Y. Yang, M. King, and M. I. Luster, "The comparative immunotoxicity of five selected compounds following developmental or adult exposure," *Journal of Toxicology and Environmental Health B*, vol. 9, no. 1, pp. 1–26, 2006.

[17] C. Heilmann, E. Budtz-Jørgensen, F. Nielsen, B. Heinzow, P. Weihe, and P. Grandjean, "Serum concentrations of antibodies against vaccine toxoids in children exposed perinatally to immunotoxicants," *Environmental Health Perspectives*, vol. 118, no. 10, pp. 1434–1438, 2010.

[18] M. M. Leijs, J. G. Koppe, K. Olie, W. M. C. Van Aalderen, P. De Voogt, and G. W. Ten Tusscher, "Effects of dioxins, PCBs, and PBDEs on immunology and hematology in adolescents," *Environmental Science and Technology*, vol. 43, no. 20, pp. 7946–7951, 2009.

[19] A. N. Colebatch and C. J. Edwards, "The influence of early life factors on the risk of developing rheumatoid arthritis," *Clinical and Experimental Immunology*, vol. 163, no. 1, pp. 11–16, 2011.

[20] P. Langer, "The impacts of organochlorines and other persistent pollutants on thyroid and metabolic health," *Frontiers in Neuroendocrinology*, vol. 31, no. 4, pp. 497–518, 2010.

[21] US Environmental Protection Agency, *Third National Health and Nutrition Examination Survey*, U. S. Environmental Protection Agency, Washington, DC, USA, 1994.

[22] G. L. Gist and J. A. R. Burg, "Trichloroethylene—a review of the literature from a health effects perspective," *Toxicology and Industrial Health*, vol. 11, no. 3, pp. 253–307, 1995.

[23] J. M. Griffin, S. J. Blossom, S. K. Jackson, K. M. Gilbert, and N. R. Pumford, "Trichloroethylene accelerates an autoimmune response by Th1 T cell activation in MRL+/+ mice," *Immunopharmacology*, vol. 46, no. 2, pp. 123–137, 2000.

[24] J. M. Griffin, K. M. Gilbert, L. W. Lamps, and N. R. Pumford, "$CD4^+$ T-cell activation and induction of autoimmune hepatitis following trichloroethylene treatment in MRL+/+ mice," *Toxicological Sciences*, vol. 57, no. 2, pp. 345–352, 2000.

[25] K. M. Gilbert, N. R. Pumford, and S. J. Blossom, "Environmental contaminant trichloroethylene promotes autoimmune disease and inhibits T-cell apoptosis in MRL+/+ mice," *Journal of Immunotoxicology*, vol. 3, no. 4, pp. 263–267, 2006.

[26] K. M. Gilbert, B. Przybyla, N. R. Pumford et al., "Delineating liver events in trichloroethylene-induced autoimmune hepatitis," *Chemical Research in Toxicology*, vol. 22, no. 4, pp. 626–632, 2009.

[27] S. J. Blossom and J. C. Doss, "Trichloroethylene alters central and peripheral immune function in autoimmune-prone MRL+/+ mice following continuous developmental and early life exposure," *Journal of Immunotoxicology*, vol. 4, no. 2, pp. 129–141, 2007.

[28] T. L. Bunn, P. J. Parsons, E. Kao, and R. R. Dietert, "Exposure to lead during critical windows of embryonic development: differential immunotoxic outcome based on stage of exposure and gender," *Toxicological Sciences*, vol. 64, no. 1, pp. 57–66, 2001.

[29] R. R. Dietert, J.-E. Lee, and T. L. Bunn, "Developmental immunotoxicology: emerging issues," *Human and Experimental Toxicology*, vol. 21, no. 9-10, pp. 479–485, 2002.

[30] S. J. Blossom and J. C. Doss, "Trichloroethylene alters central and peripheral immune function in autoimmune-prone MRL+/+ mice following continuous developmental and early life exposure," *Journal of Immunotoxicology*, vol. 4, no. 2, pp. 129–141, 2007.

[31] K. M. Gilbert, B. Przybyla, N. R. Pumford et al., "Use of transcriptomics and metabolomics to delineate liver events associated with trichloroethylene-induced autoimmune hepatitis," Submitted 2008.

[32] S. J. Blossom, J. C. Doss, and K. M. Gilbert, "Chronic exposure to a trichloroethylene metabolite in autoimmune-prone MRL+/+ mice promotes immune modulation and alopecia," *Toxicological Sciences*, vol. 95, no. 2, pp. 401–411, 2007.

[33] J. M. Griffin, K. M. Gilbert, and N. R. Pumford, "Inhibition of CYP2E1 reverses $CD4^+$ T-cell alterations in trichloroethylene-treated MRL+/+ mice," *Toxicological Sciences*, vol. 54, no. 2, pp. 384–389, 2000.

[34] K. M. Gilbert, B. Reisfeld, and T. Zurlinden, "Modeling mechanism by which trichloroethylene inhibits liver repair in mouse model of autoimmunity," 2013.

[35] T. Takabatake, H. Ishihara, Y. Ohmachi et al., "Microarray-based global mapping of integration sites for the retrotransposon, intracisternal A-particle, in the mouse genome," *Nucleic Acids Research*, vol. 36, no. 10, p. e59, 2008.

[36] X. Zhang, R. Fu, J. Yu, and X. Wu, "DNA demethylation: where genetics meets epigenetics," *Current Pharmaceutical Design*, 2013.

[37] C. A. Chougnet, P. Tripathi, C. S. Lages et al., "A major role for Bim in regulatory T cell homeostasis," *Journal of Immunology*, vol. 186, no. 1, pp. 156–163, 2011.

[38] Z. Xing, E. M. Conway, C. Kang, and A. Winoto, "Essential role of survivin, an inhibitor of apoptosis protein, in T cell development, maturation, and homeostasis," *Journal of Experimental Medicine*, vol. 199, no. 1, pp. 69–80, 2004.

[39] X. S. He, A. A. Ansari, and M. E. Gershwin, "Xenobiotic considerations for the development of autoimmune liver diseases: bad genes and bad luck," *Reviews on Environmental Health*, vol. 16, no. 3, pp. 191–202, 2001.

[40] K. Skarstein, A. C. Johannessen, R. Holmdahl, and R. Jonsson, "Effects on sialadenitis after cellular transfer in autoimmune MRL/lpr mice," *Clinical Immunology and Immunopathology*, vol. 84, no. 2, pp. 177–184, 1997.

[41] W. M. Qu, T. Miyazaki, M. Terada et al., "A novel autoimmune pancreatitis model in MRL mice treated with polyinosinic:polycytidylic acid," *Clinical and Experimental Immunology*, vol. 129, no. 1, pp. 27–34, 2002.

[42] A. Mustafa, S. D. Holladay, M. Goff et al., "Developmental exposure to 2,3,7,8-tetrachlorodibenzo-p-dioxin alters postnatal T cell phenotypes and T cell function and exacerbates autoimmune lupus in 24-week-old SNF1 mice," *Birth Defects Research A*, vol. 85, no. 10, pp. 828–836, 2009.

[43] J. Bodin, B. A. Kocbach, R. Becher, F. Kuper, M. Lovik, and U. C. Nygaard, "Transmaternal bisphenol A exposure accelerates diabetes type 1 development in NOD mice," *Toxicological Sciences*, 2013.

[44] Y. Zhang, V. J. Bolivar, and D. A. Lawrence, "Maternal exposure to mercury chloride during pregnancy and lactation affects the immunity and social behavior of offspring," *Toxicological Sciences*, vol. 133, no. 1, pp. 101–111, 2013.

[45] ATSDR, *Progress Report: Survey of Specific Childhood Cancers and Birth Defects Amoung Children Whose Mothers Were Pregnant While Living at U.S. Marine Corps Base Camp Lejeune, North Carolina, 1968–1985*, Agency for Toxic Substances and Disease Registry, Atlanta, Ga, USA, 2003.

[46] L. J. Lee, C. Chan, C. Chung, Y. Yee-Chung, G. Wang, and J. Wang, "Health risk assessment on residents exposed to chlorinated hydrocarbons contaminated in groundwater of a hazardous waste site," *Journal of Toxicology and Environmental Health A*, vol. 65, no. 3-4, pp. 219–235, 2002.

[47] S. D. Holladay and R. J. Smialowicz, "Development of the murine and human immune system: differential effects of immunotoxicants depend on time of exposure," *Environmental Health Perspectives*, vol. 108, supplement 3, pp. 463–473, 2000.

[48] B. R. Winders, R. H. Schwartz, and D. Bruniquel, "A distinct region of the murine IFN-$\gamma$ promoter is hypomethylated from early T cell development through mature naive and Th1 cell differentiation, but is hypermethylated in Th2 cells," *Journal of Immunology*, vol. 173, no. 12, pp. 7377–7384, 2004.

[49] D. Bruniquel and R. H. Schwartz, "Selective, stable demethylation of the interleukin-2 gene enhances transcription by an active process," *Nature Immunology*, vol. 4, no. 3, pp. 235–240, 2003.

[50] S. Floess, J. Freyer, C. Siewert et al., "Epigenetic control of the foxp3 locus in regulatory T cells," *PLoS Biology*, vol. 5, no. 2, p. e38, 2007.

[51] R. Yung, D. Powers, K. Johnson et al., "Mechanisms of drug-induced lupus II. T cells overexpressing lymphocyte function-associated antigen 1 become autoreactive and cause a lupuslike disease in syngeneic mice," *Journal of Clinical Investigation*, vol. 97, no. 12, pp. 2866–2871, 1996.

[52] M. A. Jeffries, M. Dozmorov, Y. Tang, J. T. Merrill, J. D. Wren, and A. H. Sawalha, "Genome-wide DNA methylation patterns in $CD4^+$ T cells from patients with systemic lupus erythematosus," *Epigenetics*, vol. 6, no. 5, pp. 593–601, 2011.

[53] B. M. Javierre, A. F. Fernandez, J. Richter et al., "Changes in the pattern of DNA methylation associate with twin discordance in systemic lupus erythematosus," *Genome Research*, vol. 20, no. 2, pp. 170–179, 2010.

[54] K. M. Gilbert, A. B. Whitlow, and N. R. Pumford, "Environmental contaminant and disinfection by-product trichloroacetaldehyde stimulates T cells in vitro," *International Immunopharmacology*, vol. 4, no. 1, pp. 25–36, 2004.

[55] D. Choudhary, I. Jansson, I. Stoilov, M. Sarfarazi, and J. B. Schenkman, "Expression patterns of mouse and human CYP orthologs (families 1–4) during development and in different adult tissues," *Archives of Biochemistry and Biophysics*, vol. 436, no. 1, pp. 50–61, 2005.

[56] T. H. Lipman, L. E. Levitt Katz, S. J. Ratcliffe et al., "Increasing incidence of type 1 diabetes in youth: twenty years of the Philadelphia pediatric diabetes registry," *Diabetes Care*, vol. 36, no. 6, pp. 1597–1603, 2013.

[57] G. W. Wong and P. S. Cheng, "Increasing incidence of childhood Graves' disease in Hong Kong: a follow-up study," *Clinical Endocrinology*, vol. 54, no. 4, pp. 547–550, 2001.

[58] K. H. Costenbader, A. Desai, G. S. Alarcón et al., "Trends in the incidence, demographics, and outcomes of end-stage renal disease due to lupus nephritis in the US from 1995 to 2006," *Arthritis and Rheumatism*, vol. 63, no. 6, pp. 1681–1688, 2011.

[59] A. M. Branum and S. L. Lukacs, "Food allergy among U.S. children: trends in prevalence and hospitalizations," *NCHS Data Brief*, no. 10, pp. 1–8, 2008.

[60] P. J. Landrigan and L. R. Goldman, "Chemical safety, health care costs and the affordable care act," *American Journal of Industrial Medicine*, vol. 57, no. 1, pp. 1–3, 2013.

[61] T. J. Woodruff, A. R. Zota, and J. M. Schwartz, "Environmental chemicals in pregnant women in the united states: NHANES 2003-2004," *Environmental Health Perspectives*, vol. 119, no. 6, pp. 878–885, 2011.

# 21

# Increased Whole Blood Viscosity is Associated with the Presence of Digital Ulcers in Systemic Sclerosis

**Peter Korsten,[1] Timothy B. Niewold,[2] Michael Zeisberg,[1] Tammy O. Utset,[3] Daniel Cho,[4] Lawrence S. Zachary,[5] Nadera J. Sweiss,[6,7] and Suncica Volkov[6]**

[1] *Department of Nephrology and Rheumatology, University Medical Center Goettingen, Goettingen, Germany*
[2] *Division of Rheumatology and Department of Immunology, Mayo Clinic, Rochester, MN, USA*
[3] *Department of Rheumatology, University of Chicago, Chicago, IL, USA*
[4] *Rheovector LLC, King of Prussia, PA, USA*
[5] *Section of Plastic and Reconstructive Surgery, Department of Surgery, University of Chicago, Chicago, IL, USA*
[6] *Division of Rheumatology, University of Illinois at Chicago, Chicago, IL, USA*
[7] *Division of Pulmonary, Critical Care, Sleep and Allergy, University of Illinois at Chicago, Chicago, IL, USA*

Correspondence should be addressed to Peter Korsten; peter.korsten@med.uni-goettingen.de

Academic Editor: Ricard Cervera

*Objective.* To investigate the role of whole blood viscosity in digital ulcer (DU) development in patients with diffuse and limited Systemic sclerosis. *Methods.* A convenience sample of patients with Systemic sclerosis (SSc) was selected from the adult Rheumatology clinic at the University of Chicago. The study group consisted of patients with SSc (with ulcers present, a history of ulcers, and no ulcers); the control group consisted of matched healthy Rheumatology clinic staff. WBV was measured using a scanning capillary viscometer at different shear rates (1–1000 1/s). *Results.* Whole blood viscosity as measured by a scanning capillary viscometer was increased in patients with SSc compared to healthy controls ($p < 0.0001$). Additionally, patients with present DU had significantly higher whole blood viscosity when compared to patients with a history of DU and patients with no history of DU ($p < 0.0001$). These findings were most pronounced at lower shear rates between 1 and 10 1/s. *Conclusion.* Whole blood viscosity might be a contributing factor in DU development in patients with SSc. Further studies with larger patient cohorts are required to fully evaluate how increased WBV contributes to the development of DU and whether the currently available treatment options improve the microcirculation by influencing WBV.

## 1. Introduction

Systemic sclerosis (SSc) is an autoimmune connective tissue disease characterized by cutaneous and visceral fibrosis, but also diffuse vascular pathology [1]. A majority of SSc patients have Raynaud's phenomenon (RP), which is an exaggerated vascular response to stimuli, such as cold temperature or emotional stress. Up to 60% of SSc patients with RP develop digital ulcers (DU) in the course of their disease [2].

The pathogenesis of DU in SSc is incompletely understood. Obliterating vasculopathy and inflammatory mediators may play a role [1]. Changes of hemorheological properties (whole blood viscosity (WBV)) in patients with secondary RP (including SSc) were already reported previously [3]. However, few studies have further investigated these findings.

Elevated WBV has been recognized as a risk factor for adverse cardiovascular events in the general population, even after adjusting for traditional risk factors such as age, male gender, obesity, hypertension, diabetes, and smoking [4]. Also, cardiovascular events in patients with chronic kidney disease have been found to be associated with increased whole blood viscosity [5].

WBV is determined by hematocrit, plasma viscosity, red blood cell aggregation, and deformability. It is influenced by shear stress and other factors. Plasma viscosity is the intrinsic flow resistance of plasma and depends on plasma protein concentrations, predominantly fibrinogen.

Rotational viscometers have been the standard technique by which blood viscosity was measured for clinical studies [6]. Disadvantages of these systems are the inability to produce viscosity data at multiple shear rates and the need to treat blood samples with anticoagulation during viscosity testing. Anticoagulated blood inhibits cell-cell interactions altering (decreasing) WBV at low shear rates [6]. Plasma and serum viscosity as well as their components can be examined by rotational viscometers, but a more reliable and reproducible way to measure WBV would help to better understand what occurs in the vessel under different conditions in terms of shear rates.

The scanning capillary viscometer (SCV Rheolog™ by Rheovector, Exton, PA, USA) used in this study is able to quickly measure WBV at a wider range of shear rates. To examine WBV with the SCV, blood components do not have to be separated (in contrast to serum or plasma viscosity) and therefore reflect physiological conditions in the blood vessel more appropriately. Increased shear rates lead to a decrease in viscosity. In areas of low shear rates, such as the digits, WBV is therefore higher. If WBV increases at a constant systolic blood pressure, peripheral vascular resistance increases, thus reducing blood flow. This could lead to development of DU in SSc. When WBV decreases, circulation improves which results in increased perfusion, particularly in the microvasculature. A pathogenic role of WBV in DU development in SSc is therefore likely. The validity of the SCV to measure WBV has been established in several studies [7].

The present study is the first study using the SCV to investigate WBV at different shear rates in relation to the presence or absence of DU in patients with SSc and healthy controls.

## 2. Patients and Methods

*2.1. Study Population.* We prospectively included 33 patients with SSc and 13 matched control subjects between October 2005 and April 2006. All subjects were 18 years or older and SSc patients met the 2013 American College of Rheumatology (ACR)/European League Against Rheumatism classification criteria for SSc [8] as well as the 1980 ACR classification criteria, which were in use at the time of study conduction.

"Presence of digital ulcer" was defined as break in the skin on the fingertip, with or without granulation tissue, which had not completed the healing process. Patients were recruited during regular office visits to the adult Rheumatology clinic at the University of Chicago. Control subjects were recruited from healthy university personnel and were matched to the SSc group. The Institutional Review Board at the University of Chicago approved the study and all subjects gave written informed consent.

Epidemiological data on all 46 subjects was obtained by routine use of structured documentation; measurements of whole blood viscosity were performed in all patients. Disease activity was assessed by physical examination and digital ulcer assessment.

*2.2. Capillary Viscometer.* 4 to 6 mL of blood with standard venipuncture were obtained and immediately processed. We used a scanning capillary viscometer (SCV, Rheovector LLC, Exton, PA) to measure WBV.

The SCV has a Food and Drug Administration Investigational Device Exempt status. It was developed in 2001 and has been validated to measure WBV (mPa × second) at incremental shear rates from 1 to 1000 seconds$^{-1}$. The SCV is a portable device that maintains blood samples in a closed system. This system is coated with biocompatible material and is temperature controlled, simulating in vivo conditions. The blood is led into a U-formed capillary, filling one of the vertical columns higher than the other, before permitting the columns to equilibrate through gravity forces. The flow occurs rapidly at first, slowing down over time until the blood levels in the two tubes are nearly equal. While the blood is flowing, the system records the height of the two columns over a defined time period (3 minutes). The flow rate (determined by the rate of change in height of the columns of blood) is directly related to the pressure drop across the capillary tube, from which the shear rate, viscosity, and shear stress of the sample can be mathematically derived. The raw data are presented graphically and then numerically on an attached computer.

The determination of a full profile (from a shear rate of 1 to 1000 s$^{-1}$) is important for the evaluation of blood properties, as variations of viscosity at low shear rates may be especially important in the pathophysiology of digital ulcer DU formation.

*2.3. Statistical Analysis.* All data were analyzed using GraphPad Prism version 6.0 for Mac OS X (GraphPad Software, La Jolla California USA, https://www.graphpad.com). Fisher's exact, Chi-square, Student's $t$-test, or Mann–Whitney test was used to compare the demographic characteristics between patients and controls as appropriate for parametric or nonparametric data.

WBV values were log-transformed and plotted against shear rates in $X$-$Y$ plots. The data were analyzed using curve-fit methods, and a strong fit was achieved using a one-phase exponential decay curve to model the WBV data at various shear rates. WBV versus shear rate curves were compared between SSc patients and the control group as well as within SSc with ulcers versus SSc with a history of ulcers versus SSc without ulcers. To test for differences between the curves, an extra sum-of-squares $F$ test was used, and $p$ values shown on the graph are derived from this test. This tests the hypothesis that the data points from each condition (for ex. patients versus control) represent the same curve or a different curve. Low $p$ values allow for the null hypothesis (same curve) to be rejected.

## 3. Results

*3.1. Patients and Controls.* The demographic characteristics of 33 SSc patients and 13 control subjects are presented in

Table 1: Characteristics of the studied patients.

| | Systemic sclerosis ($n = 33$) | Controls ($n = 13$) | $p$ value |
|---|---|---|---|
| Gender | 31 women (94%)<br>2 men (6%) | 12 women (92%)<br>1 man (8%) | 1.0 |
| Race | 20 Caucasians (60.6%)<br>10 African Americans (30.3%)<br>3 Hispanics (9.1%) | 8 Caucasians (61.5%)<br>3 African Americans (23.1%)<br>2 Hispanics (15.4%) | 0.9309 |
| Age range | 48.76 ± 12.66 | 41.15 ± 13.27 | 0.0772 |
| Disease type | Diffuse SSc ($n = 19$, 57%)<br>Limited SSc ($n = 14$, 43%) | — | |
| Disease duration | 1–29 years | — | |
| Digital ulcers | Present ulcers ($n = 4$, 12.1%)<br>History of ulcers ($n = 17$, 51.5%)<br>No history of ulcers ($n = 12$, 36.4%) | — | |

BMI: body mass index, CRP: C-reactive protein, and SSc: Systemic sclerosis.

Table 1. There were 31 women and two men in the SSc group (10 African Americans, 20 Caucasians, and 3 Hispanics). The control group consisted of twelve women and one man (8 African Americans, 3 Caucasians, and 2 Hispanics). Mean age was 48.76 ± 12.66 for SSc patients and 41.15 ± 13.27 for controls. There were no significant differences in terms of age, gender, body mass index (BMI), and ethnicity between groups.

*3.2. Characteristics of the Systemic Sclerosis Group.* Type (diffuse or limited SSc), disease duration, and digital ulcer assessment of the Systemic sclerosis group were recorded (Table 1). 19 patients (57%) had diffuse SSc while 14 patients (43%) had limited SSc. Disease duration ranged from 1 to 29 years. Presence or absence of ulcers was assessed by history and physical examination. Four patients (12.1%) had DU at the time of the study, 17 had a history of DU (51.5%), and 12 (36.4%) had no prior history of DU (36%).

*3.3. Comparison of Whole Blood Viscosity Measured at Different Shear Rates between SSc Patients and Control Group.* First, we compared WBV of the whole patient cohort with healthy control patients. Shear rates were measured ranging from 1 to 1000 $s^{-1}$. Values were significantly higher in SSc patients versus controls ($p < 0.0001$). The absolute difference was greatest at low share rates (between 1 and 10 $s^{-1}$) (Figure 1).

*3.4. Comparison of Whole Blood Viscosity between Systemic Sclerosis Patients with Ulcers, a History of Ulcers, and a Negative History for Ulcers.* Next, we investigated whether there were any detectable differences between patients with DU, a history of DU, and those with a negative history of DU (Figure 2). We found that WBV was highest for patients with ulcers compared to those with a history of DU and no history of DU ($p < 0.0001$). There was no difference between patients with a history of DU compared to patients with no history of DU ($p = 0.24$), suggesting that an increase in WBV is pathophysiologically important in DU formation.

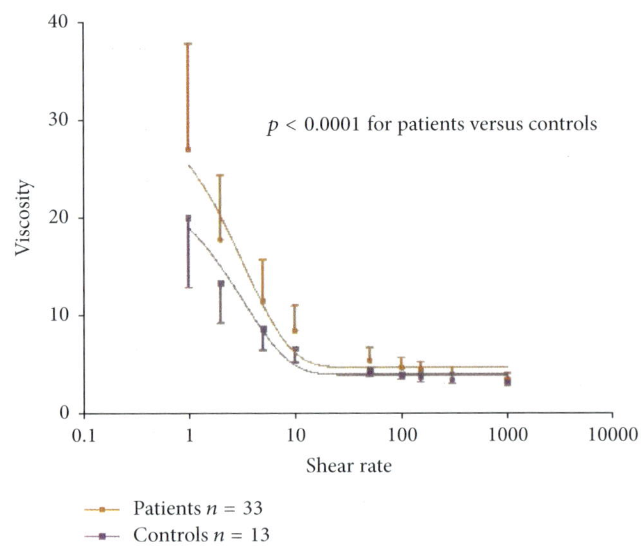


Figure 1: *Whole blood viscosity compared between patients (red) and controls (blue).* WBV was significantly higher in the Systemic sclerosis group compared to healthy controls ($p < 0.0001$). This difference was most pronounced at shear rates between 1 and 10 $s^{-1}$; however, shear rates were significantly different at all rates.

## 4. Discussion

The present study is the first examining WBV related to DU in patients with SSc using a SCTV. There are several important limitations of our study: First, the number of individuals studied was small. Second, only four patients had ulcers at the time of the examination. Also, we did not follow the patients for a longer period, which is why we cannot make any recommendations whether an increase in WBV from baseline in an individual patient translates into a higher risk for the development of DU. Despite these limitations, our study is the first to show that WBV might play a critical role in the development of active DU in patients with SSc.

The concept of altered hemorheological variables in various disease states has been studied for over 40 years. An

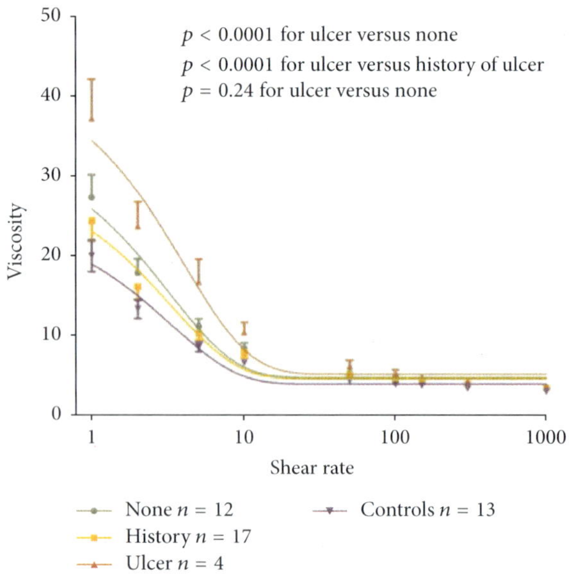


FIGURE 2: *Whole blood viscosity in Systemic sclerosis patients.* WBV was compared between patients with ulcers (red), a history of ulcers (yellow), and no history of ulcers (green). Control patients are also depicted (purple). WBV was significantly higher in patients with ulcers versus patients with a history of ulcers ($p < 0.0001$) and versus patients with no history of ulcers ($p < 0.0001$). By contrast, there was no difference between patients with a history of ulcers versus patients with no history of ulcers ($p = 0.24$).

early study by Goyle and Dormandy investigated patients with primary RP versus controls and found an increase in blood viscosity in persons with RP [9]. Nevertheless, other investigators postulated that blood viscosity is different between patients with primary RP and secondary RP [10]. Of note, these studies used different methods of WBV measurements and findings may not directly apply to our cohort. The primary purpose of this study was to analyze WBV in relation to presence or absence of DU in SSc patients, which is why we did not include other control groups. In our experience, persons with primary RP show no statistically different WBV measurements compared to healthy controls (data not shown).

Based on the results of our pilot study, studies investigating WBV in Systemic sclerosis should be performed prospectively over a longer time to assess patients at different time points during the course of their disease. Our study was a cross-sectional study intended as a hypothesis-generating study. We therefore did not make any measurements of WBV after ulcers have healed, which is another limitation. We would nevertheless suppose that WBV would be comparable to levels observed in the group with a history of ulcers, which served as comparator within the SSc group (see Figure 2).

It is hypothesized that immune-mediated inflammation in connective tissue diseases may initiate or promote atherosclerosis, which may partially explain higher incidence of cardiovascular events in this group of patients. Acute phase reactants, such as fibrinogen or increased levels of immunoglobulins, influence whole blood viscosity in autoimmune diseases, such as rheumatoid arthritis (RA) or systemic lupus erythematosus (SLE) [11]. Patients with SLE, for example, who have increased WBV, were found to have a higher incidence of arterial thromboembolic events [12]. In rheumatoid arthritis, citrullinated fibrinogen might contribute to the observed increase in WBV and has been implicated in special situations such as Felty's syndrome (reviewed by [11]). The concept of alterations in blood rheology is therefore not specific for Systemic sclerosis. Investigations of blood rheology have gained interest in cardiovascular diseases. In the recent studies by Peters et al. [4] and Celik et al. [5], WBV was measured at higher share rates and by slightly different methods because these were macrovascular studies. In these studies, higher WBV correlated with the incidence of cardiovascular events. These findings show that an increase in WBV is not specific for any disease but rather reflects a distinct pathology in a given situation.

The main finding of our study, although it is based on a low number of subjects, is that WBV is increased in SSc compared with healthy controls and was also different within the SSc group depending on the presence or absence of DU. These latter findings may have some implications. Currently, standard treatments for RP/DU in SSc include vasodilatory substances, such as calcium antagonists or, in more severe cases, iloprost infusion therapy. Bosentan, an endothelin-receptor antagonist, is recommended for the prevention of new ulcers in patients who have had DU [13]. After the results of the RAPIDS-1 and RAPIDS-2 and SEDUCE trials [14–16], the main focus in treatment and prevention of critical or refractory DU therefore relies on endothelin-1 antagonists or phosphodiesterase inhibitors.

Taken together, evidence-based treatment options are quite limited for this manifestation. It may be interesting to incorporate measurements of blood rheology in future treatment studies on RP/DU in SSc patients since not every medication might exert the same effect on blood viscosity. It is clear that other treatments are required since not all patients respond to standard treatment.

Earlier studies by Jacobs et al. [17] found that plasma viscosity was significantly lower in patients with RP after plasmapheresis and was associated with enhanced skin capillary blood flow, improvement in symptoms, and healing of the skin ulcers. Overall, plasma exchange in RP or DU has been investigated in only few studies despite seemingly promising results [3, 17, 18] and is often not mentioned in the current literature [19]. Even though therapeutic apheresis is invasive, in our experience, it is a safe and well tolerated procedure with few side effects or complications and it might be considered as a therapeutic option in refractory ulcers. While we cannot draw any conclusions on the effectiveness of plasmapheresis in refractory DU based on our data, it may be an option in recalcitrant cases.

In conclusion, despite the aforementioned limitations, our study shows that WBV is increased in SSc patients versus healthy controls and also in patients with active DU. Future studies of WBV in SSc should aim to follow a larger cohort of patients for a longer period of time to measure WBV at times of active DU and after healing and also to assess treatment effects on blood viscosity.

## Disclosure

Daniel Cho served as president of Rheologics Inc. from 2005 to 2009. He currently serves as Director of Rheovector LLC, the successor to Rheologics Inc., which closed in 2010. In this role, he provides viscometers as well as blood viscosity laboratory services to researchers.

## Conflicts of Interest

The authors declare that they have no conflicts of interest.

## References

[1] A. Gabrielli, E. V. Avvedimento, and T. N. Krieg, "Scleroderma," *The New England Journal of Medicine*, vol. 360, no. 19, pp. 1989–2003, 2009.

[2] V. Steen, C. P. Denton, J. E. Pope, and M. Matucci-Cerinic, "Digital ulcers: overt vascular disease in systemic sclerosis," *Rheumatology*, vol. 48, no. 3, pp. iii19–iii24, 2006.

[3] A. J. Dodds, P. T. Flute, M. J. G. O'Reilly, L. T. Cotton, C. J. P. Yates, and J. A. Dormandy, "Haemorrheological response to plasma exchange in Raynaud's syndrome," *British Medical Journal*, vol. 2, no. 6199, pp. 1186-1187, 1979.

[4] S. A. E. Peters, M. Woodward, A. Rumley, H. D. Tunstall-Pedoe, and G. D. O. Lowe, "Plasma and blood viscosity in the prediction of cardiovascular disease and mortality in the Scottish Heart Health Extended Cohort Study," *European Journal of Preventive Cardiology*, vol. 24, no. 2, pp. 161–167, 2017.

[5] T. Celik, M. I. Yilmaz, S. Balta et al., "The relationship between plasma whole blood viscosity and cardiovascular events in patients with chronic kidney disease," *Clinical and Applied Thrombosis/Hemostasis*, vol. 23, no. 6, pp. 663–670, 2017.

[6] R. S. Rosenson and D. Wolff, "Comparison of two whole blood viscometers: implications for cardiovascular and thrombosis research," *Thrombosis and Haemostasis*, vol. 92, pp. 225-226, 2004.

[7] T. Alexy, E. Pais, R. B. Wenby et al., "Measurement of whole blood viscosity profiles via an automated viscometer: technical details and clinical relevance," *Clinical Laboratory*, vol. 51, pp. 523–529, 2005.

[8] F. van den Hoogen, D. Khanna, J. Fransen et al., "2013 classification criteria for systemic sclerosis: an american college of rheumatology/European league against rheumatism collaborative initiative," *Arthritis & Rheumatism*, vol. 65, no. 11, pp. 2737–2747, 2013.

[9] K. B. Goyle and J. A. Dormandy, "Abnormal blood viscosity in Raynaud's phenomenon," *The Lancet*, vol. 307, no. 7973, pp. 1317-1318, 1976.

[10] C. Lacombe, J. M. Mouthon, C. Bucherer, J. C. Lelievre, O. Bletry, and P. Godeau, "Raynaud's phenomenon and blood viscosity," *Journal des Maladies Vasculaires*, vol. 17, supplement B, pp. 132–135, 1992.

[11] H. C. Kwaan, "Role of plasma proteins in whole blood viscosity: a brief clinical review," *Clinical Hemorheology and Microcirculation*, vol. 44, pp. 167–176, 2010.

[12] S. Booth, S. Chohan, J. C. Curran, T. Karrison, A. Schmitz, and T. O. Utset, "Whole blood viscosity and arterial thrombotic events in patients with systemic lupus erythematosus," *Arthritis Care & Research*, vol. 57, no. 5, pp. 845–850, 2007.

[13] O. Kowal-Bielecka, J. Fransen, J. Avouac, M. Becker, A. Kulak, Y. Allanore et al., "Update of EULAR recommendations for the treatment of systemic sclerosis," *Annals of the Rheumatic Diseases*, vol. 76, pp. 1327–1339, 2017.

[14] E. Hachulla, P.-Y. Hatron, P. Carpentier et al., "Efficacy of sildenafil on ischaemic digital ulcer healing in systemic sclerosis: the placebo-controlled SEDUCE study," *Annals of the Rheumatic Diseases*, vol. 75, no. 6, pp. 1009–1015, 2016.

[15] M. Matucci-Cerinic, C. P. Denton, D. E. Furst et al., "Bosentan treatment of digital ulcers related to systemic sclerosis: results from the RAPIDS-2 randomised, double-blind, placebo-controlled trial," *Annals of the Rheumatic Diseases*, vol. 70, no. 1, pp. 32–38, 2011.

[16] J. H. Korn, M. Mayes, M. Matucci Cerinic et al., "Digital ulcers in systemic sclerosis: prevention by treatment with bosentan, an oral endothelin receptor antagonist," *Arthritis & Rheumatology*, vol. 50, no. 12, pp. 3985–3993, 2004.

[17] M. J. Jacobs, P. J. Jörning, E. J. Van Rhede van der Kloot, P. J. Kitslaar, H. A. Lemmens, D. W. Slaaf et al., "Plasmapheresis in Raynaud's phenomenon in systemic sclerosis: a microcirculatory study," *International Journal of Microcirculation, Clinical and Experimental*, vol. 10, pp. 1–11, 1991.

[18] F. Cozzi, P. Marson, M. Rosada et al., "Long-term therapy with plasma exchange in systemic sclerosis: effects on laboratory markers reflecting disease activity," *Transfusion and Apheresis Science*, vol. 25, no. 1, pp. 25–31, 2001.

[19] A. L. Herrick, "Management of Raynaud's Phenomenon and Digital Ischemia," *Current Rheumatology Reports*, vol. 15, article 303, 2013.

# 22

# CD8+DR+ T-Cells and C3 Complement Serum Concentration as Potential Biomarkers in Thrombotic Antiphospholipid Syndrome

**Elizabeth Sarmiento, Jonathan Dale, Mauricio Arraya, Antonio Gallego, Nallibe Lanio, Joaquin Navarro, and Javier Carbone**

*Clinical Immunology Department, Hospital General Universitario Gregorio Marañon, 28007 Madrid, Spain*

Correspondence should be addressed to Javier Carbone; javier.carbone@salud.madrid.org

Academic Editor: Andras Perl

*Purpose.* To assess complement factors and T lymphocyte activation subset abnormalities in patients with thrombotic antiphospholipid syndrome (APS) as potential biomarkers for development of clinical complications. *Methods.* We assessed C3, C4, factor B concentrations (nephelometry), complement haemolytic functional activity (CH100, radial immune diffusion), and the activation status of CD4+ and CD8+ T-cells (three-colour flow cytometry) in patients with thrombotic APS. Antiphospholipid (aPL) positive patients without APS-related clinical criteria, systemic lupus erythematosus (SLE) patients, and healthy individuals were evaluated as controls. A clinical followup was performed to assess the potential relationship between the immunological parameters and development of APS-related complications. *Results.* Lower concentrations of C3 and higher levels of CD8+DR+ cells were risk factors for development of APS-related complications during followup, including rethrombosis and neuropsychiatric symptoms. Patients with diagnosed thrombotic APS had significantly lower levels of C3, C4, and CH100 as well as higher percentages of activated CD4+DR+ and of CD8+DR+ T-cells than healthy controls but similar to that observed in autoimmune disease controls. *Conclusion.* Lower C3 and C4 complement levels and higher percentages of CD8+DR+ T-cells were observed in thrombotic APS patients. The potential role of these abnormalities as biomarkers of clinical outcome warrants further evaluation in a multicenter study.

## 1. Introduction

Antiphospholipid syndrome (APS) is an autoimmune systemic disease characterized by one or more clinical episodes of venous or arterial thrombosis and obstetric complications, together with antiphospholipid antibodies (aPL) in serum [1]. Clinical complications may occur in these patients during followup. There is a lack of biomarkers to identify patients at risk for development of these clinical complications. To identify a biomarker the first step is the identification of a potential pathogenic role of the biomarker in the evaluated disease. Then the association between the biomarker and clinical outcomes should be assessed.

Activation of complement proteins by pathogen-associated and danger-associated molecular patterns induces generation of distinct effector molecules [2]. An association between aPL-induced morbidity during pregnancy and complement activation has been reported [3–5]. In murine models, complement plays an important role in fetal injury in animals with APS [6]. Serum complement proteins and function are commonly assessed to establish the degree of activation of this system in specific clinical conditions, although they have not been extensively assessed in patients with thrombotic APS [7]. Activation of T-cells has also been reported to play a role in the pathogenesis of specific models of thrombotic disease [8, 9]. Interestingly enough, the most common therapeutic interventions in thrombotic

APS, such as warfarin or heparin, have the potential to decrease lymphocyte activation and complement activation, respectively [10, 11]. Recent research supports a role for the complement system in the regulation of T-cell responses [12]. In this study, we assessed specific complement system parameters and lymphocyte activation subsets to assess their relationship with thrombotic APS and to set up the hypothesis about their potential role as biomarkers of clinical outcome in a prospective study.

## 2. Patients and Methods

*2.1. Patients.* The present study was performed in two parts: the first part was a cross-sectional case-control study to assess the relationship between immunological biomarkers and thrombotic APS; the second part was a prospective follow-up study that used the immunological study as baseline to assess whether the evaluated immunological biomarkers are potential candidates for identifying patients at risk of APS-related complications.

We included 38 patients with thrombotic APS. APS was diagnosed according to the Sydney classification criteria [1]. None of the patients had comorbidities associated with impaired complement levels, including full-blown systemic lupus erythematosus (SLE) or other systemic autoimmune diseases, chronic liver disease, recent opportunistic infections (last 6 months), and suspicion of a complement primary immunodeficiency (previous history of recurrent bacterial infections). The patients' blood was not examined in the acute phase of thrombosis. None of the patients had thrombotic episodes in the previous 3 months. No patients used heparin or its derivatives during the study or in the 3 months before the study; this may have modified complement activation. Most patients were given antithrombotic agents. Arterial events such as stroke, pulmonary embolism, and myocardial infarction were confirmed by computed tomography (CT) scan, magnetic resonance imaging (MRI), or angiography. Deep vein and arterial thrombosis were confirmed by Doppler echography or angiography.

*2.2. Controls.* The control groups comprised 14 aPL positive patients without APS-related clinical criteria, 16 systemic lupus erythematosus (SLE) patients, and 52 healthy individuals. Within aPL positive controls, all of them had autoimmune diseases (Table 1). None of these controls had full-blown SLE. SLE controls did not have clinical flare-ups during the 3 months before the study. None of the SLE patients had any laboratory criteria of the APS syndrome.

A questionnaire was administered to ensure that none of the healthy controls had any disease associated with altered complement levels.

*2.3. Plasma and Serum Sample Collection.* Immunological studies were performed the first time the patients were evaluated at the clinical immunology unit. Blood was extracted by venipuncture and collected into serum or plasma tubes. For serum extraction, the sample was left to coagulate for 30 minutes before being centrifuged at 1800 rpm for 5 minutes.

*2.4. aPL Determination.* The levels of IgG and IgM anti-cardiolipin (aCL) and IgG and IgM anti-$\beta$2 glycoprotein ($\beta$2GPI) antibodies were determined using standard ELISA assays (Fresenius, Bad Homburg, Germany). Levels of lupus anticoagulant (LA) were measured using the assays recommended in the guidelines of the International Society on Thrombosis and Haemostasis.

*2.5. Serum Quantification and Functional Assessment of Complement Proteins.* Levels of C3, C4, and factor B were measured using nephelometry with normal ranges of 83–172 mg/dL, 17–51 mg/dL, and 19–50 mg/dL, respectively (Beckman-Coulter, California, USA). CH100 was measured using radial immune diffusion with a normal range of >70 units/mL (Sanofi-Pasteur, Paris, France). These parameters are included in the protocol of all patients who are evaluated for the first time at the clinical immunology unit.

*2.6. Evaluation of Activated CD4 and CD8 T-Cells.* We performed a substudy of 18 patients, 14 aPL positive controls, 10 SLE patients, and 30 healthy controls. This substudy was not included in routine analyses. We previously investigated the association between levels of CD4 and CD8 subsets and obstetric APS [13], unexplained recurrent miscarriage [14], and chronic infectious diseases in patients who develop thrombosis [15]. In addition to the exclusion criteria set out above, the patients were not immunized and did not have active infections during the 6 months before the immunological study. The monoclonal antibodies used were directly conjugated with fluorescein isothiocyanate (FITC; FL1), phycoerythrin (PE; FL2), or peridinin chlorophyll protein (PerCP; FL3). We enumerated T-cell subsets using FITC/PE/PerCP combinations of HLADR/CD38/CD4, HLA-DR/CD25/CD4, CD28/HLADR/CD8, and isotypical controls. Lymphocyte staining was carried out using a whole-blood lysis technique, according to the recommended methodology and quality control procedures. Stained samples were analyzed using a FACScan flow cytometer (Becton Dickinson, San Jose, CA, USA) with CellQuest Pro software (Becton Dickinson).

*2.7. Clinical Followup.* To assess the potential impact of the evaluated abnormalities on clinical outcome, patients were scheduled to return to the clinical immunology unit at 6-month intervals. The revised criteria for the classification of SLE were used [16]. The cognitive symptoms inventory was used in patients with SLE (21-item questionnaire) to screen for difficulties in daily activities involving intermediate memory, concentration, attention, and executive function. Severe cognitive dysfunction was defined as a score ≥2 standard deviation (SD) below the mean in domains of attention, memory, and psychomotor speed, as compared to normative data [17]. To evaluate the inflammatory status of patients and disease controls, C-reactive protein (CRP assessed by nephelometry), rheumatoid factor (RF assessed by nephelometry), and erythrocyte sedimentation rate (ESR) were included. The disease activity status of SLE controls was assessed by the SLE Disease Activity Index (SLEDAI) [18].

TABLE 1: Clinical characteristics of patients with thrombotic APS and controls.

| Parameter | Thrombotic APS ($n = 38$) | aPL positive controls ($n = 14$) | SLE controls ($n = 16$) | Healthy controls ($n = 52$) | $P$ |
|---|---|---|---|---|---|
| Age, y, mean (range) | 50 (29–78) | 43 (37–59) | 42 (30–69) | 48 (30–75) | 0.17 |
| Sex | | | | | |
| Men (%) | 28.9 | 21.4 | 25 | 36.5 | 0.87 |
| Women (%) | 71.1 | 78.6 | 75 | 63.5 | |
| Risk factors of thrombosis | 15 (39) | 0 | 0 | 0 | — |
| Thrombotic event | | | | | |
| Stroke | 7 (18.42%) | 0 | 0 | 0 | — |
| DVT | 4 (10.53%) | 0 | 0 | 0 | — |
| CRVT | 4 (10.53%) | 0 | 0 | 0 | — |
| Pulmonary embolism | 3 (7.89%) | 0 | 0 | 0 | — |
| Hepatic vein thrombosis | 1 (2.63%) | 0 | 0 | 0 | — |
| Thrombophlebitis | 1 (2.63%) | 0 | 0 | 0 | — |
| Different combinations of thrombotic events | 12 (31.58%) | 0 | 0 | 0 | — |
| Thrombotic events and miscarriage | 4 (10.53%) | 0 | 0 | 0 | — |
| Other | 2 (5.26%) | 0 | 0 | 0 | — |
| Baseline disease | | | | | |
| Lupus like disease | 0 | 4 (28.6%) | 0 | 0 | — |
| Sjogren's syndrome | 0 | 1 (7.1%) | 0 | 0 | — |
| Systemic vasculitis | 0 | 1 (7.1%) | 0 | 0 | — |
| Rheumatoid arthritis | 0 | 1 (7.1%) | 0 | 0 | — |
| Thrombocytopenia | 9 (23.7%) | 3 (21.4%) | 4 (25%) | 0 | — |
| Cutaneous lupus | 0 | 1 (7.1%) | 0 | 0 | — |
| UCTD | 0 | 3 (21.4%) | 0 | 0 | — |
| Clinical and biological markers | | | | | |
| CRP (mg/dL) | 2.24 ± 6.84 | 0.32 ± 0.34 | 1.47 ± 2.82 | — | 0.55 |
| ESR (mm/hour) | 20.5 ± 24.8 | 9.9 ± 9.9 | 14.3 ± 8.9 | — | 0.28 |
| RF (IU/mL) | 26.4 ± 20.4 | 75.4 ± 183.9 | 23.4 ± 11.9 | — | 0.42 |
| SLEDAI index | — | — | 2.3 ± 1.8 | — | — |

CRP: C-reactive protein; CRVT: central retinal vein thrombosis; DVT: deep vein thrombosis; ESR: erythrocyte sedimentation rate; RF: rheumatoid factor; UDCD: undifferentiated connective-tissue disease.

*2.8. Statistics.* We compared the means using ANOVA test. A chi-square test was used to compare the frequencies of qualitative variables. Logistic regression was used to assess the relationship between immunological abnormalities and clinical outcome. Spearman's correlation test was used to assess the relationship between variables. We used a database constructed in Microsoft Excel, and the statistical analysis was performed using SPSS.

*2.9. Ethics.* The procedures followed in this study were in accordance with the ethical standards of our hospital ethics committee and with the Helsinki Declaration of 1975. Informed consent was obtained before the performance of the studies.

## 3. Results

*3.1. Distribution of aPL.* The distribution of aPL was as follows: IgG aCL only, $n = 8$ (21.1%); IgG aCL and IgG anti-$\beta$2GPI, $n = 7$ (18.4%); IgM aCL and IgM anti-$\beta$2GPI, $n = 1$ (2.6%); triple positivity (LA, aCL, and anti-$\beta$2GPI positive), $n = 20$ (52.6%); other, $n = 2$ (5.3%).

*3.2. Serum Complement Levels and Hypocomplementemia in Patients with Thrombotic APS.* The demographic and clinical characteristics of patients and controls are shown in Table 1. Patients with thrombotic APS showed significantly lower levels of C3, C4, and CH100 than healthy controls (Table 2). The prevalence of lower levels of C3 and C4 (defined as a concentration below the lower limit of normal) was higher in patients than in healthy controls (Table 2). Factor B concentrations were similar in patients and healthy controls. Only one patient had lower serum concentrations of factor B. Mean serum complement concentrations and prevalence of hypocomplementemia were similar in thrombotic APS patients as compared with aPL positive controls (Table 2). SLE controls disclosed significantly lower C3 concentrations than thrombotic APS patients.

TABLE 2: Concentration and functional activity of complement proteins in patients with thrombotic APS and healthy controls.

| Parameter | Patients ($n$ = 38) | aPL positive controls ($n$ = 14) | SLE controls ($n$ = 16) | Healthy controls ($n$ = 52) | $P$ |
|---|---|---|---|---|---|
| C3, mean ± SD mg/dL (range) | 97.7 ± 26.3 (58–156) | 108.8 ± 39 (61–202) | 77 ± 20 (27–106) | 113.4 ± 40.6 (61–305) | $0.35^a$, $0.05^b$, $0.04^c$ |
| Low C3 (%)[1] | 41.2 | 30.8 | 43.8 | 19.2 | $0.74^a$, $0.76^b$, $0.04^c$ |
| C4, mean ± SD mg/dL (range) | 16.9 ± 8.5 (2–41) | 21 ± 7 (12–35) | 15 ± 6 (5–27) | 23.9 ± 9.6 (12.8–74.4) | $0.19^a$, $0.58^b$, $0.001^c$ |
| Low C4 (%)[2] | 63.9 | 38.5 | 56.3 | 17.3 | $0.14^a$, $0.77^b$, $<0.01^c$ |
| FB, mean ± SD mg/dL (range) | 33 ± 7.7 (14–46.1) | 31 ± 8 (21.9–47.1) | 28 ± 6 (23–34) | 31.0 ± 8.27 (20–63) | $0.83^a$, $0.45^b$, $0.28^c$ |
| Low FB (%)[3] | 3.33 | 0 | 0 | 0 | $0.54^a$, $0.83^b$, $0.37^c$ |
| CH100, mean ± SD Units/mL (range) | 46.9 ± 17.9 (20–70) | 60 ± 27 (23–89) | 63 ± 24 (36–102) | 70.5 ± 31.5 (20–165) | $0.19^a$, $0.23^b$, $0.01^c$ |
| Low CH100 (%)[4] | 64.3 | 57.1 | 71.4 | 59.4 | $0.37^a$, $0.63^b$, $0.51^c$ |

APS: antiphospholipid syndrome; aPL positive controls: aPL+ patients without APS clinical criteria; HC: healthy controls; FB: factor B; [1]C3 normal range: 83–172 mg/dL; [2]C4 normal range: 17–51 mg/dL; [3]FB normal range: 19–50 mg/dL; [4]CH100 normal range: >70 units/mL. [a]ANOVA comparison of thrombotic APS with aPL+ controls, [b]ANOVA comparison of thrombotic APS with SLE controls, and [c]ANOVA comparison of thrombotic APS with healthy controls.

*3.3. Association between Laboratory and Clinical Abnormalities and Complement Levels.* Serum levels of C3 and C4 were significantly lower in APS patients with high titers of IgG or IgM aCL (defined as >80 units, Table 3). Patients with positive LA activity showed significantly lower C3 levels than those with negative activity (87 ± 17 versus 109 ± 30 mg/dL, $P$ = 0.014). Patients with triple positivity disclosed significantly lower serum concentrations of C3 than patients without triple positivity (86 ± 18 versus 111 ± 28 mg/dL, $P$ = 0.003).

No significant differences were observed between the concentration of the different complement proteins and CH100 when APS patients with positive antinuclear antibodies (ANA, IIF titer >160, $n$ = 8) were compared with those without positive ANA, not even when the patients were stratified by anti-DNA antibodies ($n$ = 6) (Table 3). Patients with thrombopenia showed significantly lower CH100 levels (Table 3). The presence of risk factors for thrombosis was not associated with complement levels or activity (Table 3).

*3.4. Activated Lymphocyte Subsets.* Patients with thrombotic APS had significantly higher percentages of activated CD4+DR+ and CD8+DR+ T-cells than healthy individuals but similar percentages to that observed in aPL positive and SLE controls (Figure 1). There was no association between lymphocyte activation subsets and high titer of aCL, presence of LA, or triple positivity. CD4+CD38+DR+ percentage was significantly higher in autoimmune disease controls as compared with thrombotic APS patients (Figure 1). The percentage of CD4+ cells coexpressing CD38 and HLA-DR increased progressively from thrombotic APS to SLE patients (Figure 1), while the percentage of CD4+ cells coexpressing CD25 and HLA DR tended to be higher in APS patients. Interestingly the ratio of CD4+CD25+DR+/CD4+CD38+DR+ cells was significantly higher in thrombotic APS patients as compared with disease control groups (1.3 ± 0.5, 0.83 ± 0.4, and 0.59 ± 0.36 in APS patients, aPL positive controls, and SLE patients, resp., $P$ = 0.004).

No significant correlation was observed between complement levels and T-cell subset percentages (Table 4). C4 values tended to be negatively correlated with activated CD4+DR+ and CD8+DR+ cells (Table 4).

### *3.5. Relationship between Immunological Biomarkers and Clinical Course*

*3.5.1. Complement Factors.* During the clinical followup performed after the immunological study (mean, 56 months), 11 patients (28.9%) developed APS-related clinical complications (progress to SLE ($n$ = 2), epilepsy ($n$ = 2), severe cognitive dysfunction ($n$ = 4), rethrombosis ($n$ = 1), idiopathic thrombocytopenic purpura ($n$ = 1), and premature arteriosclerosis [1]). Baseline serum concentrations of C3, C4, and CH100 were significantly lower in patients who later developed complications than in patients who were free of APS-related complications (86 ± 26 versus 107 ± 24 mg/dL ($P$ = 0.042), 13 ± 7 versus 21 ± 8 mg/dL ($P$ = 0.01), and 21 ± 17 versus 53 ± 16 U/mL ($P$ = 0.007), resp.). When we stratified the patients in two groups according to the median values of complement factors, those patients with lower C3 levels (<90 mg/dL) were at higher risk for development of complications (OR 9.99 95% CI, 1.03–97.5, $P$ = 0.047).

In APS patients C3 levels disclosed a significantly negative correlation with rheumatoid factor (2-tailed Spearman's correlation coefficient ($R$): −0.56, $P$ = 0.036). C4 levels also correlated with rheumatoid factor ($R$: −0.60, $P$ = 0.02). CH100 levels negatively correlated with CRP ($R$: −0.69, $P$ = 0.006) and with rheumatoid factor ($R$: −0.57, $P$ = 0.035). In aPL positive controls we found a positive correlation between C4 levels and serum CRP ($R$: +0.63, $P$ = 0.028). In SLE controls we did not find significant correlations between complement levels and rheumatoid factor, CRP, or ESR.

In SLE patients, CH100 levels disclosed a significantly negative correlation with the SLEDAI index ($R$: −0.75, $P$ = 0.013).

Table 3: Serum concentration and functional activity of complement proteins in thrombotic APS patients with specific laboratory and clinical abnormalities.

| Parameter | | C3 (mg/dL) | C4 (mg/dL) | FB (mg/dL) | CH100 (U/mL) |
|---|---|---|---|---|---|
| aCL titer | High | 87.6 ± 21.1 | 14.1 ± 7.7 | 30 ± 10.1 | 35.2 ± 23.7 |
| | Medium | 108.3 ± 28.6 | 20.7 ± 8.8 | 33.5 ± 7.3 | 48 ± 13.1 |
| | *P* | 0.027 | 0.026 | 0.32 | 0.31 |
| ANA | Positive | 84.3 ± 27.5 | 16.1 ± 11.9 | 27.3 ± 12.6 | 35.4 ± 24.8 |
| | Negative | 103.2 ± 24.2 | 17.13 ± 7.1 | 33.9 ± 7.7 | 37.8 ± 21.22 |
| | *P* | 0.54 | 0.76 | 0.09 | 0.85 |
| Anti-DNA | Positive | 86.6 ± 22.2 | 11.9 ± 6.1 | 34 ± 5 | 24.8 ± 3.8 |
| | Negative | 100 ± 26.9 | 18.1 ± 8.6 | 31.6 ± 10.3 | 41.8 ± 24.1 |
| | *P* | 0.26 | 0.08 | 0.62 | 0.19 |
| Thrombocytopenia | Yes | 90.9 ± 28.6 | 14.95 ± 8.3 | 25.6 ± 13.8 | 15.3 ± 13.6 |
| | No | 99.4 ± 25.9 | 17.4 ± 8.6 | 33.5 ± 7.9 | 42.8 ± 19.8 |
| | *P* | 0.46 | 0.48 | 0.07 | 0.046 |
| Risk factors for thrombosis | Yes | 97.5 ± 27.9 | 17.1 ± 8.9 | 33.4 ± 7.9 | 31.7 ± 24 |
| | No | 106 ± 28.2 | 19.3 ± 5.5 | 32.9 ± 8.9 | 47.0 ± 15.6 |
| | *P* | 0.526 | 0.55 | 0.89 | 0.42 |

High-titer aCL, IgG, or IgM anticardiolipin antibodies >80 U/mL. High-titer antinuclear antibodies (ANA) >1/160. High anti-DNA >20 IU/mL. Thrombocytopenia, platelet count < 100,000/$\mu$L. Risk factors include arterial hypertension, portal hypertension, atrial fibrillation, dyslipidemia, homocysteinemia, hypergammaglobulinemia, and smoking.

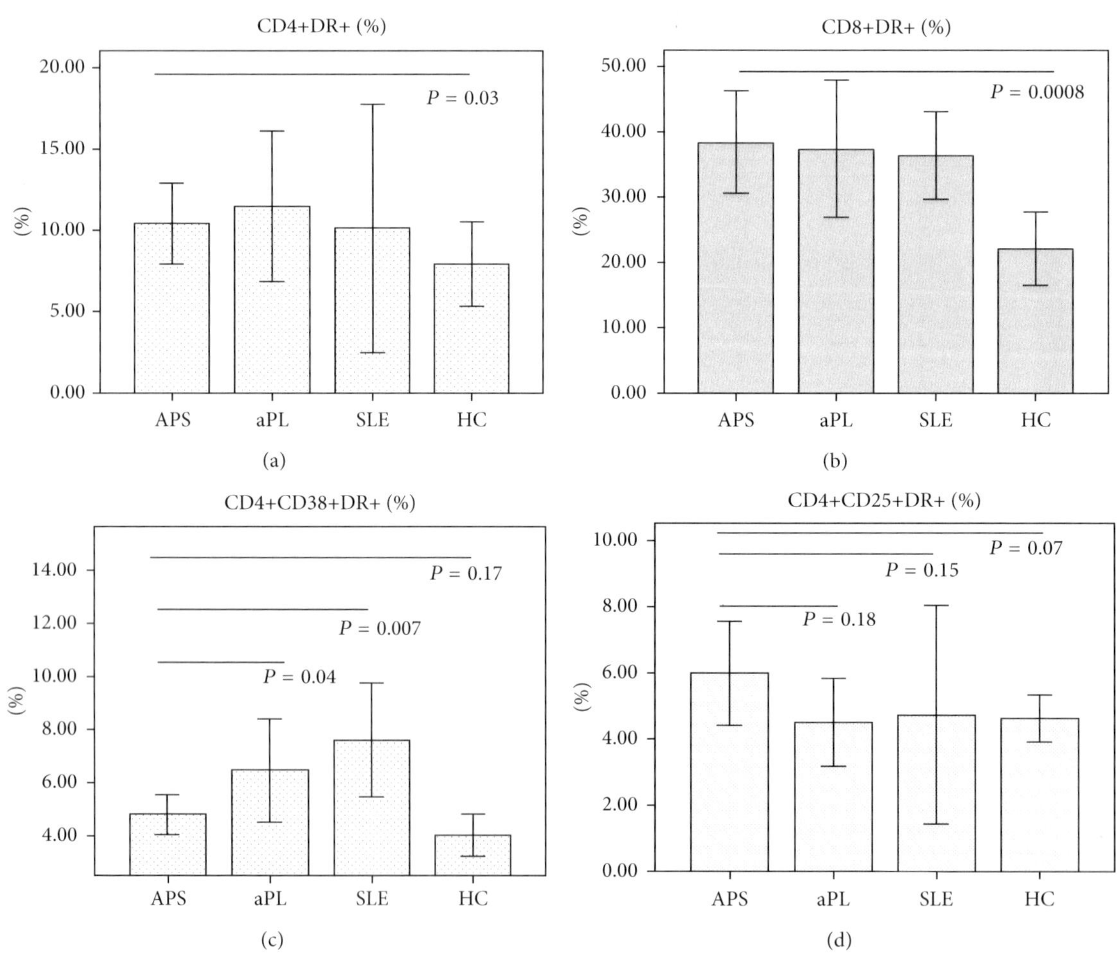


Figure 1: Activated lymphocyte subsets. CD4+ and CD8+ activated T-cell subsets in APS patients and controls. APS: thrombotic APS; aPL: aPL positive controls without APS clinical criteria; HC: healthy controls; SLE: systemic lupus erythematosus controls. Subsets are expressed as percentages over total CD4+ or CD8+ T-cells.

TABLE 4: Bivariate correlation between complement levels and lymphocyte subsets in thrombotic APS patients.

| | C3 | C4 | Factor B | CH100 |
|---|---|---|---|---|
| CD4+ DR+ | −0.23 (0.45) | −0.48 (0.09) | −0.55 (0.12) | 0.06 (0.84) |
| CD4+ CD38+ DR+ | 0.02 (0.94) | −0.03 (0.94) | −0.51 (0.16) | 0.23 (0.47) |
| CD4+ CD25+ DR+ | −0.17 (0.58) | −0.27 (0.36) | −0.52 (0.16) | −0.04 (0.91) |
| CD8+ DR+ | −0.12 (0.70) | −0.54 (0.05) | −0.42 (0.26) | −0.37 (0.23) |

Pearson's correlation.

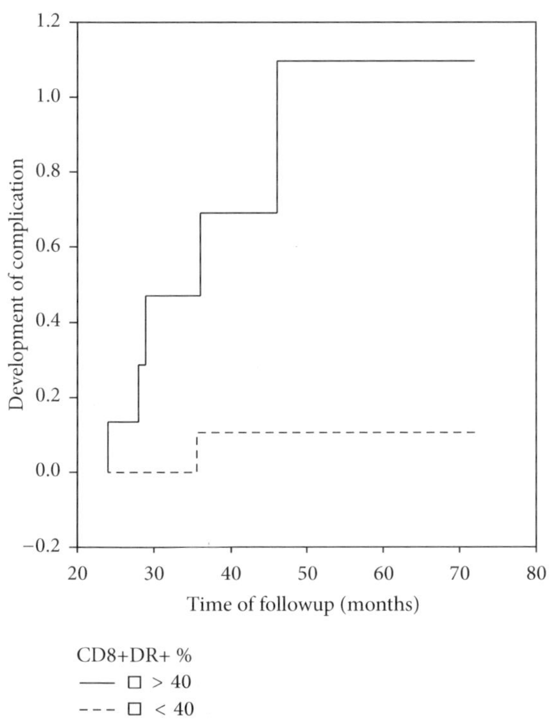


FIGURE 2: Kaplan Meier curves for development of clinical complications in thrombotic APS patients according to baseline CD8+DR+ percentages. Log Rank 5.43, $P = 0.019$.

*3.5.2. T-Cell Subsets.* During the clinical followup, 6 patients (33.3%) developed APS-related complications (progress to SLE ($n = 1$), epilepsy ($n = 2$), severe cognitive dysfunction ($n = 1$), and rethrombosis ($n = 2$)). This subgroup of patients had significantly higher percentages of CD8+DR+ T-cells ($51 \pm 20$ versus $32 \pm 8\%$, $P = 0.0007$) in the baseline study. When we stratified the patients in two groups according to the median values of lymphocyte subsets, those patients with higher CD8+DR+ levels (>40%) were at higher risk for development of complications (OR 14.9, 95% CI 1.21–185.2, $P = 0.034$) (Figure 2).

None of the evaluated clinical variables (sex (male versus female), age (>50 years versus <50 years), presence of risk factors of thrombosis, presence of triple aPL positivity, and presence of high titer antiphospholipid antibodies) were associated with development of complications (data not shown). In multivariate logistic analysis, higher percentages of CD8+DR+ (>40%) cells remained as a risk factor for development of complications (OR 14.9, 95% CI 1.21–185.2, $P = 0.034$).

CD8+DR+ percentages were not significantly correlated with CRP ($R$: +0.40, $P = 0.15$), rheumatoid factor ($R$: 0.39, $P = 0.17$), or ESR ($R$: −0.030, $P = 0.91$).

## 4. Discussion

In this study, we aimed to explore whether there was an association between levels of complement factors and of T-cell activation and clinical events. We took advantage of a long term followup of our patients in the clinical immunology unit of our hospital. In the baseline evaluation, we detected lower C3 and C4 levels in patients with high titers of aCL or triple positivity. This association supports the hypothesis of complement activation in thrombotic APS. More interestingly, in the prospective follow-up phase of the study, lower C3 complement levels and increased CD8+DR+ T-cell values were risk factors for the development of APS-related clinical complications. Even if our study was performed in few patients, higher CD8+DR+ T-cell percentages were an independent risk factor for development of complications. Poor pregnancy outcomes have been described among primary APS pregnancies with hypocomplementemia [19]. The percentage of circulating CD8+DR+ T-cells has been suggested as a biological marker which accurately reflects disease activity in SLE patients [20]. Given the lack of useful biomarkers to assess the risk of clinical progression in thrombotic APS patients, these parameters are good candidates for further evaluation in a future multicenter prospective study with greater number of patients and greater power to predict APS-related complications.

In the evaluation of the relationship of the biomarkers with thrombotic APS, we found lower concentrations of complement factors in patients with thrombotic APS as compared with healthy controls. Infections, injuries, and other types of biological stress can activate the complement system [2]. We excluded patients with known causes of low complement activity at the time of sample collection. In our study, the complement activation status of these patients was similar to that observed in aPL positive patients with distinct autoimmune conditions who lacked APS clinical criteria and in SLE patients. In thrombotic APS, no association was detected between the presence of other tested autoantibodies and complement factors, suggesting that hypocomplementemia might be aPL dependent. It has been suggested that a proinflammatory state may coexist with thrombotic

APS. In fact, accumulated evidence indicates that tissular ischemia or platelet aggregation may induce complement activation [8, 9]. The hypocomplementemia pattern that we observed affected C3 and C4, indicating that complement activation in thrombotic APS is produced mainly via the classic pathway. It was recently reported that patients with aPL had significantly increased levels of complement activation products [21]. Hypocomplementemia can be associated with increased immune complex formation. Oku et al. [7] found high immune complex levels in patients with primary APS. Carbone et al. [3] reported that 91% of women diagnosed with obstetric APS had high levels of circulating immune complex. Recently, complement activation affecting platelets was shown to be involved in vascular inflammation and thrombosis [22]. Interestingly, in our study, the relationship between complement values and inflammatory markers was better observed in APS patients than in aPL positive and SLE controls. The role of complement-mediated inflammation in reproductive failure in APS and the potential role of the immune modulation of the complement system (i.e., by the use of complement inhibitor therapies) in future studies have been discussed in recent publications of the 14th International Congress on Antiphospholipid Antibodies Task Force Reports [23, 24].

A limitation of our study is that complement split products were not evaluated. These products, rather than C3 and C4 levels, reflect more accurately complement activation. Complement activation products (C3a, C5a, and C5b-9) are able to activate endothelial cells, which result in loss of their antiinflammatory and antithrombotic potential. Direct determination of complement split products should be included in future studies.

We previously described increased levels of activated T-cell subsets in women with obstetric APS [13]. We also reported that higher levels of activated T-cells were associated with thrombosis in patients with HIV disease [15]. Although we performed the immunophenotypic study in only a small subgroup of patients, the results suggest that thrombotic APS is also associated with increased levels of T-cell activation. This hyperactivation status might be associated with reactivity against beta-2-glycoprotein-I, which has been previously demonstrated in APS [25]. On the other hand, higher percentages of T-cell activated subsets in thrombotic APS patients were similar to that described in patients with other systemic autoimmune diseases including SLE [26]. This immunophenotypic pattern of immune activation in thrombotic APS patients involved a higher expression of HLA class II (HLA-DR) molecules on CD4 and CD8 lymphocytes. A distinctive characteristic of thrombotic APS patients was the presence of a normal ratio of CD4+ cells coexpressing the alpha chain of the IL-2 receptor (CD25) over CD4+ cells coexpressing CD38 as compared with healthy controls, but higher than that observed in both disease control groups. As CD38 expression by CD4+ cells has been associated with low IL-2 production [27], these later results support the hypothesis that a proinflammatory Th1 immunophenotypic profile is predominant in thrombotic APS patients [28].

An interesting finding was the observation of the highest coexpression of CD38 and HLA-DR on CD4+ cells in SLE patients in agreement with recent studies describing that increased CD38 expression in T-cells was more prevalent in clinically active SLE [29]. A bias for IL-13 secretion has been described in CD4+CD38+ cells [27]. Th2 cytokines are involved in promoting humoral immunity including induction of IgE synthesis and promoting MHC class II expression. Increased autoreactive IgE autoantibodies have been recently described in SLE patients [30].

## Conflict of Interests

The authors declare that there is no conflict of interests regarding the publication of this paper.

## Acknowledgments

The authors acknowledge Juan Rodriguez-Molina for quality control of immunochemistry parameters. They are indebted to Paloma Sanchez-Mateos for the use of the flow cytometer. The authors wish to thank Eduardo Fernandez-Cruz, Head of the Immunology Department, for the use of the laboratory area. This study was funded by Fundación Salud 2000; Serono Prize 2005 was awarded to Javier Carbone.

## References

[1] S. Miyakis, M. D. Lockshin, T. Atsumi et al., "International consensus statement on an update of the classification criteria for definite antiphospholipid syndrome (APS)," *Journal of Thrombosis and Haemostasis*, vol. 4, no. 2, pp. 295–306, 2006.

[2] D. Ricklin and J. D. Lambris, "Complement in immune and inflammatory disorders: pathophysiological mechanisms," *Journal of Immunology*, vol. 190, no. 8, pp. 3831–3838, 2013.

[3] J. Carbone, M. Orera, M. Rodríguez-Mahou et al., "Immunological abnormalities in primary APS evolving into SLE: 6 years follow-up in women with repeated pregnancy loss," *Lupus*, vol. 8, no. 4, pp. 274–278, 1999.

[4] M. Sugiura-Ogasawara, K. Nozawa, T. Nakanishi, Y. Hattori, and Y. Ozaki, "Complement as a predictor of further miscarriage in couples with recurrent miscarriages," *Human Reproduction*, vol. 21, no. 10, pp. 2711–2714, 2006.

[5] J. Alijotas-Reig, "The complement system as a main actor in the pathogenesis of obstetric antiphospholipid syndrome," *Medicina Clinica*, vol. 134, no. 1, pp. 30–34, 2010.

[6] Z. Romay-Penabad, X. Liu X, G. Montiel-Manzano, E. P. De Martínez, and S. S. Pierangeli, "C5a receptor-deficient mice are protected from thrombophilia and endothelial cell activation induced by some antiphospholipid antibodies," *Annals of the New York Academy of Sciences*, vol. 1108, pp. 554–566, 2007.

[7] K. Oku, T. Atsumi, M. Bohgaki et al., "Complement activation in patients with primary antiphospholipid syndrome," *Annals of the Rheumatic Diseases*, vol. 68, no. 6, pp. 1030–1035, 2009.

[8] K. J. Woollard, "Immunological aspects of atherosclerosis," *Clinical Science*, vol. 125, no. 5, pp. 221–235, 2013.

[9] E. Falk, M. Nakano, J. F. Bentzon, A. V. Finn, and R. Virmani, "Update on acute coronary syndromes: the pathologists' view," *European Heart Journal*, vol. 34, no. 10, pp. 719–728, 2013.

[10] O. Bruserud and K. Lundin, "The effect of drugs used in anticoagulation therapy on T lymphocyte activation in vitro. II.

Warfarin inhibits T lymphocyte activation," *Journal of Clinical and Laboratory Immunology*, vol. 23, no. 4, pp. 169–173, 1987.

[11] G. Girardi, "Heparin treatment in pregnancy loss: potential therapeutic benefits beyond anticoagulation," *Journal of Reproductive Immunology*, vol. 66, no. 1, pp. 45–51, 2005.

[12] M. Kolev, G. Le Friec, and C. Kemper, "The role of complement in CD4+ T cell homeostasis and effector functions," *Seminars in Immunology*, vol. 25, no. 1, pp. 12–19, 2013.

[13] J. Carbone, A. Gallego, N. Lanio et al., "Quantitative abnormalities of peripheral blood distinct T, B, and natural killer cell subsets and clinical findings in obstetric antiphospholipid syndrome," *Journal of Rheumatology*, vol. 36, no. 6, pp. 1217–1225, 2009.

[14] J. Carbone, A. Gallego, N. Lanio, C. Chean, J. Navarro, and E. Sarmiento, "Peripheral blood CD8+DR+ T-cell count: a potential new immunologic marker of unexplained recurrent abortion," *Fertility and Sterility*, vol. 94, no. 1, pp. 360–361, 2010.

[15] J. Carbone, "Immune activation and increased prevalence of thrombosis in HIV infection," *Journal of Acquired Immune Deficiency Syndromes*, vol. 46, no. 3, pp. 375–376, 2007.

[16] M. C. Hochberg, "Updating the American College of Rheumatology revised criteria for the classification of systemic lupus erythematosus," *Arthritis and rheumatism*, vol. 40, no. 9, p. 1725, 1997.

[17] G. S. Alarcón, L. Cianfrini, L. A. Bradley et al., "Systemic lupus erythematosus in three ethnic groups. X: measuring cognitive impairment with the cognitive symptoms inventory," *Arthritis Care and Research*, vol. 47, no. 3, pp. 310–319, 2002.

[18] D. D. Gladman, C. H. Goldsmith, M. B. Urowitz et al., "Sensitivity to change of 3 systemic lupus erythematosus disease activity indices: international validation," *Journal of Rheumatology*, vol. 21, no. 8, pp. 1468–1471, 1994.

[19] R. Reggia, T. Ziglioli, L. Andreoli et al., "Primary antiphospholipid syndrome: any role for serum complement levels in predicting pregnancy complications?" *Rheumatology*, vol. 51, no. 12, Article ID kes225, pp. 2186–2190, 2012.

[20] J. F. Viallard, C. Bloch-Michel, M. Neau-Cransac et al., "HLA-DR expression on lymphocyte subsets as a marker of disease activity in patients with systemic lupus erythematosus," *Clinical and Experimental Immunology*, vol. 125, no. 3, pp. 485–491, 2001.

[21] K. A. Breen, P. Seed, K. Parmar, G. W. Moore, S. E. Stuart-Smith, and B. J. Hunt, "Complement activation in patients with isolated antiphospholipid antibodies or primary antiphospholipid syndrome," *Thrombosis and Haemostasis*, vol. 107, no. 3, pp. 423–429, 2012.

[22] C. Lood, S. Eriksson, B. Gullstrand et al., "Increased C1q, C4 and C3 deposition on platelets in patients with systemic lupus erythematosus-a possible link to venous thrombosis?" *Lupus*, vol. 21, no. 13, pp. 1423–1432, 2012.

[23] G. R. de Jesus, N. Agmon-Levin, C. A. Andrade et al., "14th International Congress on Antiphospholipid Antibodies: task force report on obstetric antiphospholipid syndrome," *Autoimmunity Reviews*, 2014.

[24] D. Erkan, C. L. Aguiar, D. Andrade et al., "14th International Congress on Antiphospholipid Antibodies: task force report on antiphospholipid syndrome treatment trends," *Autoimmunity Reviews*, vol. 13, no. 6, pp. 685–696, 2014.

[25] H. Torres-Aguilar, M. Blank, S. Kivity et al., "Tolerogenic dendritic cells inhibit antiphospholipid syndrome derived effector/memory CD4+ T cell response to $\beta$2GPI," *Annals of the Rheumatic Diseases*, vol. 71, no. 1, pp. 120–128, 2012.

[26] D. Erkan, R. Willis, G. Basra et al., "A prospective open-label pilot study of fluvastatin on proinflammatory and prothrombotic biomarkers in antiphospholipid antibody positive patients," *Annals of the Rheumatic Diseases*, vol. 73, no. 6, pp. 1176–1180, 2014.

[27] K. Scalzo-Inguanti and M. Plebanski, "CD38 identifies a hypoproliferative IL-13-secreting CD4+ T-cell subset that does not fit into existing naive and memory phenotype paradigms," *European Journal of Immunology*, vol. 41, no. 5, pp. 1298–1308, 2011.

[28] M. Karakantza, G. L. Theodorou, N. Meimaris et al., "Type 1 and type 2 cytokine-producing CD4+ and CD8+ T cells in primary antiphospholipid syndrome," *Annals of Hematology*, vol. 83, no. 11, pp. 704–711, 2004.

[29] E. J. Pavón, E. Zumaquero, A. Rosal-Vela et al., "Increased CD38 expression in T cells and circulating anti-CD38 IgG autoantibodies differentially correlate with distinct cytokine profiles and disease activity in systemic lupus erythematosus patients," *Cytokine*, vol. 62, no. 2, pp. 232–243, 2013.

[30] B. Dema, C. Pellefigues, S. Hasni et al., "Autoreactive IgE is prevalent in systemic lupus erythematosus and is associated with increased disease activity and nephritis," *PLoS ONE*, vol. 9, no. 2, Article ID e90424, 2014.

# 23

# Presence of DQ2.2 Associated with DQ2.5 Increases the Risk for Celiac Disease

**Lucas Malta Almeida,[1,2] Lenora Gandolfi,[1,2,3] Riccardo Pratesi,[1,2,3] Rosa Harumi Uenishi,[2,3] Fernanda Coutinho de Almeida,[1,2] Nicole Selleski,[2,3] and Yanna Karla de Medeiros Nóbrega[1,2,3,4]**

[1]*Graduate Program in Medical Sciences, University of Brasília School of Medicine, 70.900.910 Brasília, DF, Brazil*
[2]*Research Laboratory for Celiac Disease, University of Brasília School of Medicine, 70.900.910 Brasília, DF, Brazil*
[3]*Graduate Program in Health Sciences, University of Brasília School of Health Sciences, 70.900.910 Brasília, DF, Brazil*
[4]*Department of Pharmaceutical Sciences, University of Brasília School of Health Sciences, 70.900.910 Brasília, DF, Brazil*

Correspondence should be addressed to Yanna Karla de Medeiros Nóbrega; yannanobrega@gmail.com

Academic Editor: Rizgar Mageed

*Background.* Celiac disease (CD) is a genetically determined immune-mediated disorder in which gluten immunogenic peptides are presented to CD4 T cells by HLA-DQ2.5, DQ8, DQ2.2, and their combinations. Our aim is to establish a risk gradient for celiac disease based on HLA-DQ profile in a brazilian representative population and the relevance of DQ2.2 in celiac disease development. *Materials and Methods.* 237 celiac patients and 237 controls (both groups with 164 females and 73 males) were included. All samples were tested for the presence of predisposing HLA-DQ alleles using the PCR-SSP method. Results were considered significant when $p < 0.05$. Disease risk was expressed as 1 : $N$ for each HLA-DQ category described at this study. *Results.* DQ2.5 and/or DQ8 were detected in 224 celiac patients (94.5%) and 84 controls (35.4%). Eight celiac patients (3.4%) and 38 controls (16%) disclosed only DQ2.2. Even though DQ2.2 ($\beta2/\beta2$ or $\beta2$/x) showed a low CD risk of 1 : 251 and 1 : 550, respectively, the genotype DQ2.5/DQ2.2 ($\beta2/\beta2$) showed high CD risk of 1 : 10 ($p < 0.0001$). The disease risk gradient ranged from 1 : 3014 to 1 : 7. *Conclusion.* Our study allowed the determination of a risk gradient for celiac disease development in at-risk population, showing that DQ2.2 variant was relevant when associated with DQ2.5.

## 1. Introduction

Celiac disease (CD) is a genetically determined immune-mediated disorder, in which individuals carrying specific HLA haplotypes (DQ2 and/or DQ8) mount an immunologic response to the ingestion of gluten that leads to a broad range of clinical signs and symptoms. Gastrointestinal disorders are the most common manifestations and include chronic diarrhea, abdominal distention, and nutrients malabsorption. However, extraintestinal manifestations are also frequent and include numerous conditions such as dermatitis herpetiformis, anemia, dental enamel hypoplasia, osteoporosis, and neurologic problems [1].

CD activity is characterized by the production of IgA anti-endomysial antibody (IgA-EmA) and IgA anti-transglutaminase antibody (IgA-tTG), which are good markers of the active phase of the disease and are usually used as a first step in its diagnosis. In most cases, a definitive diagnosis requires a jejunal biopsy showing typical histologic abnormalities such as villous atrophy, crypt hyperplasia, and lymphocytic infiltration [2].

In the general population of Europe, United States, and countries predominantly populated by individuals of European origin, the prevalence of CD is approximately 1%. In Brazil, several prevalence studies performed to date revealed significant differences around the country, probably consequent to genetic and environmental factors and possibly also due to interlaboratory assay variability [3–7]. Although multicenter epidemiological studies that could yield reliable information on CD prevalence in Brazil are still lacking, the existing reports suggest that the disease prevalence in this country is similar to the general prevalence found in other areas of the world [2, 4, 5, 7].

Virtually all CD patients carry the alleles that code for DQ2 and/or DQ8 molecules or at least for one chain of the DQ2 heterodimer, normally $\beta$ chain, encoded by DQB1*02 allele. The occurrence of CD in the absence of these at-risk DQ factors is extremely rare [8]. The presence of these molecules does not predict with accuracy that CD will develop, since they are present in 25 to 50% of the general population, although the vast majority of these individuals will never develop the disease [9].

Consequently, in view of the nearly 100% negative predictive value, the HLA typing has been used as a screening tool in high-risk population such as carriers of type 1 diabetes, Down syndrome, or Turner syndrome [10]. HLA typing has also been used as a prognostic factor of the disease severity [11, 12] and sex distribution [13] and as an accessory element in the diagnosis of difficult cases [14]. Finally, the HLA-DQ typing to determine the future risk of CD has been extensively discussed, although its practical usage remains not clinically defined. Genetic testing of individuals could eliminate more than 60% of the population considered to have a low CD-risk (DQ2 or DQ8 negative) from future antibody testing, and the identification of high-risk individuals would allow a prospective screening, enabling an early therapeutic intervention [15].

As far as we know, no previous study has focused on the frequency of CD predisposing HLA genotypes in affected and nonaffected individuals in a Brazilian population. Consequently, our aim in the present study is to determine the frequency of CD predisposing DQ genotypes in celiac and nonceliac subjects and establish a CD-risk gradient focusing on the prevalence of DQ2.2, in Brazil.

## 2. Material and Methods

*2.1. Celiac Patients and Ethics Committee.* This retrospective study included celiac patients followed during the period of 2006 to 2014 at the Celiac Disease Outpatient Clinic of the Brasilia University Hospital. The diagnosis was achieved according to the criteria of the European Society of Pediatric Gastroenterology and Nutrition (ESPGAN) [16] and the revised guidelines of the European Society of Pediatric Gastroenterology, Hepatology and Nutrition (ESPGHAN) [17]. The study was approved by the School of Health Sciences Ethic Committee in Human Research (project number 070/06) and is in accordance with the latest Declaration of Helsinki. Written informed consent for participation was obtained from all participants prior to their enrollment in the study, including consent to publish.

*2.2. Patients and Controls.* 237 serologically and biopsy confirmed celiac patients were included in the study (164 females and 73 males, age range: 1 to 75, mean age 21.5 ± 16.2 years at sample collection). Control group included 237 unrelated, gender and age matched, healthy individuals (164 women and 73 males, age range: 1 to 75 years, mean age 18.5 ± 16.14 years at sample collection), without history of autoimmune diseases and from the same geographic area and socioeconomic stratum as the celiac patients. All controls underwent serologic tests: IgA anti-transglutaminase antibodies (QUANTA Lite™ h-tTG IgA ELISA, INOVA Diagnostic, Inc., San Diego, CA, USA) and IgA anti-endomysium antibodies (NOVA Lite® Monkey Oesophagus IFA Kit, INOVA Diagnostic, Inc., San Diego, CA, USA) and disclosed negative results.

*2.3. HLA Alleles Genotyping.* Whole blood was obtained from celiac patients and controls in EDTA containing tubes following the H3-A6 criteria of Clinical and Laboratory Standards Institute (CLSI). DNA extraction was performed using commercial kit (Illustrat™ Blood Genomic Prep Mini Kit, GE Healthcare, Buckinghamshire, UK), and quantified with a NanoVue spectrophotometer (GE Healthcare, Buckinghamshire, UK). The final concentration of DNA was adjusted to 20 ng/$\mu$L.

The amplification of the alleles DQA1*05, DQA1*02:01, DQB1*02, DQA1*03, and DQB1*03:02 was performed utilizing the commercial DQ-CD Typing Plus Kit (BioDiagene®, Palermo, Italy), which also allows the detection of homozygosis of the DQB1*02 allele.

*2.4. Statistical Analysis.* Celiac patients and controls were categorized according to their HLA-DQ profile. Fisher's exact and $\chi^2$ tests were applied to compare the frequencies of predisposing HLA-DQ alleles between celiac patients and controls. Results were considered significant when $p < 0.05$. The risk assessment calculations was based on the study by Megiorni et al. [18], in which the degree of risk was represented by 1 : $N$, where $N$ was the number of healthy individuals among which one patient is present. The analysis was performed considering a presumed prevalence of 1 : 100 in the general Brazilian population. For each HLA-DQ category, $N$ was calculated as a percentage of controls with a distinct HLA-DQ multiplied by 100 and divided by the percentage of patients with the same DQ typing.

*2.5. Nomenclature.* The DQ2.5 HLA heterodimer is encoded by the allelic variants DQA1*05 and DQB1*02. These two variants may be present either in *cis* (haplotype DR3) or in *trans* conformation (haplotype DR5/DR7). The HLA heterodimer DQ2.2 is encoded by the alleles DQA1*02:01 and DQB1*02:02, which may be found in both heterozygosis (haplotype DR7/X) and homozygosis (haplotype DR7/DR7).

Considering that previous studies have shown that the dose-dependent effect of the allele DQB1*02 significantly increases the degree of risk, we classified as $\beta 2$/x those individuals with only one copy of the DQB1*02 allele (heterozygosis) and as $\beta 2/\beta 2$ those with two copies of the same allele (homozygosis). Individuals classified as $\beta 2$/x may show either DR3/X, DR5/DR7, X/DR7, or DR7/DR4 haplotypes. Individuals pertaining to the group $\beta 2/\beta 2$ may show haplotypes DR3/DR3 or DR3/DR7 and DR7/DR7.

The HLA-DQ8 molecule is encoded by allelic variants DQA1*03 and DQB1*03:02 which are in linkage disequilibrium and consequently are commonly present in *cis*-conformation in the DR4 haplotype. This haplotype can be

TABLE 1: CD predisposing HLA-DQ frequencies in CD patients and controls and general genetic risk.

| Genotypes | DQB1*02 status | CD% ($n = 237$) | Control ($n = 237$) | $p$CD/control | General risk 1:100 |
|---|---|---|---|---|---|
| DQ2.5/DQ2.5 | ($\beta 2/\beta 2$) | 6.33% (15) | 0.42% (1) | 0.0004 | 1:7 |
| DQ2.5/DQ2.2 | ($\beta 2/\beta 2$) | 25.31% (60) | 2.53% (6) | <0.0001 | 1:10 |
| DQ2.5/DQ8 | ($\beta 2$/x) | 8.86% (21) | 1.68% (4) | 0.0007 | 1:19 |
| DQ2.5 | ($\beta 2$/x) *trans* | 10.54% (25) | 2.11% (5) | 0.0002 | 1:20 |
| | ($\beta 2$/x) *cis* | 32.91% (78) | 11% (26) | <0.0001 | 1:30 |
| DQ2.2/DQ8 | ($\beta 2$/x) | 6.33% (15) | 2.53% (6) | 0.0718 | 1:40 |
| DQ2.2/DQ2.2 | ($\beta 2/\beta 2$) | 0.84% (2) | 2.11% (5) | 0.4496 | 1:251 |
| DQ8 | — | 3.8% (9) | 10.97% (26) | 0.0043 | 1:289 |
| DQ2.2 | ($\beta 2$/x) | 2.53% (6) | 13.92% (33) | 0.0001 | 1:550 |
| DQ8/$\alpha 5$ | — | 0.42% (1) | 4.22% (10) | 0.0108 | 1:1005 |
| $\alpha 5$ | — | 1.3% (3) | 20.25% (48) | <0.0001 | 1:1594 |
| Absent | — | 0.84% (2) | 25.31% (60) | <0.0001 | 1:3014 |
| $\alpha 8$ | — | 0.0% (0) | 2.95% (7) | 0.0149 | ND |

ND: risk not determined; CD: celiac disease; $\beta 2$ refers to DQB1*02; $\alpha 5$ refers to DQA1*05; $\alpha 8$ refers to DQA1*03:01; x denotes not determined allele; $\beta 2/\beta 2$ refers to DQB1*02 homozygosis; $\beta 2$/x refers to DQB1*02 heterozygosis; $p$ value.

found either in association with DQ2.5 (DR3/DR4), DQ2.2 (DR7/DR4) or with DQA1*05 ($\alpha 5$/DR4).

The $\alpha 5$ individuals carry the allele DQA1*05 and $\alpha 8$ individuals carry the allele DQA1*03, without any other CD predisposing allele. Individuals without any CD predisposing alleles were designed as absent. "X" refers to undetermined haplotypes and "x" to undetermined alleles.

## 3. Results

The presence of HLA-DQ2.5/DQ8/DQ2.2 genotypes was categorized according to the presence of CD predisposing HLA alleles (Table 1). The HLA-DQ2.5 and/or DQ8 were detected in 224 celiac patients (94.5%) and in 84 (35.4%) controls. Eight celiac patients (3.4%) and 38 controls (16%) disclosed the HLA-DQ2.2 either in homozygosis or in heterozygosis.

The genotype DQ2.5/DQ2.5, which confers an increased risk of developing CD, was found in 15 (6.33%) celiac patients and in a single control (0.42%), while the genotype DQ2.5/DQ2.2 was found in 60 (25.31%) celiac patients and 6 controls (2.53%).

The DQ2.5 genotype, when not associated with DQ8, was present in 178 (75.1%) celiac patients and 38 (16%) controls. Ten celiac patients (4.2%) and 36 controls (15.2%) disclosed only DQ8 alone, unaccompanied by DQ2.5 nor DQ2.2.

Celiac patients and controls, who did not disclose any of the risk variants (DQ2.5, DQ2.2, or DQ8), were explored for the presence of alleles that could confer low risk for the development of CD. The frequency and absence of these alleles, in celiac patients and controls, are shown in Table S1 (see Supplementary Material available online at http://dx.doi.org/10.1155/2016/5409653).

The comparison between the frequency of CD HLA predisposing alleles in celiac patients and controls was used to establish a disease risk gradient that, in our sample, ranged from 1:7 to 1:3014 (Figure 1).

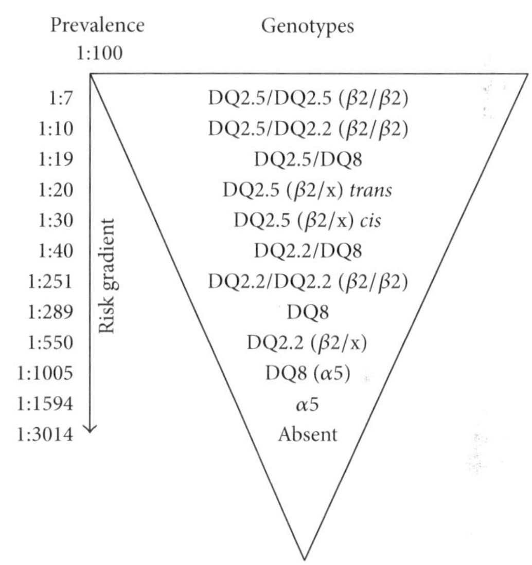


FIGURE 1: Risk gradient according to HLA haplotype combinations, considering a disease prevalence of 1:100. $\beta 2$ refers to DQB1*02; $\alpha 5$ refers to DQA1*05; "x" denotes corresponding allele not determined; individuals with only one copy of the DQB1*02 allele were classified as $\beta 2$/x (heterozygosis); individuals with two copies of the DQB1*02 allele were classified as $\beta 2/\beta 2$ (homozygosis); *trans* and *cis* indicate, respectively, $\alpha 5$ and $\beta 2$ position in different or in the same chromosome 6 pair.

The highest risks findings (1:7) were for the genotype DQ2.5/DQ2.5 ($\beta 2/\beta 2$) positive subjects ($p = 0.0004$, OR 15.95 95%, CI 2.08–121.8) and DQ2.5/DQ2.2 ($\beta 2/\beta 2$) (1:10) with $p < 0.0001$, OR 13.05 95%, CI 5.51–30.9.

The risk related to the concomitant presence of DQ2.5 and DQ8 was 1:19 ($p = 0.0007$; OR 5.66 95% CI 1.91 to 16.77). The category DQ2.5 ($\beta 2$/x) in either *trans*- (DR5/DR7) or *cis*-configuration (DR3/X) disclosed different risk values

1 : 20 ($p = 0.0002$; OR 5.47 95% CI 2.05 to 14.55) and 1 : 30 ($p < 0.0001$; 4.35 OR 95% CI 2.59 to 7.30), respectively.

The presence of DQ2.2/DQ8 was associated with a risk of 1 : 40 ($p = 0.0718$; OR 2.60 95% CI 0.991 to 6.826), while the presence of DQ2.2/DQ2.2 ($\beta 2/\beta 2$) was associated with a risk of 1 : 251 ($p = 0.4496$; OR 0.39 95% CI 0.085 to 2.06). The DQ2.2 ($\beta 2$/x) showed a risk of 1 : 550 ($p < 0.0001$; OR 0.16 95% CI 0.08–0.39), while DQ8 without any other CD predisposing allele disclosed a risk of 1 : 289 ($p = 0.0043$; OR 0.32 95%, CI 0.146 to 0.699).

The association of DQ8 and $\alpha 5$ disclosed a significant decrease in disease risk of 1 : 1005 ($p = 0.0108$; OR 0.096 95% 0.0122–0.758), when compared to the presence of DQ8 alone. Finally, the exclusive presence of $\alpha 5$ showed a risk of 1 : 1594 ($p < 0.0001$; OR 0.050 95% CI 0.015–0.165), while the complete absence of any CD-HLA-DQ predisposing alleles was associated with a risk of 1 : 3014 ($p < 0.0001$; OR 0.024 95% CI 0.006–0.101). The risk for the presence of $\alpha 8$ was undetermined.

## 4. Discussion

The onset of CD is strongly associated with the presence of HLA-DQ2 and DQ8, which are considered to account for up to 40% of the genetic risk for the disease development. Other non-HLA genes are involved in CD susceptibility, although their genetic contribution to CD is weak and is not generally considered in the calculation of the disease risk [19, 20]. Consequently, CD risk calculation, based on the presence of these HLA alleles, will allow a practical evaluation of the need for subsequent periodic tests on subjects included in the at-risk group. On the other hand, in view of the high negative predictive value of their absence, the need of further serologic testing is practically excluded in negative subjects.

Data obtained in the present study regarding the distribution of haplotypes containing DQ2.5/DQ8/DQ2.2 and their corresponding alleles, in a representative sample of Brazilian celiac patients and of presumably healthy controls, were used to calculate the risk gradient for future development of celiac disease in our population.

The Brazilian population has a high degree of genetic heterogeneity resulting from more than 500 years of interbreeding among three main ethnicities: Europeans, Amerindians, and Africans. In addition, during the last two centuries, successive migratory waves of Italians, Spaniards, Germans, Japanese, Lebanese, and Syrian further increased our population racial miscegenation. The analysis of ancestry informative markers of a representative sample of the Brazilian population disclosed a major contribution of Europeans (0.771%), followed by Africans (0.143%), and Amerindians (0.085%) [21]. The current population of Brasilia can be considered representative of the Brazilian population, since, during more than fifty years from its foundation, this city, presently with more than 2,500,000 inhabitants [22], has hosted people from all over the country.

Despite the great ethnical diversity of the distinct macroregions of Brazil, the frequency of different haplotypes in Brazilian celiac patients is relatively stable. Previous studies performed in small series of celiac patients revealed that HLA-DQ2.5 and/or DQ8 were present in 93.1% of celiac patients in the Northeastern region of Brazil, where the miscegenation with Africans and Amerindians is more intense [23]. In the Southern region, where Caucasian ancestry predominates, the frequency of 91.1% was found [24]. In this study, conducted in the Midwestern region of the country, the frequency of these genotypes was 94.5%. It is of interest that these frequencies are very similar to those found in Europe, where over 90% of the celiac patients carry the DQ2 heterodimer, the remaining being mostly characterized by the presence of DQ8 [8]. Only a small number of celiacs carry neither the DQ2 nor the DQ8 genotypes, although several have been reported to have just one chain of the DQ2 heterodimer [8].

Additionally, in our study, when considering the presence of the DQ2.5 variant without association with DQ8, the frequency found in celiac patients was 75.1%, while in previous studies performed in the Southern and Northeastern regions of Brazil was 65.3% [24] and 68.5%, respectively [23]. The presence of DQ8 alone (i.e., without the concomitant presence of DQ2.5) among our celiac patients was 10.5%. Comparatively, the frequency in the previously cited regions was, respectively, 11.9% and 17.8% [23, 24].

Interestingly, when comparing celiac patients and controls for the presence of DQ8, alone or in combination with other genotypes or alleles (Table 1), the same frequency of 19.4% was detected in both groups. The only differences between groups were the DQ8 allelic combinations and their related risks. The association of DQ8 with DQB1*02 (DQ2.5/DQ8 or DQ2.2/DQ8) is predominantly observed in celiac patients and in a minor degree in controls. The presence of this association increases 7 to 15 times the risk of developing the disease compared to DQ8 alone. These data are in agreement with the fact that the presence of DQB1*02 is associated with an increased risk of CD due to its higher antigenic repertoire, a fact which does not occur with an uncombined DQ8 [8, 18, 25, 26].

The low frequency of DQ2.2 ($\beta 2$/x and $\beta 2/\beta 2$) (Table 1) found among celiac patients ($n = 8$, 3.4%) when compared to controls ($n = 38$, 16%) shows that although this variant is a predisposing factor for CD, it has a minor capacity to trigger an autoimmune process. This fact is in accordance with low binding stability of DQ2.2 heterodimer with gluten antigens decreasing the inflammatory response [27, 28]. However, its genotyping is recommended in at-risk groups; since the genotype DQ2.2 is present in association with DQ2.5 and DQ8, it becomes a major risk factor significantly increasing the risk for CD onset [29].

In the present study, the highest risk for CD was associated with the presence of the HLA genotypes DQ2.5/DQ2.5 ($\beta 2/\beta 2$), DQ2.5/DQ2.2 ($\beta 2/\beta 2$), and DQ2.5/DQ8 that disclosed a risk of 1 : 7, 1 : 10, and 1 : 19, respectively. In comparison, in the Italian population the risk for CD was due to the presence of the HLA genotypes DQ2.5/DQ2.5 ($\beta 2/\beta 2$) and DQ2.5/DQ2.2 ($\beta 2/\beta 2$) and DQ2.5/DQ8, which were associated with a respective risk of 1 : 10 and 1 : 7 [18].

In our study, the DQ2.5 heterodimer disclosed a risk of 1 : 20 (in *trans*) and 1 : 30 (in *cis*), showing statistically significant differences. However, when *cis*- and *trans*-conformations of DQ2.5 were considered together, the resulting risk was 1:30 (data not shown), similar to the risk found in the literature [18, 30].

The combination DQ8/$\alpha$5 showed 3.5 times decreased risk of developing CD than that reported for isolated DQ8 (Figure 1). Similar relationship was found in Southern Spain [30]. Both patients and controls with this combination disclosed a DR5/DR4 haplotype configuration. It could be possible that the *trans*-conformations (DQA1*05/DQB1*03:02 and DQA1*03/DQB1*03:01) lead to the production of not very efficient heterodimers regarding to the presentation of some major immunogenic gluten peptides, since there is a lack of evidence for these events in the current study [26]. Consequently, we suggest that the association of DQA1*05/DQB1*03:02 and DQA1*03/DQB1*03:01 reduces the binding of immunogenic epitopes of gluten and transglutaminase 2, therefore not triggering an effective immune response mediated by lymphocytes B and T.

Individuals belonging to at-risk groups that only show the $\alpha$5 allele or do not disclose any CD predisposing HLA alleles could be excluded from periodical follow-ups in view of their extremely low risk of developing CD [8, 18] (Figure 1).

## 5. Conclusion

The present study showed, in a representative population of celiac patients and controls, the frequency of HLA-DQ variants DQ2.5/DQ2.2/DQ8, determining the probability of developing CD and establishing a risk gradient for the future onset of the disease. These data are useful for the screening of subjects included in at-risk groups for CD, discriminating subjects that are unlikely to develop the disease from those who must be monitored for a possible future development of CD. Additionally, this study demonstrated that although the HLA-DQ2.2 allele has a negligible risk factor when alone, its importance for the onset of CD will significantly increase when associated with DQ2.5.

## Competing Interests

The authors declare no competing interests regarding the publication of this paper.

## Authors' Contributions

Lucas Malta Almeida performed HLA genotyping of all celiac patients and controls. Lenora Gandolfi performed the clinical evaluation of all patients and revised and organized all the biopsy pathological data. Riccardo Pratesi conceived the study design and revised the manuscript. Rosa Harumi Uenishi collected blood and serum samples from patients and controls and organized all their clinical data. Fernanda Coutinho de Almeida performed the DNA extraction, quantification, and analysis. Nicole Selleski performed all the patients and controls anti-transglutaminase and anti-endomysium tests. Yanna Karla de Medeiros Nóbrega performed the statistical analysis and wrote the manuscript. All authors read and approved the final manuscript.

## Acknowledgments

The authors thank "Coordenação de Aperfeiçoamento de Pessoal de Nível Superior" (CAPES) for financial support and BioDiagene S.r.l. Molecular Diagnostic (Palermo, Italy) for the generous donation of several DQ-CD Typing Plus kits.

## References

[1] P. H. R. Green and B. Jabri, "Celiac disease," *Annual Review of Medicine*, vol. 57, pp. 207–221, 2006.

[2] J. C. Bai, M. Fried, G. R. Corazza et al., "World gastroenterology organisation global guidelines on celiac disease," *Journal of Clinical Gastroenterology*, vol. 47, no. 2, pp. 121–126, 2013.

[3] L. Gandolfi, R. Pratesi, J. C. M. Cordoba, P. L. Tauil, M. Gasparin, and C. Catassi, "Prevalence of celiac disease among blood donors in Brazil," *The American Journal of Gastroenterology*, vol. 95, no. 3, pp. 689–692, 2000.

[4] R. Pratesi, L. Gandolfi, S. G. Garcia et al., "Prevalence of coeliac disease: unexplained age-related variation in the same population," *Scandinavian Journal of Gastroenterology*, vol. 38, no. 7, pp. 747–750, 2003.

[5] S. B. C. Melo, M. I. M. Fernandes, L. C. Peres, L. E. A. Troncon, and L. C. Galvão, "Prevalence and demographic characteristics of celiac disease among blood donors in Ribeirão Preto, State of São Paulo, Brazil," *Digestive Diseases and Sciences*, vol. 51, no. 5, pp. 1020–1025, 2006.

[6] M. A. G. Pereira, C. L. Ortiz-Agostinho, I. Nishitokukado et al., "Prevalence of celiac disease in an urban area of Brazil with predominantly European ancestry," *World Journal of Gastroenterology*, vol. 12, no. 40, pp. 6546–6550, 2006.

[7] R. P. Oliveira, V. L. Sdepanian, J. A. Barreto et al., "High prevalence of celiac disease in Brazilian blood donor volunteers based on screening by IgA antitissue transglutaminase antibody," *European Journal of Gastroenterology and Hepatology*, vol. 19, no. 1, pp. 43–49, 2007.

[8] K. Karell, A. S. Louka, S. J. Moodie et al., "HLA types in celiac disease patients not carrying the DQA1*05-DQB1*02 (DQ2) heterodimer: results from the European genetics cluster on celiac disease," *Human Immunology*, vol. 64, no. 4, pp. 469–477, 2003.

[9] L. M. Sollid and B. A. Lie, "Celiac disease genetics: current concepts and practical applications," *Clinical Gastroenterology and Hepatology*, vol. 3, no. 9, pp. 843–851, 2005.

[10] I. D. Hill, M. H. Dirks, G. S. Liptak et al., "Guideline for the diagnosis and treatment of celiac disease in children: recommendations of the North American Society for Pediatric Gastroenterology, Hepatology and Nutrition," *Journal of Pediatric Gastroenterology and Nutrition*, vol. 40, no. 1, pp. 1–19, 2005.

[11] J. A. Murray, S. B. Moore, C. T. Van Dyke et al., "HLA DQ gene dosage and risk and severity of celiac disease," *Clinical Gastroenterology and Hepatology*, vol. 5, no. 12, pp. 1406–1412, 2007.

[12] F. Biagi, P. I. Bianchi, C. Vattiato et al., "Influence of HLA-DQ2 and DQ8 on severity in celiac disease," *Journal of Clinical Gastroenterology*, vol. 46, no. 1, pp. 46–50, 2012.

[13] F. Megiorni, B. Mora, M. Bonamico et al., "HLA-DQ and susceptibility to celiac disease: evidence for gender differences and parent-of-origin effects," *American Journal of Gastroenterology*, vol. 103, no. 4, pp. 997–1003, 2008.

[14] M. Hadithi, B. M. E. Von Blomberg, J. B. A. Crusius et al., "Accuracy of serologic tests and HLA-DQ typing for diagnosing celiac disease," *Annals of Internal Medicine*, vol. 147, no. 5, pp. 294–302, 2007.

[15] E. Liu, M. Rewers, and G. S. Eisenbarth, "Genetic testing: who should do the testing and what is the role of genetic testing in the setting of celiac disease?" *Gastroenterology*, vol. 128, no. 4, supplement 1, pp. S33–S37, 2005.

[16] J. A. Walker-Smith, S. Guandalini, J. Schmitz, D. H. Shmerling, and J. K. Visakorpi, "Revised criteria for diagnosis of celiac disease. Report of working group of European Society of Paediatric Gastroenterology and Nutrition," *Archives of Disease in Childhood*, vol. 65, no. 8, pp. 909–911, 1990.

[17] S. Husby, S. Koletzko, I. R. Korponay-Szabó et al., "European Society for Pediatric Gastroenterology, Hepatology, and Nutrition guidelines for the diagnosis of coeliac disease," *Journal of Pediatric Gastroenterology and Nutrition*, vol. 54, no. 1, pp. 136–160, 2012.

[18] F. Megiorni, B. Mora, M. Bonamico et al., "HLA-DQ and risk gradient for celiac disease," *Human Immunology*, vol. 70, no. 1, pp. 55–59, 2009.

[19] G. J. Tack, W. H. M. Verbeek, M. W. J. Schreurs, and C. J. J. Mulder, "The spectrum of celiac disease: epidemiology, clinical aspects and treatment," *Nature Reviews Gastroenterology & Hepatology*, vol. 7, no. 4, pp. 204–213, 2010.

[20] V. Kumar, C. Wijmenga, and S. Withoff, "From genome-wide association studies to disease mechanisms: celiac disease as a model for autoimmune diseases," *Seminars in Immunopathology*, vol. 34, no. 4, pp. 567–580, 2012.

[21] T. C. Lins, R. G. Vieira, B. S. Abreu, D. Grattapaglia, and R. W. Pereira, "Genetic composition of Brazilian population samples based on a set of twenty-eight ancestry informative SNPs," *American Journal of Human Biology*, vol. 22, no. 2, pp. 187–192, 2010.

[22] Instituto Brasileiro de Geografia e Estatística (IBGE), February 2016, http://www.ibge.gov.br/home/.

[23] M. M. Castro-Antunes, S. Crovella, L. A. C. Brandão, R. L. Guimarães, M. E. F. A. Motta, and G. A. P. da Silva, "Fequency distribution of HLA DQ2 and DQ8 in celiac patients and first-degree relatives in Recife, northeastern Brazil," *Clinics*, vol. 66, no. 2, pp. 227–231, 2011.

[24] L. M. da Silva Kotze, R. Nisihara, S. R. da Rosa Utiyama, and L. R. Kotze, "Absence of HLA-DQ2 and HLA-DQ8 does not exclude celiac disease in Brazilian patients," *Revista Espanola de Enfermedades Digestivas*, vol. 106, no. 8, pp. 561–562, 2014.

[25] H. Karinen, P. Kärkkäinen, J. Pihlajamäki et al., "Gene dose effect of the DQB1*0201 allele contributes to severity of coeliac disease," *Scandinavian Journal of Gastroenterology*, vol. 41, no. 2, pp. 191–199, 2006.

[26] S. Tollefsen, H. Arentz-Hansen, B. Fleckenstein et al., "HLA-DQ2 and -DQ8 signatures of gluten T cell epitopes in celiac disease," *The Journal of Clinical Investigation*, vol. 116, no. 8, pp. 2226–2236, 2006.

[27] M. Bodd, C. Kim, K. E. A. Lundin, and L. M. Sollid, "T-cell response to gluten in patients with HLA-DQ2.2 reveals requirement of peptide-MHC stability in celiac disease," *Gastroenterology*, vol. 142, no. 3, pp. 552–561, 2012.

[28] L.-E. Fallang, E. Bergseng, K. Hotta, A. Berg-Larsen, C.-Y. Kim, and L. M. Sollid, "Differences in the risk of celiac disease associated with HLA-DQ2.5 or HLA-DQ2.2 are related to sustained gluten antigen presentation," *Nature Immunology*, vol. 10, no. 10, pp. 1096–1101, 2009.

[29] M. J. van Belzen, B. P. C. Koeleman, J. B. A. Crusius et al., "Defining the contribution of the HLA region to cis DQ2-positive coeliac disease patients," *Genes and Immunity*, vol. 5, no. 3, pp. 215–220, 2004.

[30] M. J. Fernández-Cavada-Pollo, M. I. Alcalá-Peña, M. L. Vargas-Pérez et al., "Celiac disease and HLA-DQ genotype: diagnosis of different genetic risk profiles related to the age in Badajoz, southwestern Spain," *Revista Espanola de Enfermedades Digestivas*, vol. 105, no. 8, pp. 469–476, 2013.

# 24

# Anti-Myeloperoxidase Antibodies Associate with Future Proliferative Lupus Nephritis

**S. W. Olson,[1] J. J. Lee,[2] M. Poirier,[3] D. J. Little,[1] L. K. Prince,[1] T. P. Baker,[1] J. D. Edison,[1] and K. C. Abbott[4]**

[1] *Walter Reed National Military Medical Center, 8901 Wisconsin Avenue, Bethesda, MD 20889, USA*
[2] *Naval Medical Center San Diego, 34800 Bob Wilson Drive, San Diego, CA 92134, USA*
[3] *San Antonio Military Medical Center, 3551 Roger Brooke Dr., Fort Sam Houston, TX 78234, USA*
[4] *The National Institute of Diabetes and Digestive and Kidney Diseases (NIDDK), NIH, 6707 Democracy Blvd, Bethesda, MD 20892, USA*

Correspondence should be addressed to S. W. Olson; stephen.w.olson.mil@mail.mil

Academic Editor: Ricard Cervera

*Background.* The subclinical pathophysiology of proliferative lupus nephritis (PLN) has not been fully elucidated. Myeloperoxidase anti-neutrophil cytoplasmic antibody (MPO-ANCA) is associated with PLN, but prediagnostic levels have not been reported. *Methods.* We performed a retrospective case-control Department of Defense Serum Repository (DoDSR) study comparing MPO-ANCA levels in longitudinal prediagnostic serum samples for 23 biopsy confirmed proliferative lupus nephritis (PLN) patients to DoDSR identified age, sex, race, and age of serum matched healthy and SLE without LN disease controls. We also compared the temporal relationship of MPO-ANCA to anti-double stranded DNA antibodies (dsDNAab). *Results.* A greater proportion of PLN patients had prediagnostic MPO-ANCA levels above ≥3 U/mL and ≥6 U/mL compared to SLE without LN (91% versus 43%, $p < 0.001$; 57% versus 5%, $p < 0.001$, resp.). In subgroup analysis, the MPO-ANCA threshold of ≥3 U/mL was significant at <1 year (88% versus 39%, $p = 0.007$) and 1–4 years (87% versus 38%, $p = 0.009$) prior to diagnosis. Statistically significant subclinical MPO-ANCA levels (≥3 U/mL) occurred prior to statistically significant dsDNAab ≥ 3 IU/ml (89% versus 11%, $p = 0.003$). *Conclusions.* Subclinical MPO-ANCA levels could distinguish future PLN from SLE without LN. MPO-ANCA manifests prior to clinical disease and subclinical dsDNAab to suggest that it may contribute directly to PLN pathogenicity.

## 1. Introduction

Systemic Lupus Erythematosus (SLE) is a morbid autoimmune disease with multisystem organ involvement [1, 2]. Lupus Nephritis (LN) occurs in approximately half of SLE patients. The pathogenesis of SLE and LN is much better understood but not yet fully elucidated [3]. More than one mechanism of disease, each with multiple required deficits, may exist. Numerous autoantibodies are associated with both SLE and LN to include antineutrophil cytoplasmic antibodies (ANCA) [4, 5]. Perinuclear antineutrophil cytoplasmic antibodies (pANCA) and specifically anti-myeloperoxidase antibody (MPO-ANCA) are the predominant ANCA reported [5]. Simultaneous overt clinical manifestation of both ANCA associated vasculitis (AAV) and SLE has been reported [6–9]. Even without clinical evidence of AAV, ANCA is positive in 16%–42% of SLE patients [10–15]. A variable number of LN patients may have caused this wide range. ANCA is positive in 37%–53% of LN patients and more common in LN patients than SLE patients without LN [16–19]. ANCA is also more strongly associated with diffuse proliferative LN (PLN) than other types of LN, as well as more common in crescentic PLN than PLN without crescents [19, 20]. While the contribution of ANCA to AAV has been well described, it is unclear if ANCA directly contributes to LN pathogenesis or is simply a passive marker of disease [21–23]. SLE relapse is associated with positive ANCA levels [24]. But only presence, and not absolute level of ANCA, has been correlated with disease severity. No previous studies have evaluated prediagnostic ANCA levels or their temporal relationship with other biomarkers to provide insight into subclinical SLE and LN pathophysiology. Arbuckle et al. described the evolution of prediagnostic autoantibodies in a general SLE population but did not evaluate MPO-ANCA [22]. We recently reported that dsDNAab more frequently became elevated before PLN than before SLE without LN [23]. Subclinical ANCA levels were measured in the same Department of Defense Serum Repository (DoDSR) serum samples. We hypothesized that ANCA would be elevated in a larger percent of PLN subjects prior to diagnosis than SLE patients without LN and healthy controls. Based on our previous discovery that ANCA is present prior to anti-GBM antibody in anti-GBM disease, we also hypothesized that ANCA levels would be elevated prior to both dsDNAab and CRP to suggest a direct contribution to PLN pathophysiology [24, 25].

## 2. Materials and Methods

We performed a retrospective case-control serum bank study comparing MPO-ANCA and PR3-ANCA levels years prior to PLN diagnosis to matched healthy and SLE without LN disease controls. We previously reported preclinical dsDNAab and CRP levels for these same patients and serum samples.

As described previously, we identified 23 cases of biopsy proven PLN (WHO class III or WHO class IV) from the Walter Reed Army Medical Center renal biopsy database from 1993 to 2009. A comprehensive electronic data base review was performed for each PLN case to populate a clinical background data collection sheet. None of the cases had medications in their record that were associated with drug-induced lupus.

The Department of Defense Serum Repository (DoDSR) identified 23 age, sex, race, and age of serum sample matched healthy and 21 SLE without LN disease controls [23]. Each disease control had at least one hospitalization or three outpatient ICD-9 codes for SLE (711.0) without an ICD-9 code for lupus nephritis (583.81) or any other urinary abnormalities to suggest undiagnosed LN. The more rigorous selection criteria minimized the chance of including false positive cases that were erroneously coded during an ultimately negative SLE workup. The DoDSR also provided a list of all other ICD-9 codes for each matching disease control to document comorbidities. Walter Reed specific SLE without LN disease controls would not have been matched effectively for age, sex, race, and age of serum sample. This could have introduced insurmountable confounders into the final data set.

The DoDSR then pulled the oldest, the second most recent, and the most recent 0.5 mL serum samples prior to PLN or SLE without LN diagnosis and sent them to Quest Diagnostics Nichols Institute (Chantilly, VA).

### 2.1. Laboratory Assays

*2.1.1. Measurement of MPO-ANCA.* Quantitative measurement of MPO-ANCA antibody serum concentration was performed using the Varelisa™ MPO-ANCA EIA kit (Phadia GmbH, Freiburg, Germany). Serum aliquots from the subjects were diluted 1:101 with sample diluent and run in duplicate. Microwells were precoated with purified human MPO. 100 microliters each of calibrators (0, 3, 7, 16, 40, and 100 U/ml), controls, and diluted subject serum samples were dispensed into the wells, and the assay was performed as described in the instructions for use. The secondary antibody was a horseradish peroxidase-labeled anti-human IgG conjugate, and detection was achieved using TMB stopped with phosphoric acid solution. Absorbance was determined at 450 nm. The results are reported in U/ml, with a measuring range of 1.0 to 100 U/ml, and a detection limit of 1.0 U/ml. A clinically negative result was indicated by <6.0 U/ml. Intra-assay variability was 4.8 to 9.5 CV, and interassay variability was 3.5 to 10.7 CV over the range of the standards. The frequency distribution in 432 healthy subjects was 1.5 U/ml (95th percentile, 3.4 U/ml).

*2.1.2. Measurement of PR3-ANCA.* Quantitative measurement of PR3-ANCA antibody serum concentration was performed using the Varelisa™ PR3 ANCA EIA kit (Phadia GmbH, Freiburg, Germany). Serum aliquots from the subjects were diluted 1:101 with sample diluent and run in duplicate. The microwells were precoated with purified human neutrophil PR3. 100 microliters each of calibrators (0, 3, 7, 16, 40, and 100 U/ml), controls, and diluted subject serum samples were dispensed into the wells, and the assay was performed as described in the instructions for use. The secondary antibody was a horseradish peroxidase-labeled anti-human IgG conjugate, and detection was achieved using TMB stopped with phosphoric acid solution. Absorbance was determined at 450 nm. The results are reported in U/ml, with a measuring range of 0.5 to 100 U/ml and a detection limit of 0.5 U/ml. A clinically negative result was indicated by <6.0 U/ml. Intra-assay variability was 4.8 to 5.9% CV, and interassay variability was 2.4 to 9.3% CV over the range of the standards. The frequency distribution in 432 healthy subjects was 0.7 U/ml (95th percentile, 1.2 U/ml). For all three assays, the results were rounded to and reported in whole numbers.

*2.2. Statistical Analysis.* The percent of PLN subjects with MPO-ANCA above selected threshold values prior to diagnosis was compared to healthy and SLE without LN disease controls using the Fisher exact probability test. Odds ratios and 95% confidence intervals were also calculated. The same statistical analysis was used for all secondary outcomes and subgroup analysis. Conditional logistic regression and ROC curves were performed using STATA 12.0. Absolute MPO-ANCA change per year was calculated by dividing the difference between last MPO-ANCA (MPO-ANCA$l$) minus the index MPO-ANCA (MPO-ANCA$i$) by the difference in days ($T$) between the two samples ($Tl - Ti$) and multiplying the total by 365 days/year (MPO-ANCA$l$ − MPO-ANCA$i$)/($Tl - Ti$) $*$ 365. Infinite odds ratio values were estimated by adding 1 to the numerator (if 0 controls were positive) or denominator (if all study participants were positive) of both the disease and control groups.

The DoDSR was not able to assign a matching disease control for one case. Serum samples for a second disease control were accidently destroyed at Quest leaving two less disease control subjects for analysis of the entire time period prior to diagnosis. Not all subjects had samples available for each subgroup time period. If multiple serum samples were present for a subject in a specific subgroup analysis time period, the highest antibody level dictated group assignment. Only 20 study subjects had multiple serum samples for evaluation of change in MPO-ANCA levels over time. Antecedent rise in MPO-ANCA versus dsDNAab or CRP was established only for patients with a clear initial biomarker elevation. If both became elevated in the same sample or if neither was elevated in any sample prior to diagnosis, there was no antecedent elevation determined.

This study was approved by the Human Use Committee at Walter Reed National Military Medical Center and informed consent was waived.

## 3. Results

*3.1. Demographics.* As previously reported, this study population consisted of predominantly African American females less than 40 years old. Joint, hematologic, and dermatologic involvement was most common (Table 1). Only three of the study patients had ANCA labs at diagnosis and all were negative. The majority of PLN subjects had an elevated dsDNAab, hematuria and/or proteinuria, and WHO class IV LN on biopsy at diagnosis (Table 1). There was no statistically significant difference of joint, skin, cardiac, pulmonary, or hematologic involvement between the PLN group and the SLE without LN disease control group (Table 1).

*3.2. MPO-ANCA and PR3-ANCA.* A greater percentage of PLN cases had an elevated MPO-ANCA level (≥6 U/mL) compared to both matched healthy and SLE without LN disease controls at any time prior to diagnosis (57% versus 0%, $p < 0.001$; 57% versus 5%, $p < 0.001$, resp.) and in the subgroup less than one year prior to diagnosis (59% versus 0%, <0.001; 59% versus 8%, $p = 0.006$, resp.). There was no significant difference found in the subgroups of 1–4 years and >4 years prior to diagnosis (Table 2). More PLN patients had an MPO-ANCA level ≥ 3 U/mL compared to matched healthy and disease controls at any time (91% versus 26%, $p < 0.001$; 91% versus 43%, $p < 0.001$, resp.), less than one year prior to diagnosis (88% versus 19%, $p < 0.001$; 88% versus 39%, $p = 0.007$, resp.), 1–4 years (87% versus 13%, $p < 0.001$; 87% versus 38%, $p = 0.009$, resp.), and >4 years (69% versus 25%, $p = 0.03$; 69% versus 44%, $p = 0.29$, resp.) prior to diagnosis (Table 2). Conditional logistic regression demonstrated that each incremental U/ml rise of MPO-ANCA increased the odds of future PLN diagnosis compared to both healthy controls and SLE without LN disease controls (OR 9.1 [3.4–24.5], $p < 0.001$; OR 1.5 [1.2–1.8], $p < 0.001$, resp.; Table 3).

The MPO-ANCA ROC area under the curve was greater than 0.7 at less than 1 year, 1–4 years, and greater than 4 years for analysis of PLN cases with both healthy controls (Figure 1) and SLE without LN disease controls (Figure 2).

Neither the PLN cases, nor the disease and healthy controls had an elevated PR3-ANCA level in any serum sample. A greater percentage of PLN cases had a PR3-ANCA level ≥ 2 U/ml compared to both matched healthy and disease controls at any time prior to diagnosis (30% versus 4%, $p = 0.04$ for both).

*3.3. Time Course of Antibody Development.* In the PLN patients, MPO-ANCA became elevated a median of 139 days (25%, 75%; 63, 258 days) prior to diagnosis. MPO-ANCA was ≥3 U/mL a median of 5.75 years prior to diagnosis (25%, 75%; 1.3, 7.5 years) which is an underestimation because this level was present oldest index sample in 81% of the patients. PR3-ANCA ≥ 2 U/mL was only present in serum samples with a concurrent elevated MPO-ANCA.

A greater percentage of PLN cases had a rise in MPO-ANCA over time in comparison to both healthy and SLE without LN disease controls (70% versus 10%, $p = 0.001$; 70% versus 16%, $p < 0.001$, resp.; Table 4). Only PLN cases had a MPO-ANCA rate of rise greater than 0.5 U/mL/year (45% versus 0%, $p = 0.001$) or an absolute rise greater than 3 U/mL (30% versus 0%, $p = 0.02$; Table 4). In addition, a MPO-ANCA of ≥3 that rose more than 1 U/ml over time was highly specific for PLN (45% versus 0%, $p = 0.001$)

*3.4. MPO-ANCA versus dsDNAab and CRP.* The lowest statistically significant subclinical MPO-ANCA level (≥3 U/mL), 50% of the threshold for clinical disease, was present prior to the lowest statistically significant subclinical dsDNAab level (≥3 U/mL), as well as the dsDNAab level that is 50% of the threshold for clinical disease (≥5 U/mL) when it was possible to ascertain an antecedent antibody (89% versus 11%, $p = 0.003$; 100% versus 0%, $p < 0.001$, resp.; Table 5). It was not possible to determine temporal relationship of antibodies in cases in which both antibodies crossed threshold values in the same serum sample or did not cross the threshold in any samples.

There was no association between elevated dsDNAab and elevated MPO-ANCA (Supplemental Table 1). DsDNA antibody was as high as 640 IU/ml in the setting of a low normal MPO-ANCA level ≤ 3 U/mL. MPO-ANCA was as elevated as high as 16 in the setting of a low normal dsDNA ≤ 5 U/mL.

More PLN patients had an MPO-ANCA level ≥ 3 U/mL prior to an elevated CRP of >0.8 mg/dL (100% versus 0%, $p < 0.001$)

## 4. Discussion

In addition to SLE, MPO-ANCA has been described at diagnosis in subpopulations of multiple autoimmune and inflammatory diseases to include anti-GBM disease, IgA nephropathy, and inflammatory bowel disease [24–30]. It is not clear if MPO-ANCA contributes directly upstream to immune dysregulation or is simply a passive marker of disease. Prediagnostic autoantibody trends and temporal relationships help to address this question. Previously MPO-ANCA was detected both before anti-GBM antibody and anti-GBM diagnosis. We describe the natural history of subclinical ANCA in PLN and SLE without LN for the first time. Subclinical MPO-ANCA ≥ 3 U/mL was associated with PLN but not SLE without LN. A rising prediagnostic MPO-ANCA was also associated with future PLN. A prediagnostic

Table 1

(a) Proliferative lupus nephritis (PLN) background information on based on electronic medical record chart review. Medians presented with 25% and 75% values in parentheses for continuous data because they were not normally distributed. Some percentages are accompanied by *n*/*n* in parentheses. Prednisone dose was <10 mg/d. Other immunosuppression was discontinued at least 6 months before confirmatory kidney biopsy. Not all patients had information available for each laboratory measurement. SLE, systemic lupus erythematosus; PLN, progressive lupus nephritis; LN, lupus nephritis; CNS, central nervous system; RBC, red blood cell; dsDNA, double-stranded DNA; SM, smooth muscle; RNP, ribonucleoprotein; CRP, C-reactive protein; NIH, National Institutes of Health.

| Average age (range) | 36 years old (18–60) |
|---|---|
| Race | |
| Caucasian | 15% |
| African American | 60% |
| Other | 25% |
| Gender | |
| Female | 65% |
| History of HTN | 83 (19/23) |
| History of DM | 0 (0/23) |
| Arthralgia | 70 (16/23) |
| Dermatologic | 48 (11/23) |
| Hematologic | 53 (12/23) |
| Cardiac involvement | 35 (8/23) |
| CNS involvement | 9 (2/23) |
| Lung involvement | 35 (8/23) |
| Liver involvement | 9 (2/23) |
| Hematuria (>3 RBC phf) | 100 (23/23) |
| Proteinuria (>300 mg) | 100 (23/23) |
| Nephrotic range proteinuria (>3.5 gm) | 35 (8/23) |
| Proteinuria Quantification (average in gm) | 2.36 (0.380–4.61) |
| Serum Creatinine (average mg/dl) | 1.13 (0.6–2.4) |
| ANA (% positive) | 96 (22/23) |
| dsDNA antibody (% positive) | 82 (18/22) |
| Average (titer) | 1:320 |
| Average (U/mL peak; $n = 6$) | 189 (130–228) |
| dsDNA antibody OR ANA (% positive) | 100 (23/23) |
| ANCA (% positive) | 0 (0/3) |
| Anti-phospholipid antibody (% positive) | 38 (8/23) |
| Anti-SM antibody (% positive) | 38 (6/16) |
| Anti-RNP antibody (% positive) | 50 (8/16) |
| CRP | |
| (Average mg/dL) | 2.1 (0.1–6.6) |
| (% >0.8 mg/dL) | 79 (11/14) |
| Biopsy (%) | |
| WHO Class III | 22 (5/23) |
| WHO Class IV | 78 (18/23) |
| WHO Class IV + V | 35 (8/23) |
| Crescent Formation | 23 (6/23) |
| Median NIH activity index | 8 (5, 10) |
| Median NIH chronicity index | 3 (1, 3) |
| Median SLE disease activity index | 16 (12, 22) |
| Immunosuppression before biopsy (%) | |
| Prednisone | 22 (5/23) |
| Hydroxychloroquine | 39 (9/23) |
| Other (cyclophosphamide, mycophenolate mofetil, rituximab) | 9 (2/23) |

(b) Systemic lupus erythematosus (SLE) without lupus nephritis (LN) disease control background information on based on ICD-9 codes provided by the Department of Defense Serum Repository (DoDSR). Laboratory data were not available for these disease control patients.

| Average age (range) | 36 years old (18–60) |
|---|---|
| Race | |
| Caucasian | 15% |
| African American | 60% |
| Other | 25% |

TABLE 1: Continued.

| | |
|---|---|
| Gender | |
| Female | 65% |
| History of HTN | 36% |
| History of DM | 9% |
| Renal involvement | 0% |
| Arthralgia | 73% |
| Dermatologic | 46% |
| Hematologic | 41% |
| Anti-phospholipid positive | 23% |
| Cardiac involvement | 9% |
| CNS involvement | 9% |
| Lung involvement | 18% |
| Liver involvement | 5% |
| Median SLE disease activity index | 10 (4, 14) |

TABLE 2: The percent PLN patients with MPO-ANCA above specific thresholds compared to matching healthy and SLE without LN disease controls. The Department of Defense Serum Repository could not assign a matching disease control for one patient. The samples for a second control were lost in processing. Not all patients had samples available for each subgroup time period. If multiple serum samples were present for a patient in a specific subgroup analysis time period, the highest antibody level dictated group assignment. *Estimated due to actual infinite value.

(a)

| MPO-ANCA | Cases (%) | Healthy controls (%) | OR (odds ratio) | CI (confidence interval) | *p* value (Fisher's exact) |
|---|---|---|---|---|---|
| (≥3 U/mL): | | | | | |
| All | 91 (21/23) | 26 (6/23) | 30 | 5.3–167 | <0.001 |
| <1 year | 88 (15/17) | 19 (3/16) | 33 | 4.7–226 | <0.001 |
| 1–4 years | 87 (13/15) | 13 (2/15) | 42 | 5.2–347 | <0.001 |
| >4 years | 69 (11/16) | 25 (4/16) | 6.6 | 1.4–31 | 0.03 |
| (≥6 U/mL) | | | | | |
| All | 57 (13/23) | 0 (0/23) | 34* | 3.9–300* | <0.001 |
| <1 year | 59 (10/17) | 0 (0/16) | 28* | 2.9–262* | <0.001 |
| 1–4 years | 7 (1/15) | 0 (0/15) | 1.1* | 0.1–20* | 1.0 |
| >4 years | 19 (3/16) | 0 (0/16) | 3.9* | 0.4–42* | 0.23 |

(b)

| MPO-ANCA | Cases (%) | Disease controls (%) | OR (odds ratio) | CI (confidence interval) | *p* value (Fisher's exact) |
|---|---|---|---|---|---|
| (≥3 U/mL): | | | | | |
| All | 91 (21/23) | 43 (9/21) | 14 | 2.6–76 | <0.001 |
| <1 year | 88 (15/17) | 39 (5/13) | 12 | 1.9–76 | 0.007 |
| 1–4 years | 87 (13/15) | 38 (6/16) | 11 | 1.8–66 | 0.009 |
| >4 years | 69 (11/16) | 44 (7/16) | 2.8 | 0.7–12 | 0.29 |
| (≥6 U/mL) | | | | | |
| All | 57 (13/23) | 5 (1/21) | 26 | 3.0–228 | <0.001 |
| <1 year | 59 (10/17) | 8 (1/13) | 17 | 1.8–164 | 0.006 |
| 1–4 years | 7 (1/15) | 6 (1/16) | 1.1 | 0.1–19 | 1.0 |
| >4 years | 19 (3/16) | 0 (0/16) | 4.9* | 0.5–50* | 0.23 |

Table 3: Conditional logistic regression (CLR) for PLN MPO-ANCA by unit versus healthy controls, SLE without LN disease controls, and all controls together.

| CLR for MPO-ANCA by unit: PLN versus controls | OR (odds ratio) | CI (confidence interval) | $p$ value |
|---|---|---|---|
| Healthy controls | 9.1 | 3.4–24.5 | <0.001 |
| Disease controls | 1.5 | 1.2–1.8 | <0.001 |
| All controls | 7.1 | 1.2–44.2 | <0.001 |

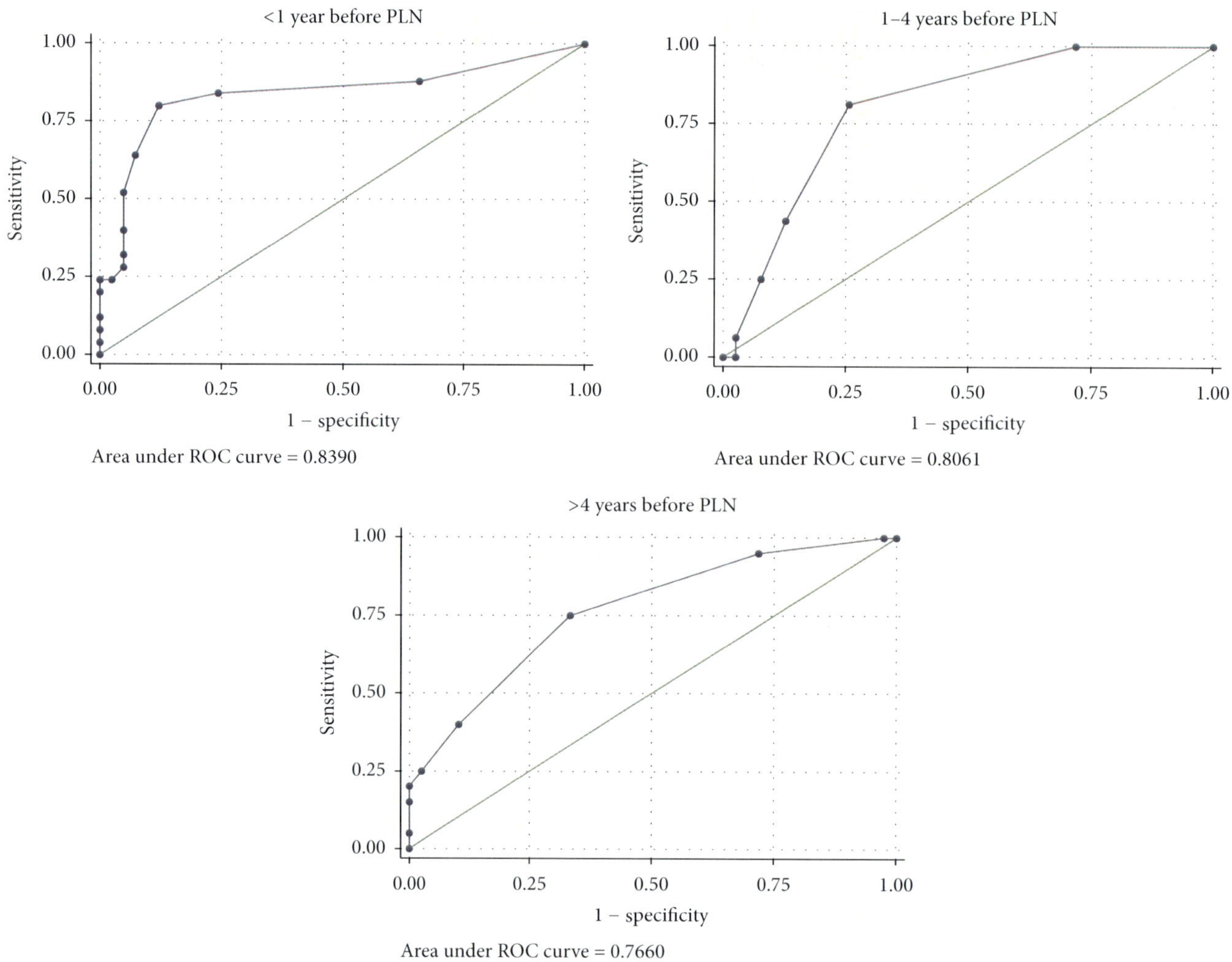


Figure 1: MPO-ANCA receiver operating curves for PLN cases versus healthy controls for <1 year, 1–4 years, and >4 years before PLN diagnosis.

MPO-ANCA that was both above 3 U/mL and continued to rise over time was most specific for developing PLN. These associations may be even stronger if the few SLE without LN disease controls with MPO-ANCA develop LN in the future. 3 U/mL is 50% of the upper limit of normal for the MPO-ANCA assay. But, abnormal ANCA levels were established in cohorts of patients with active vasculitis and not PLN or SLE without LN. It is reasonable that abnormal subclinical thresholds for other disease processes are different. Previous autoimmune disease studies have also established statistically significant prediagnostic thresholds within the normal diagnostic range consistent with these results.

Improved knowledge about subclinical MPO-ANCA trends could have prognostic implications. Overall, even low but significant MPO-ANCA may portend future PLN in SLE patients without LN. And up to 35% of SLE patients will manifest LN after initial diagnosis [31]. Closer follow-up in high risk MPO-ANCA positive SLE without LN patients could facilitate a more prompt diagnosis with earlier intervention to better preserve residual renal function. But, prospective

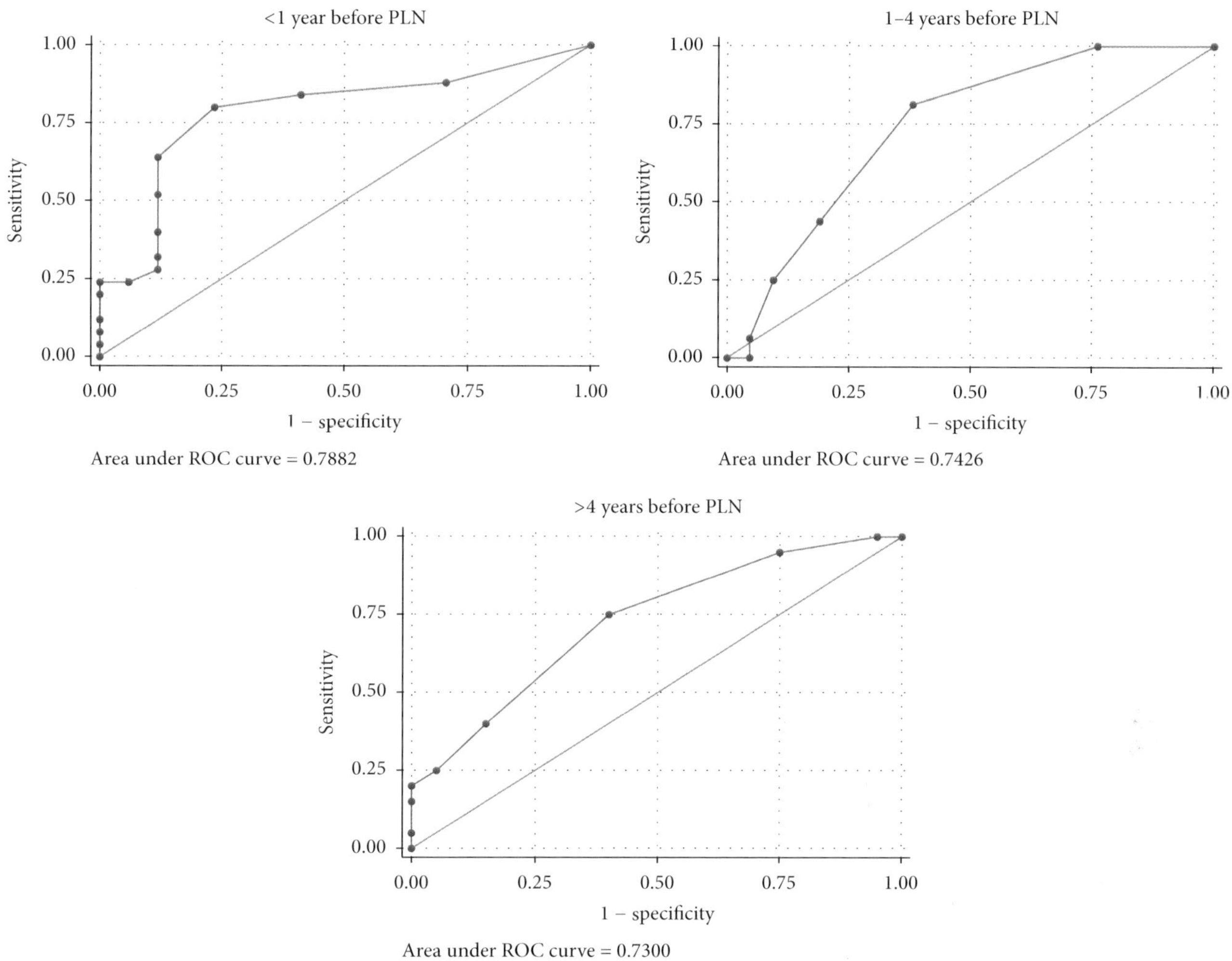


FIGURE 2: MPO-ANCA receiver operating curves for PLN cases versus SLE without LN disease controls for <1 year, 1–4 years, and >4 years before PLN diagnosis.

confirmation in a cohort of SLE without LN is required before any formal clinical implementation.

Improved knowledge about subclinical MPO-ANCA trends could also broaden our understanding of PLN pathophysiology. There is a strong correlation between ANCA and dsDNAab at diagnosis, but the subclinical relationship was previously unknown [11, 17, 19]. We found that statistically significant subclinical MPO-ANCA levels preceded statistically significant subclinical dsDNAab levels (determined on the same samples and reported in a previous publication) when a clear antecedent antibody could be determined. And both autoantibodies are present before elevated CRP, a surrogate inflammatory marker for early subclinical disease. The summation of this data suggests that MPO-ANCA may participate upstream in the pathogenesis of PLN.

MPO-ANCA seropositivity has been previously attributed to cross reactive dsDNAab, but there is a body of evidence which suggests that this is not the only contribution [32, 33]. Jethwa et al. reported compelling in vitro evidence that DNA/dsDNAab complexes from active SLE patient sera can bind cationic MPO in ANCA immunoassays to cause a "false positive" test. However, disassociation of the DNA from the dsDNAab binding site reduced but did not normalize, subsequent MPO-ANCA levels to suggest that MPO-ANCA may indeed have been present. In addition, in our study, elevated dsDNAab was not associated with elevated MPO-ANCA levels. There were examples of profoundly elevated dsDNAab with nearly undetectable MPO-ANCA as well as significantly elevated MPO-ANCA with nearly undetectable dsDNAab. These findings do not support the theory that MPO-ANCA positivity is solely explained by dsDNAab cross reactivity. Cross reacting dsDNAab would result in a strong correlation between MPO-ANCA and dsDNA seropositivity and titer, because all assays were run on the same day on the same platform. Moreover, by evaluating preclinical quantitative MPO-ANCA, we were able to demonstrate statistically significant MPO-ANCA levels occurred before dsDNAab was present to bind MPO consistent with true antibody production. Finally, Falk et al. have identified the most pathogenic epitope specific MPO-ANCA (anti-MPO 1 antibody) which was elevated in 17% of the SLE disease controls [34, 35]. It is possible and likely that both real

TABLE 4: The percent of PLN patients with MPO-ANCA absolute change and rate of rise over time above specific thresholds compared to matching healthy and SLE without LN disease controls. Only 20 cases and healthy controls and 19 SLE without LN disease controls had multiple samples to evaluate change over time. *Estimated due to actual infinite value.

(a)

| Change in MPO-ANCA (U/mL/year) | Cases (%) | Healthy controls (%) | OR (odds ratio) | CI (confidence interval) | $p$ value (Fisher's exact) |
|---|---|---|---|---|---|
| >0 U/mL | 70 (14/20) | 10 (2/20) | 21 | 3.7–120 | <0.001 |
| >0.3 U/mL | 60 (12/20) | 0 (0/20) | 32* | 3.6–291* | <0.001 |
| >0.5 U/mL | 45 (9/20) | 0 (0/20) | 18* | 2.1–161* | 0.001 |
| >1 U/mL | 20 (4/20) | 0 (0/20) | 6.3* | 0.7–59* | 0.10 |

(b)

| Absolute rise in MPO-ANCA (U/mL) | Cases (%) | Healthy controls (%) | OR (odds ratio) | CI (confidence interval) | $p$ value (Fisher's exact) |
|---|---|---|---|---|---|
| >0 U/mL | 70 (14/20) | 10 (2/20) | 21 | 3.7–120 | <0.001 |
| >1 U/mL | 55 (11/20) | 0 (0/20) | 27* | 3.0–237* | <0.001 |
| >2 U/mL | 35 (7/20) | 0 (0/20) | 12* | 1.4–110* | 0.008 |
| >3 U/mL | 30 (6/20) | 0 (0/20) | 10* | 1.1–91* | 0.02 |

(c)

| Change in MPO-ANCA (U/mL/year) | Cases (%) | Disease controls (%) | OR (odds ratio) | CI (confidence interval) | $p$ value (Fisher's exact) |
|---|---|---|---|---|---|
| >0 U/mL | 70 (14/20) | 16 (3/19) | 12 | 2.6–59 | 0.001 |
| >0.3 U/mL | 60 (12/20) | 5 (1/19) | 27 | 3.0–49 | <0.001 |
| >0.5 U/mL | 45 (9/20) | 0 (0/19) | 20* | 2.2–179 | 0.001 |
| >1 U/mL | 20 (4/20) | 0 (0/19) | 5* | 0.5–49 | 0.10 |

(d)

| Absolute rise in MPO-ANCA (U/mL) | Cases (%) | Disease controls (%) | OR (odds ratio) | CI (confidence interval) | $p$ value (Fisher's exact) |
|---|---|---|---|---|---|
| >0 U/mL | 70 (14/20) | 16 (3/19) | 12 | 2.6–59 | 0.001 |
| >1 U/mL | 55 (11/20) | 11 (2/19) | 10 | 1.9–57 | 0.006 |
| >2 U/mL | 35 (7/20) | 5 (1/19) | 10 | 1.1–89 | 0.04 |
| >3 U/mL | 30 (6/20) | 0 (0/30) | 10* | 1.1–93* | 0.02 |

TABLE 5: Temporal relationship of detectable autoantibodies. Patients without a clear antecedent antibody above the designated threshold were not included in analysis. OR, odds ratio; CI, confidence interval.

| Comparison thresholds | Antecedent MPO-ANCA (%) | Antecedent dsDNAab (%) | OR | CI | $p$ value (Fisher's exact) |
|---|---|---|---|---|---|
| MPO-ANCA ≥ 3U/ml versus dsDNAab ≥ 3 IU/ml | 89 (8/9) | 11 (1/9) | 64 | 3.4–1211 | 0.003 |
| MPO-ANCA ≥ 3 U/ml versus dsDNAab ≥ 5 IU/ml | 100 (10/10) | 0 (0/10) | 100* | 5.5–1831* | <0.001 |

MPO-ANCA and DNA/dsDNAab bound MPO complexes may contribute to MPO-ANCA seropositivity.

MPO-ANCA stimulation of NETosis, the externalization of cellular chromatin and cytoplasmic protein containing fibers that capture pathogens or stimulate autoantibody production, is one intriguing hypothesis for MPO-ANCA directed pathogenicity. While NETosis has not been specifically evaluated previously, previous literature supports the hypothesis. MPO-ANCA triggers neutrophil NET deployment in vitro. There is increased NET formation in both MPO-ANCA vasculitis and SLE. NET burden can serve as a nidus for dsDNAab, ANA, C1q, and additional MPO-ANCA production to induce a deleterious positive feedback cycle. Both NET and autoantibody containing immune complexes can then cause end organ damage to include LN [36–41]. There is evidence that NETosis has a stronger association with LN than SLE without LN. Persistence of NET burden is associated with LN as well as elevated dsDNAab and anti-NET antibodies [37]. Netting neutrophils present in kidney biopsies are specifically associated with PLN and increased disease activity on kidney biopsy [40].

DoDSR study limitations inherent to the retrospective case-control design have been reported previously [23, 24]. For this specific study, the relatively low sample size limited power for subgroup analysis. Additional mesangial and membranous lupus nephritis disease controls were lacking. MPO-ANCA change over time calculations assume a linear rise which has not been proven. Absent comparison literature for preclinical MPO-ANCA evaluation below diagnostic thresholds was initially a concern. But, percent of healthy controls with MPO-ANCA $\geq 3$ U/ml in this study was similar to that found in our anti-GBM disease study (23% versus 17%). And now we have reported significant differences between the percent of disease and control patients with subclinical biomarkers above thresholds within the normal diagnostic range in multiple studies [23, 24, 42, 43]. A final limitation is that small number of prediagnostic samples from PLN cases may have dated between SLE and PLN diagnosis. But, similar to the general population, the majority of PLN cases were diagnosed simultaneously or within a year of SLE diagnosis and when prediagnostic MPO-ANCA was positive, it was most often also positive in the earliest available sample. Because of these limitations, this data does not prove that MPO-ANCA directly contributes to the pathogenicity in a subpopulation of PLN. The data simply adds to our understanding of the complex and not fully elucidated pathophysiology of PLN.

Follow-up studies are required to more fully describe the subclinical pathophysiology of PLN. Preclinical presence, trajectory, and temporal relationship of anti-Smith, anti-RNP, anti-DNAase, anti-C1q, anti-lactoferin, anti-Cathepsin G, anti-elastase, and anti-NET antibody levels need to be evaluated in a larger cohort of PLN. Additional mesangial and membranous LN disease control comparison groups will strengthen analysis. Mesangial LN is a particularly important comparison group because it can have a similar clinical presentation to early PLN. In addition, we need to better characterize the prediagnostic MPO-ANCA to include epitope specificity, Fc glycosylation patterns, and avidity [34, 44–46]. Evaluation of the in vitro capability of PLN prediagnostic MPO-ANCA to trigger NET release from neutrophils would be needed to confirm pathogenic characteristics. MPO-ANCA may play a general role in autoimmune pathogenesis and at least partially explain observed subclinical and clinical autoimmune overlap syndromes.

MPO-ANCA may help delineate the SLE patients that are at risk for future PLN and may also directly contribute to the PLN pathogenesis. A more precise understanding of preclinical SLE pathogenesis may provide more specific future therapeutic targets for research.

## Disclosure

The views expressed in this manuscript are those of the authors and do not reflect the official policy of the Department of the Army, Department of Defense, or the US Government.

## Conflicts of Interest

The authors declare that they have no conflicts of interest.

## Supplementary Materials

Supplemental Table 1: a comparison of the percent of PLN cases with an elevated dsDNAab that have a concurrent elevated MPO-ANCA versus those that have a normal MPO-ANCA. *(Supplementary Materials)*

## References


[1] G. C. Tsokos, "Systemic lupus erythematosus," *The New England Journal of Medicine*, vol. 365, no. 22, pp. 2110–2121, 2011.

[2] A. Rahman and D. A. Isenberg, "Systemic lupus erythematosus," *The New England Journal of Medicine*, vol. 358, no. 9, pp. 929–939, 2008.

[3] M. Lech and H.-J. Anders, "The pathogenesis of lupus nephritis," *Journal of the American Society of Nephrology*, vol. 24, no. 9, pp. 1357–1366, 2013.

[4] P. Alba, L. Bento, M. J. Cuadrado et al., "Anti-dsDNA, anti-Sm antibodies, and the lupus anticoagulant: significant factors associated with lupus nephritis," *Annals of the Rheumatic Diseases*, vol. 62, no. 6, pp. 556–560, 2003.

[5] D. Sen and D. A. Isenberg, "Antineutrophil cytoplasmic autoantibodies in systemic lupus erythematosus," *Lupus*, vol. 12, no. 9, pp. 651–658, 2003.

[6] N. N. Masani, L. J. Imbriano, V. D. D'Agati, and G. S. Markowitz, "SLE and rapidly progressive glomerulonephritis," *American Journal of Kidney Diseases*, vol. 45, no. 5, pp. 950–955, 2005.

[7] B. Hervier, M. Hamidou, J. Haroche, C. Durant, A. Mathian, and Z. Amoura, "Systemic lupus erythematosus associated with ANCA-associated vasculitis: an overlapping syndrome?" *Rheumatology International*, vol. 32, no. 10, pp. 3285–3290, 2012.

[8] S. H. Nasr, V. D. D'Agati, H.-R. Park et al., "Necrotizing and crescentic lupus nephritis with antineutrophil cytoplasmic antibody seropositivity," *Clinical Journal of the American Society of Nephrology*, vol. 3, no. 3, pp. 682–690, 2008.

[9] M. Isono, H. Araki, T. Haitani et al., "Diffuse alveolar hemorrhage in lupus nephritis complicated by microscopic polyangiitis," *Clinical and Experimental Nephrology*, vol. 15, no. 2, pp. 294–298, 2011.

[10] R. Pauzner, M. Urowitz, D. Gladman, and J. Gough, "Antineutrophil cytoplasmic antibodies in systemic lupus erythematosus," *The Journal of Rheumatology*, vol. 21, no. 9, pp. 1670–1673, 1994.

[11] M. Galeazzi, G. Morozzi, G. D. Sebastiani et al., "Antineutrophil cytoplasmic antibodies in 566 European patients with systemic lupus erythematosus: prevalence, clinical associations and correlation with other autoantibodies," *Clinical and Experimental Rheumatology*, vol. 16, no. 5, pp. 541–546, 1998.

[12] P. A. Merkel, R. P. Polisson, Y. Chang, S. J. Skates, and J. L. Niles, "Prevalence of antineutrophil cytoplasmic antibodies in a large inception cohort of patients with connective tissue disease," *Annals of Internal Medicine*, vol. 126, no. 11, pp. 866–873, 1997.

[13] A. Schnabel, E. Csernok, D. A. Isenberg, C. owka, and W. L. Gross, "Antineutrophil cytoplasmic antibodies in systemic lupus erythematosus," *Arthritis & Rheumatism*, vol. 38, no. 5, pp. 633–637, 1995.

[14] K. Nishiya, H. Chikazawa, S. Nishimura, N. Hisakawa, and K. Hashimoto, "Anti-neutrophil cytoplasmic antibody in patients with systemic lupus erythematosus is unrelated to clinical features," *Clinical Rheumatology*, vol. 16, no. 1, pp. 70–75, 1997.

[15] I. Manolova, M. Dancheva, and K. Halacheva, "Antineutrophil cytoplasmic antibodies in patients with systemic lupus erythematosus: prevalence, antigen specificity, and clinical associations," *Rheumatology International*, vol. 20, no. 5, pp. 197–204, 2001.

[16] R. J. Falk and J. C. Jennette, "Anti-neutrophil cytoplasmic autoantibodies with specificity for myeloperoxidase in patients with systemic vasculitis and idiopathic necrotizing and crescentic glomerulonephritis," *The New England Journal of Medicine*, vol. 318, no. 25, pp. 1651–1657, 1988.

[17] H.-F. Pan, X.-H. Fang, G.-C. Wu et al., "Anti-neutrophil cytoplasmic antibodies in new-onset systemic lupus erythematosus and lupus nephritis," *Inflammation*, vol. 31, no. 4, pp. 260–265, 2008.

[18] V. D. Pradhan, S. S. Badakere, L. S. Bichile, and A. F. Almeida, "Anti-neutrophil Cytoplasmic Antibodies (ANCA) in systemic lupus erythematosus: Prevalence, clinical associations and correlation with other autoantibodies," *Journal of the Association of Physicians of India*, vol. 52, pp. 533–537, 2004.

[19] H. J. Chin, C. Ahn, C. S. Lim et al., "Clinical implications of antineutrophil cytoplasmic antibody test in lupus nephritis," *American Journal of Nephrology*, vol. 20, no. 1, pp. 57–63, 2000.

[20] F. Yu, Y. Tan, G. Liu, S.-X. Wang, W.-Z. Zou, and M.-H. Zhao, "Clinicopathological characteristics and outcomes of patients with crescentic lupus nephritis," *Kidney International*, vol. 76, no. 3, pp. 307–317, 2009.

[21] P. E. Spronk, H. Bootsma, G. Horst et al., "Antineutrophil cytoplasmic antibodies in systemic lupus erythematosus," *British Journal of Rheumatology*, vol. 35, no. 7, pp. 625–631, 1996.

[22] M. R. Arbuckle, M. T. McClain, M. V. Rubertone et al., "Development of autoantibodies before the clinical onset of systemic lupus erythematosus," *The New England Journal of Medicine*, vol. 349, no. 16, pp. 1526–1533, 2003.

[23] S. W. Olson, J. J. Lee, L. K. Prince et al., "Elevated subclinical double-stranded DNA antibodies and future proliferative lupus nephritis," *Clinical Journal of the American Society of Nephrology*, vol. 8, no. 10, pp. 1702–1708, 2013.

[24] S. W. Olson, C. B. Arbogast, T. P. Baker et al., "Asymptomatic autoantibodies associate with future anti-glomerular basement membrane disease," *Journal of the American Society of Nephrology*, vol. 22, no. 10, pp. 1946–1952, 2011.

[25] A. J. Roth and R. J. Falk, "Autoantibodies: what's in their teeth?" *Journal of the American Society of Nephrology*, vol. 22, no. 10, pp. 1783-1784, 2011.

[26] C. Bantis, M. Stangou, C. Schlaugat et al., "Is presence of ANCA in crescentic IgA nephropathy a coincidence or novel clinical entity? A case series," *American Journal of Kidney Diseases*, vol. 55, no. 2, pp. 259–268, 2010.

[27] J. G. M. C. Damoiseaux, B. Bouten, A. M. L. W. Linders et al., "Diagnostic value of anti-Saccharomyces cerevisiae and antineutrophil cytoplasmic antibodies for inflammatory bowel disease: high prevalence in patients with celiac disease," *Journal of Clinical Immunology*, vol. 22, no. 5, pp. 281–288, 2002.

[28] C. Roozendaal, A. W. M. Van Milligen De Wit, E. B. Haagsma et al., "Antineutrophil cytoplasmic antibodies in primary sclerosing cholangitis: defined specificities may be associated with distinct clinical features," *American Journal of Medicine*, vol. 105, no. 5, pp. 393–399, 1998.

[29] J. Broekroelofs, A. H. L. Mulder, G. F. Nelis, B. D. Westerveld, J. W. Cohen Tervaert, and C. G. M. Kallenberg, "Anti-neutrophil cytoplasmic antibodies (ANCA) in sera from patients with inflammatory bowel disease (IBD): relation to disease pattern and disease activity," *Digestive Diseases and Sciences*, vol. 39, no. 3, pp. 545–549, 1994.

[30] M. Haas, J. Jafri, S. M. Bartosh, S. L. Karp, S. G. Adler, and S. M. Meehan, "ANCA-associated crescentic glomerulonephritis with mesangial IgA deposits," *American Journal of Kidney Diseases*, vol. 36, no. 4, pp. 709–718, 2000.

[31] H. M. Bastian, J. M. Roseman, G. McGwin, G. S. Alarcón, B. J. Fessler, and J. D. Reveille, "Systemic lupus erythematosus in three ethnic groups. XII. Risk factors for lupus nephritis after diagnosis," *Lupus*, vol. 11, no. 3, pp. 152–160, 2002.

[32] H. S. Jethwa, P. H. Nachman, R. J. Falk, and J. C. Jennette, "False-positive myeloperoxidase binding activity due to DNA/anti-DNA antibody complexes: a source for analytical error in serologic evaluation of anti-neutrophil cytoplasmic autoantibodies," *Clinical and Experimental Immunology*, vol. 121, no. 3, pp. 544–550, 2000.

[33] J. W. C. Tervaert, "Autoantibodies in systemic vasculitis," *Australian and New Zealand Journal of Medicine*, vol. 22, no. 2, pp. 171-172, 1992.

[34] A. J. Roth, J. D. Ooi, J. J. Hess et al., "Epitope specificity determines pathogenicity and detectability in anca-associated vasculitis," *The Journal of Clinical Investigation*, vol. 123, no. 4, pp. 1773–1783, 2013.

[35] K. G. Stember, J. Hess, C. D. Henderson, S. Mallal, C. Jennette, R. J. Falk et al., "Detecting autoreactive cells and pathogenic epitopes in MPO-ANCA vasculitis," *Journal of the American Society of Nephrology*, vol. 28, no. 117, 2017.

[36] D. Nakazawa, H. Shida, U. Tomaru et al., "Enhanced formation and disordered regulation of NETs in myeloperoxidase-ANCA-associated microscopic polyangiitis," *Journal of the American Society of Nephrology*, vol. 25, no. 5, pp. 990–997, 2014.

[37] A. Hakkim, B. G. Fürnrohr, K. Amann et al., "Impairment of neutrophil extracellular trap degradation is associated with lupus nephritis," *Proceedings of the National Acadamy of Sciences of the United States of America*, vol. 107, no. 21, pp. 9813–9818, 2010.

[38] D. Nakazawa, U. Tomaru, and A. Ishizu, "Possible implication of disordered neutrophil extracellular traps in the pathogenesis of MPO-ANCA-associated vasculitis," *Clinical and Experimental Nephrology*, vol. 17, no. 5, pp. 631–633, 2013.

[39] J. Leffler, M. Martin, B. Gullstrand et al., "Neutrophil extracellular traps that are not degraded in systemic lupus erythematosus activate complement exacerbating the disease," *The Journal of Immunology*, vol. 188, no. 7, pp. 3522–3531, 2012.

[40] E. Villanueva, S. Yalavarthi, C. C. Berthier et al., "Netting neutrophils induce endothelial damage, infiltrate tissues, and expose immunostimulatory molecules in systemic lupus erythematosus," *The Journal of Immunology*, vol. 187, no. 1, pp. 538–552, 2011.

[41] A. Bodaño, J. Amarelo, A. González, J. J. Gómez-Reino, and C. Conde, "Novel DNASE I mutations related to systemic lupus erythematosus," *Arthritis & Rheumatology*, vol. 50, no. 12, pp. 4070-4071, 2004.

[42] S. W. Olson, D. Owshalimpur, C. M. Yuan et al., "Relation between asymptomatic proteinase 3 antibodies and future granulomatosis with polyangiitis," *Clinical Journal of the American Society of Nephrology*, vol. 8, no. 8, pp. 1312–1318, 2013.

[43] B. M. Weiss, J. Hebreo, D. V. Cordaro et al., "Increased serum free light chains precede the presentation of immunoglobulin light chain amyloidosis," *Journal of Clinical Oncology*, vol. 32, no. 25, pp. 2699–2704, 2014.

[44] Z. Cui, M.-H. Zhao, M. Segelmark, and T. Hellmark, "Natural autoantibodies to myeloperoxidase, proteinase 3, and the glomerular basement membrane are present in normal individuals," *Kidney International*, vol. 78, no. 6, pp. 590–597, 2010.

[45] M. Holland, K. Takada, T. Okumoto et al., "Hypogalactosylation of serum IgG in patients with ANCA-associated systemic vasculitis," *Clinical & Experimental Immunology*, vol. 129, no. 1, pp. 183–190, 2002.

[46] M. Holland, H. Yagi, N. Takahashi et al., "Differential glycosylation of polyclonal IgG, IgG-Fc and IgG-Fab isolated from the sera of patients with ANCA-associated systemic vasculitis," *Biochimica et Biophysica Acta (BBA) - General Subjects*, vol. 1760, no. 4, pp. 669–677, 2006.

# 25

# Increased Circulating Th17 Cells, Serum IL-17A, and IL-23 in Takayasu Arteritis

**Durga Prasanna Misra, Smriti Chaurasia, and Ramnath Misra**

*Department of Clinical Immunology, Sanjay Gandhi Post Graduate Institute of Medical Sciences, Rae Bareily Road, Lucknow, Uttar Pradesh 226 014, India*

Correspondence should be addressed to Ramnath Misra; rnmisra2000@gmail.com

Academic Editor: Andras Perl

*Introduction.* Th17, $\gamma\delta$T, NK, and NKT cells in peripheral blood and serum IL-17 and IL-23 in Takayasu arteritis (TA) were measured and correlated with disease activity. *Methods.* Th17 (anti-CD3APC, CD4PECy7, and IL-17PE), NKT, NK (anti-CD3APC, CD56FITC), and $\gamma\delta$T (anti-CD3FITC and $\gamma\delta$TCRAPC) cells were enumerated by flow cytometry in peripheral blood of 30 patients with TA (ACR1990 criteria) and 20 healthy controls, serum IL-17 and IL-23 measured by ELISA. Relation with disease activity (NIH criteria, ITAS2010) was analyzed (using nonparametric tests, median with interquartile range). *Results.* Mean age of patients was $33.47 \pm 11.78$ years (25 females); mean symptom duration was $7.1 \pm 5.3$ years. 13 were not on immunosuppressants; 12 were active (ITAS2010 $\geq 4$). The percentage of Th17 cells was significantly expanded in TA (patients 2.1 (1.5–3.2) versus controls 0.75 (0.32–1.2); $p < 0.0001$) with no differences in other cell populations. Serum IL-17 and IL-23 (pg/mL) in patients (6.2 (4.6–8.5) and 15 (14.9–26.5), resp.) were significantly higher ($p < 0.001$) than controls (3.9 (3.9–7.3) and undetectable median value, resp.). Subgroup analysis revealed no correlation of Th17 cells, serum IL-17, and IL-23 with disease activity or medications, nor any significant difference before and after medication. *Conclusions.* There is significant expansion of Th17 cells and elevated serum IL-17 and IL-23 levels in TA patients compared to healthy controls.

## 1. Introduction

Takayasu arteritis (TA) is a rare granulomatous large vessel vasculitis (LVV) of unknown etiology. The pathogenesis of TA has not yet been clearly elucidated; both innate and adaptive immunity are involved. Innate immune cells, gamma delta ($\gamma\delta$) T lymphocytes and natural killer cells, are increased in aortic tissue biopsies of TA [1]. Adaptive immunity also plays a role in TA peripheral blood of patients having an increased ratio of $CD4^+/CD8^+$ T cells [2]. T-helper cells producing IFN-$\gamma$ (Th1 cells) promote granulomatous inflammation in TA. Studies in Giant Cell Arteritis (GCA), the other variant of LVV, have shown increased Th1 and Th17 (T-helper 17 cells, producing IL-17A) in peripheral blood and also elevated serum IFN-$\gamma$ and IL-17A [3]. Recent studies have shown efficacy of IL-6 receptor blockade (tocilizumab) in refractory TA [4]. IL-6 skews naïve T-helper cells to a Th17 phenotype, maintained by IL-23 secreted by antigen presenting cells [5, 6]. Natural killer (NK) cells, natural killer T (NKT) cells, and $\gamma\delta$ T cells also produce IL-17A [5, 7]. Since the role of IL-17A has not yet been clearly defined in TA, we proposed to study cell populations that are producers of IL-17A in peripheral blood, that is, Th17 cells, NK cells, NKT cells, and $\gamma\delta$ T cells, and serum levels of IL-17A and IL-23 in patients with TA, and looked for their relationship with clinical disease activity.

## 2. Materials and Methods

The study was approved by the Institute Ethics Committee, SGPGIMS, Lucknow (Ethics committee number 2013-24-DM-Exp) and performed in accordance with the ethical standards laid down in the 1964 Declaration of Helsinki and its later amendments. Thirty consecutive patients fulfilling 1990 American College of Rheumatology criteria for TA [8] were included after seeking informed consent. For comparison, 20 healthy controls of similar age and sex were included after obtaining informed consent. Erythrocyte sedimentation rate (ESR) was measured by Westergren's method for all patients at time of sampling. Clinical activity was assessed using ITAS2010, ITAS-A [9], and NIH criteria [10]. 1.0 mL of heparinized whole blood was collected and flow cytometry performed immediately to enumerate cell populations under study. Serum was stored at −80°C for IL-17A and IL-23 estimation. 10 patients presented to us for the first time and were diagnosed with Takayasu arteritis (TA); hence they were not on treatment before (i.e., treatment-naïve). Clinical assessment of active disease merited starting immunosuppressive treatment. They were treated as per the standard practice at our clinic with oral weekly methotrexate (15–25 mg/week) and prednisolone (1 mg/kg/day for 6 weeks followed by gradual taper to 7.5 mg/day over 3 to 6 months). For these patients, repeat blood sampling was done after 3 months for comparison with baseline sample after receiving immunosuppressant. All analyses were done using nonparametric tests using Graph Pad Prism software version 6.0e (values represented as median with interquartile range in brackets with Mann-Whitney test used for intergroup comparison).

### 2.1. Cell Subsets Analysis by FACS

*2.1.1. Th17 Cells.* Heparinized whole blood cultured with complete RPMI medium and 10% FCS in the ratio of 1 : 1 was activated with 50 ng/mL phorbol myristate acetate (PMA; Sigma, St. Louis, USA) and 1 $\mu$g/mL ionomycin (Sigma, St. Louis, USA) for 6 hours and Golgi Plug 2 $\mu$M monensin (Sigma, St. Louis, USA) was added for the last 4 four hours of activation. Cells were surface-stained with PECy7-labeled monoclonal anti-CD4 and APC-labeled monoclonal anti-CD3 antibodies (BD Biosciences, Franklin Lakes, New Jersey, USA) followed by red blood cells (RBC) lysis using FACS lysing solution (BD Biosciences, Franklin Lakes, New Jersey, USA). After washing with phosphate buffered saline (PBS), the cells were fixed using a fixation buffer (Leucoperm, ABD Serotech, San Diego, CA, USA) and washed twice with PBS (pH7.2, 0.15 M). The cells were then permeabilized with permeabilization buffer (Leucoperm, ABD Serotech, San Diego, CA, USA) and intracellularly stained with phycoerythrin-(PE-) labeled monoclonal antibodies against IL-17A. Cells were washed and resuspended in PBS.

*2.1.2. $\gamma\delta$ T Cells.* 100 microlitre of heparinized whole blood was surface-stained with FITC-labeled anti-CD3 antibodies and APC-conjugated anti-$\gamma\delta$ TCR (BD Bioscience, Franklin Lakes, New Jersey, USA) and lysed and washed as mentioned above.

*2.1.3. NK and NKT Cells.* 100 microlitre of heparinized whole blood was surface-stained with APC-labeled anti-CD3 and FITC-labeled anti-CD56 antibodies (BD Bioscience, Franklin Lakes, New Jersey, USA) and lysed and washed as mentioned above. In each assay, markers were drawn based on data from isotype-specific IgG antibodies.

Table 1: Demographic details of patients and controls.

| | Patients | Controls | $p$ value |
|---|---|---|---|
| Total number | 30 | 20 | |
| Mean age | 33.5 (±11.8) | 34.2 (±11.3) | 0.84* |
| Sex (female : male) | 25 : 5 | 13 : 7 | 0.137** |
| On any immunosuppressant | 17 | — | — |
| Median prednisolone dose (mg/day) | 7.5 (6.9–20) ($n$ = 14) | — | — |
| Median oral methotrexate dose (mg/week) | 17.5 (15–20) ($n$ = 11) | — | — |
| Median azathioprine dose (mg/day) | 100 (100–150) ($n$ = 3) | — | — |
| Angiographic type (Numano's) | V – 66.7%<br>I – 23.3%<br>IIb - 6.7%<br>IIa – 3.3% | — | — |

*Mann-Whitney $U$ test.
**$z$-statistic.

A total of 100,000 events for Th17 cells and 50,000 events each for $\gamma\delta$ T cells, NK, and NKT cells were acquired. NK cells were identified as $CD3^-CD56^+$, NKT cells were identified as $CD3^+CD56^+$ (in lymphocyte gate), $\gamma\delta$ T cells were $\gamma\delta$-TCR and $CD3^+$ (in CD3 gate), and $CD3^+CD4^+$ cells positive for IL-17 were identified as Th17 cells (in CD3 gate). Acquisition of cells was done on Beckman coulter flow cytometer and analyzed by Navios software.

*2.1.4. Serum IL-17A and IL-23.* IL-17A and IL-23 were measured by ELISA as per manufacturer instructions (eBiosciences, San-Diego, USA) (sensitivity for serum IL-17A, 4 pg/mL, serum IL-23, 15 pg/mL).

## 3. Results

Demographic characteristics of patients and controls are detailed in Table 1. Both were comparable for age and gender distribution.

There was no significant difference in NK, NKT (Figure 1), or $\gamma\delta$ T cells (Figure 2) between patients and control. However, Th17 cells were significantly expanded in patients with TA (3.1-fold higher in patients versus controls (2.69 ± 2.07 versus 0.87 ± 0.61%, resp.), $p < 0.0001$). Similarly serum IL-17A levels showed a significant elevation in patients compared to controls (1.62-fold higher in patients versus controls (8.60 ± 8.07 versus 5.32 ± 1.75 pg/mL, resp.), $p < 0.0001$). Serum IL-23 was detectable in 14 patients and in none of the controls, and the levels in patients were significantly higher than controls (1.75-fold higher in patients versus controls (26.17 ± 29.01 versus 14.9 ± 0.0 pg/mL, resp.), $p = 0.0007$) (Figure 3). Th17 cells, serum IL-17 A, or IL-23 did not correlate significantly with ESR (Pearson's correlation coefficient −0.08, −0.34, and −0.21, resp., $p > 0.05$ for all), ITAS2010 (Pearson's correlation

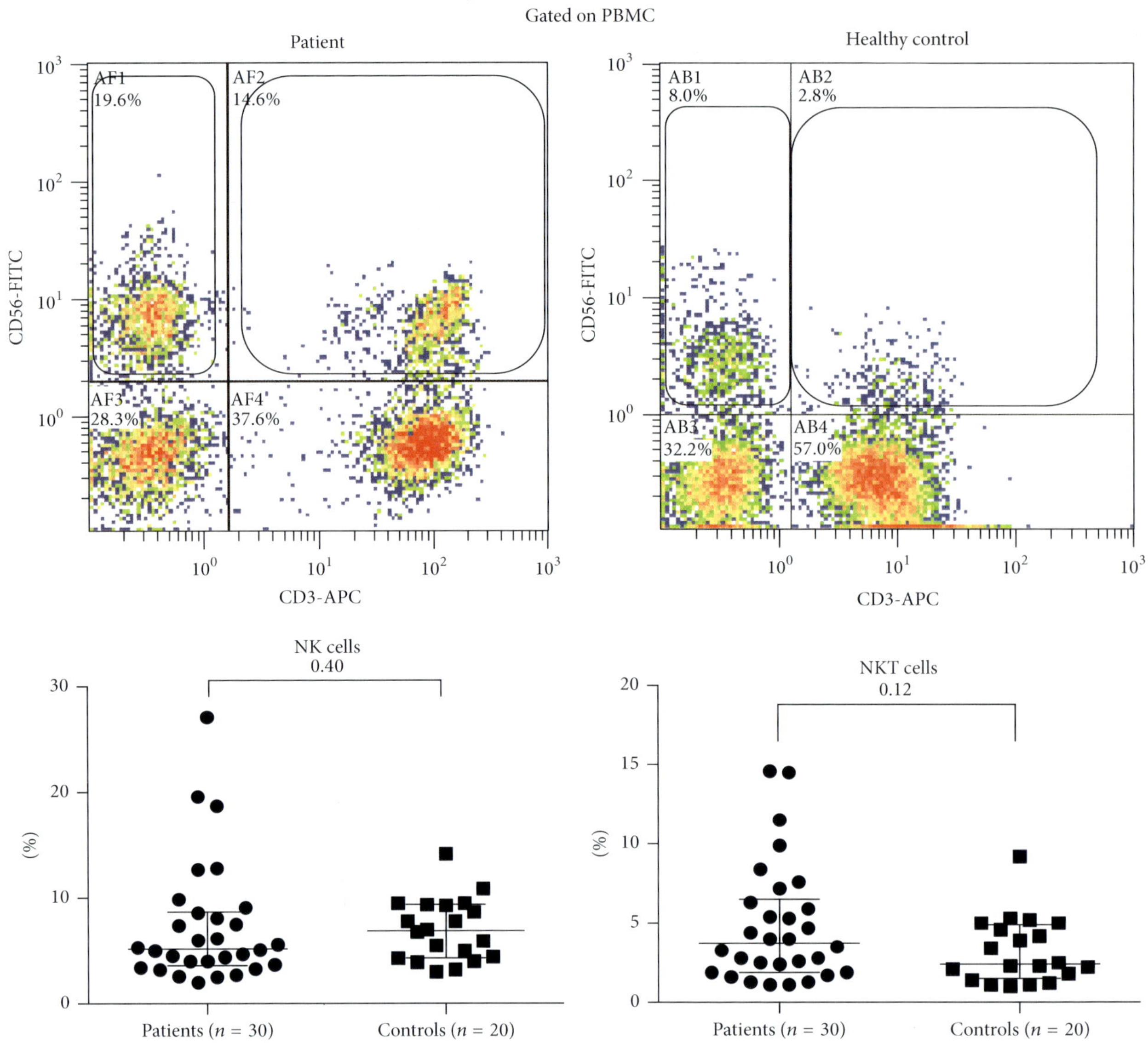


FIGURE 1: In peripheral blood of 30 patients and 20 controls, natural killer (NK) and natural killer T (NKT) cells were identified by gating on PBMCs and surface staining for CD3 and CD56. NK cells were $CD3^-CD56^+$ and NKT cells were $CD3^+CD56^+$. Bars represent median with interquartile range. $p$ value (Mann-Whitney test) is mentioned in each figure.

coefficient −0.23, +0.05, and −0.25, resp., $p > 0.05$ for all), or ITAS-A (Pearson's correlation coefficient −0.25, −0.02, and −0.26, resp., $p > 0.05$ for all). There was no significant correlation demonstrable between Th17 cells and serum IL-17 (Pearson's correlation coefficient −0.11, $p = 0.58$) or IL-23 (Pearson's correlation coefficient +0.37, $p = 0.052$). Thirteen patients were active as assessed by NIH criteria, and 12 were active as assessed by ITAS2010 ≥ 4. There was no significant difference in populations of Th17 cells or serum levels of IL-17A and IL-23 in between active or inactive patients. Thirteen patients were not on immunosuppressive medications, and comparing Th17 cells and serum IL-17A and IL-23 in them versus patients on immunosuppression revealed no significant difference (Table 2).

Furthermore, we compared proportions of patients active (by NIH criteria) and on immune suppressive medications as well as ITAS2010, ITAS-A, and serum levels of IL-17A and IL-23, in subgroups of patients with Th17 cell expansion (defined as levels of Th17 cells greater than 2 SD of the mean value of controls) versus those who did not and could not demonstrate any differences between these two subgroups (Table 3).

For the 10 patients for whom we had paired samples before and 3 months after immunosuppression (prednisolone and methotrexate), there was a decline in Th17 cells following treatment. Serum IL-17A levels remained similar, and serum IL-23 was detectable in 3 patients before and none after immunosuppression. None of these differences reached statistical significance (Figure 4). However, post hoc power analysis revealed that the study was not sufficiently powered to distinguish the effect of medication on the levels of Th17 cells and serum IL-17 and IL-23 levels.

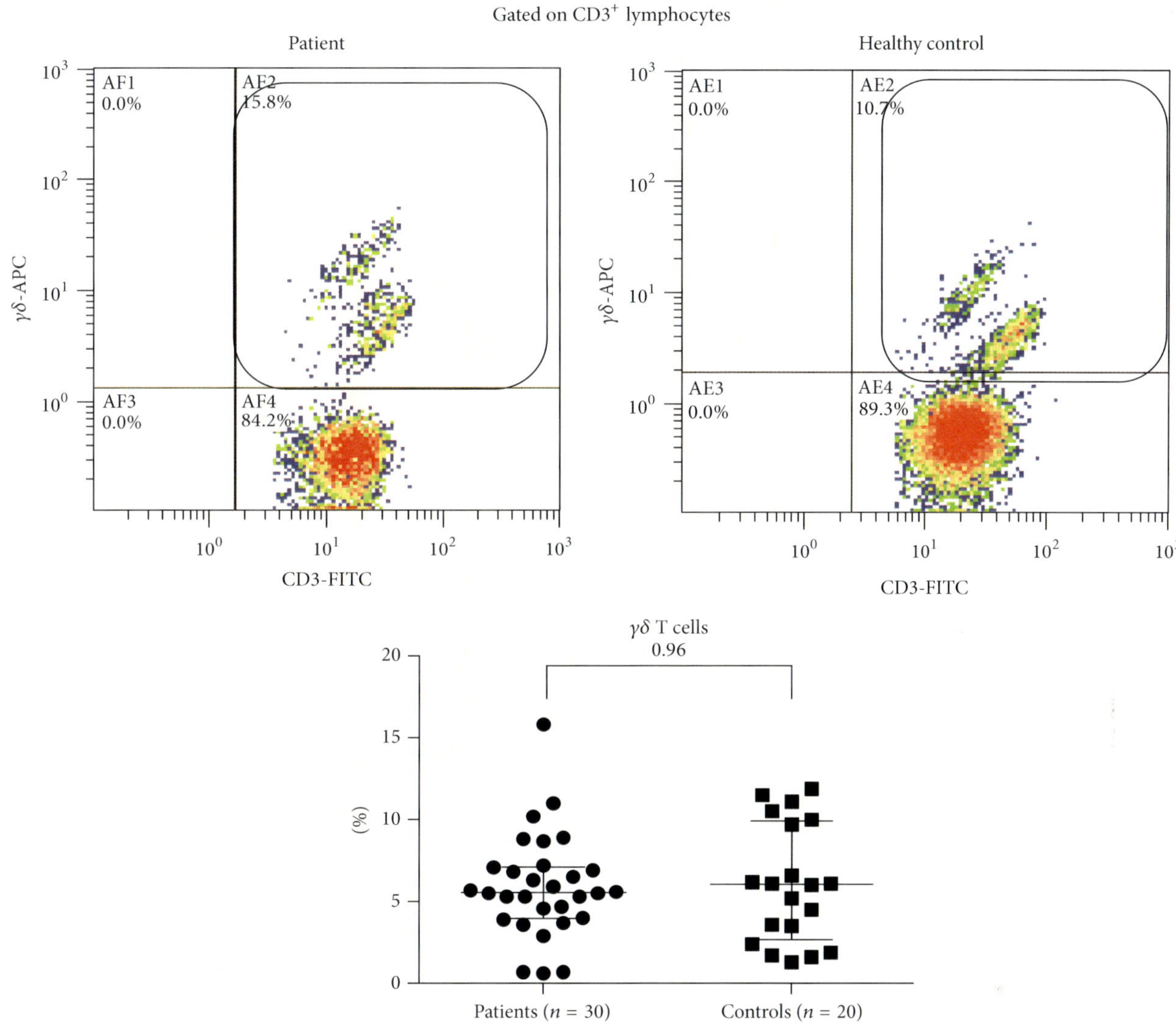


FIGURE 2: In peripheral blood of 30 patients and 20 controls, $\gamma\delta$ T cells were identified by $\gamma\delta$ TCR+ cells on CD3 gate. Bars represent median with interquartile range. $p$ value (Mann-Whitney test) is mentioned in each figure.

## 4. Discussion

We found an increase in serum levels of IL-17A and IL-23 in patients with TA compared with controls. The increased levels neither correlated with overall disease activity state nor became normal with immunosuppressive therapy. We also found increased expansion of Th17 cells, which produce IL-17 A, but not with NK, NKT, or gamma delta T cells (which are other producers of IL-17A) in the peripheral blood. In a subset of immunosuppressive-naïve patients, there seemed to be no differences before or after immunosuppression in Th17 cells, serum-IL-17A, or IL-23.

Our findings corroborate a recent publication by Saadoun et al. studying T cell populations and cytokines which showed increased Th17 cells in TA patients [11], which on in vitro stimulation showed increased IL-17A and IL-23 levels compared to healthy controls. However, they demonstrated higher in vitro production of IL-17A in patients with active TA (as assessed by NIH criteria) compared with those in remission, in contrast to our findings. There were no differences in Th17 cells, serum IL-17A, and IL-23 in patients on immunosuppression. Alibaz-Oner et al. explored serum levels of cytokines in patients with TA, and contrary to our findings, they failed to demonstrate an increase in serum IL-23 levels compared to healthy controls [12]. They had not studied serum IL-17A in their patients. The strength of our study was that we assessed levels of Th17 cells, serum IL-17, and IL-23 in a subgroup of patients before and after immunosuppression and could not demonstrate a difference.

In GCA, expansion of Th17 cells and increased serum IL-17 compared to controls have been demonstrated, and these levels are suppressed with corticosteroid use [3]. Interestingly, our study confirms contrary findings in TA [11], wherein the circulating Th17 cells are not suppressed with immunosuppressive medication use, including corticosteroids. This may suggest that Th17 cells in TA and GCA have different responses to corticosteroid therapy, in spite of both being classified as large vessel vasculitides.

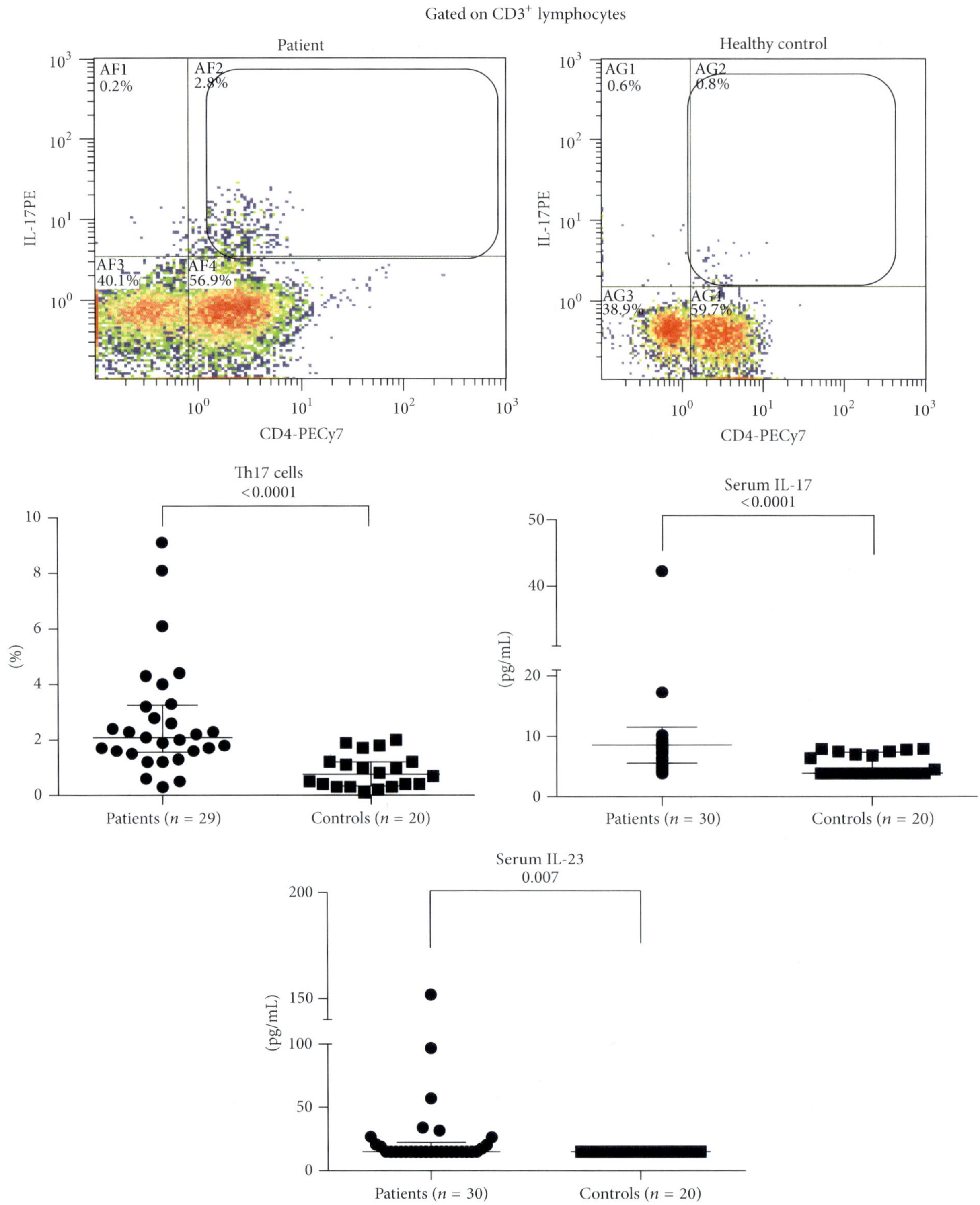


FIGURE 3: T-helper 17 (Th17) cells were measured in peripheral blood of 29 patients (could not be studied in one patient due to technical difficulties) and 20 healthy controls, after culture of whole blood for 6 hours followed by gating on $CD3^+$ lymphocytes. Th17 cells were identified by surface staining for CD4 and intracellular staining for IL-17A. Serum IL-17A and IL-23 were measured by ELISA. Bars represent median with interquartile range. $p$ value (Mann-Whitney test) is mentioned in each figure.

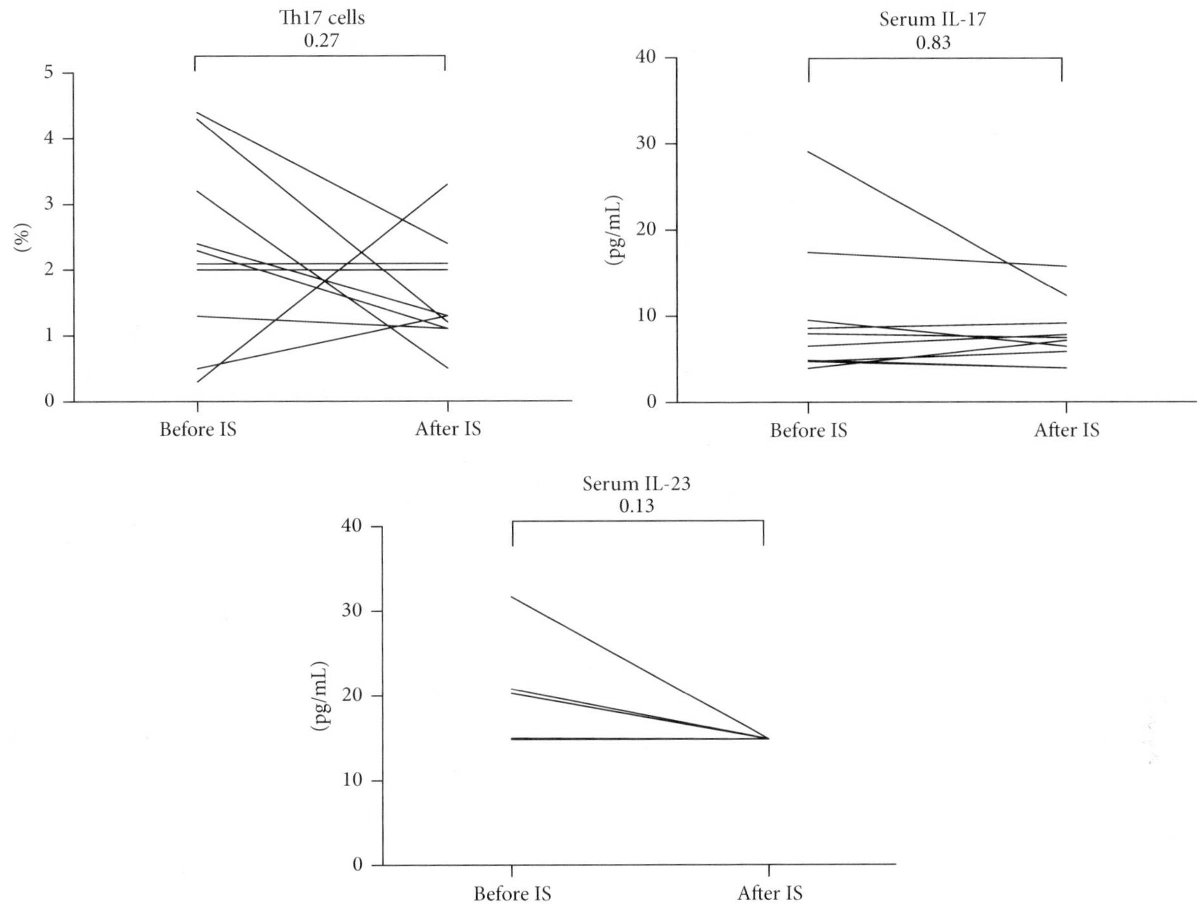


FIGURE 4: For the subgroup of 10 patients who were immunosuppressive- (IS-) naïve and were started on treatment (prednisolone and methotrexate), T-helper 17 (Th17) cells and serum IL-17A and IL-23 before and 3 months after therapy were recorded. There were no significant differences. Serum IL-23 was detectable in 3 patients prior to immunosuppression and in none of them after. $p$ value (Mann-Whitney test) is mentioned in each figure.

TABLE 2: Th17 cells, serum IL-17, and IL-23 levels with respect to disease activity parameters and immunosuppressants.

| | Activity measured by NIH criteria | | |
|---|---|---|---|
| | Active ($n$ = 13) | Inactive ($n$ = 17) | $p$ value (Mann-Whitney) |
| Th17 cells (%) | 2.1 (1.4–3) | 2.05 (1.6–4.3) ($n$ = 16*) | 0.55 |
| IL-17A (pg/mL) | 7.4 (4.7–9) | 5.3 (4.4–8.5) | 0.56 |
| IL-23 (pg/mL) | 14.9 (14.9–17.7) | 15 (14.9–30.5) | 0.07 |
| | Activity measured by ITAS2010 ≥ 4 | | |
| | Active ($n$ = 12) | Inactive ($n$ = 18) | $p$ value (Mann-Whitney) |
| Th17 cells (%) | 2.2 (1.4–3.1) | 1.9 (1.6–4.2) ($n$ = 17*) | 0.80 |
| IL-17A (pg/mL) | 7.7 (4.7–9.2) | 5.4 (4.4–8.6) | 0.54 |
| IL-23 (pg/mL) | 14.9 (14.9–19) | 15 (14.9–28.7) | 0.13 |
| | Data with respect to immunosuppressants | | |
| | Not on immunosuppressants ($n$ = 13) | On immunosuppressants** ($n$ = 17) | $p$ value (Mann-Whitney) |
| Th17 cells (%) | 2 (1.3–2.8) | 2.3 (1.6–3.8) ($n$ = 16*) | 0.30 |
| IL-17A (pg/mL) | 6.5 (4.7–9) | 6.1 (4.4–8.6) | 0.85 |
| IL-23 (pg/mL) | 14.9 (14.9–20.6) | 15 (14.9–26.6) | 0.36 |

Values represented as median with interquartile range in brackets.
*Th17 cell population could not be studied in one patient due to technical difficulties.
**14 patients were on prednisolone, 11 on oral methotrexate, and 3 on azathioprine.

TABLE 3: Comparison of Th17 expanders versus the rest.

| Parameter | Patients with expansion of Th17 cells ($n$ = 15) | Patients without expansion of Th17 cells ($n$ = 14) | $p$ value |
|---|---|---|---|
| On immunosuppression | 6/15 | 7/14 | 0.157 |
| Active by Kerr's criteria | 7/15 | 6/14 | 0.157 |
| ITAS2010 | 1 (0–8) | 1 (0–10) | 0.80 |
| ITAS-A | 3 (2–10) | 3.5 (1.75–11.5) | 0.73 |
| Serum IL-17A | 4.96 (4.72–8.39) | 7.28 (4.29–8.78) | 0.48 |
| Serum IL-23 | 14.9 (14.9–26.38) | 14.9 (14.9–19.37) | 0.52 |

Values represented as median with interquartile range in brackets.
Th17 expanders were defined as those patients with TA having percentage of Th17 cells greater than 2 SD of the mean value of controls.
$p$ = ns for all comparisons between the two groups.

A recent study showed increased IL-17 mRNA levels in temporal artery biopsy samples compared to controls in spite of peripheral blood IL-17 levels being similar to controls. Levels of IL-17 mRNA when elevated in the temporal artery actually predicted sustained responsiveness to glucocorticoid treatment [13]. IL-17 polymorphisms have been linked to GCA [14], and more recently in TA [15]. Studies on pathogenesis of TA are limited by the availability of aortic tissue samples [16]. However, a recent study shows expression of IL-17A in aortic tissue biopsies of active TA patients [11].

NK cells and gamma delta T cells (which are other producers of IL-17A) have been shown to be increased in vascular tissue biopsies from patients with TA, but we could not demonstrate NK cell or gamma delta T cell expansion in the peripheral blood compared to controls. The disease process in TA originates in the walls of large vessels. Levels of cytokines and cellular alterations in the peripheral blood are only a surrogate of these changes in the aortic tissue and may not reflect those at tissue level. This might explain why there was no demonstrable correlation between Th17 cells and serum levels of IL-17, or difference with respect to disease activity or medication intake. The clinical assessment of disease activity in TA is imperfect and is a work in progress [17]. Indeed aortic biopsies have shown active inflammation in patients with TA with a normal ESR [18].

Th17 expansion has also been demonstrated in variable vessel vasculitis, that is, Behcet's disease [19]. In small vessel vasculitides, Th17 skewing has been demonstrated in patients with inactive granulomatosis with polyangiitis (Wegener's) and active eosinophilic granulomatosis with polyangiitis [20]. Th17 cells remained elevated in patients with ANCA vasculitis both in active disease as well as in remission, similar to our findings in TA [21].

The exact pathogenic significance of Th17 cell expansion in TA is unclear. Aortic biopsies from patients with TA have shown neutrophil infiltrates in vascular lesions [1]. Th17 cells, by virtue of secreting IL-17A, can recruit neutrophils to sites of vascular inflammation, and IL-23 helps sustain the population of Th17 cells. Hence, corroboration with aortic biopsies is needed to further define the exact role of Th17 cells in the pathogenesis of TA.

Rare case reports of large vessel arteritis induced by Epstein-Barr virus [22] and coxsackie virus [23] have been described in literature. The etiology of TA is not yet clear, and one of the hypotheses, emerging from such case reports, is a viral infection triggering vasculitis. Th17 cells have been linked to viral persistence [24]; hence our findings of increased Th17 cells in TA could suggest viral persistence as one of the mechanisms driving TA.

Recent literature suggests efficacy of IL-6 receptor blockade (tocilizumab) in patients with difficult-to-treat TA [4]. IL-6, acting on IL-6 receptor, expressed on naïve T-helper cells, skews differentiation towards Th17 subset. Hence our finding of Th17 expansion and increased serum IL-17 in TA may have relevance explaining the efficacy of tocilizumab therapy in TA. In view of emerging Th17-IL-17 targeted therapies in spondyloarthropathies (ustekinumab, antibody to common p40 subunit of IL12 and IL-23; secukinumab, antibody to IL-17A; brodalumab, antibody to IL-17 receptor antagonist) [25], our findings of increased IL-17 and IL-23 in TA offer potential newer therapeutic approaches in refractory TA.

The limitations of our study were a relatively small sample size. However, this must be considered in view of the fact that TA is a rare large vessel vasculitis. Also, we did not measure serum CRP but instead measured ESR using a standardized technique. Lack of aortic biopsy samples to study Th17 cell and IL-17 and IL-23 mRNA expression is another limitation of our study.

To conclude, our finding of increased Th17 cells and serum IL-17A and IL-23 in TA offers newer insights into the pathogenesis of a rare large vessel vasculitis. The lack of suppression of Th17 cells in patients receiving immunosuppression, unlike in GCA, lends credence to the hypothesis that TA and GCA are pathogenetically different. Tissue level studies looking for both innate and adaptive immune cells and cytokines will provide further support to the role of Th17 cells in this disease.

## Disclosure

Current affiliation to Durga Prasanna Misra: Department of Clinical Immunology, Jawaharlal Institute of Postgraduate Medical Education and Research (JIPMER), Puducherry – 605006, India.

## Competing Interests

None of the authors have any competing interests to declare.

## References

[1] Y. Seko, S. Minota, A. Kawasaki et al., "Perforin-secreting killer cell infiltration and expression of a 65-kD heat-shock protein in

aortic tissue of patients with Takayasu's arteritis," *The Journal of Clinical Investigation*, vol. 93, no. 2, pp. 750–758, 1994.

[2] S. Sagar, N. K. Ganguly, M. Koicha, and B. K. Sharma, "Immunopathogenesis of Takayasu arteritis," *Heart and Vessels*, vol. 7, no. 7, pp. 85–90, 1992.

[3] J. Deng, B. R. Younge, R. A. Olshen, J. J. Goronzy, and C. M. Weyand, "Th17 and th1 T-cell responses in giant cell arteritis," *Circulation*, vol. 121, no. 7, pp. 906–915, 2010.

[4] R. Goel, D. Danda, S. Kumar, and G. Joseph, "Rapid control of disease activity by tocilizumab in 10 'difficult-to-treat' cases of Takayasu arteritis," *International Journal of Rheumatic Diseases*, vol. 16, no. 6, pp. 754–761, 2013.

[5] W. B. van den Berg and I. B. McInnes, "Th17 cells and IL-17 a—focus on immunopathogenesis and immunotherapeutics," *Seminars in Arthritis and Rheumatism*, vol. 43, no. 2, pp. 158–170, 2013.

[6] J. P. Sherlock, P. C. Taylor, and C. D. Buckley, "The biology of IL-23 and IL-17 and their therapeutic targeting in rheumatic diseases," *Current Opinion in Rheumatology*, vol. 27, no. 1, pp. 71–75, 2015.

[7] S. Zhu and Y. Qian, "IL-17/IL-17 receptor system in autoimmune disease: mechanisms and therapeutic potential," *Clinical Science*, vol. 122, no. 11, pp. 487–511, 2012.

[8] A. W. S. de Souza and J. F. de Carvalho, "Diagnostic and classification criteria of Takayasu arteritis," *Journal of Autoimmunity*, vol. 48-49, pp. 79–83, 2014.

[9] R. Misra, D. Danda, S. M. Rajappa et al., "Development and initial validation of the Indian Takayasu Clinical Activity Score (ITAS2010)," *Rheumatology*, vol. 52, no. 10, pp. 1795–1801, 2013.

[10] G. S. Kerr, C. W. Hallahan, J. Giordano et al., "Takayasu arteritis," *Annals of Internal Medicine*, vol. 120, no. 11, pp. 919–929, 1994.

[11] D. Saadoun, M. Garrido, C. Comarmond et al., "Th1 and Th17 cytokines drive inflammation in takayasu arteritis," *Arthritis & Rheumatology*, vol. 67, no. 5, pp. 1353–1360, 2015.

[12] F. Alibaz-Oner, S. P. Yentur, G. Saruhan-Direskeneli, and H. Direskeneli, "Serum cytokine profiles in Takayasu's arteritis: search for biomarkers," *Clinical and Experimental Rheumatology*, vol. 33, no. 2, supplement 89, pp. S-32–S-35, 2015.

[13] G. Espígol-Frigolé, M. Corbera-Bellalta, E. Planas-Rigol et al., "Increased IL-17A expression in temporal artery lesions is a predictor of sustained response to glucocorticoid treatment in patients with giant-cell arteritis," *Annals of the Rheumatic Diseases*, vol. 72, no. 9, pp. 1481–1487, 2013.

[14] A. Márquez, J. Hernández-Rodríguez, M. C. Cid et al., "Influence of the *IL17A* locus in giant cell arteritis susceptibility," *Annals of the Rheumatic Diseases*, vol. 73, no. 9, pp. 1742–1745, 2014.

[15] D. Danda, M. Hindhumathi, G. Ruchika et al., "Cytokine gene polymorphisms in Asian Indian patients with Takayasu's Arteritis (TA)—a single center study," *Indian Journal of Rheumatology*, vol. 9, article S2, 2014.

[16] L. Arnaud, J. Haroche, A. Mathian, G. Gorochov, and Z. Amoura, "Pathogenesis of Takayasu's arteritis: a 2011 update," *Autoimmunity Reviews*, vol. 11, no. 1, pp. 61–67, 2011.

[17] P. Bacon, R. Sivakumar, D. Danda, and R. Misra, "Vasculitis assessment and Takayasu aorto-arteritis," *Indian Journal of Rheumatology*, vol. 7, no. 3, pp. 153–158, 2012.

[18] G. S. Hoffman, "Takayasu arteritis: lessons from the American National Institutes of Health experience," *International Journal of Cardiology*, vol. 54, supplement, pp. S99–102, 1996.

[19] J. Kim, J. A. Park, E. Y. Lee, Y. J. Lee, Y. W. Song, and E. B. Lee, "Imbalance of Th17 to Th1 cells in Behcet's disease," *Clinical and Experimental Rheumatology*, vol. 28, no. 4, supplement 60, pp. S16–S19, 2010.

[20] B. Wilde, M. Thewissen, J. Damoiseaux, P. van Paassen, O. Witzke, and J. W. C. Tervaert, "T cells in ANCA-associated vasculitis: what can we learn from lesional versus circulating T cells?" *Arthritis Research and Therapy*, vol. 12, article 204, 2010.

[21] E. Nogueira, S. Hamour, D. Sawant et al., "Serum IL-17 and IL-23 levels and autoantigen-specific Th17 cells are elevated in patients with ANCA-associated vasculitis," *Nephrology Dialysis Transplantation*, vol. 25, no. 7, pp. 2209–2217, 2010.

[22] K. Murakami, M. Ohsawa, S.-X. Hu, H. Kanno, K. Aozasa, and M. Nose, "Large-vessel arteritis associated with chronic active Epstein-Barr virus infection," *Arthritis and Rheumatism*, vol. 41, no. 2, pp. 369–373, 1998.

[23] V. Di Giacomo, F. Meloni, M. G. Transi, G. Mastroberardino, G. Iannucci, and V. Sciacca, "An uncommon systemic arteritis—a case report," *Angiology*, vol. 37, no. 1, pp. 63–71, 1986.

[24] N. E. Martinez, F. Sato, E. Kawai, S. Omura, R. P. Chervenak, and I. Tsunoda, "Regulatory T cells and Th17 cells in viral infections: implications for multiple sclerosis and myocarditis," *Future Virology*, vol. 7, no. 6, pp. 593–608, 2012.

[25] N. Yeremenko, J. E. Paramarta, and D. Baeten, "The interleukin-23/interleukin-17 immune axis as a promising new target in the treatment of spondyloarthritis," *Current Opinion in Rheumatology*, vol. 26, no. 4, pp. 361–370, 2014.

26

# Understanding and Managing Pregnancy in Patients with Lupus

**Guilherme Ramires de Jesus,[1] Claudia Mendoza-Pinto,[2,3] Nilson Ramires de Jesus,[1] Flávia Cunha dos Santos,[1] Evandro Mendes Klumb,[4] Mario García Carrasco,[2,3] and Roger Abramino Levy[4]**

[1]*Department of Obstetrics, Universidade do Estado do Rio de Janeiro, Rio de Janeiro, Brazil*
[2]*Systemic Autoimmune Diseases Research Unit, Hospital General Regional No. 36-CIBIOR, Instituto Mexicano del Seguro Social, Puebla, Mexico*
[3]*Department of Immunology and Rheumatology, Medicine School, Benemérita Universidad Autónoma de Puebla, Puebla, Mexico*
[4]*Department of Rheumatology, Universidade do Estado do Rio de Janeiro, Rio de Janeiro, Brazil*

Correspondence should be addressed to Guilherme Ramires de Jesus; guilhermedejesus@gmail.com

Academic Editor: Juan-Manuel Anaya

Systemic lupus erythematosus (SLE) is a chronic, multisystemic autoimmune disease that occurs predominantly in women of fertile age. The association of SLE and pregnancy, mainly with active disease and especially with nephritis, has poorer pregnancy outcomes, with increased frequency of preeclampsia, fetal loss, prematurity, growth restriction, and newborns small for gestational age. Therefore, SLE pregnancies are considered high risk condition, should be monitored frequently during pregnancy and delivery should occur in a controlled setting. Pregnancy induces dramatic immune and neuroendocrine changes in the maternal body in order to protect the fetus from immunologic attack and these modifications can be affected by SLE. The risk of flares depends on the level of maternal disease activity in the 6–12 months before conception and is higher in women with repeated flares before conception, in those who discontinue useful medications and in women with active glomerulonephritis at conception. It is a challenge to differentiate lupus nephritis from preeclampsia and, in this context, the angiogenic and antiangiogenic cytokines are promising. Prenatal care of pregnant patients with SLE requires close collaboration between rheumatologist and obstetrician. Planning pregnancy is essential to increase the probability of successful pregnancies.

## 1. Introduction

Systemic lupus erythematosus (SLE) is a chronic, multisystemic autoimmune disease that occurs predominantly in women of fertile age. The risk of obstetric complications in pregnant SLE patients is significant, with an increased risk of spontaneous abortion, intrauterine fetal death, preeclampsia (PE), intrauterine growth restriction (IUGR), and preterm birth. In addition, pregnancy may be associated with disease flares requiring immunosuppressive therapy. Therefore, pregnancies in SLE patients are considered a high risk condition. Maternal health and fetal development should be monitored frequently during pregnancy. If possible, delivery should occur in a controlled setting. An obstetrician with experience in high-risk pregnancies should follow pregnant women with SLE, including a multidisciplinary approach with rheumatologic and neonatal team. Fortunately, due to medical advances the number of SLE patients who become pregnant has increased worldwide and most pregnancies are successful [1, 2].

Although these patients have fewer live births with more pregnancy complications, they may have subsequent uncomplicated pregnancies after a poor outcome. Recent studies have analyzed novel markers of poor pregnancy outcomes and new approaches to the management of SLE during pregnancy and SLE activity during pregnancy remains an ongoing problem, since major organ involvement can negatively affect outcomes [3]. Adverse fetal outcomes in obstetric SLE include fetal loss (spontaneous abortion and intrauterine fetal death), IUGR, premature birth, premature rupture of membranes, neonatal lupus, and perinatal mortality. Maternal complications in SLE patients include SLE activity, PE, and arterial hypertension, especially in patients with renal involvement [4].

A recent population-based study by Vinet et al. followed 1334 women with SLE through the Quebec administrative databases and found that SLE women have fewer live births than the general population. Over a 9-year period, 559 live births occurred in SLE patients compared with the 708 that would have been expected in the general population (standardized incidence ratio 0.79; 95% confidence interval (CI) 0.73–0.86) [5].

In the United States, there are an estimated 4500 pregnancies in SLE women each year and pregnancy complications are common: one-third of the pregnancies result in a caesarean section, the birth is preterm in 33% of all gestations, and over 20% of all women will develop by PE [2].

Studies suggest that fetal loss may be decreasing in recent years. In 1960 to 1965, the mean rate of fetal loss was 43%, compared with 17% in 2000 to 2003 [4]. However, in a multiethnic population with SLE in North America, the fetal loss rate may be related to comorbidities and disease activity before pregnancy [6]. Thus, the risk of fetal loss is higher in women with hypertension, active SLE [7], lupus nephritis (LN) [8, 9], hypocomplementemia, elevated levels of anti-DNA antibodies, antiphospholipid antibodies (aPL), or thrombocytopenia [10, 11]. Further research is required to confirm this correlation in lupus pregnancy; several factors may predict fetal death, such as SLE activity, active LN, and the presence of aPL [6].

An optimistic finding from a population-based study in New South Wales, Australia, which looked at 675 women with SLE and 1058 deliveries, suggested that women whose first pregnancies result in perinatal death could nevertheless expect a live birth in subsequent pregnancies [12]. However, it is not clear whether parity increases the risk of SLE, as high-quality studies of large datasets have produced conflicting results [13].

## 2. Interaction of Pregnancy and Systemic Lupus Erythematosus

Pregnancy induces dramatic immune and neuroendocrine abnormalities in the maternal body in order to protect the foetus from immunologic attack by the mother. Instead of general immunosuppression, which would weaken maternal defense against infection, there is a modulation of the composition and function of immune-competent cells and immune-modulatory molecules in the maternal system during pregnancy [14]. The fetus promotes tolerance to paternal antigens by migration of fetal cells and cell-free fetal DNA to the maternal circulation during normal pregnancy. Fetal cells remain in the mother for decades, creating a state of microchimerism [15, 16].

After delivery, the maternal body adjusts to a nonpregnant state, which is not simply a return to the condition before conception, but occurs under the influence of immune activation at parturition [17]. The profound immunologic adaptations necessary for maternal tolerance of the foetus in pregnancy and the immunologic reset to a nonpregnant state thereafter, influence maternal autoimmune rheumatic diseases in several ways. Figure 1 shows the main elements interacting in SLE and pregnancy.

The activity of immunocompetent cells is regulated by cytokines and chemokines with T helper cells as key effectors. Cytokines are important mediators acting in concert with other factors to support successful pregnancy. One of the most important immunological modifications during pregnancy is the Th1/Th2 cytokine shift. Th1 includes interferon (IFN)-$\gamma$, interleukin- (IL-) 1, IL-2, IL-12, and tumor necrosis factor- (TNF-) alpha, which stimulate cellular immunity, and Th2 includes IL-4, IL-5, IL-6, and IL-10, which induce humoral immunity and antibody production. Since SLE is mainly a Th2-mediated disease, during pregnancy a predominance of the Th2 response may be expected, making disease exacerbation more likely. However, lower levels of estrogens, progesterone, and Th2 cytokines were found in the third trimester of pregnancy in SLE patients compared with healthy pregnant women [18].

Besides Th1 and Th2 cells, there is a third subset of CD4+T helper cells, Th17 cells, which activate the immune system and interleukin-17 (IL-17) family [19–21]. IL-17 has a proinflammatory effect and drives the development of Th17 cells, whereas a milieu of tolerance promotes the development of Treg cells [19, 22]. Increased numbers of Th17 cells are also found in conditions linked to pregnancy, such as preeclampsia and recurrent pregnancy loss (Figure 1) [23, 24].

SLE is characterized by a loss of tolerance in both the T cell and B cell compartments, resulting in B cell hyperreactivity with pathogenic autoantibody formation. One important factor that has emerged is the response of SLE to sex steroid hormones [25]. Estrogens enhance antibody production, T helper type 2 immune responses, and B cell immunity. At high concentrations, such as those found in pregnancy, estrogens and gestagens stimulate the secretion of IL-4, IL10, TGF-$\beta$, and IFN-$\gamma$ while simultaneously suppressing production of TNF-$\alpha$ [26].

In SLE patients, IL-6 serum levels remained low and did not increase in the third trimester of pregnancy, as they did in healthy controls. The absence of a rise in IL-6 is interesting in the context of cytokine function: IL-6 is necessary for T cell help for B cells [27]. IL-10 did rise progressively during pregnancy in healthy women [18]. In contrast, IL-10 levels were already significantly higher at conception in SLE patients and remained elevated throughout pregnancy and postpartum. IL-10 was originally thought to be a Th2 cytokine but is now known to be a pleiotropic cytokine with both immune stimulatory and immune suppressive functions that place it outside the Th1-Th2 paradigm [27]. Persistent high levels of IL-10 indicate a constitutional overproduction in SLE, resulting in continuous B cell stimulation.

No significant differences between SLE patients and controls were found in either sTNFR I or II levels or profiles before and during pregnancy. sTNFR I levels were significantly higher during pregnancy and postpartum in SLE patients with active disease compared with healthy controls [18]. Studies of regulatory T cells in SLE patients have shown

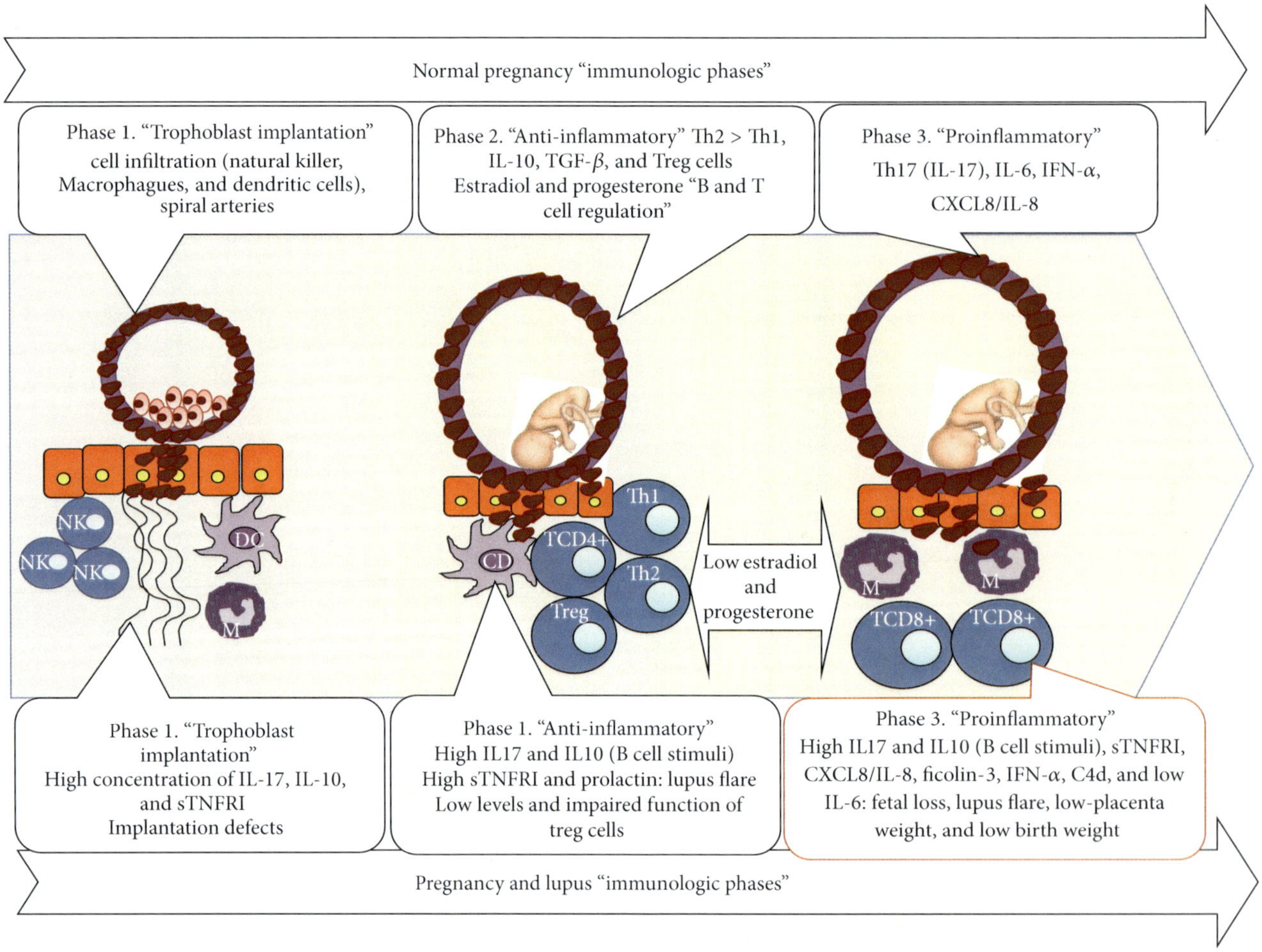


Figure 1: Pathogenesis in normal and SLE pregnancy.

reduced numbers in active SLE and impaired suppressive function of Treg cells [28]. A pilot study indicates that there is an imbalance between Treg and Th17 numbers in pregnant SLE patients [29].

During and after pregnancy, women with SLE have increased serum concentrations of CXCL8/IL-8, CXCL9/MIG, CXCL10/IP-10, and IL-10 chemokines compared with normal pregnancies, especially during active disease (Figure 1) [30].

Ficolins are soluble molecules of the innate immune system that recognize carbohydrate molecules on microbial pathogens and apoptotic and necrotic cells. Elevated ficolin-3 in specific manifestations may indicate a pathogenetic role of ficolin-3 in SLE. Ficolin-2 may be involved in the direct removal of trophoblast-derived material from the maternal circulation. Low levels of circulating ficolin-2 might impair the clearance of shed apoptotic and necrotic placental material [31, 32]. Genetic and functional alterations in ficolins should be investigated as risk factors for lupus flares in pregnant women.

A recent study has identified a new mechanism by which IFN-$\alpha$ induces an antiangiogenic milieu, increasing the sensitivity of endothelial cells to soluble vascular endothelial growth factor (VEGF), also known as fms-like tyrosine kinase-1 (sFlt1), and suggesting that elevated IFN-$\alpha$ may contribute to the pathogenesis of preeclampsia in some SLE pregnancies [33].

SLE and pregnancy-induced hypertension (PIH) share histological findings in the placenta, complement dysregulation, and fetal outcomes. Placentas of patients with SLE (50%) and PIH (35%) showed a higher $H$-score (range 0–300) for C4d immunoreactivity than control cases with linear staining on the membrane of the syncytiotrophoblast. High C4d groups were significantly associated with low-placental weights and low birth weight in both SLE and PIH. C4d might be utilized as a biomarker for a subsequent risk for IUGR and control during the gestation period in pregnant SLE patients [34].

Pregnancy induces substantial changes in hormone levels [35]. High prolactin (PRL) levels seem to be associated with active SLE during pregnancy. PRL, a cytokine, can influence immune responses. High PRL has been found in 20–30% of SLE patients and seems to be associated with clinical activity during pregnancy [36].

Anti-PRL autoantibodies have been found in 13.1% of pregnant SLE patients. Pregnant SLE women with anti-PRL autoantibodies had fewer adverse outcomes of pregnancy. This suggests PRL may play a role in pregnancy outcomes [37]. Table 1 summarized the main hormonal and immune responses are present in normal pregnancy and lupus pregnancy.

## 3. Lupus Flares during Pregnancy

An important aspect of pregnancy in SLE patients is the risk of disease flares. It is not simple to quantify the incidence of these complications because many clinical studies were performed using individual definitions of flare. Recently, efforts have been made to create a "pregnancy-version" of existing activity indexes, such as the ECLAM, SLEDAI, SLAM, and LAI, aimed at making studies more comparable [38]. The British Isles Lupus Assessment Group (BILAG) 2004-Pregnancy index has been shown to be reliable for the assessment of disease activity in pregnant SLE patients [39].

The results of prospective, controlled observational studies show some discordancy: some studies found that women are at increased risk of lupus flares when pregnant, while other studies found the rate of flares was unchanged as compared to nonpregnant SLE patients [38]. This discrepancy may be explained by disease heterogeneity, the limited number of patients enrolled in SLE-pregnancy studies, the lack of homogeneous criteria for defining lupus flares, and the different SLE treatments used during pregnancy. In addition, several manifestations secondary to pregnancy may be wrongly attributed to lupus flares, including arthralgia, myalgia, facial and palmar rash, hearing loss, and edema in the face, hands, and lower limbs. Likewise, serological abnormalities used to define lupus flares may be physiologically altered during pregnancy, that is, complement and erythrocyte sedimentation rate.

A disease flare may occur at any time, but there may be a trend towards flares in the third trimester. As the timing of flares is unpredictable, regular follow-up is indicated throughout pregnancy and postpartum. There seems to be a consensus that the risk of flares depends on the level of maternal disease activity in the 6–12 months before conception and is higher in women with repeated flares before conception [38], in those who discontinue useful medications (in particular hydroxychloroquine) [40] and, in particular, in women with active glomerulonephritis at conception [41].

Poor control of disease activity before pregnancy may also have detrimental effects on pregnancy outcomes. A study showed that disease activity in the 6 months before conception was associated with an increase in the rate of pregnancy loss [7]. Patients with a combination of high SLE activity and low complement or positive anti-dsDNA had the highest rate of pregnancy loss and preterm birth [42] and hence the importance of a careful evaluation of the maternal condition before and during pregnancy. In fact, patients who started a pregnancy in a stable remission period and continued on medications experienced fewer flares, which were mostly mild and generally well managed with a temporary increase in the prednisone dose [40].

In a recent study, 132 pregnancies in 96 SLE patients were prospectively followed by monthly clinical and laboratory evaluations. Predictors of SLE flares during pregnancy were identified by stepwise logistic regression analysis. Maternal lupus flares occurred in 57% of pregnancies and were best predicted by the number of flares before conception. Table 2 depicts the types of flares and the respective predictors. The same features of previous manifestations were the best predictors of further manifestations: dermatological flares by previous skin rash, renal flares by previous nephritis, and haematological flares by previous haematological abnormalities [43].

Thrombocytopenia in SLE during pregnancy indicates higher disease activity, severe organ damage, early onset preeclampsia, and higher pregnancy loss. Central nervous system (CNS) lupus in pregnancy represents an especially severe manifestation of SLE and may involve great maternal and fetal risks [44]. Compared with nonpregnant active female SLE patients, active pregnant-related lupus, including new-onset lupus and flare lupus, had a higher incidence of renal and hematological involvement but less mucocutaneous and musculoskeletal involvement [44].

*3.1. Lupus Nephritis (LN).* The presence of renal disease (of any cause) is a significant risk factor for obstetric complications [41, 45–47], and even small reductions in the glomerular filtration rate (GFR) may increase the chance of pregnant women to develop PE [48]. LN is among the findings that most often induces increased morbidity and mortality during pregnancy. Patients with LN more frequently use high doses of corticosteroids and immunosuppressive agents have a higher frequency of severe infections and hospital admission and also have an increased mortality rate [49]. Active LN shows positive association with premature delivery, increased frequency of hypertension, and of PE [50].

To distinguish clinical indicators of LN activity from pregnancy physiological manifestations and those related to PE can be a challenge. In the first trimester of pregnancy, maternal systemic circulation suffers remarkable physiological vasodilation and relaxin, a hormone produced by the corpus luteum, is a major contributor. One of the results of these changes is a physiological elevation of the GFR and consequent serum creatinine reduction, so values of 0.9 mg/dL may suggest an underlying renal disease requiring further investigation. Protein excretion in the urine is also increased and rates equal to or above 300 mg/24 hours are considered pathological [51, 52]. Therefore, during pregnancy patients with LN may have isolated elevation of proteinuria that is not necessarily indicative of active nephritis.

The patients with LN have 2-3 times higher chance of flare when compared to patients without LN, both systemic and renal disease activity [53]. On the other hand, the use of azathioprine during pregnancy by patients with LN was associated with a lower frequency of flare [54].

Varying results have been reported on pregnancy outcomes in SLE women with preexisting LN. The rate of successful pregnancies ranged between 65% and 92% and the incidence of flares ranged between 8% and 30% [41, 42, 48, 55–57]. A systematic review and meta-analysis of pregnancy outcomes showed a significant association between active LN

Table 1: Hormonal and immune response differences between normal pregnancies.

| Immune and hormonal response | Normal pregnancy | Lupus and pregnancy | Clinical manifestation associated |
|---|---|---|---|
| Th17: IL-17 | High | Higher increase | Preeclampsia and pregnancy loss |
| Estradiol and progesterone | Higher in second and third trimester | Lower in second and third trimester | Impaired placental function and fetal loss |
| IL-6 | Low at first trimester but high in the third trimester | Low in the three trimesters | Altered immune regulation from T cell to B cell |
| IL-10 | Low in the trimester but high in the last trimester | High since preconception throughout pregnancy and still postpartum | Continuous B cell stimulation |
| Treg cells | High | Low number and impaired function | Lupus activity |
| Chemokines<br>CXCL8/IL-8<br>CXCL9/MIG<br>CXCL10/IP-10 | Low | Higher serum concentrations | Increase pregnancy complications and lupus flares |
| Ficolin-3 | Low | Increase | Haemolysis |
| IFN-$\alpha$ | Low | Higher concentration | Contribution to preeclampsia |
| C4d | Low | Higher concentration | Low placenta weight and low birth weight |
| Prolactin | Low | Higher concentration | Lupus activity |

IL: interleukin; Treg cells: T regulatory cells; CXCL: chemokine ligand; MIG: monokine induced by gamma interferon; IP-10: interferon gamma-induced protein 10; INF-$\alpha$: interferon alpha; C4d: complement component.

Table 2: Type of SLE flare during pregnancy, manifestations, risk factor, and conduction.

| Type of SLE flare during pregnancy | Manifestations | Risk factor | Management |
|---|---|---|---|
| Mucocutaneous | High inflammatory rash often sparing the nasolabial folds | Anti-Ro/SSA, previous involvement | Topical corticosteroids or oral prednisone, HCQ |
| Articular | Arthralgia, arthritis, carpal tunnel syndrome (related to pregnancy edema) | Anti-dsDNA positivity | HCQ, NSAID until 28th week, prednisone throughout |
| Hematological | Cytopenias | aPL, Coombs, previous involvement | Leukopenia: discard drug-related;<br>hemolytic anemia: high dose prednisone and azathioprine;<br>thrombocytopenia: high dose prednisone and azathioprine may use IVIG and rituximab |
| Renal | Hypertension, edema, proteinuria | aDNA, low C3 and C4 differentiate between APS microangiopathy and preeclampsia, previous involvement | Immunosuppressive treatment with corticosteroids;<br>pulse-methyl prednisolone |
| CNS | Wide range including depression and psychosis | CNS manifestation provided pregnancy | Antidepressants; pulse-methyl prednisolone |
| Vascular | Cutaneous vasculitis | Previous involvement | Prednisone and azathioprine |

aPL: antiphospholipid antibodies; APS: antiphospholipid syndrome; CNS: central nervous system; HCQ: hydroxychloroquine; IVIG: intravenous immunoglobulin.

and both the onset of maternal hypertension during pregnancy and the rate of premature birth [50].

PE, which is more common in women with SLE, detected in up to 20% versus 7.6% in healthy pregnant controls. This obstetric complication have clinical and laboratory manifestations that can be fully superimposable to the active LN, which is in turn a risk factor for the development of PE [50, 51, 58]. Furthermore, patients with LN tend to develop PE earlier compared with women with SLE without nephritis [48].

Table 3: Features differentiating preeclampsia and lupus nephritis.

| Clinical and laboratory features | Preeclampsia | Lupus nephritis |
|---|---|---|
| Hypertension | After 20 weeks of gestation | Any time during pregnancy |
| Platelets | Low-normal | Low-normal |
| Complements | Normal-low | Rising titres |
| Anti-dsDNA | Absent or unchanged | Normal to raised |
| Creatinine | Normal to raised | Normal to raised |
| Serum uric acid | Elevated | Normal |
| 24-hour urine calcium | <195 mg/dL | >195 mg/dL |
| Urinary sediment | Inactive | Active |
| Other organs involved | Occasionally CNS or HELLP | Evidence of active nonrenal SLE |
| Response to steroids | No | Yes |

One of the most complex and challenging aspects during a pregnancy of a woman with lupus is the precise characterization of the LN activity and the differentiation of PE. In both complications hypertension, proteinuria and edema are present. The differential diagnosis is essential, as the treatment varies significantly: in PE, delivery should be considered, while immunosuppressive drugs should be administered to patients with SLE nephritis. LN is likely to be associated with positive anti-dsDNA antibodies (especially in high titers), serum complement consumption, and dysmorphic hematuria and/or red blood cell cylinders. In this scenario, the probable diagnosis is a proliferative kidney disease [59]. During clinical evaluation, the onset of fever, presence of discoid or subacute cutaneous lupus lesions, vasculitis, oral ulcers, polyserositis, lymphadenomegaly, positive direct Coombs, myocarditis, and pneumonitis also indicate lupus flare. In contrast, if the gestational age is greater than 22 weeks, with no signs of SLE activity and hyperuricemia is present, we can state the diagnosis of PE with relative precision. Some features, if present, may help to distinguish between the two conditions (Table 3). However, in many circumstances the patients' manifestations are not complete.

Renal biopsy is a valuable research tool for accurate characterization of LN, but it is usually avoided during pregnancy considering technical difficulties of this procedure in pregnant women. Either way, a recent study found that renal biopsy provides useful information for the management of patients with LN during pregnancy [60].

Complementary elements, such as some angiogenic (VEGF and placental growth factor (PlGF)) and antiangiogenic cytokines (sFlt-1 and soluble endoglin), may help to differentiate between LN and PE [61]. Recent papers have shown that patients with nonpregnant LN, regardless of flares, have increased values of angiogenic cytokines compared to women without SLE, [62] while levels of the antiangiogenic cytokine sFlt-1 is higher in women with active LN compared to patients without flares [63]. Patients with PE have progressive reduction of the amounts of angiogenic cytokines, the opposite expression identified in patients with SLE and LN, and also rising antiangiogenic titers. These results are preliminary and more research is needed before we can employ these citokines to differentiate between these two conditions in routine clinical practice.

## 4. Maternal Outcome

*4.1. Organ Involvement and Pregnancy.* Patients with a high degree of irreversible organ damage are more likely to suffer complications or worsening of previous damage during and after pregnancy [64]. LN is a major manifestation of SLE and, therefore, it is common to have a pregnancy in SLE women with a biopsy-proven diagnosis of renal disease. SLE patients with active LN are at higher risk for pregnancy complications than those without and should be advised against pregnancy until they have renal remission of at least 6 months, and if possible, 12–18 months, according to recommendations [55]. Women with quiescent disease (proteinuria <500 mg/day and inactive urinary sediment) and unaffected renal function are at reasonably low risk during pregnancy but should be closely monitored.

In normal pregnancy, the glomerular filtration rate increases by 30–50% and creatinine clearance rises to <100 mL/min, causing a decrease in serum creatinine. Tubular reabsorption of protein is decreased during pregnancy, and this is why an increase in the normal proteinuria level to 150–180 mg/24 h is possible. However, new-onset proteinuria >300 mg/24 h may be considered pathological in pregnant patients without proteinuria at baseline. Varying results have been reported on pregnancy outcomes in SLE women with preexisting LN. The rate of successful pregnancies ranged between 65% and 92%, and the incidence of flares ranged between 8% and 30% [7, 41, 42, 48, 55–57].

A systematic review and meta-analysis of pregnancy outcomes showed a significant association between active LN and both the onset of maternal hypertension during pregnancy and the rate of premature birth. A history of LN was also associated with preeclampsia. It should be noted that during pregnancy renal flare may determine further loss of kidney function in the short and the long term, with potential accelerated progression to end stage renal disease [50].

Apart from renal involvement, other organs may be negatively influenced by pregnancy. Patients with restrictive pulmonary disease may worsen during pregnancy due to thoracic compression by the growing uterus. Likewise, women with cardiac disease may be at risk of heart failure due to volume overload caused by the normal increase in circulating volume [65, 66]. Contraindications to pregnancy are shown in the following part.

Contraindications to pregnancy in SLE patients are as follows: severe pulmonary hypertension (estimated systolic PSAP > 50 mmHg or symptomatic); advanced heart failure; severe restrictive lung disease; moderate/severe chronic renal failure (creatinine > 2,8 mg/dL); current use of cyclophosphamide, mycophenolate mofetil, methotrexate, leflunomide, statins and angiotensin converting enzyme inhibitor; active renal (24 h urinary protein > 0.5 g) or CNS disease in the past 6 months; recent major thrombosis (<2 years).

Cardiovascular disease (CVD) is a leading cause of morbidity and mortality in SLE. Whether pregnancy acts as a vascular stress test that unmasks endothelial vulnerability to injury that manifests as PE or whether PE itself causes damage that is responsible for future CVD is not clear. A recent preliminary study found that SLE patients with a history of PE had an almost fourfold increase in the rate of subclinical CVD, although there was no association with the presence of plaque [67].

*4.2. Morbidity and Mortality.* A recent US study of pregnancy-related admissions, using information derived from discharge codes, found that women with SLE may be at increased risk of serious medical complications and mortality in comparison with non-SLE pregnant women [58]. At conception, SLE patients had more comorbidities than healthy women. Specifically, SLE patients had more pregestational diabetes, arterial hypertension, pulmonary hypertension, renal failure, and thrombophilia [58]. Moreover, SLE patients tended to become pregnant at an older age compared with the general population. Even after adjustment for increased age, the risk of maternal complications in women with SLE remained higher than in healthy pregnant women. There was an estimated 2–4-fold increase in the rate of caesarean section, PE, and eclampsia, especially in women with preexisting hypertension and/or renal insufficiency taking high-dose prednisone. The risk of sepsis and pneumonia was greatly increased, due to both disease-related immune dysregulation and immunosuppressive therapy. The risk of sepsis and pneumonia was greatly increased, due to both disease-related immune dysregulation and immunosuppressive therapy [58]. Hematological complications requiring transfusion, such as postpartum haemorrhage, antepartum bleeding, anaemia at delivery, and thrombocytopenia were more common in SLE patients [68].

The risk for both venous thromboembolism and stroke was 6.5- fold higher than that of healthy pregnant women, and the excess maternal mortality rate was estimated at 20 times higher than in the general population. These data, collected using the discharge diagnosis, may be not comparable with those derived from tertiary referral centres in which careful multidisciplinary management of pregnant women with SLE allows better maternal and fetal outcomes. However, the data underline the potential risk of increased maternal morbidity and mortality and suggest the need for a high level of vigilance during SLE pregnancies [69]. Several clinical and biochemical factors have been associated with adverse maternal and fetal outcomes in patients with SLE as shown in the following part.

*Clinical, Serological, and Biochemical Factors Associated with Adverse Maternal and Fetal Outcomes in SLE*

Clinical factors are as follows: active disease within 6 months prior to conception and during pregnancy, SLE onset during pregnancy, active lupus nephritis or chronic kidney disease (creatinine > 2.8 mg/dL), maternal hypertension, previous fetal loss.

Serological factors are as follows: antiphospholipid antibodies, anti-double-stranded DNA antibodies.

Biochemical factors are as follows: low complement levels, proteinuria, thrombocytopenia.

Catastrophic antiphospholipid syndrome (CAPS) is a rare complication that occurs in less than 1% of patients with APS but is a life-threatening variant of that thrombophilia. The analysis of 409 catastrophic events included in the CAPS Registry showed that nineteen (4.6%) of were presented during pregnancy or puerperium and nine (47%) of those patients also had SLE [70].

## 5. Pregnancy and Neonatal Outcome

*5.1. Pregnancy Outcome.* Despite major improvement in the last decades, the risk of obstetric and neonatal complications in SLE pregnancy is greater than in general population. It has been estimated that women with SLE have fewer live births compared with the general population, in particular those with high disease activity [17]. Maternal lupus activity and the presence of concomitant antiphospholipid syndrome (APS) were found to be associated with major obstetrical complications [7, 17], being estimated that about 20% of pregnancies in women with SLE end with a fetal wastage [10].

The risk of PE, IUGR, fetal loss, and preterm delivery is greater in patients with SLE compared to general population, especially in those with active nephritis [71]. In a systematic review of 2751 pregnancies in 1842 patients with SLE, reactivation of the disease was identified in 25.6% of cases, hypertension in 16.3%, nephritis in 16.1%, PE in 7.6%, eclampsia in 0.8%, and prematurity in 39.4% of births. There was a positive association between preterm birth and active nephritis and between hypertension and active nephritis or nephritis history [50]. The PROMISSE study, a multicenter study of large-scale, reported that 15% of SLE patients without severe disease developed PE, rising to 22% if there were also positive aPL [68].

The EUROAPS registry reported on the obstetrical results of 247 women recently. Recurrent first trimester miscarriage followed by fetal loss was the most common obstetric morbidities in this mostly Caucasian cohort. Several types of obstetric complications appeared in 52% of the cases; most did not lead to fetal death. Prematurity was the most common finding (47%), followed by stillbirth and fetal loss (22.5%), miscarriage (16%), fetal growth restriction (14%), and early

(13%) and late onset PE (12%). All laboratory categories of aPL distributions are represented in the registry. The presence of lupus anticoagulant (LAC), isolated or in combination with anticardiolipin (aCL) and/or anti-beta2-glycoprotein I (anti-$\beta$2GPI), was the strongest marker related to poor obstetric outcomes. Low complement levels were found in almost 50% of the complicated cases, showing classic complement pathway activation. Maternal and fetal outcomes were good when the currently accepted treatment was given; however, no effort should be spared to improve these recommendations. Thrombosis and progression to SLE in mothers with obstetric APS were uncommon compared with "classical APS." Showing that differences between classical APS and obstetric APS may exist, the authors conclude that more studies have to be done to understand the laboratory subsets and obstetric outcome [72]. With the use of the Global APS Score (GAPSS) it was demonstrated that, in the SLE population, the presence of LAC is the strongest risk factor for thrombosis. In addition to that, the higher the number of positive tests (single versus double or triple positivity), the stronger the association with thrombosis [73].

The review of 76 pregnancies in 63 lupus patients at the Hospital Universitário Pedro Ernesto-UERJ found similar results. Fifteen percent of patients developed PE, 30% hypertension, and 27% of fetuses had chronic fetal distress and 14 patients needed to increase the dosage of corticosteroids during pregnancy. The birth occurred in a mean gestational age of 35 weeks and fetal death was more frequent in patients with nephritis when compared to patients without nephritis (37% versus 12.2%) [47]. Similarly, Clowse et al. reported that, regardless of clinical activity, both low complement and presence of anti-DNA in the second trimester were associated with higher rate of fetal loss and preterm delivery. When combined with clinical activity, the presence of these parameters was more strongly predictive of fetal loss and prematurity [42].

In a cohort of 96 patients, Borella et al. evaluated prospectively 132 pregnancies and reported 12% of PE, 8% of premature rupture of membranes, and 12% of preterm premature rupture of membranes. Twenty-two percent of live births were preterm, while 17% of the patients suffered pregnancy loss. Fetal loss was best predicted by hypertension at conception, while preterm birth was associated with coexistence of APS and the title of anti-ds DNA before pregnancy. Interestingly, the presence of APS was not associated with pregnancy loss, the fact that could be explained by the use of low dose aspirin and heparin in patients with APS and/or positive aPL [43].

As it can be noted, there is a high incidence of preterm delivery. It can be spontaneous, usually related to premature rupture of membranes, or iatrogenic as an option to protect the health of the mother and/or the fetus, like in cases of PE or fetal distress [74]. Other risk factors for preterm delivery include disease activity prior to and during pregnancy (including serological activity, i.e., high title anti-DNA antibodies, low serum complement levels) [42], higher prednisone dose, and hypertension [7]. Neonatal death, long-term medical complications, and cognitive impairment are more frequent in babies born before 28-week gestation [75], so voluntary interruption of pregnancy before this point should be carefully discussed between physicians and the family. Regarding the birth of babies with low weight (<2500 g) or small for gestational age (birth weight less than the 10th percentile for gestational age), these conditions are more common in SLE pregnancies, ranging from 6 to 35% [76]. This finding is not surprising because placental insufficiency, which is frequent in lupus pregnancies [77], leads to IUGR and to the birth of small for gestational age infants.

*5.2. Neonatal Lupus Syndromes.* Neonatal lupus syndromes refer to a clinical spectrum of cutaneous, cardiac, and systemic abnormalities observed in newborn infants whose mothers have Ro/SSA and La/SSB autoantibodies. The condition is rare, usually benign and self-limited, but may sometimes have serious consequences. It is due to passive transfer of anti-Ro/SSA and/or anti-La/SSB antibodies in some babies of mothers with autoimmune disease [78].

These autoantibodies may damage the developing tissue and increase the risk of bearing infants with neonatal lupus erythematosus (NLE). Approximately 98% of affected infants have maternal transfer of autoantibodies against Ro/SSA, La/SSB, and, less commonly, U1-RNP. However, only 1-2% of mothers with these autoantibodies have neonates with NLE, regardless of whether the mothers are symptomatic or not [79].

The diagnosis is usually made based on the clinical features and the demonstration of neonatal lupus-associated antibodies in the serum of the mother or affected infant. The most common clinical manifestations of NLE are, in decreasing order of frequency, dermatologic, cardiac, and hepatic abnormalities. Some infants may also have hematologic, neurologic, or splenic abnormalities. The most serious complication in the neonate is complete heart block (CHB), which occurs in approximately 2% of such pregnancies. CHB can be devastating for these babies: over 60% require a pacemaker (and recurrent changes as the child grows), 10% will develop cardiomyopathy late after birth despite pacemaker placement, and the 10-year mortality rate is 20–35% [79].

*5.3. Pregnancy in Mothers with Anti-Ro Antibodies.* The high risk of CHB is the most important issue related to the presence of anti-Ro antibodies during pregnancy. CHB normally develops between 18 and 24 weeks of gestation and is usually preceded by lesser degrees of conduction delays, which may be reversed with early treatment [80]. However, conduction abnormalities may progress very rapidly and CHB is often the first rhythm abnormality detected. Various tools have been developed for the early detection of lesser degrees of heart block, including fetal Doppler echocardiography, fetal kinetocardiogram, and transabdominal fetal electrocardiogram [81, 82], although fetal Doppler echocardiography remains the most commonly used modality. All fetuses exposed should be monitored weekly between 16 and 26 weeks of gestation and biweekly thereafter [83]. Detection of an early conduction defect such as a prolonged PR interval should be considered a danger signal.

Although some early blocks are transient, progression to CHB remains unpredictable. Prophylactic treatment should be discussed if the PR interval remains persistently prolonged. Maternal administration of fluorinated corticosteroids has shown benefits on fetal survival in some studies. However, the results are not consistent and the benefits must be weighed against the higher risk of IUGR and preterm birth [81]. Treatment of established CHB remains even more unsatisfactory. Improved fetal outcomes were reported after transplacental treatment with dexamethasone and beta-adrenergic stimulants in one study, but these findings were not replicated [84]. Hydroxychloroquine during pregnancy, on the other hand, reduces the risk of cardiac NLS in at-risk fetuses [85, 86].

The risk of recurrence of CHB in subsequent pregnancies after an affected pregnancy is much greater, but hydroxychloroquine reduced this risk by 65% in one study [85]. Open label data also showed beneficial effects for intravenous immunoglobulin (IVIG), but two large randomized controlled trials showed negative results [87, 88]. The study design, the dose of IVIG used, and the differing composition of IVIG may have contributed to the negative outcomes [89]. In summary, there is no satisfactory current treatment for established CHB [90].

There is consensus on the prognostic factors of poor outcomes associated with neonatal CHB: detection of CHB at gestational age < 20 weeks, ventricular rate < 50 bpm, fetal hydrops, changes in the fetal echocardiogram, carditis, impaired left ventricular function, endocardial fibroelastosis, and a maternal diagnosis of SLE or Sjögren's syndrome [91, 92].

## 6. Prenatal Care

Ideally, all patients with SLE that desire to get pregnant should have a preconception visit, when the physician evaluates the risks associated to the pregnancy, medications that are contraindicated during pregnancy and if the patient is in the best moment to get pregnant according to underlying disease activity and complications (Figure 2). Planned pregnancies have demonstrated reduced flare rates and better obstetric outcomes in women with SLE [1].

After conception, antenatal management of pregnant patients with SLE requires close collaboration between rheumatologist and obstetrician [1]. The woman with SLE who gets pregnant should be submitted to clinical and laboratory evaluations during the first visit, in order to identify SLE disease activity and situations that increase risk of fetal complications. Recommended visits, laboratory tests, and ultrasound evaluations are listed on the following part.

*Visits, Laboratory Tests, and Ultrasound Evaluation Recommended during Prenatal Care of Patients with Lupus*

*Visits*

(i) Obstetrician visits are as follows:

(a) monthly until 20 weeks,
(b) every two weeks until 28 weeks,
(c) weekly after 28 weeks until delivery.

(ii) Rheumatologist visits are as follows:

(a) ideally, a rheumatologist should support the obstetrician during prenatal care;
(b) if not possible, the rheumatologist should see the patient every 4–6 weeks.

*Laboratory Tests*

(i) First visit tests are as follows:

(a) complete blood count, platelet count, prothrombin activation time, and partial thromboplastin time;
(b) lupus anticoagulant; anticardiolipin antibody IgG and IgM; and anti-$\beta 2$ glycoprotein I IgG and IgM (which must be repeated in 12 weeks if positive);
(c) anti-Ro/SS-A, anti-La/SS- B, anti-Sm, and anti-RNP;
(d) blood glucose, BUN, creatinine, uric acid, AST, and ALT;
(e) anti-DNA, C3, C4, and CH50;
(f) urinary sediment; 24-hour proteinuria or protein/creatinine ratio in a single urine sample; dysmorphic research erythrocyte in urine, creatinine clearance and urine culture.

(ii) Quarterly visit tests are as follows:

(a) complete blood count, platelet count;
(b) anti-DNA, C3, C4, and CH50;
(c) blood glucose, BUN, creatinine, uric acid, AST, and ALT;
(d) 24-hour proteinuria or protein/creatinine ratio in a single urine sample if preeclampsia or lupus nephritis is suspected, as well as research erythrocyte dysmorphism.

*Ultrasound and Doppler Velocimetry Studies.* They include the following:

(i) monthly after 24 weeks: evaluation of fetal growth, amniotic fluid, and umbilical artery (fetal-placental flow),
(ii) uterine artery evaluation at 24 weeks: screening tests for preeclampsia and intrauterine growth restriction.

Intervals of the visits and frequency of laboratory tests may be smaller in case of disease activity or suspected PE.

Laboratory tests should be interpreted in the light of the knowledge of the changes imposed by pregnancy itself. Despite being used as a marker of inflammatory disease

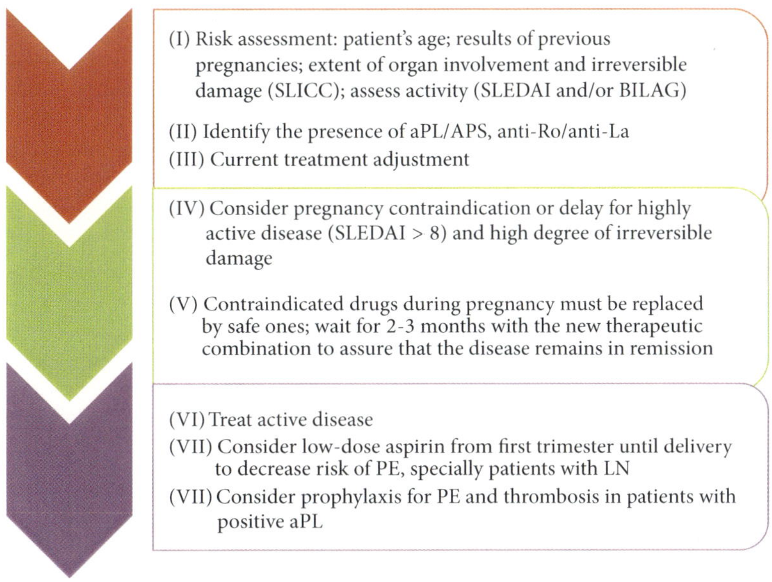


FIGURE 2: Counselling and pregnancy planning for patients with lupus.

activity, erythrocyte sedimentation rate (ESR) rises by pregnancy itself, so it should not be used in pregnant women with SLE. Serum complement levels tend to increase during pregnancy and its fall should be assessed relative to a baseline test. Incidentally thrombocytopenia may occur in about 10% of pregnant women and it becomes difficult to distinguish from lupus activity. The urinary excretion of proteins, which normally rises during pregnancy, can reach about 300 mg/24 hours without having clinical significance [1]. Also, pregnant women generally tend to have urinary tract infections, and the use of immunosuppressants agents may inhibit cellular deviation and leukocytosis.

Renal function should be assessed even in patients without nephritis history as it can be asymptomatic or start during pregnancy, as well as the need for a baseline for comparison in the case of kidney injury during the course of pregnancy. Hepatic involvement is uncommon in patients with SLE, but the evaluation of their role is required especially in patients taking azathioprine because of its hepatotoxicity, with repeat tests at least every 3 months.

Regarding the mentioned antibodies, aPL (LAC, aCL, and anti-$\beta$2GPI) is markers of adverse pregnancy outcomes and may be helpful in the case of a thrombotic event during pregnancy. It should be remembered that the presence of aPL in lupus patients without obstetric (recurrent spontaneous abortion, fetal loss) or thrombotic events (deep vein thrombosis, arterial thrombosis) does not provide the diagnosis of APS or even justifies the prescription of heparin to these patients. Most of authors recommend the use of low dose aspirin during pregnancy for patients with SLE and positive aPL [93].

Lupus flares are likely to be associated with hypocomplementemia and increased titers of anti-DNA antibodies; in comparison, complement levels are usually (but not always) increased in patients with preeclampsia. The anti-Ro/SSA and anti-La/SSB are responsible for neonatal lupus and anti-Sm is the antibody specific for SLE. Patients with positive anti-Ro/SSA or anti-La/SSB should perform fetal echocardiography weekly from 16 to 26 weeks and biweekly thereafter [1]. ANA, anti-Ro/SS-A, anti-La/SS-B, anti-Sm, and anti-RNP do not change with disease activity and therefore do not need to be repeated later.

Current standard of care in SLE pregnancy includes Doppler studies of uterine arteries and umbilical artery, which are helpful to assess placental function and to exclude the occurrence of complications such as PE and fetal distress [40]. Uterine Doppler studies are useful as screening test for PE and the 24th week is the best moment for the evaluation. Abnormal uterine artery Doppler studies have been identified in patients with SLE with posterior fetal loss, PE, IUGR, and preterm labor [94, 95].

Umbilical Doppler ultrasound gives a more accurate definition of the placental function, showing various degrees of impairment such as increased resistance, absent or even reverse diastolic flow, which is a clear sign of placental insufficiency and fetal distress [41, 96]. Follow-up with monthly ultrasound and Doppler velocimetry studies starting at 24 weeks to assess fetal growth, amniotic fluid, and fetal-placental flow is recommended considering the high incidence of fetal growth restriction and chronic distress [96]. Alterations of umbilical artery Doppler velocimetry should be managed similarly to those patients without SLE. Normal evaluation of these tests has a high negative predictive value for fetal death. It is important to notice that these previously cited fetal complications may be related to the presence of aPL.

## 7. Treatment

As already discussed, SLE can reactivate during pregnancy, situation that requires proper handling of antirheumatic drugs. The use of hydroxychloroquine during pregnancy is accepted and recommended by members of the American College of Rheumatology and the European League against Rheumatism (EULAR) [97, 98]. Hydroxychloroquine use during pregnancy in patients with SLE reduces the number of flares and hypertensive disorders [99], so its use should be continued during pregnancy or prescribed for those that are not using. Its use during pregnancy is safe, without reported malformations, growth restriction and ocular, auditory, or neurological toxicity in exposed fetus [2, 40]. Chloroquine has smaller data when compared to hydroxychloroquine, but no long-term sequel was also demonstrated [100]. In addition, a systematic review did not report any ocular abnormality in children born from mothers treated with chloroquine or hydroxychloroquine during gestation [101]. Both are secreted in breast-milk, but there was no report of adverse effects in breastfed children whose mothers used hydroxychloroquine [100].

Corticosteroids represent the treatment of choice in cases of reactivation of SLE during pregnancy and can be used as prednisone or prednisolone. These compounds are inactivated by the enzyme 11-$\beta$-hydroxysteroid dehydrogenase 2 and reduce fetal exposure to approximately 10% of maternal dosage [102]. Therefore, the use of these drugs does not replace the use of betamethasone or dexamethasone when they are indicated for fetal lung maturation. The dose should be the minimum necessary and depends on the impaired organ, using the same criteria recommended for nonpregnant women, with great parsimony as possible in order to minimize adverse events. The use of doses above 10 mg/day of prednisone is associated with increased risk of developing arterial hypertension, dyslipidemia, fluid retention, and maternal hyperglycemia. Intravenous pulses of methylprednisolone can be used safely if indicated for severe activity [40]. Corticosteroids do not enter breast milk in large quantities and there is no contraindication to breastfeeding in women who are on corticosteroid therapy [103]. Women that are breastfeeding and using higher doses of corticosteroids should wait 4 hours after taking the pill to breast-feed, reducing the drug concentration in the breast-milk [100].

There is no evidence that the prophylactic use of corticosteroids in SLE pregnant women without active disease prevents exacerbations during pregnancy, so this conduct is considered inappropriate.

The nonsteroidal anti-inflammatory drugs can be administered to management arthralgia or serositis in the lowest dose possible for a short time and it is recommended to be completely discontinued after the 32th week. After this time, there is high risk of fetal and maternal hemorrhage in addition to fetal renal dysfunction, oligodramnia, and premature closure of arterial duct [100].

Azathioprine in doses up to 2.5 mg/kg/day remains one of the therapeutic resources available in cases of SLE activation during pregnancy, being the immunosuppressant of choice for the treatment of severe maternal disease or refractory to isolated use of corticosteroids. This immunosuppressant and steroid sparing agent is not associated with teratogenicity in humans, as the fetal liver is not capable of metabolizing azathioprine into its active form [100], although teratogenicity has been reported in animal studies [104]. The treatment with azathioprine is compatible with breastfeeding, with no risks for the child [100].

Cyclophosphamide, mycophenolate mofetil, leflunomide, and methotrexate have teratogenic effects and should not be used during pregnancy [104]. Mycophenolate mofetil should be stopped at least 6 months prior to conception and changed to azathioprine, with a small risk of flare during this period [54]. Table 4 summarizes recommendations for the use of medications during pregnancy and lactation of patients with SLE.

## 8. Contraception and Assisted Reproduction

Pregnancy outcomes are optimized when pregnancy is planned in patients with SLE and APS. Contraception in SLE/APS patients goes beyond the simple need to avoid unwanted pregnancies. Several conditions may require effective contraception: early stage of the disease, very active disease, severe organ involvement or damage, and the use of embryotoxic/foetotoxic drugs. Therefore, contraceptive counselling is essential in clinical rheumatology, although many women still do not receive adequate information in clinical practice [105].

Effective contraception is underused in patients with rheumatic diseases. In a study of 97 SLE patients at risk of pregnancy, 55% had unprotected sex occasionally and 23% "most of the time" [106]. In another study of 86 patients, 55% of those using contraceptives regularly were using less-effective barrier methods only, even when being on teratogenic medications [105].

A common misconception among women with SLE is that they "cannot use birth control," since the "classical" estrogen-containing pill is generally contraindicated. The message should be that women with SLE should be considered good candidates for many contraceptive methods, including hormonal contraceptives, and the most suitable choice should be made individually [107].

The three main types of contraceptives are barrier methods, intrauterine devices (IUD), and hormonal methods. Barrier methods are an effective, cheap method of preventing pregnancy, and sexually transmitted disease. However the unintended pregnancy rate remains at around 17% for condoms and diaphragms. IUD are available in nonmedicated or medicated (progesterone) forms. With typical use, the rate of unplanned pregnancy is around 2%. Complications include irregular bleeding after placement, the risk of expulsion (5% falling out over the 5-year life of the device), and the risk of infection after insertion that may lead to pelvic inflammatory disease (PID). Current IUD devices are actually safer in high-risk groups [108], but the risk of infections should be continuously monitored. It may be preferable to use IUD in patients with a single sexual partner and mild treatment (no immunosuppressive drugs, prednisone < 10 mg per day). The use of estrogen-containing oral contraceptives (OC) has been discouraged due to initial reports of lupus flares due to hormonal treatment and subsequently supported by growing experimental evidence of the role of estrogens in the pathogenesis of SLE [109]. However, two recent randomized clinical trials [110, 111] supported the safety of low dose combined

TABLE 4: Recommendations for the use of medications for pregnancy planning.

| Medication | Recommendation for pregnancy planning | Indication during pregnancy | FDA 1979 class | Comment for using during pregnancy | Maternal adverse reactions | Fetal/neonatal adverse reactions | Lactation |
|---|---|---|---|---|---|---|---|
| Aspirin (low dose) | Start before conception | Obstetric APS | B/C | 80–100 mg/d used isolated or in combination with LMWH | Bleeding | No | Allowed |
| Azathioprine | Without stopping | Used in cases requiring immunosuppression and to save corticoid | D* | 1–2,5 mg/Kg/d | Liver toxicity and bone marrow toxicity | No | Allowed |
| Belimumab | Not start during pregnancy Not stop during pregnancy | Arthritis, other inflammatory | C | 10 mg/kg IV q2 weeks ×3 doses, Maintenance: 10 mg/kg IV q4 weeks | Reactivation of tuberculosis | No | Not allowed |
| Cyclosporine A | | | C | Blood pressure monitor | Increase of blood pressure | Low birth weight | Not allowed |
| Cyclophosphamide | Stop > 6 months before conception | Not allowed | X | | | | Not allowed |
| Fluorinated corticosteroids | It will be used in more advanced pregnancy | NLE and maturity of fetal lungs | B | Use betamethasone 12 mg/d for two days | Uncontrolled glycemic | No | Allowed |
| Hydroxychloroquine | Keep the drug to prevent reactivation of lupus | Lupus, arthritis | N | 200–400 mg/d | Maternal skin hyperpigmentation | No | Allowed |
| Leflunomide | Stop 3–6 months before conception | Not allowed | X | | | | Not allowed |
| Low-molecular weight heparin | Generally used | Obstetric APS | C | Used in prophylactic dose of 0.5 mg/Kg QID for OBAPS and in full dose 1 mg/Kg BID for thrombotic APS | Osteoporosis, thrombocytopenia | No | Allowed |
| NSAID | Avoid since it may decrease | Arthritis, other inflammatory | C/D | Avoid in the 3rd trimester | Gastric bleeding | Premature closure of the ductus arteriosus, oligohydramnios | Allowed |
| Methotrexate | Stop 3–6 months before conception | Not allowed | X | | | | Not allowed |
| Mycophenolate mofetil | Stop before conception | Not allowed | X | | | | Not allowed |
| Prednisone/prednisolone | Try to minimize dose due to maternal AEs | Lupus, arthritis, other inflammatory diseases | C | Inactivated in the placenta, minimize dose due to maternal AEs | Increase of blood pressure, osteopenia, gestational diabetes, immunosuppression, grooves. | Cleft lip sporadically Low birth weight Premature birth | Allowed (if more than 40 mg, wait for 3 hours) |
| Rituximab | Not start during pregnancy Not stop during pregnancy | Arthritis, other inflammatory | C | 375 $mg/m^2$/IV q4 weeks | Reactivation of tuberculosis | No | Not allowed |

Table 4: Continued.

| Medication | Recommendation for pregnancy planning | Indication during pregnancy | FDA 1979 class | Comment for using during pregnancy | Maternal adverse reactions | Fetal/neonatal adverse reactions | Lactation |
|---|---|---|---|---|---|---|---|
| Statins | Stop before conception | Not allowed | X | | | | Not Allowed |
| ACEi | Stop before conception | Not allowed | D | | | Fetal death, renal dysfunction and oligohydramnios | Allowed |
| Tacrolimus | | Used in cases requiring immunosuppression | C | 0,1–0,2 mg/kg/d | Diabetes, increase of blood pressure, reactivation of tuberculosis | Increase of blood pressure, diarrhea, headache, renal dysfunction | Not allowed |
| Warfarin | Stop at conception | Not allowed | X | | | | Allowed |

AEs: adverse events; APS: antiphospholipid syndrome; OBAPS: obstetric APS; ACEi: angiotensin converting enzyme inhibitor.

OC in a well-defined population of stable SLE patients with inactive or stable active disease with respect to the risk of lupus flares. However, the presence of aPL remains a major contraindication to combined OC due to the increased risk of thrombosis. Progestin-only preparations (daily oral pill, depot medroxyprogesterone, and subcutaneous implants) do not appear to increase immune activity and are not associated with increased rates of flares, and the dose of progestin does not increase the risk of thrombosis; a recent large study in SLE patients showed good gynaecological tolerability (low rate of discontinuation due to breakthrough bleeding or hypoestrogenia) [112]. A major concern about the use of progesterone is its effects on bone health; however, the reduction in bone mineral density has been shown to be reversible after discontinuation of treatment [113].

Women affected by SLE have an overall fertility rate similar to that of the normal obstetric population, with a mean of two live births [114]. However, there are some conditions in which fertility may be impaired [115], like presence of chronic renal failure [116] and use of cyclophosphamide. The risk of infertility is related to the cumulative dose of the drug and the patient's age, with older women having a lower ovarian reserve at higher risk for premature ovarian failure. Protection of ovarian function can be provided by treatment with gonadotropin-releasing hormone analogues [117]. Women should be informed that NSAIDs may inhibit ovulation and that these should be stopped at day 8 of the menstrual cycle when they want to conceive [118].

Whatever the cause of infertility, whether being disease-related or not, patients with SLE may need medically assisted reproductive techniques (ARTs). The technique most-frequently used is in vitro fertilization and embryo transfer (IVF-ET), which requires ovarian stimulation for oocyte pick-up. Ovarian stimulation may create concern in SLE/APS women for several reasons, both theoretical and due to results from small studies [119]: (1) high dose estrogens may induce a disease flare; (2) the enhanced hormonal milieu may increase the risk of thrombosis, especially in women with aPL; (3) these complications may become life threatening in the case of ovarian hyperstimulation syndrome; (4) there may be a trend towards a worse prognosis for both pregnancy rates and live-birth rates after ARTs. Antithrombotic prophylaxis should be carried out in women with aPL, with particular attention paid to women with a prior thrombosis [120].

ARTs may be considered for patients with SLE and APS as these procedures do not appear to increase the risk of disease flares or thrombosis. In addition, the presence of aPL does not independently predict the outcome of IVF pregnancies. As with natural pregnancies, it is recommended that candidates for ART should have quiescent disease for at least six months prior to attempting to become pregnant, to ensure the best possible outcome for mother and child [121].

Recent studies consistently state that screening ART candidates for autoantibodies and treating for positive findings is not justified [122–125]. The US Practice Committee of the American Society for Reproductive Medicine has published guidelines to this effect [126]. Blindly testing for and identifying these autoantibodies in otherwise asymptomatic women may cause undue anxiety given the prognostic uncertainty of the findings.

## 9. Conclusions

SLE pregnancies are considered high risk condition and recent studies reinforce the importance of planning the pregnancy. As suggested by several authors, the association of SLE and pregnancy, mainly with active disease, especially nephritis, has poorer pregnancy outcomes, with increased frequency of PE, fetal loss, prematurity, growth restriction, and newborns small for gestational age. The differential diagnosis from PE and LN remains a challenge. Antenatal management of pregnant patients with SLE requires close monitoring and collaboration between rheumatologist and obstetrician. With better treatments and preservation of renal function, combined with current recommendations for planning pregnancy during the quiescent period, a better maternal and fetal prognosis can be expected in pregnancies of patients with SLE.

## Conflict of Interests

The authors declare that there is no conflict of interests regarding the publication of this paper.

## Acknowledgment

Guilherme Ramires de Jesus, Evandro Mendes Klumb, and Roger Abramino Levy have received support from Fundação Carlos Chagas Filho de Amparo à Pesquisa do Estado do Rio de Janeiro (FAPERJ).

## References


[1] A. Lateef and M. Petri, "Managing lupus patients during pregnancy," *Best Practice and Research: Clinical Rheumatology*, vol. 27, no. 3, pp. 435–447, 2013.

[2] M. E. B. Clowse, "Lupus activity in pregnancy," *Rheumatic Disease Clinics of North America*, vol. 33, no. 2, pp. 237–252, 2007.

[3] E. Peart and M. E. B. Clowse, "Systemic lupus erythematosus and pregnancy outcomes: an update and review of the literature," *Current Opinion in Rheumatology*, vol. 26, no. 2, pp. 118–123, 2014.

[4] C. A. Clark, K. A. Spitzer, and C. A. Laskin, "Decrease in pregnancy loss rates in patients with systemic lupus erythematosus over a 40-year period," *Journal of Rheumatology*, vol. 32, no. 9, pp. 1709–1712, 2005.

[5] É. Vinet, J. Labrecque, C. A. Pineau et al., "A population-based assessment of live births in women with systemic lupus erythematosus," *Annals of the Rheumatic Diseases*, vol. 71, no. 4, pp. 557–559, 2012.

[6] R. Andrade, M. L. Sanchez, G. S. Alarcón et al., "Adverse pregnancy outcomes in women with systemic lupus erythematosus from a multiethnic US cohort: LUMINA (LVI) [corrected]," *Clinical and Experimental Rheumatology*, vol. 26, no. 2, pp. 268–274, 2008.

[7] M. E. B. Clowse, L. S. Magder, F. Witter, and M. Petri, "The impact of increased lupus activity on obstetric outcomes," *Arthritis and Rheumatism*, vol. 52, no. 2, pp. 514–521, 2005.

[8] M. D. Lockshin, "Pregnancy does not cause systemic lupus erythematosus to worsen," *Arthritis & Rheumatism*, vol. 32, no. 6, pp. 665–670, 1989.

[9] G. Ruiz-Irastorza, F. Lima, J. Alves et al., "Increased rate of lupus flare during pregnancy and the puerperium: a prospective study of 78 pregnancies," *British Journal of Rheumatology*, vol. 35, no. 2, pp. 133–138, 1996.

[10] M. E. B. Clowse, L. S. Magder, F. Witter, and M. Petri, "Early risk factors for pregnancy loss in lupus," *Obstetrics and Gynecology*, vol. 107, no. 2, pp. 293–299, 2006.

[11] K.-L. Wong, F.-Y. Chan, and C.-P. Lee, "Outcome of pregnancy in patients with systemic lupus erythematosus. A prospective study," *Archives of Internal Medicine*, vol. 151, no. 2, pp. 269–273, 1991.

[12] A. W. Shand, C. S. Algert, L. March, and C. L. Roberts, "Second pregnancy outcomes for women with systemic lupus erythematosus," *Annals of the Rheumatic Diseases*, vol. 72, no. 4, pp. 547–551, 2013.

[13] K. T. Jørgensen, B. V. Pedersen, N. M. Nielsen, S. Jacobsen, and M. Frisch, "Childbirths and risk of female predominant and other autoimmune diseases in a population-based Danish cohort," *Journal of Autoimmunity*, vol. 38, no. 2-3, pp. J81–J87, 2012.

[14] M. Ostensen and M. Clowse, "Pathogenesis of pregnancy complications in systemic lupus erythematosus," *Current Opinion in Rheumatology*, vol. 25, no. 5, pp. 591–596, 2013.

[15] A. Munoz-Suano, A. B. Hamilton, and A. G. Betz, "Gimme shelter: the immune system during pregnancy," *Immunological Reviews*, vol. 241, no. 1, pp. 20–38, 2011.

[16] D. W. Bianchi, G. K. Zickwolf, G. J. Weil, S. Sylvester, and M. A. Demaria, "Male fetal progenitor cells persist in maternal blood for as long as 27 years postpartum," *Proceedings of the National Academy of Sciences of the United States of America*, vol. 93, no. 2, pp. 705–708, 1996.

[17] E. Vinet, A. E. Clarke, C. Gordon et al., "Decreased live births in women with systemic lupus erythematosus," *Arthritis Care and Research*, vol. 63, no. 7, pp. 1068–1072, 2011.

[18] A. Doria, A. Ghirardello, L. Iaccarino et al., "Pregnancy, cytokines, and disease activity in systemic lupus erythematosus," *Arthritis Care & Research*, vol. 51, no. 6, pp. 989–995, 2004.

[19] M. Østensen, F. Förger, and P. M. Villiger, "Cytokines and pregnancy in rheumatic disease," *Annals of the New York Academy of Sciences*, vol. 1069, pp. 353–363, 2006.

[20] S. Q. Crome, A. Y. Wang, and M. K. Levings, "Translational mini-review series on Th17 cells: function and regulation of human T helper 17 cells in health and disease," *Clinical & Experimental Immunology*, vol. 159, no. 2, pp. 109–119, 2010.

[21] M. H. Nyirenda, L. Sanvito, P. J. Darlington et al., "TLR2 stimulation drives human naive and effector regulatory T cells into a Th17-like phenotype with reduced suppressive function," *The Journal of Immunology*, vol. 187, no. 5, pp. 2278–2290, 2011.

[22] A. B. Pernis, "Th17 cells in rheumatoid arthritis and systemic lupus erythematosus," *Journal of Internal Medicine*, vol. 265, no. 6, pp. 644–652, 2009.

[23] E. Bettelli, M. Oukka, and V. K. Kuchroo, "$T_H$-17 cells in the circle of immunity and autoimmunity," *Nature Immunology*, vol. 8, no. 4, pp. 345–350, 2007.

[24] V. Saini, S. Arora, A. Yadav, and J. Bhattacharjee, "Cytokines in recurrent pregnancy loss," *Clinica Chimica Acta*, vol. 412, no. 9-10, pp. 702–708, 2011.

[25] A. Doria, L. Iaccarino, P. Sarzi-Puttini et al., "Estrogens in pregnancy and systemic lupus erythematosus," *Annals of the New York Academy of Sciences*, vol. 1069, pp. 247–256, 2006.

[26] M. Cutolo, A. Sulli, S. Capellino et al., "Sex hormones influence on the immune system: basic and clinical aspects in autoimmunity," *Lupus*, vol. 13, no. 9, pp. 635–638, 2004.

[27] P. Conti, D. Kempuraj, K. Kandere et al., "IL-10, an inflammatory/inhibitory cytokine, but not always," *Immunology Letters*, vol. 86, no. 2, pp. 123–129, 2003.

[28] R. K. Chowdary Venigalla, T. Tretter, S. Krienke et al., "Reduced CD4+,CD25- T cell sensitivity to the suppressive function of CD4+,CD25$^{high}$,CD127$^{-/low}$ regulatory T cells in patients with active systemic lupus erythematosus," *Arthritis & Rheumatism*, vol. 58, no. 7, pp. 2120–2130, 2008.

[29] C. Tower, I. Crocker, D. Chirico, P. Baker, and I. Bruce, "SLE and pregnancy: the potential role for regulatory T cells," *Nature Reviews Rheumatology*, vol. 7, no. 2, pp. 124–128, 2011.

[30] S. Björkander, K. Bremme, J.-O. Persson, R. F. van Vollenhoven, E. Sverremark-Ekström, and U. Holmlund, "Pregnancy-associated inflammatory markers are elevated in pregnant women with systemic lupus erythematosus," *Cytokine*, vol. 59, no. 2, pp. 392–399, 2012.

[31] T. Andersen, L. Munthe-Fog, P. Garred, and S. Jacobsen, "Serum levels of ficolin-3 (Hakata antigen) in patients with systemic lupus erythematosus," *Journal of Rheumatology*, vol. 36, no. 4, pp. 757–759, 2009.

[32] A. Halmos, J. Rigó, J. Szijártó, G. Füst, Z. Prohászka, and A. Molvarec, "Circulating ficolin-2 and ficolin-3 in normal pregnancy and pre-eclampsia," *Clinical & Experimental Immunology*, vol. 169, no. 1, pp. 49–56, 2012.

[33] D. Andrade, M. Kim, L. P. Blanco et al., "Interferon-$\alpha$ and angiogenic dysregulation in pregnant lupus patients destined for preeclampsia," *Arthritis & Rheumatology*, vol. 67, no. 4, pp. 977–987, 2015.

[34] S. Minamiguchi, Y. Mikami, N. Nakajima et al., "Complement split product C4d deposition in placenta in systemic lupus erythematosus and pregnancy-induced hypertension," *Pathology International*, vol. 63, no. 3, pp. 150–157, 2013.

[35] D. N. Burns, P. Nourjah, D. J. Wright et al., "Changes in immune activation markers during pregnancy and postpartum," *Journal of Reproductive Immunology*, vol. 42, no. 2, pp. 147–165, 1999.

[36] L. Jara-Quezada, A. Graef, and C. Lavalle, "Prolactin and gonadal hormones during pregnancy in systemic lupus erythematosus," *Journal of Rheumatology*, vol. 18, no. 3, pp. 349–353, 1991.

[37] A. Leaños-Miranda, G. Cárdenas-Mondragón, A. Ulloa-Aguirre, I. Isordia-Salas, A. Parra, and J. Ramírez-Peredo, "Anti-prolactin autoantibodies in pregnant women with systemic lupus erythematosus: maternal and fetal outcome," *Lupus*, vol. 16, no. 5, pp. 342–349, 2007.

[38] A. Doria, A. Tincani, and M. Lockshin, "Challenges of lupus pregnancies," *Rheumatology*, vol. 47, supplement 3, pp. iii9–iii12, 2008.

[39] C.-S. Yee, M. Akil, M. Khamashta et al., "The BILAG2004-pregnancy index is reliable for assessment of disease activity in pregnant SLE patients," *Rheumatology*, vol. 51, no. 10, pp. 1877–1880, 2012.

[40] G. Ruiz-Irastorza and M. A. Khamashta, "Lupus and pregnancy: integrating clues from the bench and bedside," *European Journal of Clinical Investigation*, vol. 41, no. 6, pp. 672–678, 2011.

[41] E. Imbasciati, A. Tincani, G. Gregorini et al., "Pregnancy in women with pre-existing lupus nephritis: predictors of fetal and maternal outcome," *Nephrology Dialysis Transplantation*, vol. 24, no. 2, pp. 519–525, 2009.

[42] M. E. B. Clowse, L. S. Magder, and M. Petri, "The clinical utility of measuring complement and anti-dsDNA antibodies during pregnancy in patients with systemic lupus erythematosus," *Journal of Rheumatology*, vol. 38, no. 6, pp. 1012–1016, 2011.

[43] E. Borella, A. Lojacono, M. Gatto et al., "Predictors of maternal and fetal complications in SLE patients: a prospective study," *Immunologic Research*, vol. 60, no. 2-3, pp. 170–176, 2014.

[44] H. Yang, H. Liu, D. Xu et al., "Pregnancy-related systemic lupus erythematosus: clinical features, outcome and risk factors of disease flares—a case control study," *PLoS ONE*, vol. 9, no. 8, Article ID e104375, 2014.

[45] T. J. Stanhope, W. M. White, K. G. Moder, A. Smyth, and V. D. Garovic, "Obstetric nephrology: lupus and lupus nephritis in pregnancy," *Clinical Journal of the American Society of Nephrology*, vol. 7, no. 12, pp. 2089–2099, 2012.

[46] S. M. Ramin, A. C. Vidaeff, E. R. Yeomans, and L. C. Gilstrap III, "Chronic renal disease in pregnancy," *Obstetrics & Gynecology*, vol. 108, no. 6, pp. 1531–1539, 2006.

[47] E. M. Klumb, L. M. S. Barros, L. Romeiro, N. R. de Jesús, R. A. Levy, and E. M. N. Albuquerque, "The impact of nephritis on gestational results in women with systemic lupus erythematosus," *Revista Brasileira de Reumatologia*, vol. 45, no. 3, pp. 107–113, 2005.

[48] K. Bramham, B. J. Hunt, S. Bewley et al., "Pregnancy outcomes in systemic lupus erythematosus with and without previous nephritis," *Journal of Rheumatology*, vol. 38, no. 9, pp. 1906–1913, 2011.

[49] C. K. Li and D. A. Isenberg, "Systemic lupus erythematosus," *Medicine*, vol. 34, no. 11, pp. 445–452, 2006.

[50] A. Smyth, G. H. M. Oliveira, B. D. Lahr, K. R. Bailey, S. M. Norby, and V. D. Garovic, "A systematic review and meta-analysis of pregnancy outcomes in patients with systemic lupus erythematosus and lupus nephritis," *Clinical Journal of the American Society of Nephrology*, vol. 5, no. 11, pp. 2060–2068, 2010.

[51] J. P. Buyon, "Updates on lupus and pregnancy," *Bulletin of the NYU Hospital for Joint Diseases*, vol. 67, no. 3, pp. 271–275, 2009.

[52] K. P. Conrad and J. M. Davison, "The renal circulation in normal pregnancy and preeclampsia: is there a place for relaxin?" *The American Journal of Physiology—Renal Physiology*, vol. 306, no. 10, pp. F1121–F1135, 2014.

[53] M. A. Saavedra, C. Cruz-Reyes, O. Vera-Lastra et al., "Impact of previous lupus nephritis on maternal and fetal outcomes during pregnancy," *Clinical Rheumatology*, vol. 31, no. 5, pp. 813–819, 2012.

[54] R. Fischer-Betz, C. Specker, R. Brinks, M. Aringer, and M. Schneider, "Low risk of renal flares and negative outcomes in women with lupus nephritis conceiving after switching from mycophenolate mofetil to azathioprine," *Rheumatology*, vol. 52, no. 6, pp. 1070–1076, 2013.

[55] F. Z. Rahman, J. Rahman, S. A. Al-Suleiman, and M. S. Rahman, "Pregnancy outcome in lupus nephropathy," *Archives of Gynecology and Obstetrics*, vol. 271, no. 3, pp. 222–226, 2005.

[56] E. Oviasu, J. Hicks, and J. S. Cameron, "The outcome of pregnancy in women with lupus nephritis," *Lupus*, vol. 1, no. 1, pp. 19–25, 1991.

[57] G. Moroni, S. Quaglini, G. Banfi et al., "Pregnancy in lupus nephritis," *American Journal of Kidney Diseases*, vol. 40, no. 4, pp. 713–720, 2002.

[58] M. E. Clowse, M. Jamison, E. Myers, and A. H. James, "A national study of the complications of lupus in pregnancy," *The American Journal of Obstetrics & Gynecology*, vol. 199, no. 2, pp. 127.e1–127.e6, 2008.

[59] E. M. Klumb, C. A. Silva, C. C. Lanna et al., "Consensus of the Brazilian Society of Rheumatology for the diagnosis, management and treatment of lupus nephritis," *Revista Brasileira de Reumatologia*, vol. 55, no. 1, pp. 1–21, 2015.

[60] T. K. Chen, A. C. Gelber, F. R. Witter, M. Petri, and D. M. Fine, "Renal biopsy in the management of lupus nephritis during pregnancy," *Lupus*, vol. 24, no. 2, pp. 147–154, 2015.

[61] R. J. Levine, S. E. Maynard, C. Qian et al., "Circulating angiogenic factors and the risk of preeclampsia," *The New England Journal of Medicine*, vol. 350, no. 7, pp. 672–683, 2004.

[62] G. de Jesus, N. de Jesus, R. Levy, and E. Klumb, "The use of angiogenic and antiangiogenic factors in the differential diagnosis of pre-eclampsia, antiphospholipid syndrome nephropathy and lupus nephritis," *Lupus*, vol. 23, no. 12, pp. 1299–1301, 2014.

[63] G. R. de Jesus, C. S. Oliveira, F. C. Santos et al., "Angiogenic and antiangiogenic factors in patients with systemic lupus erythematosus," *Arthritis & Rheumatology*, vol. 66, supplement, p. S1157, 2014.

[64] C. E. Kleinrouweler, M. M. J. Wiegerinck, C. Ris-Stalpers et al., "Accuracy of circulating placental growth factor, vascular endothelial growth factor, soluble fms-like tyrosine kinase 1 and soluble endoglin in the prediction of pre-eclampsia: a systematic review and meta-analysis," *BJOG*, vol. 119, no. 7, pp. 778–787, 2012.

[65] C. Oakley and C. A. Warnes, *Heart Disease in Pregnancy*, Blackwell Publishing, Malden, Mass, USA, 2nd edition, 2007.

[66] M. Bonnin, F. J. Mercier, O. Sitbon et al., "Severe pulmonary hypertension during pregnancy: mode of delivery and anesthetic management of 15 consecutive cases," *Anesthesiology*, vol. 102, no. 6, pp. 1133–1137, 2005.

[67] P. Lin, E. Rhew, R. B. Ness et al., "Adverse pregnancy outcomes and subsequent risk of cardiovascular disease in women with systemic lupus erythematosus," *Lupus Science & Medicine*, vol. 1, no. 1, Article ID e000024, 2014.

[68] J. E. Salmon, C. Heuser, M. Triebwasser et al., "Mutations in complement regulatory proteins predispose to preeclampsia: a genetic analysis of the PROMISSE cohort," *PLoS Medicine*, vol. 8, no. 3, Article ID e1001013, 2011.

[69] A. Tincani, C. Bazzani, S. Zingarelli, and A. Lojacono, "Lupus and the antiphospholipid syndrome in pregnancy and obstetrics: clinical characteristics, diagnosis, pathogenesis, and treatment," *Seminars in Thrombosis and Hemostasis*, vol. 34, no. 3, pp. 267–273, 2008.

[70] J. A. Gómez-Puerta, G. Espinosa, and R. Cervera, "Catastrophic antiphospholipid syndrome: diagnosis and management in pregnancy," *Clinics in Laboratory Medicine*, vol. 33, no. 2, pp. 391–400, 2013.

[71] M. Østensen, L. Andreoli, A. Brucato et al., "State of the art: reproduction and pregnancy in rheumatic diseases," *Autoimmunity Reviews*, vol. 14, no. 5, pp. 376–386, 2015.

[72] J. Alijotas-Reig, R. Ferrer-Oliveras, A. Ruffatti et al., "The European Registry on Obstetric Antiphospholipid Syndrome (EUROAPS): a survey of 247 consecutive cases," *Autoimmunity Reviews*, vol. 14, no. 5, pp. 387–395, 2015.

[73] S. Sciascia, G. Sanna, V. Murru, D. Roccatello, M. A. Khamashta, and M. L. Bertolaccini, "GAPSS: the global anti-phospholipid syndrome score," *Rheumatology*, vol. 52, no. 8, Article ID ket388, pp. 1397–1403, 2013.

[74] C. A. Clark, K. A. Spitzer, J. N. Nadler, and C. A. Laskin, "Preterm deliveries in women with systemic lupus erythematosus," *Journal of Rheumatology*, vol. 30, no. 10, pp. 2127–2132, 2003.

[75] M. J. Johnson, M. Petri, F. R. Witter, and J. T. Repke, "Evaluation of preterm delivery in a systemic lupus erythematosus pregnancy clinic," *Obstetrics and Gynecology*, vol. 86, no. 3, pp. 396–399, 1995.

[76] S. Y. Yuen, A. Krizova, J. M. Ouimet, and J. E. Pope, "Pregnancy outcome in systemic lupus erythematosus (SLE) is improving: Results from a case control study and literature review," *The Open Rheumatology Journal*, vol. 2, no. 1, pp. 89–98, 2009.

[77] M. S. Magid, C. Kaplan, L. R. Sammaritano, M. Peterson, M. L. Druzin, and M. D. Lockshin, "Placental pathology in systemic lupus erythematosus: a prospective study," *The American Journal of Obstetrics and Gynecology*, vol. 179, no. 1, pp. 226–234, 1998.

[78] K. Lun Hon and A. K. C. Leung, "Neonatal lupus erythematosus," *Autoimmune Diseases*, vol. 2012, Article ID 301274, 6 pages, 2012.

[79] P. M. Izmirly, M. Y. Kim, C. Llanos et al., "Evaluation of the risk of anti-SSA/Ro-SSB/La antibody-associated cardiac manifestations of neonatal lupus in fetuses of mothers with systemic lupus erythematosus exposed to hydroxychloroquine," *Annals of the Rheumatic Diseases*, vol. 69, no. 10, pp. 1827–1830, 2010.

[80] P. M. Izmirly, C. Llanos, L. A. Lee, A. Askanase, M. Y. Kim, and J. P. Buyon, "Cutaneous manifestations of neonatal lupus and risk of subsequent congenital heart block," *Arthritis and Rheumatism*, vol. 62, no. 4, pp. 1153–1157, 2010.

[81] D. M. Friedman, M. Y. Kim, J. A. Copel, C. Llanos, C. Davis, and J. P. Buyon, "Prospective evaluation of fetuses with autoimmune-associated congenital heart block followed in the PR Interval and Dexamethasone Evaluation (PRIDE) study," *The American Journal of Cardiology*, vol. 103, no. 8, pp. 1102–1106, 2009.

[82] A. J. J. T. Rein, D. Mevorach, Z. Perles et al., "Early diagnosis and treatment of atrioventricular block in the fetus exposed to maternal anti-SSA/Ro-SSB/La antibodies a prospective, observational, fetal kinetocardiogram-based study," *Circulation*, vol. 119, no. 14, pp. 1867–1872, 2009.

[83] J. P. Buyon, R. M. Clancy, and D. M. Friedman, "Cardiac manifestations of neonatal lupus erythematosus: guidelines to management, integrating clues from the bench and bedside," *Nature Clinical Practice Rheumatology*, vol. 5, no. 3, pp. 139–148, 2009.

[84] E. T. Jaeggi, J.-C. Fouron, E. D. Silverman, G. Ryan, J. Smallhorn, and L. K. Hornberger, "Transplacental fetal treatment improves the outcome of prenatally diagnosed complete atrioventricular block without structural heart disease," *Circulation*, vol. 110, no. 12, pp. 1542–1548, 2004.

[85] P. M. Izmirly, N. Costedoat-Chalumeau, C. N. Pisoni et al., "Maternal use of hydroxychloroquine is associated with a reduced risk of recurrent anti-SSA/ro-antibody—associated cardiac manifestations of neonatal lupus," *Circulation*, vol. 126, no. 1, pp. 76–82, 2012.

[86] R. D. Tunks, M. E. B. Clowse, S. G. Miller, L. R. Brancazio, and P. C. A. Barker, "Maternal autoantibody levels in congenital heart block and potential prophylaxis with antiinflammatory agents," *American Journal of Obstetrics & Gynecology*, vol. 208, no. 1, pp. 64.e1–64.e7, 2013.

[87] D. M. Friedman, C. Llanos, P. M. Izmirly et al., "Evaluation of fetuses in a study of intravenous immunoglobulin as preventive therapy for congenital heart block: results of a multicenter, prospective, open-label clinical trial," *Arthritis and Rheumatism*, vol. 62, no. 4, pp. 1138–1146, 2010.

[88] C. N. Pisoni, A. Brucato, A. Ruffatti et al., "Failure of intravenous immunoglobulin to prevent congenital heart block: findings of a multicenter, prospective, observational study," *Arthritis and Rheumatism*, vol. 62, no. 4, pp. 1147–1152, 2010.

[89] J. G. Routsias, N. C. Kyriakidis, D. M. Friedman et al., "Association of the idiotype: antiidiotype antibody ratio with the efficacy of intravenous immunoglobulin treatment for the prevention of recurrent autoimmune-associated congenital heart block," *Arthritis & Rheumatism*, vol. 63, no. 9, pp. 2783–2789, 2011.

[90] M. Østensen, "Intravenous immunoglobulin does not prevent recurrence of congenital heart block in children of SSA/Ro-positive mothers," *Arthritis and Rheumatism*, vol. 62, no. 4, pp. 911–914, 2010.

[91] H. Eliasson, S.-E. Sonesson, G. Sharland et al., "Isolated atrioventricular block in the fetus: a retrospective, multinational, multicenter study of 175 patients," *Circulation*, vol. 124, no. 18, pp. 1919–1926, 2011.

[92] P. M. Izmirly, A. Saxena, M. Y. Kim et al., "Maternal and fetal factors associated with mortality and morbidity in a multi-racial/ethnic registry of anti-SSA/Ro-associated cardiac neonatal lupus," *Circulation*, vol. 124, no. 18, pp. 1927–1935, 2011.

[93] G. R. R. de Jesus, F. C. Dos Santos, C. S. Oliveira, W. Mendes-Silva, N. R. de Jesus, and R. A. Levy, "Management of obstetric antiphospholipid syndrome," *Current Rheumatology Reports*, vol. 14, no. 1, pp. 79–86, 2012.

[94] R. Madazli, M. A. Yuksel, M. Oncul, M. Imamoglu, and H. Yilmaz, "Obstetric outcomes and prognostic factors of lupus pregnancies," *Archives of Gynecology and Obstetrics*, vol. 289, no. 1, pp. 49–53, 2014.

[95] G. Pagani, R. Reggia, L. Andreoli et al., "The role of second trimester uterine artery Doppler in pregnancies with systemic lupus erythematosus," *Prenatal Diagnosis*, vol. 35, no. 5, pp. 447–452, 2015.

[96] D. Le Thi Huong, B. Wechsler, D. Vauthier-Brouzes et al., "The second trimester Doppler ultrasound examination is the best predictor of late pregnancy outcome in systemic lupus erythematosus and/or the antiphospholipid syndrome," *Rheumatology*, vol. 45, no. 3, pp. 332–338, 2006.

[97] B. H. Hahn, M. A. McMahon, A. Wilkinson et al., "American College of Rheumatology guidelines for screening, treatment, and management of lupus nephritis," *Arthritis Care and Research*, vol. 64, no. 6, pp. 797–808, 2012.

[98] G. K. Bertsias, M. Tektonidou, Z. Amoura et al., "Joint European League Against Rheumatism and European Renal Association-European Dialysis and Transplant Association (EULAR/ERA-EDTA) recommendations for the management of adult and paediatric lupus nephritis," *Annals of the Rheumatic Diseases*, vol. 71, no. 11, pp. 1771–1782, 2012.

[99] R. A. Levy, V. S. Vilela, M. J. Cataldo et al., "Hydroxychloroquine (HCQ) in lupus pregnancy: double-blind and placebo-controlled study," *Lupus*, vol. 10, no. 6, pp. 401–404, 2001.

[100] A. Makol, K. Wright, and S. Amin, "Rheumatoid arthritis and pregnancy: safety considerations in pharmacological management," *Drugs*, vol. 71, no. 15, pp. 1973–1987, 2011.

[101] A. Osadchy, T. Ratnapalan, and G. Koren, "Ocular toxicity in children exposed in utero to antimalarial drugs: review of the literature," *Journal of Rheumatology*, vol. 38, no. 12, pp. 2504–2508, 2011.

[102] V. Jain and C. Gordon, "Managing pregnancy in inflammatory rheumatological diseases," *Arthritis Research and Therapy*, vol. 13, no. 1, article 206, 2011.

[103] R. M. Ward, B. A. Bates, W. E. Benitz et al., "The transfer of drugs and other chemicals into human milk," *Pediatrics*, vol. 108, no. 3, pp. 776–789, 2001.

[104] J. M. W. Hazes, P. G. Coulie, V. Geenen et al., "Rheumatoid arthritis and pregnancy: evolution of disease activity and pathophysiological considerations for drug use," *Rheumatology*, vol. 50, no. 11, pp. 1955–1968, 2011.

[105] J. Yazdany, L. Trupin, R. Kaiser et al., "Contraceptive counseling and use among women with systemic lupus erythematosus: a gap in health care quality?" *Arthritis Care and Research*, vol. 63, no. 3, pp. 358–365, 2011.

[106] E. B. Schwarz and S. Manzi, "Risk of unintended pregnancy among women with systemic lupus erythematosus," *Arthritis Care & Research*, vol. 59, no. 6, pp. 863–866, 2008.

[107] K. R. Culwell, K. M. Curtis, and M. del Carmen Cravioto, "Safety of contraceptive method use among women with systemic lupus erythematosus: a systematic review," *Obstetrics and Gynecology*, vol. 114, no. 2, part 1, pp. 341–353, 2009.

[108] E. M. Stringer, C. Kaseba, J. Levy et al., "A randomized trial of the intrauterine contraceptive device vs hormonal contraception in women who are infected with the human immunodeficiency virus," *The American Journal of Obstetrics and Gynecology*, vol. 197, no. 2, pp. 144.e1–144.e8, 2007.

[109] M. Cutolo, S. Capellino, and R. H. Straub, "Oestrogens in rheumatic diseases: friend or foe?" *Rheumatology*, vol. 47, supplement 3, pp. iii2–iii5, 2008.

[110] J. Sánchez-Guerrero, A. G. Uribe, L. Jiménez-Santana et al., "A trial of contraceptive methods in women with systemic lupus erythematosus," *The New England Journal of Medicine*, vol. 353, no. 24, pp. 2539–2549, 2005.

[111] M. Petri, M. Y. Kim, K. C. Kalunian et al., "Combined oral contraceptives in women with systemic lupus erythematosus," *The New England Journal of Medicine*, vol. 353, no. 24, pp. 2550–2558, 2005.

[112] N. Chabbert-Buffet, Z. Amoura, P.-Y. Scarabin et al., "Pregnane progestin contraception in systemic lupus erythematosus: a longitudinal study of 187 patients," *Contraception*, vol. 83, no. 3, pp. 229–237, 2011.

[113] A. M. Kaunitz, R. Arias, and M. McClung, "Bone density recovery after depot medroxyprogesterone acetate injectable contraception use," *Contraception*, vol. 77, no. 2, pp. 67–76, 2008.

[114] C. J. Hardy, B. P. Palmer, S. J. Morton, K. R. Muir, and R. J. Powell, "Pregnancy outcome and family size in systemic lupus erythematosus: a case-control study," *Rheumatology*, vol. 38, no. 6, pp. 559–563, 1999.

[115] R. A. Hickman and C. Gordon, "Causes and management of infertility in systemic lupus erythematosus," *Rheumatology*, vol. 50, no. 9, pp. 1551–1558, 2011.

[116] C. A. Silva, E. Bonfa, and M. Østensen, "Maintenance of fertility in patients with rheumatic diseases needing antiinflammatory and immunosuppressive drugs," *Arthritis Care & Research*, vol. 62, no. 12, pp. 1682–1690, 2010.

[117] Z. Blumenfeld, O. Mischari, N. Schultz, N. Boulman, and A. Balbir-Gurman, "Gonadotropin releasing hormone agonists may minimize cyclophosphamide associated gonadotoxicity in SLE and autoimmune diseases," *Seminars in Arthritis and Rheumatism*, vol. 41, no. 3, pp. 346–352, 2011.

[118] M. C. Micu, R. Micu, and M. Ostensen, "Luteinized unruptured follicle syndrome increased by inactive disease and selective cyclooxygenase 2 inhibitors in women with inflammatory arthropathies," *Arthritis Care and Research*, vol. 63, no. 9, pp. 1334–1338, 2011.

[119] N. Guballa, L. Sammaritano, S. Schwartzman, J. Buyon, and M. D. Lockshin, "Ovulation induction and in vitro fertilization in systemic lupus erythematosus and antiphospholipid syndrome," *Arthritis & Rheumatism*, vol. 43, no. 3, pp. 550–556, 2000.

[120] L. C. Udoff and D. W. Branch, "Management of patients with antiphospholipid antibodies undergoing in vitro fertilization," *Journal of Autoimmunity*, vol. 15, no. 2, pp. 209–211, 2000.

[121] A. Levine and M. Lockshin, "Assisted reproductive technology in SLE and APS," *Lupus*, vol. 23, no. 12, pp. 1239–1241, 2014.

[122] K. L. Buckingham and L. W. Chamley, "A critical assessment of the role of antiphospholipid antibodies in infertility," *Journal of Reproductive Immunology*, vol. 80, no. 1-2, pp. 132–145, 2009.

[123] C. Coughlan, X. Yuan, T. Nafee, J. Yan, N. Mariee, and T. Li, "The clinical characteristics of women with recurrent implantation failure," *Journal of Obstetrics and Gynaecology*, vol. 33, no. 5, pp. 494–498, 2013.

[124] A. Steinvil, R. Raz, S. Berliner et al., "Association of common thrombophilias and antiphospholipid antibodies with success rate of in vitro fertilisation," *Thrombosis and Haemostasis*, vol. 108, no. 6, pp. 1192–1197, 2012.

[125] C. Chighizola and G. de Jesus, "Antiphospholipid antibodies and infertility," *Lupus*, vol. 23, no. 12, pp. 1232–1238, 2014.

[126] Practice Committee of American Society for Reproductive Medicine, "Anti-phospholipid antibodies do not affect IVF success," *Fertility and Sterility*, vol. 90, no. 5, supplement, pp. S172–S173, 2008.

# 27

# Cardiovascular Disease in Latin American Patients with Systemic Lupus Erythematosus

**Jenny Amaya-Amaya, Juan Camilo Sarmiento-Monroy, Julián Caro-Moreno, Nicolás Molano-González, Rubén D. Mantilla, Adriana Rojas-Villarraga, and Juan-Manuel Anaya**

*Center for Autoimmune Diseases Research (CREA), School of Medicine and Health Sciences, Universidad del Rosario, Carrera 24 No. 63C-69, 111221 Bogotá, Colombia*

Correspondence should be addressed to Jenny Amaya-Amaya; jecamaya@gmail.com

Academic Editor: Yehuda Shoenfeld

*Objective.* This study was performed to determine the prevalence of and associated risk factors for cardiovascular disease (CVD) in Latin American (LA) patients with systemic lupus erythematosus (SLE). *Methods.* First, a cross-sectional analytical study was conducted in 310 Colombian patients with SLE in whom CVD was assessed. Associated factors were examined by multivariate regression analyses. Second, a systematic review of the literature on CVD in SLE in LA was performed. *Results.* There were 133 (36.5%) Colombian SLE patients with CVD. Dyslipidemia, smoking, coffee consumption, and pleural effusion were positively associated with CVD. An independent effect of coffee consumption and cigarette on CVD was found regardless of gender and duration of disease. In the systematic review, 60 articles fulfilling the eligibility criteria were included. A wide range of CVD prevalence was found (4%–79.5%). Several studies reported ancestry, genetic factors, and polyautoimmunity as novel risk factors for such a condition. *Conclusions.* A high rate of CVD is observed in LA patients with SLE. Awareness of the observed risk factors should encourage preventive population strategies for CVD in patients with SLE aimed at facilitating the suppression of cigarette smoking and coffee consumption as well as at the tight control of dyslipidemia and other modifiable risk factors.

## 1. Introduction

Systemic lupus erythematosus (SLE) is a complex systemic autoimmune disease (AD), characterized by the production of numerous pathogenic autoantibodies [1]. Diverse heritable, hormonal, and environmental factors and immune-system aberrations contribute to the clinical expression of the disease [2]. The heterogeneous nature of SLE explains the broad spectrum of clinical manifestations (i.e., subphenotypes). SLE affects predominantly women (female-to-male ratio 9 : 1) of child-bearing age [3]. The annual incidence and prevalence range from 1.4 to 11 cases per 100,000 population, and from 7.4 to 159.4 cases per 100,000 population, respectively [4] depending on a variety of factors, including age, gender, and ancestry. African, Hispanic, and Asian ancestry significantly influence both the risk of developing the disorder and outcome [4]. A bimodal mortality was described by Urowitz et al. [5] characterized by an early peak in the first 3 years after diagnosis due to active disease, infections and glomerulonephritis, and a second peak, 4–20 years after SLE diagnosis, in which cardiovascular disease (CVD) is the main feature and cause of death. Although overall mortality for patients with SLE has improved over the past 30 years, mortality due to CVD has remained almost the same [6].

CVD is the leading cause of mortality, responsible for about 30% of deaths worldwide. Globally, 80% of total CVD deaths occur in developing countries [7]. In addition, there is strong epidemiologic evidence that CVD risk among SLE patients compared to the general population is at least doubled [8]. Noteworthy, the excessive cardiovascular (CV) events observed in SLE individuals are not fully explained by classic risk factors. Several SLE-specific factors, including disease activity and duration, and possibly specific manifestations and therapies, further increase CV risk [8]. In fact, SLE *per se* seems to be an independent risk factor for the development of accelerated atherosclerosis [9].

SLE is not uncommon in Latin America (LA), the geographical area defined by Mexico, Central America, South America, and the islands of the Caribbean, a rapidly growing region with almost 600 million inhabitants [10]. Latin Americans are considered a highly admixed population due to a mixed ethnicity (so called *mestizos*) that is mainly derived from a European and Amerindian inheritance [11]. The increased prevalence of chronic diseases in LA has been attributed to diverse causes including the ageing of the population and lifestyle factors such as smoking, physical inactivity, and excess alcohol intake [12]. Despite important advances in recent decades, LA remains one of the world's most unequal regions [13]. Enormous cultural differences in health perceptions in LA exist, correlating with individuals' economic and health conditions [12]. So far, some studies regarding SLE have documented differences in health status, disease prevalence, treatment outcomes, and healthcare use among different ethnic groups, suggesting that minorities influence SLE health disparities [14–19]. Thus, this study was performed to determine the prevalence and associated risk factors for CVD in Latin American patients with SLE.

## 2. Material and Methods

*2.1. Study Population.* First, a cross-sectional analytical study was conducted in 310 Colombian patients with SLE in whom CVD was assessed. The subjects were seen at the Center for Autoimmune Diseases Research (CREA) in Bogota, Colombia. All of them fulfilled the 1997 update American College of Rheumatology classification criteria for SLE [20]. This study was done in compliance with Act 008430/1993 by Ministry of Health of the Republic of Colombia, which classified it as a minimal-risk research. The institutional review board of the Universidad del Rosario approved the study design.

Information on patient socio-demographic and cumulative clinical and laboratory data, as well as household description, were obtained by interview, standardized report form, physical examination and chart review. All data were collected in an electronic and secure database. Socio-demographic variables included age at SLE onset, disease duration, educational and socioeconomic status, current occupation, smoking habits, coffee consumption, expositional factors and physical activity. Age at onset of the disease was defined as the first subjective experience of the symptom(s) and/or sign(s) described in any of the items of the classification criteria [21]. Duration of disease was considered as the difference between age at onset and the date of first participation in the study. Educational level was recorded as the number of years of education and was divided into two groups (more or less than 9 years) of education based on the "General Law of Education" in Colombia [22, 23]. Socioeconomic status was categorized on the basis of national legislation and was divided into low (1 and 2) and high (3–6) status. Smoking habits was assessed as ever; 1–6, 6–15, and >15 packages/year; or quitter cigarette consumption. Coffee intake was asked as yes or not, and measured in cups per day (1-2, 2–4, >4). Several expositional factors were also questioned, including the use of silicone implants, hair dyes, pesticides and organic solvents [24].

*2.2. Clinical Variables.* Clinical and laboratory variables were registered as present or absent at any time during the course of the disease. Clinical features of the disease were included taking into account the revised American College of Rheumatology criteria [20] and others manifestations as follows: polyautoimmunity (coexistence of an additional AD in the same individual on the basis of international criteria) [25, 26], multiple autoimmune syndrome (presence of more than two AD in the same patient) [26–28]; familial autoimmunity, and familial autoimmune disease were also registered as the presence of any other AD and SLE in first degree relatives (FDR) respectively [27–29]. Regarding pharmacological treatment, current or past use of azathioprine, mycophenolate mofetil, cyclophosphamide, methotrexate, antimalarials (i.e., clhoroquine, hydroxychloroquine), glucocorticoids (i.e., prednisolone, metilprednisolone, and deflazacort), and biological therapy (i.e., Rituximab) were recorded.

*2.3. Cardiovascular Assessment.* Five subphenotypes were defined and assessed: first, hypertension, defined as having a blood pressure ≥140/90 mm Hg or using any antihypertensive medication [30]: systolic and diastolic blood pressures were measured twice with at least a 15-minute interval between and the averages were recorded. Second, history of stroke, third, coronary event (i.e., unstable angina, myocardial infarction (MI)), fourth, thrombotic event (other than coronary disease and carotid involvement, requiring anticoagulant treatment), fifth, carotid disease (doppler criteria or intima-media thickness ≥0.9).

*2.4. Laboratories Measurements.* Relevant laboratory variables associated with SLE were recorded. Antinuclear antibodies, antidouble strand DNA antibodies, precipitating antibodies to extractable nuclear antigens (Sm, U1-RNP, Ro/SS-A, La/SS-B), anticardiolipin IgG and IgM, antibeta 2-glycoprotein 1 IgG and IgM antibodies, and lupus anticoagulant were extracted from the patient's clinical record. Other autoantibodies including rheumatoid factor, anticyclic citrullinated peptide, -thyroperoxidase enzyme, -thyroglobulin, -Scl 70, -centromere, -mitochondrial, and -smooth muscle antibodies were also recorded. Inflammatory biomarkers, including erythrocyte sedimentation rate (ESR), and serum high sensitive C-reactive protein (CRP) levels, as well as white blood cell and platelet count, hemoglobin levels, mean corpuscular volume, coombs test, complement (i.e., C3 and C4 levels), TSH, tetraiodothyronine T4, venereal disease research laboratory, and creatinine were extracted from patient's clinical record. Likewise, serum levels of total cholesterol (TC), triglycerides (TGL), high-density lipoprotein cholesterol (HDL), low-density lipoprotein cholesterol (LDL), and glycemia were determined by blood tests provided by every patient.

*2.5. Assessment of Traditional Risk Factors for CVD.* Patients were assessed for traditional CVD risk factors including current age (≥45 and ≥55 years for men and women, resp.) [31–34]. Type 2 diabetes mellitus (T2DM) was defined as having a fasting plasma glucose level ≥7 mmol/L (126 mg/dL), or taking any antidiabetic agents at the time of assessment [35]. A diagnosis of dyslipidemia was given if the patient had (a) hypercholesterolemia, defined as taking lipid-lowering medication as a surrogate, or having a fasting plasma TC ≥200 mg/dL (b) HDL ≤40 mg/dL, (c) hypertriglyceridemia (TGL ≥150 mg/dL), or (d) elevated LDL (≥100 mg/dL) [31, 36]. Current hemoglobin ≤12 g/dL established a diagnosis of anemia and current levels of creatinine (abnormal defined as ≥1.2 mg/dL) were evaluated as well. History of premature CAD in FDR was also assessed [37]. Patients and their past medical records were evaluated for the current or past use of aspirin or hormone replacement therapy.

*2.6. Statistical Analysis.* First, univariate analyses were done. Categorical variables were analyzed by frequencies. Kolmogorov-Smirnov normality test was done to evaluate normality for quantitative continuous variables. Parametric data are expressed as the mean and standard deviation, and nonparametric data are described as the median and interquartile range. Second, associations between traditional and nontraditional CVD risk factors were assessed by bivariate analyses. The presence of CVD was assessed through chi square tests or Fisher's exact tests when the variable was dichotomous. Parametric values were analyzed by *t* student test. Nonparametric values were analyzed by Mann-Whitney *U* test. Clinical variables with a $P \leq 0.25$ were included in a multivariable model. Finally, a multivariate binomial logistic regression model having CVD as the dependent variable was fit. As independent factors, the model included the traditional and nontraditional associations that were statistically significant in bivariate analyses and those variables that were biologically plausible. Moreover, other logistic regression models were made, including interactions between independent factors. In both circumstances, the models were adjusted by gender and duration of the disease. Adequacies of logistic models were assessed using the Hosmer-Lemeshow goodness-of-fit test. The Nagelkerke $R^2$ (i.e., pseudo-$R^2$) was used to estimate the percentage of variance explained by the models. Adjusted odds ratios (AOR) were calculated with 95% confidence intervals (CI). The Wald statistic test was used to evaluate the significance of individual logistic regression coefficients for each independent variable. Statistical analyses were done by the Statistical Package for the Social Sciences (SPSS, v.20, Chicago, IL, USA).

*2.7. Systematic Review of Literature.* The Preferred reporting items for Systematic Reviews and Meta-analyses guidelines were followed [38] to systematically search in the following databases: PubMed, EMBASE, Scopus, SciELO, and Virtual Health Library—which includes BIREME, LILACS and many others LA sources—about CVD and SLE in LA population. Three reviewers did the search and extraction data independently (AAJC, SMJC, and CMJ) using predefined eligibility criteria, from inception up to February 2013.

The search was done in PubMed, using the following Medical Subject Headings (MeSH terms) groups: "Lupus Erythematosus, Systemic," "Cardiovascular Diseases;" "Latin America," "Ethnic Groups," "Brazil," "Mexico," "Colombia," "Chile," "Cuba," "Panama," "Venezuela," "Bolivia," "Peru," "Argentina," "Uruguay," "Paraguay," "Ecuador," "Nicaragua," "Surinam," "French Guiana," "Guatemala," "Honduras," "Belize," "Costa Rica," "El Salvador," "Puerto Rico," "Dominican Republic," and "Haiti." Each one of them was cross-referenced with the following MeSH terms/keywords: "risk factors," "traditional risk factors," "classic risk factors," "non-traditional risk factors," "novel risk factors," "hypertension," "metabolic syndrome," "obesity," "smoking," "tobacco," "dyslipidemia," "advanced age," "menopausal status," "family history of CVD," "hyperhomocysteinemia," "sedentary lifestyle," "renal impairment," "male gender," "type 2 diabetes mellitus," "insulin resistance," "hormone replacement therapy," "coffee," "ancestry," "polymorphism, genetic," "poliautoimmunity," "autoantibodies," "antibodies, antiphospholipid," "lupus coagulation inhibitor," "circulation anticoagulants," "antibodies, anticardiolipins," "beta 2-glycoprotein I," "endothelial cells antibodies," "systemic inflammation," "c-reactive protein," "blood sedimentation," "tumor necrosis factor," "cytokines," "immune complex," "disease activity," "SLEDAI," "organ damage," "SDI," "duration of illness," "immune cells aberrations," "glucocorticoids," "steroids," "DMARD," "antirheumatic agents," "methotrexate," "biological therapy," "rituximab," "anti-Inflammatory agents, non-steroidal," "azathioprine," "vasculopathy," "lupus nephritis," "premature menopause," "endogenous dyslipidemia," "sociodemographic factors," "hypovitaminosis D," "vitamin D deficiency," "low vitamin D," "osteoporosis," "biomarkers," "antiphospholipid syndrome," "thyroiditis, autoimmune," "Graves Disease," "Hashimoto Disease," "scleroderma," "Sjögren's syndrome," "rheumatoid arthritis," "hypertension," "ischemic heart disease," "coronary artery disease," "acute coronary syndrome," "congestive heart failure," "myocardial infarction," "stroke," "angina," "thrombosis," "deep vein thromboses," "pulmonary embolism," "periphery arterial disease," and "atherosclerosis." Each term was cross-referenced for the greatest number of results. No limits regarding language, period of publication, or publication type were used.

The same terms were used for searching in EMBASE and Scopus databases. Each MeSH term and keyword was translated into DeCS (Health Sciences Descriptors) in order to explore sources of information in Spanish, Portuguese, and English through SciELO and Virtual Health Library databases.

*2.8. Study Selection, Data Extraction, and Quality Assessment.* Reviewers screened all titles and abstracts and applied the eligibility criteria in order to identify studies that were appropriate for inclusion [39]. A study was included if (a) the abstract was available, (b) it contained original data, (c) it used accepted classification criteria for SLE, (d) it measured CV risk factors (traditional and/or nontraditional), (e) it examined as a clinical endpoints: hypertension, ischemic heart disease (IHD), coronary artery disease (CAD), acute coronary syndrome (ACS), MI, angina, congestive heart failure (CHF), stroke, thrombosis, peripheral arterial disease (PAD), and subclinical atherosclerosis, and (d) it includes LA population. In order to complete the systematic review, several authors were contacted by E-mail for full text and those references from the articles that seemed to be relevant to the review were hand-searched.

Articles were excluded from the analysis if they dealt with juvenile SLE or were done on animal models (i.e., murine models) instead of SLE patients. Studies were also excluded if they were reviews or case reports, or if they discussed topics not related to CVD, and/or were not done on LA population. Blinded reviewers (AAJC, SMJC, and MJC) organized selected articles on the basis of publication source, country, author, year, type of study, sample size, traditional and nontraditional risk factors, cardiovascular outcomes evaluated, and main results. Only novel risk factors with statistical significance were included. For details, see Supplementary Table S1 in the supplementary material available online at http://dx.doi.org/10.1155/2013/794383. Each record was classified based on the quality score of the studies that was assigned by applying the levels established by the Oxford Centre for Evidence-based Medicine 2011 in order to evaluate the risk of bias [40]. The search results were compared and disagreements were resolved by consensus.

## 3. Results

*3.1. Description of the Study Population.* Out of a total of 310 patients, 91.3% (283/310) were women. The median (interquartile range) of age and duration of the disease was 37 (22) and 5 (9) years, respectively. CVD was observed in 36.5% (113/310). The most frequent condition was hypertension (25.2%) (Tables 1 and 2).

*3.2. Factors Associated with CVD.* Current age, ever smoking, coffee consumption, polyautoimmunity (i.e., antiphospholipid syndrome), dyslipidemia, use of cytotoxic drugs, serositis, renal involvement (i.e., nephrotic syndrome), and thrombocytopenia were all risk factors significantly associated with CVD. Instead, ethnicity and leukopenia were factors negatively associated with CVD (Table 3).

*3.3. Adjusted Effects of Risk Factors for CVD.* Dyslipidemia, pleural effusion, polyautoimmunity, and renal compromise were variables significantly associated with CVD, regardless of gender and duration of the disease by logistic regression analysis (Table 4). The association between CVD and smoking habit remained statistically significant after establishing interaction with coffee consumption (Table 5).

*3.4. Systematic Literature Review.* There were 21,161 articles identified in PubMed, EMBASE, and Scopus databases search. Additional records identified through other sources included 814 articles (SciELO and Virtual Health Library). Therefore, the database searches provided a total of 21,975 publications. Of these, 19,729 were identified as duplicates. A total of 2,246 full text articles were assessed for eligibility. Only 115 articles were included for methodological analysis.

TABLE 1: Demographic and clinical characteristics of 310 patients with SLE.

| Characteristic | Median (IQR) |
|---|---|
| Age (y) | 37 (22) |
| Duration of disease (y) | 5.0 (9.0) |
| **Characteristic** | **Mean (SD)** |
| Age at SLE onset (y) | 38 (15.4) |
| Age of diagnosis (y) | 39.8 (15.8) |
| **Sociodemographic characteristic** | **% (*n*/*N*)** |
| Female | 91.3 (283/310) |
| High education level | 85.6 (255/298) |
| High socioeconomic status | 79.5 (236/297) |
| Mixed occupation | 23.2 (71/306) |
| Housewife | 21.2 (65/306) |
| Exposure to hair dyes | 40.6 (125/308) |
| **Clinical manifestation** | **% (*n*/*N*)** |
| Cutaneous compromise | 88.1 (273/310) |
| Arthropathy | 87.7 (272/310) |
| Neurological involvement | 10 (31/310) |
| Hematological criteria | 34.5 (107/310) |
| Immunological criteria | 78.1 (242/310) |
| Raynaud's phenomenon | 39.4 (122/310) |
| Vasculitis | 18.4 (57/310) |
| Alopecia | 47.7 (148/310) |
| Livedo reticularis | 19 (59/310) |
| Pleural effusion | 23.5 (73/310) |
| Pulmonary hypertension | 6.5 (20/310) |
| Pulmonary embolism | 2.9 (9/310) |
| Pericarditis | 14.5 (45/310) |
| Lupus nephritis | 46.5 (144/310) |
| Nephritic syndrome | 5.5 (17/310) |
| Nephrotic syndrome | 16.8 (58/310) |
| Histological pattern | |
| Normal | 8.5 (7/82) |
| Mesangial glomerulonephritis | 15.9 (13/82) |
| Focal segmental glomerulonephritis | 13.4 (11/82) |
| Proliferative glomerulonephritis | 41.5 (34/82) |
| Membranous glomerulonephritis | 11 (9/82) |
| **Autoimmune disease(s)** | **% (*n*/*N*)** |
| Polyautoimmunity | 26.1 (81/310) |
| MAS | 6.1 (19/310) |
| Familial autoimmunity in FDR | 30.3 (94/310) |
| RA | 3.9 (12/310) |
| APS | 8.7 (27/310) |
| SS | 8.7 (27/310) |
| AITD | 6.8 (21/310) |

TABLE 1: Continued.

| Characteristic | Median (IQR) |
|---|---|
| Comorbidities | % (*n*/*N*) |
| Fibromyalgia | 9.7 (30/309) |
| Depression | 21.4 (66/309) |
| Epilepsy | 3.9 (12/309) |
| Peptic ulcer disease | 38.5 (119/309) |
| Anemia | 8.1 (25/309) |
| Osteoporosis | 5.8 (18/309) |
| Malaria | 2.3 (7/303) |
| Hepatitis A | 7.1 (22/309) |
| Miscarriage | 20.2 (57/282) |
| Drugs | % (*n*/*N*) |
| Azathioprine | 33.9 (105/310) |
| Antimalarial | 80.6 (250/310) |
| Mycophenolate Mofetil | 15.8 (49/310) |
| Steroid | 78.4 (243/310) |
| Rituximab | 7.4 (23/310) |
| Cytotoxic agents | 12.3 (38/310) |
| Biological treatment | 8.4 (26/310) |
| Methotrexate | 34.8 (108/310) |
| Laboratories findings | % (*n*/*N*) |
| Anemia | 25.9 (76/293) |
| Leukopenia | 38 (114/300) |
| Lymphopenia | 78.7 (85/202) |
| Thrombocytopenia | 7.8 (23/296) |
| C-reactive protein (+) | 35.4 (57/161) |
| Erythrocyte sedimentation rate (+) | 46.2 (104/225) |
| VDRL (+) | 24.5 (26/204) |
| Abnormal serum creatinine | 9.7 (26/268) |
| Abnormal creatinine clearance | 56.6 (94/166) |
| 24 hours proteinuria (+) | 37.7 (80/212) |
| Hematuria | 57.4 (58/101) |
| Pyuria | 36.1 (56/155) |
| Antinuclear antibodies (+) | 98.6 (287/291) |
| Lupus anticoagulant (+) | 51 (52/102) |
| Anti-dsDNA antibodies (+) | 54.6 (147/269) |
| Low complement 3 (C3) | 60.8 (160/263) |
| Low complement 4 (C4) | 31.4 (83/264) |
| aCL IgG (+) | 33.8 (79/234) |
| aCL IgM (+) | 32.4 (73/225) |
| Beta 2-glycoprotein antibodies IgG (+) | 29.4 (10/34) |
| Beta 2-glycoprotein antibodies IgM (+) | 28.6 (6/21) |
| Anti-Ro antibodies (+) | 48.6 (122/251) |
| Anti-La antibodies (+) | 26.2 (64/244) |
| Anti-Sm antibodies (+) | 36 (89/247) |
| Anti-RNP antibodies (+) | 46 (109/237) |
| Rheumatoid factor (+) | 34.6 (27/78) |
| Citrullinated peptide antibodies (+) | 34.3 (12/35) |
| Thyroid stimulating hormone (+) | 51.5 (53/207) |
| Thyroid peroxidase antibodies (+) | 38.6 (17/44) |
| Thyroglobulin antibodies (+) | 20 (6/30) |

CVD: cardiovascular disease; SLE: systemic lupus erythematosus; IQR: interquartile range; SD: standard deviation; Y: years; MAS: multiple autoimmune syndrome; FDR: first-degree relatives; RA: rheumatoid arthritis; APS: antiphospholipid syndrome; SS: Sjögren's syndrome; AITD: autoimmune thyroid disease; VDRL: venereal disease research laboratory; aCL: anticardiolipin antibodies.
Arthropathy was defined as the presence of at least one of the following: arthritis, arthralgia, hands edema, or Jaccoud's arthropathy.
Cutaneous compromise was defined as the presence of at least one of the following: photosensitivity, oral ulcers, malar rash, discoid lupus, subacute lupus, and urticaria.
Neurological involvement were defined as the presence of at least one of the following: seizures, psychosis, and peripheral nerve compromise.
Hematological criteria were defined as the presence of at least one of the following: hemolytic anemia, leukopenia, lymphopenia, and thrombocytopenia.
Immunological criteria were defined as the presence of at least one of the following: anti-dsDNA, anti-Sm, anticardiolipin IgG or IgM, lupus anticoagulant, false-positive test VDRL, or fluorescent treponemal antibody absorption test.

Finally, 60 articles that had interpretable data and fulfilled the eligibility criteria were included. In 3 papers, data extraction was made from abstract [41–43]. For details, see Supplementary Table S1. There were 29 from Brazil [42, 44–71], 14 from Mexico [43, 72–84], 6 from United States of America [16–18, 85–87], 5 from Argentina [14, 41, 88–90], 4 from Puerto Rico [91–94], and 1 from Colombia [95] and Chile [96]. Five studies correspond to SLE LUMINA (LUpus in MInorities: nature versus nurture) multiethnic cohort [16–18, 85, 86]. The LUMINA cohort is comprised of patients of Hispanic (from Texas and Puerto Rico), African-American and Caucasian background. Two studies correspond to GLADEL'S (Grupo Latino Americano De Estudio de Lupus) longitudinal inception cohort [14, 97]. Thirty studies were cross-sectional, 15 were case-controls, 11 were cohort, 2 nested case-control and 2 were an inception cohort. The flowchart for systematic literature review and articles included in the analysis are shown in Figure 1.

*3.5. Prevalence, Risk Factors, and Subphenotypes of CVD.* Out of total of 60 articles that fulfilled eligibility criteria, 46 had interpretable data regarding CVD frequency, which corresponds to a prevalence range of 4%–79.5%. Several *classic* CV risk factors such as metabolic syndrome (MetS), obesity, dyslipidemia, hypertension, T2DM, sedentary lifestyle, male gender, smoking, advanced age, hyperhomocysteinemia, renal impairment, family history of CVD, and menopausal status were described. Several studies reported *nontraditional* risk factors such as ancestry, certain single-nucleotide polymorphisms, SLE *per se*, polyautoimmunity, autoantibodies (i.e., antiphospholipid), markers of systemic inflammation

TABLE 2: Cardiovascular disease characteristics of 310 patients with SLE.

| | % ($n/N$) |
|---|---|
| *Clinical manifestation* | |
| Cardiovascular disease | 36.5 (113/310) |
| Hypertension | 25.2 (78/310) |
| Stroke | 16.8 (52/310) |
| Coronary disease | 2.6 (8/310) |
| Thrombotic event | 1.6 (5/310) |
| Carotid disease | 0.6 (2/310) |
| *Risk factors* | |
| Type 2 diabetes mellitus | 1.9 (6/309) |
| Dyslipidemia | 18.1 (56/309) |
| Ever smoking | 39.21 (120/306) |
| 1 to 6 packages/year | 4.2 (13/306) |
| 6 to 15 packages/year | 2.6 (8/306) |
| More than 15 packages/year | 2.3 (7/306) |
| Quitter | 30.1 (92/306) |
| Coffee consumption | 61.5 (187/304) |
| 1 to 2 cups/day | 30.9 (94/304) |
| 2 to 4 cups/day | 22.7 (69/304) |
| More than 4 cups/day | 7.9 (24/304) |
| Never | 38.5 (117/304) |
| *Laboratories findings* | |
| Abnormal triglycerides | 34.3 (12/35) |
| Abnormal total cholesterol | 44.4 (16/22) |
| Abnormal high-density cholesterol | 58.8 (20/34) |
| Abnormal low-density cholesterol | 33.3 (8/24) |
| Abnormal glycemic | 25.7 (9/35) |

(i.e., CRP), SLE disease activity, SLE duration, organ damage, immune cells aberrations, medication (i.e., glucocorticoids), vasculopathy, lupus nephritis, endogenous dyslipidemia, bone mineral density, education level, and monthly income. A broad spectrum of CV subphenotypes including hypertension, IHD, CAD, ACS, MI, angina, CHF, stroke, thrombosis, peripheral arterial disease, subclinical atherosclerosis, and mortality due to CVD were described in LA individuals with SLE. For details, see Figure 2 and Supplementary Table S1.

## 4. Discussion

The analysis of Colombian patients with SLE discloses a high prevalence of CVD (36.5%). In contrast, prospective North Americans cohort studies showed a prevalence and annual incidence of CVD between 6 and 10%, and 1.5%, respectively [9, 98, 99]. Meanwhile, a case control study on the British General Practice Research Database showed higher risk of CVD in patients with SLE than rheumatoid arthritis [100]. Furthermore, in Italian population, Doria et al. [101] demonstrated rates of 10–40% for subclinical atherosclerosis. This inconsistency may reflect methodological obstacles such as differences in the definition of CVD outcome. Since CVD begins by endothelial dysfunction, hypertension was considered as the first subphenotype to be assessed.

*4.1. Epidemiology of Atherosclerosis among Patients with SLE.* Carotid plaque is prevalent in 21% of SLE patients under age of 35 and in up to 100% of those over age 65 [102]. The most striking example of raised risk of MI comes from the University of Pittsburgh SLE cohort, in which women with SLE aged 35–44 were >50 times more likely to experience MI than women without SLE from the Framingham Offspring study (RR 52.4; 95% CI 21.6–98.5) [8, 98].

Independent predictive risk factors for CV events had been assessed in five large prospective cohorts of patients with SLE, including Baltimore (1992, $n = 229$) [103], Pittsburg (1997, $n = 498$) [98], LUMINA (2004, $n = 546$) [17], Toronto (2007, $n = 561$) [104] and Systemic Lupus International Collaborating Clinics-Registry for Atherosclerosis (2010, $n = 637$) [105]. These cohorts found association of diverse classic risk factors (i.e., older age at diagnosis, smoking, hypercholesterolemia, male gender, and hypertension), as well as novel risk factors (i.e., longer duration of SLE and glucocorticoid use, antiphospholipid antibodies, and neuropsychiatric lupus), with CVD in SLE patients [105, 106]. In a recent meta-analysis, Schoenfeld et al. [8] showed that epidemiologic data strongly support that SLE patients are at elevated relative risk of CVD. The risks of MI, CHF, CVA, and CVD mortality are all increased among SLE patients compared to general population risks. The variability regarding the relative importance of risk factors for CVD among SLE patients in past epidemiologic studies is likely due in part to different design methods and different patient and comparison groups.

*4.2. CVD in Hispanics with SLE.* CVD has been assessed in LUMINA multiethnic cohort and GLADEL's longitudinal inception cohort, which demonstrated differences in sociodemographic, clinical (i.e., subphenotypes), immunologic, and therapeutic characteristics, in SLE patients with CV events [14–19, 85, 86, 93]. The present study adds further evidence about the high frequency of CVD in patients with SLE, their traditional risk factors (i.e., dyslipidemia, and smoking), and highlights coffee consumption as a factor for such a complication. Through the systematic review several factors and outcomes related to CVD were also identified (Table 6).

*4.3. Cigarette Smoking and Coffee Consumption Independently Influence the Risk of Developing CVD.* Several studies have assessed smoking as an independent risk factor for CV atherosclerotic disease [17, 107–111]. Gustafsson et al. [110] found that smoking may be the main traditional risk factor promoting increased CV risk in 208 SLE patients (RR 3.4, 95% CI 1.3–9.2). Previously, the same group found that smoking was predictive of MI, stroke, peripheral vascular disease (PVD) or CV mortality among the same patient population [109]. Toloza et al. [17] prospectively followed SLE patients over a median follow-up of 73.8 months and compared those who had a CVD event to those who did not as part of the LUMINA study. Current cigarette use was significantly associated with a 3.7-times increased risk of

Table 3: Characteristics associated with CVD in 310 patients with SLE.

| Characteristic | Cardiovascular disease 113/310 % (*n*/*N*) | Noncardiovascular disease 197/310 % (*n*/*N*) | OR (95% CI) | *P* |
|---|---|---|---|---|
| Sociodemographic characteristic | | | | |
| Age (y) | Median (IQR): 40 (23) | Median (IQR): 36 (21) | | 0.059 |
| Age at SLE onset (y) | Median (IQR): 30 (19) | Median (IQR): 26 (18) | | 0.175 |
| Age of diagnosis (y) | Median (IQR): 34 (22) | Median (IQR): 28 (18) | | 0.041 |
| Ever smoking | 50.9 (57/112) | 37.1 (73/194) | 1.75 (1.09–2.61) | 0.019 |
| Coffee | 70.5 (79/112) | 55.2 (108/192) | 1.94 (1.19–3.18) | 0.009 |
| Hair dye | 46 (52/113) | 37.4 (73/195) | 1.42 (0.89–2.29) | 0.139 |
| Pesticides | 3.5 (4/113) | 1 (2/197) | 3.56 (0.64–19.75) | 0.122 |
| Autoimmune disease(s) | | | | |
| MAS | 3.5 (4/113) | 7.1 (14/197) | 0.48 (0.15–1.49) | 0.196 |
| Familial autoimmunity in FDR | 19.5 (22/113) | 25.4 (50/197) | 0.71 (0.40–1.25) | 0.235 |
| RA | 0.9 (1/113) | 5.6 (11/197) | 0.15 (0.01–1.19) | 0.062 |
| APS | 16.8 (19/113) | 4.1 (8/197) | 4.77 (2.01–11.31) | 0.0001 |
| AITD | 4.4 (5/113) | 9.1 (16/197) | 0.52 (0.18–1.47) | 0.213 |
| Comorbidities | | | | |
| Type 2 diabetes mellitus | 3.5 (4/113) | 1 (2/197) | 3.56 (0.64–19.75) | 0.196 |
| Dyslipidemia | 28.3 (32/113) | 12.2 (24/197) | 2.83 (1.56–5.11) | 0.0001 |
| Fibromyalgia | 14.2 (16/113) | 7.1 (14/197) | 2.14 (1.00–4.57) | 0.045 |
| Treatment | | | | |
| Antimalarials | 77 (87/113) | 82.7 (163/197) | 0.69 (0.39–1.23) | 0.217 |
| Mycophenolate Mofetil | 19.5 (22/113) | 13.7 (27/197) | 1.52 (0.82–2.82) | 0.181 |
| Cytotoxics agents | 17.7 (20/113) | 9.1 (16/197) | 2.13 (1.07–4.23) | 0.027 |
| Clinical variable | | | | |
| Discoid lupus | 5.3 (6/113) | 9.1 (16/197) | 0.55 (0.21–1.44) | 0.225 |
| Alopecia | 41.5 (47/113) | 51.3 (101/197) | 0.67 (0.42–1.08) | 0.101 |
| Subacute | 6.2 (7/113) | 3 (6/197) | 2.10 (0.68–6.41) | 0.239 |
| Urticaria | 19.5 (22) | 10.2 (20/197) | 2.14 (1.11–4.12) | 0.021 |
| Vasculitis | 15 (17/113) | 20.3 (40/197) | 0.89 (0.37–1.29) | 0.250 |
| Neurological involvement | 13.3 (15/113) | 8.1 (16/197) | 1.73 (0.82–3.65) | 0.146 |
| Headache | 28.2 (33/113) | 18.9 (37/197) | 1.79 (1.03–3.06) | 0.035 |
| Psychosis | 7.1 (8/113) | 3.8 (7/197) | 2.08 (0.72–5.86) | 0.164 |
| Serositis | 37.2 (42/113) | 23.9 (47/197) | 1.88 (1.14–3.12) | 0.013 |
| Pleural effusion | 31.9 (36/113) | 18.9 (37/197) | 2.02 (1.18–3.44) | 0.009 |
| Hands edema | 32.7 (37/113) | 15.9 (33/197) | 2.41 (1.40–4.16) | 0.0001 |
| Renal involvement | 56.6 (84/113) | 40.9 (80/197) | 1.91 (1.19–3.05) | 0.006 |
| Nephrotic | 27.4 (31/113) | 10.7 (21/197) | 3.16 (1.71–5.84) | 0.0001 |
| Pulmonary haemorrhage | 3.5 (4/113) | 0.5 (1/197) | 7.19 (0.79–65.16) | 0.061 |
| Laboratory findings | | | | |
| Thrombocytopenia | 11.9 (13/109) | 5.3 (10/187) | 2.39 (1.01–5.67) | 0.041 |
| Leukopenia | 30.6 (34/111) | 42.3 (80/189) | 0.60 (0.36–0.98) | 0.044 |
| Lymphopenia | 71.6 (78/109) | 78.7 (148/188) | 0.68 (0.39–1.17) | 0.163 |
| Abnormal creatinine | 17 (17/100) | 5.4 (8/169) | 3.61 (1.54–8.47) | 0.002 |
| Abnormal creatinine clearance | 64.4 (38/59) | 52.3 (56/107) | 1.64 (0.85–3.17) | 0.133 |
| Proteinuria (+) | 50 (41/82) | 30 (39/130) | 2.33 (1.31–4.13) | 0.003 |
| aCLIgG (+) | 40.7 (35/88) | 29.7 (44/149) | 1.62 (0.93–2.82) | 0.087 |
| Lupus anticoagulant (+) | 58.5 (24/41) | 45.9 (29/61) | 1.66 (0.74–3.70) | 0.211 |

CVD: cardiovascular disease; SLE: systemic lupus erythematosus; OR: odds ratio; CI: confidence interval; IQR: interquartile range; SD: standard deviation; Y: years; MAS: multiple autoimmune syndrome; FDR: first-degree relatives; RA: rheumatoid arthritis; APS: antiphospholipid syndrome; AITD: autoimmune thyroid disease; aCL: anticardiolipin antibodies.

Table 4: Factors associated with CVD in patients with SLE*.

| Characteristic | $\beta$ | AOR | 95% CI | $P$ |
|---|---|---|---|---|
| Dyslipidemia | 0.971 | 2.64 | 1.32–5.28 | 0.005 |
| Pleural effusion | 0.751 | 2.12 | 1.17–3.84 | 0.013 |
| Ever smoking | 0.602 | 1.83 | 1.07–3.10 | 0.025 |
| Coffee consumption | 0.559 | 1.75 | 1.01–3.04 | 0.043 |
| Renal involvement | 0.476 | 1.61 | 0.94–3.84 | 0.081 |

CVD: cardiovascular disease; SLE: systemic lupus erythematosus; $\beta$: $\beta$ coefficient; AOR: adjusted odds ratio; 95% CI: 95% confidence interval.
*The model was adjusted by gender and duration of the disease.

Table 5: Factors associated with CVD in patients with SLE including interaction between smoking and coffee consumption*.

| Characteristic | $\beta$ | AOR | 95% CI | $P$ |
|---|---|---|---|---|
| APS | 1.55 | 4.71 | 1.81–12.2 | 0.001 |
| Dyslipidemia | 1.07 | 2.92 | 1.54–5.55 | 0.001 |
| Pleural effusion | 0.78 | 2.19 | 1.20–3.98 | 0.011 |
| Smoking and coffee | 0.60 | 1.82 | 1.05–3.13 | 0.03 |

CVD: cardiovascular disease; SLE: systemic lupus erythematosus; $\beta$: $\beta$ coefficient; AOR: adjusted odds ratio; CI: confidence interval; APS: antiphospholipid syndrome.
*Adjusted by gender and duration of the disease including interaction between smoking and coffee consumption. $P$-values persisted significant despite the evaluation of the four possible combinations (i.e., smoking, coffee, smoking and coffee, none) through the adjustment of the multivariate model.

having a CVD event. In the PROFILE population, another multicenter, multiethnic study population, Bertoli et al. [111] found that smoking acted as an independent risk factor associated with a 2-fold decrease in time to a CV event among 1,333 SLE patients over a 6.4-year follow-up period.

Several studies have evaluated the association between coffee consumption and CVD in the general population with controversial results. Two Dutch studies [112, 113] found no association between coffee intake, high blood pressure, and CVD. Despite the classification of coffee consumption differed among studies, some results suggest that habitual coffee consumption is associated with increased risk of hypertension [114]. In the same way, Klag et al. [115] demonstrated over many years of followup that coffee drinking is associated with small increases in blood pressure but appears to play a small role in the development of hypertension. When they compared with nondrinkers at baseline, coffee drinkers had a greater incidence of hypertension during follow-up (18.8% versus. 28.3%; $P = 0.03$). Relative risk (95% confidence interval) of hypertension associated with drinking 5 or more cups a day was 1.35 (0.87–2.08) for baseline intake and 1.60 (1.06–2.40) for intake over followup. Other effects attributed to coffee drinking are the increase in systemic vascular resistance, increased serum cholesterol levels, arterial stiffness, plasma rennin activity, epinephrine and norepinephrine, driving an unfavorable effect on endothelial function in healthy population [116]. On the other hand an Australia study [117] detected a negative association between coffee, hypertension, and MetS. Likewise, an increase in flow-mediated dilation and a decrease in CRP levels related to coffee drinking have been observed regardless of CAD [118, 119].

In order to isolate the interaction of smoking and coffee consumption, two regression models were made in which both the independent effect of coffee and smoking consumption on CVD as well as their interaction remains significant, demonstrating synergism between them (i.e., multiplicative effect). Otherwise, coffee consumption has not been evaluated systematically in SLE patients with CVD. However, since there is not a universal accepted tool for assessing coffee consumption, a bias concerning this variable is not precluded. Furthermore, membership bias could also exist because coffee consumption in Colombia is a well-defined tradition.

*4.4. Traditional Risk Factors for CVD in SLE.* Diverse lupus cohorts had shown the influence of advanced age, dyslipidemia, obesity, hypertension, and hyperhomocysteinemia, as classical risk factors for CVD [109, 120, 121]. Younger patients with SLE have the greatest relative risk compared to their healthy counterparts, but the absolute risk of CVD among SLE patients increases with advancing age [8]. de Souza et al. [58] observed that young Brazilian patients with SLE presented higher prevalence of carotid plaque than controls.

López-Jaramillo et al. [122] showed that the concentration of proinflammatory cytokines is higher in the LA population than in developed countries, suggesting a higher susceptibility to develop systemic low-degree inflammation at a given level of abdominal obesity, which contributes to the burden of CVD in this population. The inflammatory milieu of SLE leads to deregulation of lipid metabolism pathways, which contribute to the increased risk of atherosclerotic disease among these patients [123, 124]. Five large cohort studies have shown hypercholesterolemia as a risk factor for CVD in SLE patients [98, 103, 125–127]. Our results confirm the role of dyslipidemia as an independent risk factor for CVD in LA patients with SLE [50, 52, 53, 58, 60, 62–64, 66, 80, 81, 83, 84, 89]. For more details see Table 6.

*4.5. Nontraditional Risk Factors for CVD in SLE.* It is well known that while traditional CVD risk factors are undoubtedly important in increasing the CVD risk among SLE patients, these do not fully account for the elevated risk of CVD in this population [9]. Thereby, SLE-associated factors play an important role in the premature atherosclerosis process characteristic of these patients [128, 129]. Evidence strongly suggests that atherosclerotic plaque is largely driven

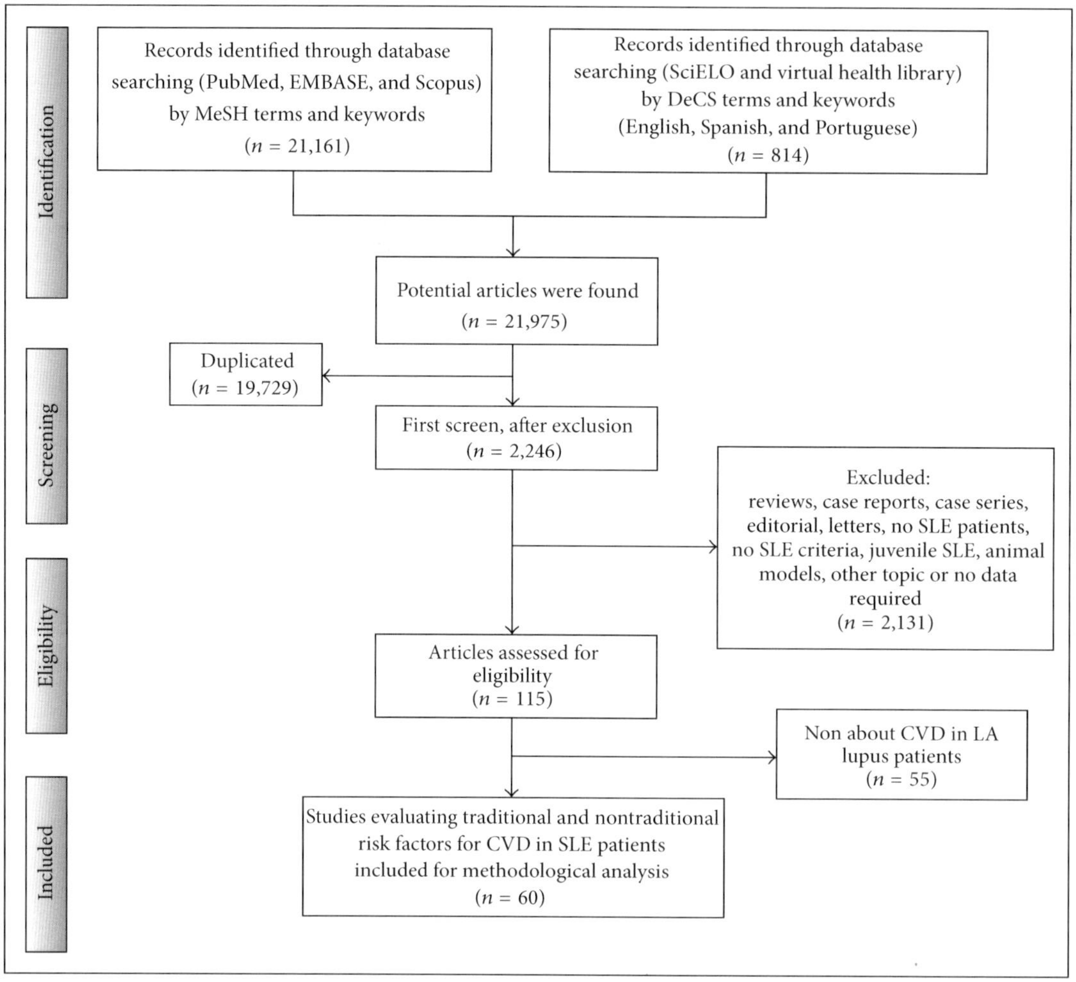


FIGURE 1: Flowchart of the systematic literature review. SLE: systemic lupus erythematosus, CVD: cardiovascular disease, LA: Latin America.

by inflammation and an active immunological response [130–132] and points to SLE itself as an independent risk factor for premature CAD [133, 134]. Nontraditional risk factors for CVD in ADs may be classified into genetics, AD-related, and miscellaneous [135, 136].

Family and twin studies have repeatedly supported a role for heredity in CAD, particularly in young individuals. Several genetic markers have been proposed as predisposing factors for CVD in SLE patients [87, 137, 138]. The SLE-associated risk factors represent a broad spectrum of conditions related to the autoimmune nature of the disease. All of these pathways may eventually converge into a shared proatherogenic phenotype [139]. Table 6 summarizes the state of the art of CVD risk factors in LA patients with SLE.

*4.6. Assessment and Management of CV Risk in SLE Patients.* Physicians often face the question of how to personalize treatment and prevention of CV events. Framingham risk score (FRS) is widely used to stratify asymptomatic patients into different CV risk categories in order to target the intensity of primary medical intervention. This score is strongly influenced by age and therefore has limited usefulness in young patients with SLE [140]. Therefore, evaluation of only traditional CAD risk factors in lupus patients may result in the underestimation of their future overall CAD risk. The contribution of inflammatory biomarkers should be also considered to gain a complete picture of the CAD risk in patients with underlying conditions that increase inflammation such as SLE [141]. The Reynolds Risk score incorporates CRP concentration in the risk model and reclassifies approximately 50% of women in the 10-year FRS 5–20% risk category into different risk categories [142]. Another proposed approach corresponds to Systematic Coronary Risk Evaluation that is recommended by the EULAR experts and is widely used for CV assessment in patients with rheumatoid arthritis and other forms of inflammatory arthritis [143]. Neither of these charts includes the broad variety of risk factors that are disease-specific and could potentially explain the increased burden due to CV events. Therefore, CV risk in SLE patients is consistently underestimated with these scales.

Recently, Petri and Magder [144] proposed a data-driven risk equation of CV risk in SLE, based on data collected in a longitudinal cohort that can better estimate 10-year CV risk than the Framingham equation. In this model an integer score is given to each variable including age over 40, male gender, systolic blood pressure over 140, TC over 160,

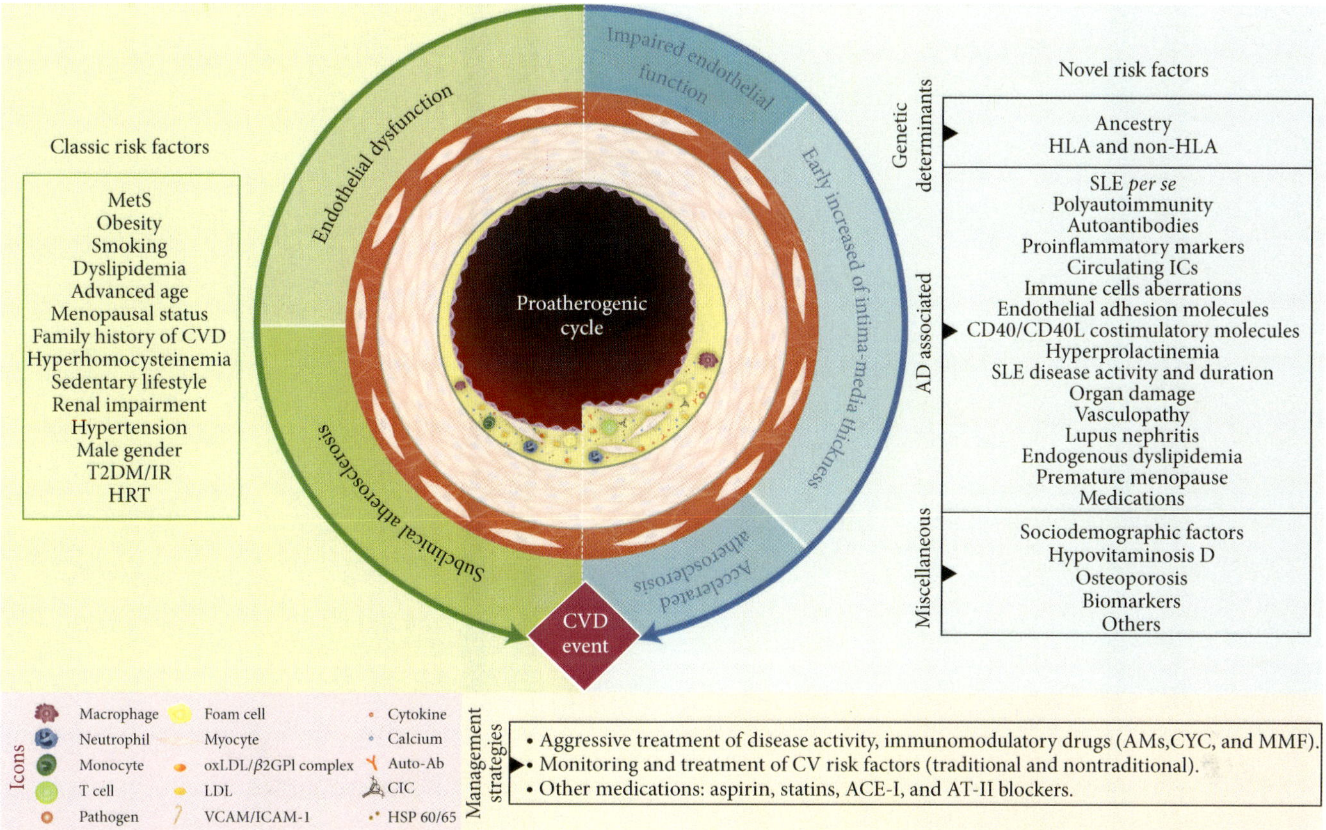


FIGURE 2: Traditional and autoimmune-related mechanisms of cardiovascular disease in systemic lupus erythematosus. A complex interaction between traditional and disease-specific traits leads to premature atherosclerotic process. Several risk factors (left) have been described since The Framingham Heart Study, known as classic risk factors, which over time conduce to endothelial dysfunction, subclinical atherosclerosis, and CV event manifest. In the autoimmune setting (right), a broad spectrum of novel risk factors contribute to development of premature vascular damage. This damage is represented by impaired endothelial function and early increased of Intima-Media Thickness which are surrogates of the accelerated atherosclerosis process, which is perpetuated by a chronic proinflammatory milieu. The cornerstone of management of CV risk include an aggressive treatment of disease activity, the continuous monitoring and treatment of modifiable CV risk factors, as well as the use of other medications in order to diminish de CV burden. CVD: cardiovascular disease, SLE: systemic lupus erythematosus, MetS: metabolic syndrome, T2DM: type 2 diabetes mellitus, IR: insulin resistance, HRT: hormone replacement therapy, CIC: Circulating Immune complex, oxLDL/B2GPI complex: oxidized-low density lipoprotein/$\beta$2 glycoprotein I, HDL: high density lipoprotein, Auto-Ab: auto-antibodies, AMs: antimalarials, CYC: cyclophosphamide, AZA: azathioprine, MMF: mycophenolate mofetil, ACE-I: angiotensin-converting enzyme inhibitors, AT-II blockers: angiotensin II receptor blockers.

smoking, T2DM, mean SLE disease activity index (SLEDAI), history of lupus anticoagulant, and low mean C3. Using this model, together in the absence of SLE-specific risk factors, the estimated risk is higher than what would be projected based on the FRS. Nevertheless, this model is not exempt: limitations on, for example, HDL and LDL are not available at all routine visits. Further validation of this model is warranted.

SLE entails a CVD equivalent to T2DM; thus, lower lipid goals, aspirin use, and an aggressive monitoring are required [145, 146]. Studies aimed to evaluate whether or not traditional treatment regimens prevent or slow atherosclerosis in SLE patients have been published [147]. The recent randomized controlled Lupus Atherosclerosis Prevention Study suggested that atorvastatin do not slow progression of subclinical atherosclerosis [148].

There are several new mechanisms of action described for antimalarials, many of them with beneficial effects in the management of CV risk in patients with SLE [149, 150]. There is evidence that antimalarials reduce serum cholesterol and LDL levels, elevate HDL cholesterol, and when taken concomitantly with steroids can reduce serum cholesterol [151]. Penn et al. [152] suggested that hydroxychloroquine use is associated with a lower fasting glucose and a decrease in the homeostasis model assessment-insulin resistance (HOMA-IR) index. Rekedal et al. [153] showed that hydroxychloroquine initiation was associated with a significantly greater reduction in HbA1c as compared to methotrexate initiation among diabetic patients with rheumatic diseases. In addition, beneficial effects of hydroxycloroquine on thrombosis formation have also been described. Multiple retrospective cohort studies have shown a reduced incidence of thrombotic events and improved overall survival in patients with SLE treated with antimalarials [154–157].

The presence of low vitamin D levels has been associated with disrupting self-tolerance. Therefore, it is tempting to speculate that vitamin D might prove useful as a preventive

TABLE 6: Traditional and nontraditional risk factors associated with cardiovascular disease and systemic lupus erythematosus in Latin America.

| Risk factor associated with CVD | Comments | Reference(s) |
|---|---|---|
| | Traditional | |
| Hypertension | Hypertension influences the risk of death by CVD in SLE patients. | [64, 89] |
| | Hypertension acts as CVD subphenotype as well as a risk factor. | [45, 49, 71, 88] |
| | Patients with SLE were at increased risk of thrombosis when it is associated with hypertension. | [17, 80, 84] |
| | Compared with patients without atherosclerotic plaque, those with plaque had higher prevalence of hypertension. | [54, 63, 66, 73] |
| | Lupus patients with abnormal myocardial scintigraphic findings and hypertension, as a risk factor for CAD, had a higher risk of abnormal findings on coronary angiography. | [52, 53] |
| | Patients with lupus had higher hypertension prevalence than controls with noninflammatory disorders. | [14, 68, 90] |
| T2DM | T2DM influence on abnormal myocardial perfusion in asymptomatic patients with SLE. | [53] |
| | Alterations in glycemic profile were associated with traditional risk factors for CHD and lupus characteristics, including CVD, damage index, and renal involvement. | [17, 68, 81] |
| | Patients with SLE and T2DM were at increased risk of thrombosis. This risk remains elevated throughout the course of the disease. | [16, 80] |
| | T2DM is an independent risk factor for atherosclerotic plaque and CAC. | [63, 71, 84] |
| Dyslipidemia | The main risk factor for death in SLE was heart involvement, which was influenced by dyslipidemia. | [50, 89] |
| | High levels of TGL were associated with myocardial perfusion abnormalities and endothelial dysfunction | [52, 53, 83] |
| | There was high prevalence of dyslipidemia as risk factor for thrombotic events. | [60, 62, 80] |
| | Alterations in lipid profile was a risk factor for premature CAC in young women with SLE. | [66, 84] |
| | CAD was more prevalent in dyslipidemic women with SLE than controls. | [64, 81] |
| | Compared with patients without atherosclerotic plaque, those with plaque had high level of TGL and LDL. | [58, 63] |
| Male gender | Male gender was a risk factor for developing severe organ damage (CVD) and mortality in SLE patients. | [16, 17, 53, 60] |
| | Males with SLE were at increased risk of thrombosis and CAC. This risk remains elevated throughout the course of the disease. | [80, 84, 85] |
| | Patients had more peripheral vascular and gonadal involvement compared with published data from non-Hispanic SLE populations. | [76] |
| MetS | SLE patients had a high prevalence of MetS that directly contributes to increasing inflammatory status and oxidative stress. | [69] |
| | MetS was associated with traditional risk factors for CHD and lupus characteristics, including CVD, damage Index, and renal involvement. | [68, 81] |
| | Presence of MetS was related to CVD in SLE patients. | [90, 94] |
| Obesity | Patients with SLE who had excess weight present distinct clinical-laboratory findings, sociodemographic characteristics, and treatment options when compared to normal weight patients. | [17, 71, 81] |
| | Excess weight is associated with some traditional risk factors for CVD and SLE poor prognosis. | [58, 65, 68] |
| | Increase weight influence on abnormal myocardial perfusion in asymptomatic patients with SLE. | [53, 64] |
| | SLE patients with high BMI have increased QT interval parameters when compared to controls. This prolongation may lead to an increased CV risk. | [55] |
| | Major values in BMI were related with the presence of CAD and carotid plaque. | [58, 63, 64] |

Table 6: Continued.

| Risk factor associated with CVD | Comments | Reference(s) |
|---|---|---|
| Smoking | Smoking is an important determinant in the occurrence of thrombotic (central and/or peripheral, arterial and/or venous) events in SLE patients. | [18, 69, 81] |
| | Smoking was an independent risk factor for atherosclerotic plaque and thrombosis. | [63, 68, 80] |
| | Smoking habit influence on abnormal myocardial perfusion in asymptomatic patients with SLE. | [53] |
| | Smoking was a risk factor for premature CAC in young women with SLE. | [66, 84] |
| Advance age | CAD was more prevalent in women with SLE. | [64, 85, 86] |
| | Several traditional risk factors, including age, appear to be important contributors to atherosclerotic CV damage. | [16, 71] |
| | The presence of CVD has been associated with older age. | [16, 59] |
| | Age was directly related with atherosclerotic plaque formation. | [63] |
| Menopausal status | High percentage of SLE patients with abnormal angiographic findings was in postmenopausal status. | [52] |
| | There is high prevalence of premature menopausal status as a risk factor for CVD. | [60] |
| | Postmenopausal status was a risk factor for premature CAC in young women with SLE. | [66, 68, 84] |
| | Postmenopausal women had a higher prevalence of subclinical AT and abnormal myocardial perfusion in asymptomatic patients with SLE. | [53, 63] |
| Family history of CVD | Familial history of CVD was an independent risk factor for atherosclerotic process. | [17, 63, 68] |
| | Family history of CVD was a risk factor for premature CAC in young women with SLE. | [66, 84] |
| | Family history of CVD influence on abnormal myocardial perfusion in asymptomatic patients with SLE. | [53] |
| HRT | HRT use was not associated with the occurrence of vascular arterial events in the LUMINA patients. HRT use in women with SLE should be individualized, but data suggest its use may be safe if aPL antibodies are not present or vascular arterial events have not previously occurred. | [17] |
| Hyperhomocysteinemia | Hyperhomocysteinemia was a risk factor for CAC in SLE patients. | [84] |
| | The presence of polyautoimmunity and hyperhomocysteinemia was risk factors for thrombotic events. | [41] |
| | Nontraditional | |
| *Genetic determinants* | | |
| Ancestry | There are several differences regarding clinical (including CVD), prognostic, socioeconomic, educational, and access to medical care features in GLADEL cohort according to ancestry (White, Mestizo, and African-LA). | [14] |
| Non-HLA | An SNP in FGG rs2066865 demonstrated association with arterial thrombosis risk in Hispanic Americans patients with SLE. | [87] |
| | The CRP GT20 variant is more likely to occur in African-American and Hispanic SLE patients than in Caucasian ones, and SLE patients carrying the GT20 allele are more likely to develop vascular arterial events (LUMINA multiethnic cohort). | [86] |
| *SLE-associated* | | |
| Poliautoimmunity | The presence of APS was the major independent contributor to the development of severe organ damage in Brazilian patients with SLE. | [54] |
| | APS and its characteristic antibodies may contribute to the development of thrombotic events in Brazilian and Mexican lupus patients. | [57, 78] |
| | APS had high impact in CVD and survival in Brazilian lupus patients. | [42] |
| | Polyautoimmunity (APS) may suggest concerted pathogenic actions with other autoantibodies in the development of thrombotic events in Mexican patients with SLE. | [78] |

Table 6: Continued.

| Risk factor associated with CVD | Comments | Reference(s) |
|---|---|---|
| SLE *per se* | SLE diagnosis was significantly associated with carotid plaque formation and development of CV event in Brazilian patients with SLE. | [58] |
| | High percentage of patients with abnormal angiographic findings had higher ACR criteria number for SLE Brazilian patients with SLE. | [52] |
| Autoantibodies | One of the independent predictors of vascular events in a multiethnic US cohort (LUMINA) was the presence of any aPL antibody. | [17] |
| | anti-$\beta$2GPI antibodies were strongly associated with thrombosis in patients with Mexicans with SLE. The decrease of anti-$\beta$2GPI levels at the time of thrombosis may indicate a pathogenic role. | [77] |
| | The higher frequency of aPT found in Mexican patients with SLE with thrombosis may suggest concerted pathogenic actions with other autoantibodies in the development of thrombotic events. | [78] |
| | Patients with aCL antibodies seem to be at an increased risk for arterial and venous thrombotic events in Puerto Ricans and Chilean patients with SLE. | [92, 96] |
| | There was correlation between lupus anticoagulant and thrombotic events in Brazilian lupus patients. | [50] |
| | aCL antibodies were associated with thrombotic events, mainly in high titers in Chilean SLE patients. | [96] |
| | aCL antibodies were significantly associated with CV events and showed an association with echocardiographic abnormalities in Brazilian patients with SLE. | [51] |
| | Mexican patients had more peripheral vascular compared with published data from non-Hispanic SLE populations. | [76] |
| Immune cells aberrations | Complement fixing activity of aCL antibodies seems to be relevant in thrombotic venous events in Brazilian patients with SLE. | [57] |
| Inflammatory markers | Increased ESR was independently associated with MetS in Puerto Ricans lupic patients. | [94] |
| | One of the independent predictors of vascular events in a multiethnic US cohort (LUMINA) was elevated serum levels of CRP. | [16, 17] |
| Endogenous dyslipidemia | HDL distribution and composition (−HDL2b, +HDL3b, and +HDL3c) were abnormal in noncomplicated Mexican SLE patients. | [79] |
| | Low HDL levels and increased TGL levels were associated with atherosclerosis by cIMT measurement in Colombian lupic patients. | [95] |
| | SLE patients have a lipid profile abnormality in Brazilian patients with SLE. This pattern of dyslipoproteinemia may increase the risk of developing CAD. | [47] |
| Disease activity | Disease activity (SLAM) is an important determinant in the occurrence of thrombotic (central and/or peripheral, arterial, and/or venous) events in the LUMINA cohort. | [18] |
| | SLEDAI scores were positively correlated with BMI and WC in Brazilian population with SLE. | [69] |
| | Higher disease activity was independently associated with MetS and thrombosis in Puerto Ricans and Mexican SLE patients. | [80, 94] |
| | Higher score of SLICC was associated with atherosclerotic plaque in Brazilian SLE patients. | [58] |
| | High scores in diseases activity index (SLEDAI and SLICC) were associated with myocardial perfusion abnormalities in Brazilian SLE patients. | [52] |
| | Brazilian SLE patients have a lipid profile abnormality which is aggravated by disease activity and may reside in a defect of VLDL metabolism. | [47] |
| | Disease activity was predictor of CAC in Mexican SLE patients. | [84] |
| | Higher disease activity was independently associated with MetS in Puerto Ricans patients with SLE. | [94] |

Table 6: Continued.

| Risk factor associated with CVD | Comments | Reference(s) |
|---|---|---|
| Organ damage | Baseline and accrued damage increase mortality risk (including due to CVD) in Brazilian patients with SLE. | [61] |
| | Mexican patients had more peripheral vascular involvement (measured by SDI), compared with published data from non-Hispanic SLE populations. | [76] |
| | In Brazilian SLE patients, MetS was associated with both traditional risk factors for CHD and lupus characteristics including damage index. | [68] |
| | There was a correlation between IMT and revised damage index (SLICC) in Brazilian SLE patients. | [58] |
| | Atherosclerotic CV damage in SLE is multifactorial, and disease-related factors (including CRP levels and SDI at baseline) appear to be important contributors to such an occurrence (LUMINA multiethnic cohort). | [16] |
| Long duration | Longer duration of SLE was associated with atherosclerotic plaque and CV events in Brazilian population. | [58, 59] |
| | A correlation between IMT and duration of the disease was found in Brazilian patients with SLE. | [63] |
| | Disease duration was independent predictor for premature CAC in young Brazilian women with SLE. | [66] |
| Medications | PDN > 10 mg/day was independently associated with MetS in Puerto Ricans SLE patients. | [94] |
| | In Brazilian SLE patients, there was a correlation between IMT and the duration of PDN use. | [63] |
| | IHD was observed in two types of Mexican SLE patients: those with long-term steroid therapy and those with frank episodes of vasculitis. | [73] |
| Vasculopathy | Current vasculitis was associated with abnormal myocardial scintigraphy in Brazilian patients with SLE. | [53] |
| | Puerto Ricans patients with SLE and RP seem to be at increased risk for arterial and venous thrombotic events. | [92] |
| | IHD was observed in two types of Mexican SLE patients: those with long-term steroid therapy and those with frank episodes of vasculitis. | [73] |
| Renal involvement | In Brazilian SLE patients, MetS was associated with traditional risk factors for CHD and lupus characteristics, including damage index and renal involvement (nephritic syndrome). | [68] |
| *Miscellaneous* | | |
| BMD | Decreased BMD was an independent predictor for premature CAC in Brazilian young women with SLE. | [66] |
| Sociodemographic factors | A low education and monthly income were associated with MetS in Mexican patients with SLE and RA. | [81] |

aCL: anticardiolipins antibodies; ACR: American College of Rheumatology; anti-$\beta$2GPI: anti-beta2 glycoprotein 1 antibodies; aPT: antiprothrombin antibodies; aPL: antiphospholipid antibodies; APS: antiphospholipid syndrome; AT: atherosclerosis; BMD: bone mineral density; BMI: body mass index; CAC: coronary artery calcification; CAD: coronary artery disease; cIMT: carotid Intimal Medial Thickness; CHD: coronary heart disease; CRP: C-reactive protein; CV: cardiovascular; CVD: cardiovascular disease; ESR: erythrocyte sedimentation rate; GLADEL: Grupo Latino Americano De Estudio de Lupus; HDL: high-density lipoprotein cholesterol; HRT: hormone replacement therapy; IHD: ischemic heart disease; IMT: intimal media thickness; LA: Latin America; LDL: low-density lipoprotein cholesterol; LUMINA: LUpus in MInorities: NAture versus nurture cohort; MetS: metabolic syndrome; PDN: prednisolone; RP: Raynaud's phenomenon; T2DM: type 2 diabetes mellitus; TGL: triglycerides; SLAM: Systemic Lupus Activity Measure; SLE: systemic lupus erythematosus; SLEDAI: systemic lupus erythematosus disease activity index; SLICC: Systemic Lupus International Collaborating Clinics score; SDI: SLICC damage index; SNP: single-nucleotide polymorphism; VLDL: very low-density lipoprotein cholesterol; WC: waist circumference.

agent by reducing the risk of developing an autoimmune response [158]. In addition, vitamin D has been found to have antithrombotic properties improving the risk of CVD. Vitamin D deficiency has been linked to the development of atherosclerosis. As a corollary, the use of vitamin D may be useful to improve microvascular endothelial function [158].

## 5. Limitations of the Study

As a cross-sectional study, it is placed at level 4 of evidence according to Oxford Evidence Based Medicine [40]. Although the study sample size is not negligible, it would have been more valuable to have had an appropirate followup to establish valid associations between CVD, novel risk factors, and SLE. This, in turn, could have improved both internal and external validities.

The diversity of parameters defining CVD in SLE precluded homogenization of analysis and assessment in the systematic review. Often, one or two CVD subphenotypes were assessed as primary outcomes but many did not consider general CVD compromise. Therefore, it was not possible to perform a meta-analysis and to establish true measures of association such as odds ratios. Finally, we acknowledge that publication bias may exist.

## 6. Final Remarks and Conclusions

CVD is a major cause of morbidity and mortality in SLE patients. SLE and CVD share common pathophysiology mechanisms (i.e., systemic and chronic inflammation) with secondary accelerated atherosclerosis. Since traditional risk factors do not completely explain the high rates of CVD in patients with SLE, novel risk factors related to autoimmunity are now recognized. In the current study classical risk factors such as dyslipidemia, coffee consumption, and smoking habit are highlighted, and SLE-related factors (i.e., SLE-antiphospholipid syndrome polyautoimmunity, pleural effusion, and renal involvement) are confirmed. In addition, several factors associated with CVD in LA patients with SLE were reviewed. Altogether, our results should encourage preventive population strategies for CVD in patients with SLE [106, 159], aimed at facilitating the suppression of cigarette smoking and coffee consumption as well as to the tight control of dyslipidemia and other modifiable risk factors.

## Conflict of Interests

The authors have indicated that they have no conflict of interests regarding the content of this paper.

## Author's Contribution

Jenny Amaya-Amaya and Juan Camilo Sarmiento-Monroy contributed equally to this work.

## Acknowledgments

The authors thank all patients for their participation in the study, José-Leonardo Pérez-Fernández, Ana Catalina Herrera Díaz, and colleagues at the Center for Autoimmune Diseases Research (CREA) for their fruitful discussions and contributions. This work was supported by the School of Medicine and Health Sciences, Universidad del Rosario, Bogotá, Colombia.

## References

[1] Z. Liu and A. Davidson, "Taming lupus—a new understanding of pathogenesis is leading to clinical advances," *Nature Medicine*, vol. 18, pp. 871–882, 2012.

[2] G. C. Tsokos, "Mechanisms of disease: systemic lupus erythematosus," *The New England Journal of Medicine*, vol. 365, no. 22, pp. 2110–2121, 2011.

[3] S. G. Guerra, T. J. Vyse, and D. S. C. Graham, "The genetics of lupus: a functional perspective," *Arthritis Research and Therapy*, vol. 14, article 211, 2012.

[4] D. P. D'Cruz, M. A. Khamashta, and G. R. Hughes, "Systemic lupus erythematosus," *The Lancet*, vol. 369, no. 9561, pp. 587–596, 2007.

[5] M. B. Urowitz, A. A. M. Bookman, B. E. Koehler, D. A. Gordon, H. A. Smythe, and M. A. Ogryzlo, "The bimodal mortality pattern of systemic lupus erythematosus," *The American Journal of Medicine*, vol. 60, no. 2, pp. 221–225, 1976.

[6] L. Björnådal, L. Yin, F. Granath, L. Klareskog, and A. Ekbom, "Cardiovascular disease a hazard despite improved prognosis in patients with systemic lupus erythematosus: results from a Swedish population based study 1964–95," *Journal of Rheumatology*, vol. 31, no. 4, pp. 713–719, 2004.

[7] A. Bitton and T. Gaziano, "The Framingham heart study's impact on global risk assessment," *Progress in Cardiovascular Diseases*, vol. 53, no. 1, pp. 68–78, 2010.

[8] S. R. Schoenfeld, S. Kasturi, and K. H. Costenbader, "The epidemiology of atherosclerotic cardiovascular disease among patients with SLE: a systematic review," *Seminars in Arthritis and Rheumatism*, vol. 43, no. 1, pp. 77–95, 2013.

[9] J. M. Esdaile, M. Abrahamowicz, T. Grodzicky et al., "Traditional Framingham risk factors fail to fully account for accelerated atherosclerosis in systemic lupus erythematosus," *Arthritis and Rheumatism*, vol. 44, no. 10, pp. 2331–2337, 2001.

[10] E. González Burchard, L. N. Borrell, S. Choudhry et al., "Latino populations: a unique opportunity for the study of race, genetics, and social environment in epidemiological research," *The American Journal of Public Health*, vol. 95, no. 12, pp. 2161–2168, 2005.

[11] A. L. Price, N. Patterson, F. Yu et al., "A genomewide admixture map for latino populations," *The American Journal of Human Genetics*, vol. 80, no. 6, pp. 1024–1036, 2007.

[12] E. Lora, "Health perceptions in Latin America," *Health Policy and Planning*, vol. 27, pp. 555–569, 2012.

[13] S. M. Barreto, J. J. Miranda, J. P. Figueroa et al., "Epidemiology in Latin America and the Caribbean: current situation and challenges," *International Journal of Epidemiology*, vol. 41, no. 2, pp. 557–571, 2012.

[14] B. A. Pons-Estel, L. J. Catoggio, M. H. Cardiel et al., "The GLADEL multinational Latin American prospective inception cohort of 1,214 patients with systemic lupus erythematosus: ethnic and disease heterogeneity among 'hispanics'," *Medicine*, vol. 83, no. 1, pp. 1–17, 2004.

[15] S. Chaiamnuay, A. M. Bertoli, M. Fernández et al., "The impact of increased body mass index on systemic lupus erythematosus: data from LUMINA, a multiethnic cohort (LUMINA XLVI) [corrected]," *Journal of Clinical Rheumatology*, vol. 13, no. 3, pp. 128–133, 2007.

[16] G. J. Pons-Estel, L. A. González, J. Zhang et al., "Predictors of cardiovascular damage in patients with systemic lupus erythematosus: data from LUMINA (LXVIII), a multiethnic US cohort," *Rheumatology*, vol. 48, no. 7, pp. 817–822, 2009.

[17] S. M. A. Toloza, A. G. Uribe, G. McGwin Jr. et al., "Systemic lupus erythematosus in a multiethnic US cohort (LUMINA): XXIII. Baseline predictors of vascular events," *Arthritis and Rheumatism*, vol. 50, no. 12, pp. 3947–3957, 2004.

[18] K. T. Ho, C. W. Ahn, G. S. Alarcón et al., "Systemic lupus erythematosus in a multiethnic cohort (LUMINA): XXVIII. Factors predictive of thrombotic events," *Rheumatology*, vol. 44, no. 10, pp. 1303–1307, 2005.

[19] P. I. Burgos, G. McGwin Jr., J. D. Reveille, L. M. Vilá, and G. S. Alarcón, "Factors predictive of thrombotic events in LUMINA, a multi-ethnic cohort of SLE patients (LXXII)," *Rheumatology*, vol. 49, no. 9, Article ID keq140, pp. 1720–1725, 2010.

[20] E. L. Smith and R. H. Shmerling, "The American college of rheumatology criteria for the classification of systemic lupus erythematosus: strengths, weaknesses, and opportunities for improvement," *Lupus*, vol. 8, no. 8, pp. 586–595, 1999.

[21] M. C. Hochberg, "Updating the American college of rheumatology revised criteria for the classification of systemic lupus erythematosus," *Arthritis and Rheumatism*, vol. 40, no. 9, p. 1725, 1997.

[22] Colombia, Law no. 30, Public Service in Higher Education, 1992.

[23] Colombia, Law no. 115, General on education, 1994.

[24] C. Barragán-Martínez, C. A. Speck-Hernández, G. Montoya-Ortiz, R. D. Mantilla, J. M. Anaya, and A. Rojas-Villarraga, "Organic solvents as risk factor for autoimmune diseases: a systematic review and meta-analysis," *PLoS ONE*, vol. 7, no. 12, Article ID e51506, 2012.

[25] Y. Shoenfeld and R. Cervera, *Diagnostic Criteria in Autoimmune Diseases*, 2008.

[26] A. Rojas-Villarraga, J. Amaya-Amaya, A. Rodriguez-Rodriguez, R. D. Mantilla, and J. M. Anaya, "Introducing polyautoimmunity: secondary autoimmune diseases no longer exist," *Autoimmune Diseases*, vol. 2012, Article ID 254319, 9 pages, 2012.

[27] J. M. Anaya, R. Corena, J. Castiblanco, A. Rojas-Villarraga, and Y. Shoenfeld, "The kaleidoscope of autoimmunity: multiple autoimmune syndromes and familial autoimmunity," *Expert Review of Clinical Immunology*, vol. 3, no. 4, pp. 623–635, 2007.

[28] J. M. Anaya, "The autoimmune tautology," *Arthritis Research and Therapy*, vol. 12, no. 6, article 147, 2010.

[29] J. Cárdenas-Roldán, A. Rojas-Villarraga, and J. M. Anaya, "How do autoimmune diseases cluster in families? A systematic review and meta-analysis," *BMC Medicine*, vol. 11, article 73, 2013.

[30] D. W. Jones and J. E. Hall, "Seventh report of the joint national committee on prevention, detection, evaluation, and treatment of high blood pressure and evidence from new hypertension trials," *Hypertension*, vol. 43, no. 1, pp. 1–3, 2004.

[31] N. J. Stone, S. Bilek, and S. Rosenbaum, "Recent national cholesterol education program adult treatment panel III update: adjustments and options," *The American Journal of Cardiology*, vol. 96, no. 4, pp. 53E–59E, 2005.

[32] P. W. F. Wilson, R. B. D'Agostino, D. Levy, A. M. Belanger, H. Silbershatz, and W. B. Kannel, "Prediction of coronary heart disease using risk factor categories," *Circulation*, vol. 97, no. 18, pp. 1837–1847, 1998.

[33] S. M. Grundy, R. Pasternak, P. Greenland, S. Smith Jr., and V. Fuster, "Assessment of cardiovascular risk by use of multiple-risk-factor assessment equations: a statement for healthcare professionals from the American heart association and the American college of cardiology," *Circulation*, vol. 100, no. 13, pp. 1481–1492, 1999.

[34] Asia Pacific Cohort Studies Collaboration, "The impact of cardiovascular risk factors on the age-related excess risk of coronary heart disease," *International Journal of Epidemiology*, vol. 35, no. 4, pp. 1025–1033, 2006.

[35] American Diabetes Association, "Standards of medical care in diabetes—2012," *Diabetes Care*, vol. 35, supplement 1, pp. S11–S63, 2012.

[36] Z. Reiner, A. L. Catapano, G. de Backer et al., "ESC/EAS Guidelines for the management of dyslipidaemias: the task force for the management of dyslipidaemias of the European society of cardiology (ESC) and the European atherosclerosis society (EAS)," *European Heart Journal*, vol. 32, no. 14, pp. 1769–1818, 2011.

[37] British Cardiac Society, British Hyperlipidaemia Association, British Hypertension Society, and British Diabetic Association, "Joint British recommendations on prevention of coronary heart disease in clinical practice: summary," *The British Medical Journal*, vol. 320, no. 7236, pp. 705–708, 2000.

[38] A. Liberati, D. G. Altman, J. Tetzlaff et al., "The PRISMA statement for reporting systematic reviews and meta-analyses of studies that evaluate health care interventions: explanation and elaboration," *Journal of Clinical Epidemiology*, vol. 62, pp. e1–34, 2009.

[39] F. J. Mateen, J. Oh, A. I. Tergas, N. H. Bhayani, and B. B. Kamdar, "Titles versus titles and abstracts for initial screening of articles for systematic reviews," *Clinical Epidemiology*, vol. 6, pp. 89–95, 2013.

[40] OCEBM Levels of Evidence Working Group, *The Oxford 2011 Levels of Evidence*, Oxford Centre for Evidence-Based Medicine, 2011.

[41] L. Onetti, S. Villafañe, E. Menso et al., "Hyperhomocystinemia as a thrombotic risk factor in patients suffering from systemic lupus erithematosus and antiphospholipid syndrome," *Revista de la Facultad de Ciencias Médicas*, vol. 62, no. 3, pp. 19–23, 2005.

[42] F. V. Signorelli, G. F. Salles, and J. A. Papi, "Antiphospholipid syndrome as predictor of mortality in Brazilian patients with systemic lupus erythematosus," *Lupus*, vol. 20, article 419, 2011.

[43] J. Cabiedes, A. R. Cabral, and D. Alarcon-Segovia, "Clinical manifestations of the antiphospholipid syndrome in patients with systemic lupus erythematosus associate move strongly with anti-$\beta$2-glycoprotein-I than with antiphospholipid antibodies," *Journal of Rheumatology*, vol. 22, no. 10, pp. 1899–1906, 1995.

[44] C. J. Bastos, A. C. Queiroz, and R. Martinelli, "Cardiac involvement in systemic lupus erythematosus: anatomo-pathological study," *Revista da Associação Médica Brasileira*, vol. 39, no. 3, pp. 161–164, 1993.

[45] W. H. Chahade, E. I. Sato, J. E. Moura Jr., L. T. L. Costallat, and L. E. C. Andrade, "Occasional series: lupus around the world. Systemic lupus erythematosus in Sao Paulo, Brazil: a clinical and laboratory overview," *Lupus*, vol. 4, no. 2, pp. 100–103, 1995.

[46] L. J. Alves, L. Hydalgo, L. F. Rolim et al., "Clinical and laboratorial diagnosis of heart disease in systemic lupus erythematosus," *Arquivos Brasileiros de Cardiologia*, vol. 68, no. 2, pp. 79–83, 1997.

[47] E. F. Borba and E. Bonfá, "Dyslipoproteinemias in systemic lupus erythematosus: influence of disease, activity, and anticardiolipin antibodies," *Lupus*, vol. 6, no. 6, pp. 533–539, 1997.

[48] L. T. L. Costallat, C. P. L. C. Lia, N. L. Neto, R. M. Yamada, and A. M. Samara, "Causes of death in systemic lupus erythematosus," *Revista Brasileira de Reumatologia*, vol. 37, no. 4, pp. 205–209, 1997.

[49] M. C. B. T. Rocha, S. S. Teixeira, C. Bueno, M. B. G. Vendramini, R. P. Martinelli, and M. B. Santiago, "Demographic, clinical, and laboratory profile of 100 patients with systemic lupus erythematosus in the State of Bahia," *Revista Brasileira de Reumatologia*, vol. 40, no. 5, pp. 221–230, 2000.

[50] A. C. Travassos, M. C. Rocha, S. Souza, C. Brandao, J. F. Silva, and M. Santiago, "Freqtiencia dos anticorpos antifosfolfpides

(aFL) em portadores de lupus eritematoso sistemico (LES) no Estado da Bahia," *Revista Brasileira de Reumatologia*, vol. 40, pp. 183–188, 2000.

[51] C. A. Falcão, I. C. Alves, W. H. Chahade, A. L. B. P. Duarte, and N. Lucena-Silva, "Echocardiographic abnormalities and antiphospholipid antibodies in patients with systemic lupus erythematosus," *Arquivos Brasileiros de Cardiologia*, vol. 79, no. 3, pp. 285–291, 2002.

[52] E. M. C. Sella, E. I. Sato, and A. Barbieri, "Coronary artery angiography in systemic lupus erythematosus patients with abnormal myocardial perfusion scintigraphy," *Arthritis and Rheumatism*, vol. 48, no. 11, pp. 3168–3175, 2003.

[53] E. M. C. Sella, E. I. Sato, W. A. Leite, J. A. O. Filho, and A. Barbieri, "Myocardial perfusion scintigraphy and coronary disease risk factors in systemic lupus erythematosus," *Annals of the Rheumatic Diseases*, vol. 62, no. 11, pp. 1066–1070, 2003.

[54] M. Soares, L. Reis, J. A. S. Papi, and C. R. L. Cardoso, "Rate, pattern and factors related to damage in Brazilian systemic lupus erythematosus patients," *Lupus*, vol. 12, no. 10, pp. 788–794, 2003.

[55] C. R. L. Cardoso, M. A. O. Sales, J. A. S. Papi, and G. F. Salles, "QT-interval parameters are increased in systemic lupus erythematosus patients," *Lupus*, vol. 14, no. 10, pp. 846–852, 2005.

[56] M. C. B.T. da Rocha, M. J. P. Vilar, E. A. M. Freire, and M. B. Santiago, "Arterial occlusion in systemic lupus erythematosus: a good prognostic sign?" *Clinical Rheumatology*, vol. 24, no. 6, pp. 602–605, 2005.

[57] M. M. Shinzato, C. Bueno, V. S. T. Viana, E. F. Borba, C. R. Gonçalves, and E. Bonfá, "Complement-fixing activity of anticardiolipin antibodies in patients with and without thrombosis," *Lupus*, vol. 14, no. 12, pp. 953–958, 2005.

[58] A. W. S. de Souza, F. S. Hatta, F. Miranda Jr., and E. I. Sato, "Atherosclerotic plaque in carotid arteries in systemic lupus erythematosus: frequency and associated risk factors," *Sao Paulo Medical Journal*, vol. 123, no. 3, pp. 137–142, 2005.

[59] B. F. A. Freire, R. C. da Silva, A. T. Fabro, and D. C. dos Santos, "Is systemic lupus erithematosus a new risk factor for atherosclerosis?" *Arquivos brasileiros de cardiologia*, vol. 87, no. 3, pp. 300–306, 2006.

[60] R. W. Telles, C. C. D. Lanna, G. A. Ferreira, M. A. P. de Carvalho, and A. Ribeiro, "Freqüência de doença cardiovascular aterosclerótica e de seus fatores de risco em pacientes com lúpus eritematoso sistêmico," *Revista Brasileira de Reumatologia*, vol. 47, pp. 165–173, 2007.

[61] C. R. L. Cardoso, F. V. Signorelli, J. A. S. Papi, and G. F. Salles, "Initial and accrued damage as predictors of mortality in Brazilian patients with systemic lupus erythematosus: a cohort study," *Lupus*, vol. 17, no. 11, pp. 1042–1048, 2008.

[62] C. R. L. Cardoso, F. V. Signorelli, J. A. Papi, and G. F. Salles, "Prevalence and factors associated with dyslipoproteinemias in Brazilian systemic lupus erythematosus patients," *Rheumatology International*, vol. 28, no. 4, pp. 323–327, 2008.

[63] R. W. Telles, C. C. D. Lanna, G. A. Ferreira, A. J. Souza, T. P. Navarro, and A. L. Ribeiro, "Carotid atherosclerotic alterations in systemic lupus erythematosus patients treated at a Brazilian university setting," *Lupus*, vol. 17, no. 2, pp. 105–113, 2008.

[64] R. A. M. Cadaval, J. E. Martinez, M. A. Mazzolin, R. G. T. Barros, and F. A. de Almeida, "Avaliação do risco coronariano em mulheres com lúpus eritematoso sistêmico," *Revista Brasileira de Reumatologia*, vol. 49, no. 6, 2009.

[65] F. D. M. M. dos Santos, M. C. Borges, M. I. T. D. Correia, R. W. Telles, and C. C. D. Lanna, "Assessment of nutritional status and physical activity in systemic lupus erythematosus patients," *Revista Brasileira de Reumatologia*, vol. 50, no. 6, pp. 631–645, 2010.

[66] G. G. Ribeiro, E. Bonfá, R. S. Neto et al., "Premature coronary artery calcification is associated with disease duration and bone mineral density in young female systemic lupus erythematosus patients," *Lupus*, vol. 19, no. 1, pp. 27–33, 2010.

[67] S. K. Shinjo, E. Bonfá, D. Wojdyla et al., "Antimalarial treatment may have a time-dependent effect on lupus survival: data from a multinational Latin American inception cohort," *Arthritis and Rheumatism*, vol. 62, no. 3, pp. 855–862, 2010.

[68] R. W. Telles, C. C. D. Lanna, G. A. Ferreira, and A. L. Ribeiro, "Metabolic syndrome in patients with systemic lupus erythematosus: association with traditional risk factors for coronary heart disease and lupus characteristics," *Lupus*, vol. 19, no. 7, pp. 803–809, 2010.

[69] M. A. B. Lozovoy, A. N. C. Simão, M. S. N. Hohmann et al., "Inflammatory biomarkers and oxidative stress measurements in patients with systemic lupus erythematosus with or without metabolic syndrome," *Lupus*, vol. 20, no. 13, pp. 1356–1364, 2011.

[70] D. C. C. Souza, A. H. Santo, and E. I. Sato, "Mortality profile related to systemic lupus erythematosus: a multiple cause-of-death analysis," *Journal of Rheumatology*, vol. 39, no. 3, pp. 496–503, 2012.

[71] F. de Miranda Moura dos Santos, M. C. Borges, R. W. Telles, M. I. T. D. Correia, and C. C. D. Lanna, "Excess weight and associated risk factors in patients with systemic lupus erythematosus," *Rheumatology International*, vol. 33, pp. 681–688, 2013.

[72] J. Gobaira Maluf, A. Zghaib Abad, and P. A. R. López, "The heart in systemic lupus erythematosus. Study in 32 non-selected patients (author's transl)," *Archivos del Instituto de Cardiologia de Mexico*, vol. 52, no. 3, pp. 223–228, 1982.

[73] E. Badui, D. Garcia-Rubi, E. Robles et al., "Cardiovascular manifestations in systemic lupus erythematosus. Prospective study of 100 patients," *Angiology*, vol. 36, no. 7, pp. 431–441, 1985.

[74] G. J. Ruiz-Arguelles, A. Ruiz-Arguelles, D. Alarcon-Segovia et al., "Natural anticoagulants in systemic lupus erythematosus. Deficiency of protein S bound to C4bp associates with recent history of venous thromboses, antiphospholipid antibodies, and the antiphospholipid syndrome," *Journal of Rheumatology*, vol. 18, no. 4, pp. 552–558, 1991.

[75] M. Salazar-Paramo, I. G. de la Torre, M. J. Fritzler, S. Loyau, and E. Anglés-Cano, "Antibodies to fibrin-bound tissue-type plasminogen activator in systemic lupus erythematosus are associated with Raynaud's phenomenon and thrombosis," *Lupus*, vol. 5, no. 4, pp. 275–278, 1996.

[76] A. Zonana-Nacach, A. Camargo-Coronel, P. Yáñez et al., "Measurement of damage in 210 Mexican patients with systemic lupus erythematosus: relationship with disease duration," *Lupus*, vol. 7, no. 2, pp. 119–123, 1998.

[77] L. Gómez-Pacheco, A. R. Villa, C. Drenkard, J. Cabiedes, A. R. Cabral, and D. Alarcón-Segovia, "Serum anti-$\beta$2-glycoprotein-I and anticardiolipin antibodies during thrombosis in systemic lupus erythematosus patients," *The American Journal of Medicine*, vol. 106, no. 4, pp. 417–423, 1999.

[78] F. Salcido-Ochoa, J. Cabiedes, D. Alarcón-Segovia, and A. R. Cabral, "Antiprothrombin antibodies in patients with systemic lupus erythematosus or with primary antiphospholipid syndrome," *Journal of Clinical Rheumatology*, vol. 8, no. 5, pp. 251–255, 2002.

[79] J. G. Juárez-Rojas, A. X. Medina-Urrutia, R. Posadas-Sánchez et al., "High-density lipoproteins are abnormal in young women with uncomplicated systemic lupus erythematosus," *Lupus*, vol. 17, no. 11, pp. 981–987, 2008.

[80] J. Romero-Díaz, I. García-Sosa, and J. Sánchez-Guerrero, "Thrombosis in systemic lupus erythematosus and other autoimmune diseases of recent onset," *Journal of Rheumatology*, vol. 36, no. 1, pp. 68–75, 2009.

[81] A. Zonana-Nacach, E. Santana-Sahagún, F. J. Jiménez-Balderas, and A. Camargo-Coronel, "Prevalence and factors associated with metabolic syndrome in patients with rheumatoid arthritis and systemic lupus erythematosus," *Journal of Clinical Rheumatology*, vol. 14, no. 2, pp. 74–77, 2008.

[82] A. G. Uribe, J. Romero-Díaz, M. Apte et al., "Impact of immigration on the clinical expression of systemic lupus erythematosus: a comparative study of Hispanic patients residing in the USA and Mexico," *Rheumatology*, vol. 48, no. 11, pp. 1392–1397, 2009.

[83] E. Alexánderson, J. M. Ochoa, R. Calleja et al., "Endothelial dysfunction in systemic lupus erythematosus: evaluation with 13N-ammonia PET," *Journal of Nuclear Medicine*, vol. 51, no. 12, pp. 1927–1931, 2010.

[84] J. Romero-Díaz, F. Vargas-Vóracková, E. Kimura-Hayama et al., "Systemic lupus erythematosus risk factors for coronary artery calcifications," *Rheumatology*, vol. 51, no. 1, pp. 110–119, 2012.

[85] S. M. A. Toloza, J. M. Roseman, G. S. Alarcón et al., "Systemic lupus erythematosus in a multiethnic US cohort (LUMINA): XXII. Predictors of time to the occurrence of initial damage," *Arthritis and Rheumatism*, vol. 50, no. 10, pp. 3177–3186, 2004.

[86] A. J. Szalai, G. S. Alarcón, J. Calvo-Alén et al., "Systemic lupus erythematosus in a multiethnic US cohort (LUMINA). XXX: association between C-reactive protein (CRP) gene polymorphisms and vascular events," *Rheumatology*, vol. 44, no. 7, pp. 864–868, 2005.

[87] R. Kaiser, Y. Li, M. Chang et al., "Genetic risk factors for thrombosis in systemic lupus erythematosus," *Journal of Rheumatology*, vol. 39, no. 8, pp. 1603–1610, 2012.

[88] S. Finkielman, N. M. Bleichmar, M. Norymberg, and A. Agrest, "Arterial hypertension in systemic lupus erythematosus," *Medicina*, vol. 29, no. 3, pp. 165–170, 1969.

[89] V. Bellomio, A. Spindler, E. Lucero et al., "Systemic lupus erythematosus: mortality and survival in Argentina. A multicenter study," *Lupus*, vol. 9, no. 5, pp. 377–381, 2000.

[90] A. Zonana-Nacach, E. Santana-Sahagún, F. J. Jiménez-Balderas et al., "Metabolic syndrome in Argentinean patients with systemic lupus erythematosus," *Lupus*, vol. 18, no. 11, pp. 1019–1025, 2009.

[91] L. M. Vilá, A. M. Mayor, A. H. Valentín, M. García-Soberal, and S. Vilá, "Clinical and immunological manifestations in 134 Puerto Rican patients with systemic lupus erythematosus," *Lupus*, vol. 8, no. 4, pp. 279–286, 1999.

[92] V. E. Rodriguez, E. N. Gonzalez-Pares, and C. Rivera, "Clinical manifestations and vascular events in patients with lupus erythematosus anticardiolipin antibodies and raynaud's phenomenon," *Puerto Rico Health Sciences Journal*, vol. 25, no. 4, pp. 307–313, 2006.

[93] M. Fernández, J. Calvo-Alén, A. M. Bertoli et al., "Systemic lupus erythematosus in a multiethnic US cohort (LUMINA L II): relationship between vascular events and the use of hormone replacement therapy in postmenopausal women," *Journal of Clinical Rheumatology*, vol. 13, no. 5, pp. 261–265, 2007.

[94] A. M. Negrón, M. J. Molina, A. M. Mayor, V. E. Rodríguez, and L. M. Vilá, "Factors associated with metabolic syndrome in patients with systemic lupus erythematosus from Puerto Rico," *Lupus*, vol. 17, no. 4, pp. 348–354, 2008.

[95] L. M. Yassin, J. Londoño, G. Montoya et al., "Atherosclerosis development in SLE patients is not determined by monocytes ability to bind/endocytose Ox-LDL," *Autoimmunity*, vol. 44, no. 3, pp. 201–210, 2011.

[96] P. Abumohor, C. Cerda, O. Neira et al., "Anticardiolipin antibodies in systemic lupus erythematosus: prevalence and clinical associations," *Revista Medica de Chile*, vol. 119, no. 5, pp. 517–523, 1991.

[97] D. Alarcón-Segovia, M. E. Alarcón-Riquelme, M. H. Cardiel et al., "Familial aggregation of systemic lupus erythematosus, rheumatoid arthritis, and other autoimmune diseases in 1,177 lupus patients from the GLADEL cohort," *Arthritis and Rheumatism*, vol. 52, no. 4, pp. 1138–1147, 2005.

[98] S. Manzi, E. N. Meilahn, J. E. Rairie et al., "Age-specific incidence rates of myocardial infarction and angina in women with systemic lupus erythematosus: comparison with the Framingham study," *The American Journal of Epidemiology*, vol. 145, no. 5, pp. 408–415, 1997.

[99] A. N. Kiani, L. Magder, and M. Petri, "Coronary calcium in systemic lupus erythematosus is associated with traditional cardiovascular risk factors, but not with disease activity," *Journal of Rheumatology*, vol. 35, no. 7, pp. 1300–1306, 2008.

[100] L. M. Fischer, R. G. Schlienger, C. Matter, H. Jick, and C. R. Meier, "Effect of rheumatoid arthritis or systemic lupus erythematosus on the risk of first-time acute myocardial infarction," *The American Journal of Cardiology*, vol. 93, no. 2, pp. 198–200, 2004.

[101] A. Doria, L. Iaccarino, A. Ghirardello et al., "Long-term prognosis and causes of death in systemic lupus erythematosus," *The American Journal of Medicine*, vol. 119, no. 8, pp. 700–706, 2006.

[102] T. Thompson, K. Sutton-Tyrrell, R. P. Wildman et al., "Progression of carotid intima-media thickness and plaque in women with systemic lupus erythematosus," *Arthritis and Rheumatism*, vol. 58, no. 3, pp. 835–842, 2008.

[103] M. Petri, S. Perez-Gutthann, D. Spence, and M. C. Hochberg, "Risk factors for coronary artery disease in patients with systemic lupus erythematosus," *The American Journal of Medicine*, vol. 93, no. 5, pp. 513–519, 1992.

[104] M. B. Urowitzx, D. Ibañez, and D. D. Gladman, "Atherosclerotic vascular events in a single large lupus cohort: prevalence and risk factors," *Journal of Rheumatology*, vol. 34, no. 1, pp. 70–75, 2007.

[105] M. B. Urowitz, D. Gladman, D. Ibañez et al., "Atherosclerotic vascular events in a multinational inception cohort of systemic lupus erythematosus," *Arthritis Care and Research*, vol. 62, no. 6, pp. 881–887, 2010.

[106] D. P. M. Symmons and S. E. Gabriel, "Epidemiology of CVD in rheumatic disease, with a focus on RA and SLE," *Nature Reviews Rheumatology*, vol. 7, no. 7, pp. 399–408, 2011.

[107] L. V. Scalzi, S. Bhatt, R. C. Gilkeson, and M. L. Shaffer, "The relationship between race, cigarette smoking and carotid intimal medial thickness in systemic lupus erythematosus," *Lupus*, vol. 18, no. 14, pp. 1289–1297, 2009.

[108] M. B. Urowitz, D. Gladman, D. Ibañez et al., "Clinical manifestations and coronary artery disease risk factors at diagnosis of systemic lupus erythematosus: data from an international inception cohort," *Lupus*, vol. 16, no. 9, pp. 731–735, 2007.

[109] J. Gustafsson, I. Gunnarsson, O. Börjesson et al., "Predictors of the first cardiovascular event in patients with systemic lupus

erythematosus—a prospective cohort study," *Arthritis Research and Therapy*, vol. 11, no. 6, article R186, 2009.

[110] J. T. Gustafsson, J. F. Simard, I. Gunnarsson et al., "Risk factors for cardiovascular mortality in patients with systemic lupus erythematosus, a prospective cohort study," *Arthritis Research and Therapy*, vol. 14, article R46, 2012.

[111] A. M. Bertoli, L. M. Vilá, G. S. Alarcón et al., "Factors associated with arterial vascular events in PROFILE: a multiethnic lupus cohort," *Lupus*, vol. 18, no. 11, pp. 958–965, 2009.

[112] M. T. Driessen, L. L. J. Koppes, L. Veldhuis, D. Samoocha, and J. W. R. Twisk, "Coffee consumption is not related to the metabolic syndrome at the age of 36 years: the Amsterdam growth and health longitudinal study," *European Journal of Clinical Nutrition*, vol. 63, no. 4, pp. 536–542, 2009.

[113] C. S. P. M. Uiterwaal, W. M. M. Verschuren, H. B. Bueno-de-Mesquita et al., "Coffee intake and incidence of hypertension," *The American Journal of Clinical Nutrition*, vol. 85, no. 3, pp. 718–723, 2007.

[114] Z. Zhang, G. Hu, B. Caballero, L. Appel, and L. Chen, "Habitual coffee consumption and risk of hypertension: a systematic review and meta-analysis of prospective observational studies," *The American Journal of Clinical Nutrition*, vol. 93, no. 6, pp. 1212–1219, 2011.

[115] M. J. Klag, N. Y. Wang, L. A. Meoni et al., "Coffee intake and risk of hypertension: the Johns Hopkins precursors study," *Archives of Internal Medicine*, vol. 162, no. 6, pp. 657–662, 2002.

[116] A. Di Castelnuovo, R. Di Giuseppe, L. Iacoviello, and G. de Gaetano, "Consumption of cocoa, tea and coffee and risk of cardiovascular disease," *European Journal of Internal Medicine*, vol. 23, no. 1, pp. 15–25, 2012.

[117] S. H. Jee, J. He, P. K. Whelton, I. Suh, and M. J. Klag, "The effect of chronic coffee drinking on blood pressure: a meta-analysis of controlled clinical trials," *Hypertension*, vol. 33, no. 2, pp. 647–652, 1999.

[118] M. Nardini, F. Natella, and C. Scaccini, "Role of dietary polyphenols in platelet aggregation. A review of the supplementation studies," *Platelets*, vol. 18, no. 3, pp. 224–243, 2007.

[119] M. Shechter, G. Shalmon, M. Scheinowitz et al., "Impact of acute caffeine ingestion on endothelial function in subjects with and without coronary artery disease," *The American Journal of Cardiology*, vol. 107, no. 9, pp. 1255–1261, 2011.

[120] E. Svenungsson, K. Jensen-Urstad, M. Heimbürger et al., "Risk factors for cardiovascular disease in systemic lupus erythematosus," *Circulation*, vol. 104, no. 16, pp. 1887–1893, 2001.

[121] M. J. Roman, J. E. Salmon, R. Sobel et al., "Prevalence and relation to risk factors of carotid atherosclerosis and left ventricular hypertrophy in systemic lupus erythematosus and antiphospholipid antibody syndrome," *The American Journal of Cardiology*, vol. 87, no. 5, pp. 663–666, 2001.

[122] P. López-Jaramillo, C. Velandia-Carrillo, J. Alvarez-Camacho, D. D. Cohen, T. Sánchez-Solano, and G. Castillo-López, "Inflammation and hypertension: are there regional differences?" *International Journal of Hypertension*, vol. 2013, Article ID 492094, 12 pages, 2013.

[123] M. McMahon, J. Grossman, B. Skaggs et al., "Dysfunctional proinflammatory high-density lipoproteins confer increased risk of atherosclerosis in women with systemic lupus erythematosus," *Arthritis and Rheumatism*, vol. 60, no. 8, pp. 2428–2437, 2009.

[124] M. McMahon, B. J. Skaggs, L. Sahakian et al., "High plasma leptin levels confer increased risk of atherosclerosis in women with systemic lupus erythematosus, and are associated with inflammatory oxidised lipids," *Annals of the Rheumatic Diseases*, vol. 70, no. 9, pp. 1619–1624, 2011.

[125] Z. Touma, D. D. Gladman, D. Ibañez, and M. B. Urowitz, "Ability of non-fasting and fasting triglycerides to predict coronary artery disease in lupus patients," *Rheumatology*, vol. 51, no. 3, Article ID ker339, pp. 528–534, 2012.

[126] J. Mikdashi, B. Handwerger, P. Langenberg, M. Miller, and S. Kittner, "Baseline disease activity, hyperlipidemia, and hypertension are predictive factors for ischemic stroke and stroke severity in systemic lupus erythematosus," *Stroke*, vol. 38, no. 2, pp. 281–285, 2007.

[127] M. Nikpour, M. B. Urowitz, D. Ibanez, P. J. Harvey, and D. D. Gladman, "Importance of cumulative exposure to elevated cholesterol and blood pressure in development of atherosclerotic coronary artery disease in systemic lupus erythematosus: a prospective proof-of-concept cohort study," *Arthritis Research and Therapy*, vol. 13, article R156, 2011.

[128] P. E. Westerweel, R. K. M. A. C. Luyten, H. A. Koomans, R. H. W. M. Derksen, and M. C. Verhaar, "Premature atherosclerotic cardiovascular disease in systemic lupus erythematosus," *Arthritis and Rheumatism*, vol. 56, no. 5, pp. 1384–1396, 2007.

[129] J. Frostegård, "Atherosclerosis in patients with autoimmune disorders," *Arteriosclerosis, Thrombosis, and Vascular Biology*, vol. 25, no. 9, pp. 1776–1785, 2005.

[130] E. Y. Rhew and R. Ramsey-Goldman, "Premature atherosclerotic disease in systemic lupus erythematosus—role of inflammatory mechanisms," *Autoimmunity Reviews*, vol. 5, no. 2, pp. 101–105, 2006.

[131] Y. Sherer and Y. Shoenfeld, "Mechanisms of disease: atherosclerosis in autoimmune diseases," *Nature Clinical Practice Rheumatology*, vol. 2, no. 2, pp. 99–106, 2006.

[132] M. McMahon, B. H. Hahn, and B. J. Skaggs, "Systemic lupus erythematosus and cardiovascular disease: prediction and potential for therapeutic intervention," *Expert Review of Clinical Immunology*, vol. 7, no. 2, pp. 227–241, 2011.

[133] M. Nikpour, M. B. Urowitz, and D. D. Gladman, "Premature atherosclerosis in systemic lupus erythematosus," *Rheumatic Disease Clinics of North America*, vol. 31, no. 2, pp. 329–354, 2005.

[134] L. E. Full, C. Ruisanchez, and C. Monaco, "The inextricable link between atherosclerosis and prototypical inflammatory diseases rheumatoid arthritis and systemic lupus erythematosus," *Arthritis Research and Therapy*, vol. 11, no. 2, article 217, 2009.

[135] J. C. Sarmiento-Monroy, J. Amaya-Amaya, J. S. Espinosa-Serna, C. Herrera-Díaz, J. M. Anaya, and A. Rojas-Villarraga, "Cardiovascular disease in rheumatoid arthritis: a systematic literature review in latin america," *Arthritis*, vol. 2012, Article ID 371909, 17 pages, 2012.

[136] J. Amaya-Amaya, J. C. Sarmiento-Monroy, R. D. Mantilla, R. Pineda-Tamayo, A. Rojas-Villarraga, and J. M. Anaya, "Novel risk factors for cardiovascular disease in rheumatoid arthritis," *Immunologic Research*, vol. 56, no. 2-3, pp. 267–286, 2013.

[137] L. N. Troelsen, P. Garred, B. Christiansen, C. Torp-Pedersen, and S. Jacobsen, "Genetically determined serum levels of mannose-binding lectin correlate negatively with common carotid intima-media thickness in systemic lupus erythematosus," *Journal of Rheumatology*, vol. 37, no. 9, pp. 1815–1821, 2010.

[138] B. Marasini, M. Massarotti, M. de Monti, M. Erario, G. Ghilardi, and M. L. Biondi, "Genetic contribution to carotid vascular disease in patients with systemic lupus erythematosus," *Journal of Clinical Immunology*, vol. 28, no. 2, pp. 131–133, 2008.

[139] J. M. Kahlenberg and M. J. Kaplan, "Mechanisms of premature atherosclerosis in rheumatoid arthritis and lupus," *Annual Review of Medicine*, vol. 64, pp. 249–263, 2013.

[140] V. K. Kawai, J. F. Solus, A. Oeser et al., "Novel cardiovascular risk prediction models in patients with systemic lupus erythematosus," *Lupus*, vol. 20, no. 14, pp. 1526–1534, 2011.

[141] P. W. F. Wilson, "Evidence of systemic inflammation and estimation of coronary artery disease risk: a population perspective," *The American Journal of Medicine*, vol. 121, no. 10, pp. S15–S20, 2008.

[142] P. M. Ridker, J. E. Buring, N. Rifai, and N. R. Cook, "Development and validation of improved algorithms for the assessment of global cardiovascular risk in women: the Reynolds risk score," *The Journal of the American Medical Association*, vol. 297, no. 6, pp. 611–619, 2007.

[143] M. J. L. Peters, D. P. M. Symmons, D. McCarey et al., "EULAR evidence-based recommendations for cardiovascular risk management in patients with rheumatoid arthritis and other forms of inflammatory arthritis," *Annals of the Rheumatic Diseases*, vol. 69, no. 2, pp. 325–331, 2010.

[144] M. Petri and L. Magder, "SLE cardiovascular risk equation," *Lupus*, vol. 22, no. 1, pp. 3–5, 2013.

[145] J. R. Elliott, S. Manzi, and D. Edmundowicz, "The role of preventive cardiology in systemic lupus erythematosus," *Current Rheumatology Reports*, vol. 9, no. 2, pp. 125–130, 2007.

[146] I. N. Bruce, "Cardiovascular disease in lupus patients: should all patients be treated with statins and aspirin?" *Best Practice and Research: Clinical Rheumatology*, vol. 19, no. 5, pp. 823–838, 2005.

[147] J. R. Elliott and S. Manzi, "Cardiovascular risk assessment and treatment in systemic lupus erythematosus," *Best Practice and Research: Clinical Rheumatology*, vol. 23, no. 4, pp. 481–494, 2009.

[148] M. A. Petri, A. N. Kiani, W. Post, L. Christopher-Stine, and L. S. Magder, "Lupus Atherosclerosis Prevention Study (LAPS)," *Annals of the Rheumatic Diseases*, vol. 70, no. 5, pp. 760–765, 2011.

[149] I. Ben-Zvi, S. Kivity, P. Langevitz, and Y. Shoenfeld, "Hydroxychloroquine: from malaria to autoimmunity," *Clinical Reviews in Allergy and Immunology*, vol. 42, no. 2, pp. 145–153, 2012.

[150] S. J. Katz and A. S. Russell, "Re-evaluation of antimalarials in treating rheumatic diseases: re-appreciation and insights into new mechanisms of action," *Current Opinion in Rheumatology*, vol. 23, no. 3, pp. 278–281, 2011.

[151] S. J. Morris, M. C. M. Wasko, J. L. Antohe et al., "Hydroxychloroquine use associated with improvement in lipid profiles in rheumatoid arthritis patients," *Arthritis Care and Research*, vol. 63, no. 4, pp. 530–534, 2011.

[152] S. K. Penn, A. H. Kao, L. L. Schott et al., "Hydroxychloroquine and glycemia in women with rheumatoid arthritis and systemic lupus erythematosus," *Journal of Rheumatology*, vol. 37, no. 6, pp. 1136–1142, 2010.

[153] L. R. Rekedal, E. Massarotti, R. Garg et al., "Changes in glycosylated hemoglobin after initiation of hydroxychloroquine or methotrexate treatment in diabetes patients with rheumatic diseases," *Arthritis and Rheumatism*, vol. 62, no. 12, pp. 3569–3573, 2010.

[154] R. Kaiser, C. M. Cleveland, and L. A. Criswell, "Risk and protective factors for thrombosis in systemic lupus erythematosus: results from a large, multi-ethnic cohort," *Annals of the Rheumatic Diseases*, vol. 68, no. 2, pp. 238–241, 2009.

[155] H. Jung, R. Bobba, J. Su et al., "The protective effect of antimalarial drugs on thrombovascular events in systemic lupus erythematosus," *Arthritis and Rheumatism*, vol. 62, no. 3, pp. 863–868, 2010.

[156] M. Petri, "Use of hydroxychloroquine to prevent thrombosis in systemic lupus erythematosus and in antiphospholipid antibody-positive patients," *Current Rheumatology Reports*, vol. 13, no. 1, pp. 77–80, 2011.

[157] G. S. Alarcón, G. McGwin, A. M. Bertoli et al., "Effect of hydroxychloroquine on the survival of patients with systemic lupus erythematosus: data from LUMINA, a multiethnic US cohort (LUMINA L)," *Annals of the Rheumatic Diseases*, vol. 66, no. 9, pp. 1168–1172, 2007.

[158] C. Perricone, N. Agmon-Levin, S. Colafrancesco, and Y. Shoenfeld, "Vitamins and systemic lupus erythematosus: to D or not to D," *Expert Review of Clinical Immunology*, vol. 9, no. 5, pp. 397–399, 2013.

[159] M. Mosca, C. Tani, M. Aringer et al., "European league against rheumatism recommendations for monitoring patients with systemic lupus erythematosus in clinical practice and in observational studies," *Annals of the Rheumatic Diseases*, vol. 69, no. 7, pp. 1269–1274, 2010.

# Permissions

All chapters in this book were first published in AD, by Hindawi Publishing Corporation; hereby published with permission under the Creative Commons Attribution License or equivalent. Every chapter published in this book has been scrutinized by our experts. Their significance has been extensively debated. The topics covered herein carry significant findings which will fuel the growth of the discipline. They may even be implemented as practical applications or may be referred to as a beginning point for another development.

The contributors of this book come from diverse backgrounds, making this book a truly international effort. This book will bring forth new frontiers with its revolutionizing research information and detailed analysis of the nascent developments around the world.

We would like to thank all the contributing authors for lending their expertise to make the book truly unique. They have played a crucial role in the development of this book. Without their invaluable contributions this book wouldn't have been possible. They have made vital efforts to compile up to date information on the varied aspects of this subject to make this book a valuable addition to the collection of many professionals and students.

This book was conceptualized with the vision of imparting up-to-date information and advanced data in this field. To ensure the same, a matchless editorial board was set up. Every individual on the board went through rigorous rounds of assessment to prove their worth. After which they invested a large part of their time researching and compiling the most relevant data for our readers.

The editorial board has been involved in producing this book since its inception. They have spent rigorous hours researching and exploring the diverse topics which have resulted in the successful publishing of this book. They have passed on their knowledge of decades through this book. To expedite this challenging task, the publisher supported the team at every step. A small team of assistant editors was also appointed to further simplify the editing procedure and attain best results for the readers.

Apart from the editorial board, the designing team has also invested a significant amount of their time in understanding the subject and creating the most relevant covers. They scrutinized every image to scout for the most suitable representation of the subject and create an appropriate cover for the book.

The publishing team has been an ardent support to the editorial, designing and production team. Their endless efforts to recruit the best for this project, has resulted in the accomplishment of this book. They are a veteran in the field of academics and their pool of knowledge is as vast as their experience in printing. Their expertise and guidance has proved useful at every step. Their uncompromising quality standards have made this book an exceptional effort. Their encouragement from time to time has been an inspiration for everyone.

The publisher and the editorial board hope that this book will prove to be a valuable piece of knowledge for researchers, students, practitioners and scholars across the globe.

# List of Contributors

**Rachna Aggarwal, Kristi A. Koelsch and Biji T. Kurien**
Department of Medicine, University of Oklahoma Health Sciences Center, Oklahoma City, OK 73104, USA
Arthritis & Immunology Program, Oklahoma Medical Research Foundation, Oklahoma City, OK 73104, USA

**Juan-Manuel Anaya**
Center for Autoimmune Diseases Research (CREA), Universidad del Rosario, Bogotá, Colombia

**R. Hal Scofield**
Department of Medicine, University of Oklahoma Health Sciences Center, Oklahoma City, OK 73104, USA
Arthritis & Immunology Program, Oklahoma Medical Research Foundation, Oklahoma City, OK 73104, USA
Medical Service, Department of Veterans Affairs Medical Center, Oklahoma City, OK 73104, USA

**Elena Bellavista**
Interdepartmental Center for Studies on Biophysics, Bioinformatics and Biocomplexity "L. Galvani" (CIG), University of Bologna, 40126 Bologna, Italy
Department of Experimental, Diagnostic and Specialty Medicine (DIMES), University of Bologna, 40126 Bologna, Italy

**Aurelia Santoro**
Department of Experimental, Diagnostic and Specialty Medicine (DIMES), University of Bologna, 40126 Bologna, Italy

**Daniela Galimberti**
Neurology Unit, Department of Pathophosiology and Transplantation, University of Milan, Centro Dino Ferrari, Fondazione IRCCS Cà Granda, Ospedale Maggiore Policlinico, 20122 Milan, Italy

**Cristoforo Comi**
Interdisciplinary Research Center of Autoimmune Diseases (IRCAD), University of Eastern Piedmont, "Amedeo Avogadro," 28100 Novara, Italy

**Fabio Luciani**
Inflammation and Infection Research Centre, School of Medical Sciences, University of New South Wales, Sydney, NSW2052, Australia

**Michele Mishto**
Institut für Biochemie, Charité Universitätsmedizin Berlin, 10117 Berlin, Germany
Centro Interdipartimentale di Ricerca sul Cancro "Giorgio Prodi," University of Bologna, 40126 Bologna, Italy

**Yaswanth Ala, Mohammed Khalid Pasha and Prasanna Latha Komaravalli**
Department of Genetics, Osmania University, Hyderabad, Telangana 500007, India

**Raja Narasimha Rao**
Central Railway Hospital, Lallaguda, Hyderabad, Telangana 500017, India

**Parveen Jahan**
Department of Genetics, Osmania University, Hyderabad, Telangana 500007, India
Department of Zoology, School of Sciences, Maulana Azad National Urdu University, Gachibowli, Hyderabad, Telangana 500032, India

**Soumya Nair**
Om Dental Clinic, No. 1554, Hebbal 2nd Stage, Mysore 570017, India

**Mohamed Faizuddin and Jayanthi Dharmapalan**
M.R. Ambedkar Dental College and Hospital, No. 1/37, Cline Road, Cooke Town, Bangalore 560005, India

**Kuniaki Terato and Christopher T. Do**
Chondrex, Inc., 2607 151st Place NE, Redmond, WA 98052, USA

**Hiroshi Shionoya**
Asama Chemicals Co., Ltd., 20-3 Nihonbashi Kodenmacho, Chuo-ku, Tokyo 103, Japan

**Martin J. Bergman**
Rheumatology Department, Drexel University College of Medicine and Taylor Hospital, 8 Morton Avenue, Suite 304, Ridley Park, Philadelphia, PA 19078-2216, USA

**William Reiss, Carol Chung, Pamela Wong and Adam Turpcu**
Genentech, Inc., 1 DNA Way, South San Francisco, CA 94080, USA

**Datis Kharrazian**
1001 Canvasback Court, Carlsbad, CA 92011, USA
Division of Sciences, Bastyr University California, 4106 Sorrento Valley Boulevard, San Diego, CA 92121, USA

**Ivana Burazor**
Cardiology Department, Institute for Rehabilitation, Sokobanjska 17, 11000 Belgrade, Serbia

**Aristo Vojdani**
Immunosciences Lab Inc, Los Angeles, CA 90035, USA

**Hend Hilal Al-Sherbeni**
Rheumatology and Rehabilitation Department, Faculty of Medicine, Cairo University, Cairo, Egypt

**Ahmed Mohamed Fahmy**
Pathology Department, National Cancer Institute (NCI), Cairo University, Cairo, Egypt

**Nadine Sherif**
Gynecology and Obstetrics Department, Faculty of Medicine, Cairo University, Cairo, Egypt

**Maria Eleftheria Evangelopoulos, Georgios Koutsis and Manolis Markianos**
Department of Neurology, Eginition Hospital, Athens University Medical School, 74 Vassilisis Sophias Avenue, 11528 Athens, Greece

**Roberto Assandri and Marta Monari**
Clinical Investigation Laboratory, Humanitas Clinical and Research Center, Rozzano, Milan, Italy

**Anna Colombo**
Humanitas Clinical and Research Center, Rozzano, Milan, Italy

**Alessandra Dossi and Alessandro Montanelli**
Humanitas Clinical and Research Center, Rozzano, Milan, Italy
Clinical Investigation Laboratory, Diagnostics Department, Spedali Civili of Brescia, Brescia, Italy

**Antonio Calabrò**
Department of Experimental and Clinical Biomedical Sciences, University of Florence, Viale Pieraccini 6, 50139 Florence, Italy
Tuscany Referral Center for Adult Coeliac Disease, Viale Pieraccini 6, 50139 Florence, Italy

**Ewa Gralka**
Magnetic Resonance Center (CERM), University of Florence, Via L. Sacconi 6, 50019 Sesto Fiorentino, Italy

**Claudio Luchinat**
Magnetic Resonance Center (CERM), University of Florence, Via L. Sacconi 6, 50019 Sesto Fiorentino, Italy
Department of Chemistry, University of Florence, Via della Lastruccia 3, 50019 Sesto Fiorentino, Italy

**Edoardo Saccenti**
Biosystems Data Analysis Group, University of Amsterdam, 904 Science Park, 1098 XH Amsterdam, The Netherlands
Laboratory of Systems and Synthetic Biology, Wageningen University and Research Center, Dreijenplein 10, 6703 HB Wageningen, The Netherlands

**Leonardo Tenori**
Magnetic Resonance Center (CERM), University of Florence, Via L. Sacconi 6, 50019 Sesto Fiorentino, Italy
FiorGen Foundation, Via L. Sacconi 6, 50019 Sesto Fiorentino, Italy

**Komenan Kassi and Kouame A. Kouassi**
Department of Dermatology and Infectiology, Training and Research Unit of Medical Sciences, F´elix Houphou¨et Boigny University (FHBU) of Abidjan-Cocody, Abidjan 21 BP 5151, Cote d'Ivoire

**Oussou Armel Mienwoley**
Training and Research Unit of Medical Sciences, University of Bouaké, Bouaké 01 BP V18, Cote d'Ivoire
Mother Maria Elisa Andreoli Health Center, Cocody Riviera Palmeraie, Cidex 3, Abijan-Riviera BP 51, Cote d'Ivoire

**Mohamed Kouyate and Sylvanus Koui**
Department of Histopathology, University Hospital of Treichville, Abidjan 01 BP V3, Cote d'Ivoire

**Edith Marie Williams**
Department of Public Health Sciences, Medical University of South Carolina, 135 Cannon Street, Suite 303, Charleston, SC 29425, USA

**Jiajia Zhang and Larisa Bruner**
University of South Carolina, Columbia, SC 29208, USA

**Judith Anderson and Laurene Tumiel-Berhalter**
State University of New York at Buffalo, Buffalo, NY 14215, USA

**Joaquin A. Pena and Timothy E. Lotze**
Baylor College of Medicine, Houston, TX 77030, USA

**Maria van der Pals, Johan Svensson and Annelie Carlsson**
Department of Pediatrics, Clinical Sciences, Skåne University Hospital, Lund University, 205 02 Lund, Sweden

**Anneli Ivarsson and Fredrik Norström**
Department of Public Health and Clinical Medicine, Epidemiology and Global Health, Umeå University, 905 85 Umeå, Sweden

**Lotta Högberg**
Division of Pediatrics, Department of Clinical and Experimental Medicine, Faculty of Health Sciences, Linköping University, 581 85 Linköping, Sweden
Department of Pediatrics in Norrköping, County Council of Östergötland, 603 79 Norrköping, Sweden

**R. Fonseca and M. Figueiredo-Braga**
1 Department of Clinical Neurosciences and Mental Health, Faculty of Medicine, University of Porto, 4200-319 Porto, Portugal

**M. Bernardes and G. Terroso**
Rheumatology Department, São João Hospital, 4200-319 Porto, Portugal

**M. de Sousa**
IBMC/GABBA, University of Porto, 4150-180 Porto, Portugal

**O. Zargari**
Department of Dermatology, Skin Research Center, Shahid Beheshti University of Medical Sciences, Tehran, Iran

**E. Kazemnezhad Leyli**
Department of Biostatistics, Guilan University of Medical Sciences, Rasht, Iran

**S. Z. Azimi**
Department of Dermatology, Skin Research Center, Guilan University of Medical Sciences, Rasht, Iran

**Edwin Liu, Kristen McDaniel, Stephanie Case, Liping Yu, and Aaron W. Michels**
Barbara Davis Center for Childhood Diabetes, School of Medicine, University of Colorado Denver, Mail Stop A140, 1775 Aurora Court, Aurora, CO 80045, USA

**Bernd Gerhartz, Nils Ostermann, Gabriela Fankhauser, Valerie Hungerford, Chao Zou, Marcel Luyten and Katherine J. Seidl**
Novartis Institutes for Biomedical Research, 4002 Basel, Switzerland

**Kathleen M. Gilbert, William Woodruff and Sarah J. Blossom**
University of Arkansas for Medical Sciences, Arkansas Children's Hospital Research Institute, 13 Children's Way, Little Rock, AR 72202, USA

**Peter Korsten and Michael Zeisberg**
Department of Nephrology and Rheumatology, University Medical Center Goettingen, Goettingen, Germany

**Timothy B. Niewold**
Division of Rheumatology and Department of Immunology, Mayo Clinic, Rochester, MN, USA

**Tammy O. Utset**
Department of Rheumatology, University of Chicago, Chicago, IL, USA

**Daniel Cho**
Rheovector LLC, King of Prussia, PA, USA

**Lawrence S. Zachary**
Section of Plastic and Reconstructive Surgery, Department of Surgery, University of Chicago, Chicago, IL, USA

**Suncica Volkov**
Division of Rheumatology, University of Illinois at Chicago, Chicago, IL, USA

**Nadera J. Sweiss**
Division of Rheumatology, University of Illinois at Chicago, Chicago, IL, USA
Division of Pulmonary, Critical Care, Sleep and Allergy, University of Illinois at Chicago, Chicago, IL, USA

**Elizabeth Sarmiento, Jonathan Dale, Mauricio Arraya, Antonio Gallego, Nallibe Lanio, Joaquin Navarro and Javier Carbone**
Clinical Immunology Department, Hospital General Universitario Gregorio Marañon, 28007 Madrid, Spain

**Lucas Malta Almeida and Fernanda Coutinho de Almeida**
Graduate Program in Medical Sciences, University of Brasília School of Medicine, 70.900.910 Brasília, DF, Brazil
Research Laboratory for Celiac Disease, University of Brasília School of Medicine, 70.900.910 Brasília, DF, Brazil

**Lenora Gandolfi and Riccardo Pratesi**
Graduate Program in Medical Sciences, University of Brasília School of Medicine, 70.900.910 Brasília, DF, Brazil
Research Laboratory for Celiac Disease, University of Brasília School of Medicine, 70.900.910 Brasília, DF, Brazil
Graduate Program in Health Sciences, University of Brasília School of Health Sciences, 70.900.910 Brasília, DF, Brazil

**Rosa Harumi Uenishi and Nicole Selleski**
Research Laboratory for Celiac Disease, University of Brasília School of Medicine, 70.900.910 Brasília, DF, Brazil
Graduate Program in Health Sciences, University of Brasília School of Health Sciences, 70.900.910 Brasília, DF, Brazil

**Yanna Karla de Medeiros Nóbrega**
Graduate Program in Medical Sciences, University of Brasília School of Medicine, 70.900.910 Brasília, DF, Brazil
Research Laboratory for Celiac Disease, University of Brasília School of Medicine, 70.900.910 Brasília, DF, Brazil
Graduate Program in Health Sciences, University of Brasília School of Health Sciences, 70.900.910 Brasília, DF, Brazil
Department of Pharmaceutical Sciences, University of Brasília School of Health Sciences, 70.900.910 Brasília, DF, Brazil

**S. W. Olson, D. J. Little, L. K. Prince, T. P. Baker and J. D. Edison**
Walter Reed National Military Medical Center, 8901 Wisconsin Avenue, Bethesda, MD 20889, USA

**J. J. Lee**
Naval Medical Center San Diego, 34800 Bob Wilson Drive, San Diego, CA 92134, USA

**M. Poirier**
San Antonio Military Medical Center, 3551 Roger Brooke Dr., Fort Sam Houston, TX 78234, USA

**K. C. Abbott**
The National Institute of Diabetes and Digestive and Kidney Diseases (NIDDK), NIH, 6707 Democracy Blvd, Bethesda, MD 20892, USA

**Durga Prasanna Misra, Smriti Chaurasia and Ramnath Misra**
Department of Clinical Immunology, Sanjay Gandhi Post Graduate Institute of Medical Sciences, Rae Bareily Road, Lucknow, Uttar Pradesh 226 014, India

**Guilherme Ramires de Jesus, Nilson Ramires de Jesus and Flávia Cunha dos Santos**
1Department of Obstetrics, Universidade do Estado do Rio de Janeiro, Rio de Janeiro, Brazil

**Claudia Mendoza-Pinto and Mario García Carrasco**
Systemic Autoimmune Diseases Research Unit, Hospital General Regional No. 36-CIBIOR, Instituto Mexicano del Seguro Social, Puebla, Mexico
Department of Immunology and Rheumatology, Medicine School, Benemérita Universidad Autónoma de Puebla, Puebla, Mexico

**Evandro Mendes Klumb and Roger Abramino Levy**
Department of Rheumatology, Universidade do Estado do Rio de Janeiro, Rio de Janeiro, Brazil

**Jenny Amaya-Amaya, Juan Camilo Sarmiento-Monroy, Julián Caro-Moreno, Nicolás Molano-González, Rubén D. Mantilla, Adriana Rojas-Villarraga and Juan-Manuel Anaya**
Center for Autoimmune Diseases Research (CREA), School of Medicine and Health Sciences, Universidad del Rosario, Carrera 24 No. 63C-69, 111221 Bogotá, Colombia

# Index